ADVENTURE THERAPY AROUND THE GLOBE

International Perspectives and Diverse Approaches

Edited by
Christine L. Norton,
Cathryn Carpenter,
and Anita Pryor

ADVENTURE THERAPY AROUND THE GLOBE

International Perspectives and Diverse Approaches

Edited by
Christine L. Norton,
Cathryn Carpenter,
and Anita Pryor

COMMON GROUND PUBLISHING 2015

First published in 2015 in Champaign, Illinois, USA
by Common Ground Publishing LLC
as part of the Health, Wellness, and Society book imprint

Library of Congress Cataloging-in-Publication Data

Adventure therapy around the globe : international perspectives and diverse approaches / edited by Christine L. Norton, Cathryn Carpenter, and Anita Pryor.
pages cm
Includes bibliographical references.
ISBN 978-1-61229-773-6 (pbk : alk. paper) -- ISBN 978-1-61229-774-3 (pdf)
1. Adventure therapy. I. Norton, Christine Lynn. II. Carpenter, Cathryn, 1962- III. Pryor, Anita.

RC489.A38A38 2015
616.89'165--dc23

2015006271

Cover photo credit: "Healing Trees" by Cathryn Carpenter

Table of Contents

Acknowledgements

This book represents a large number of the keynotes, presentations and workshops presented at the Fifth and Sixth International Adventure Therapy Conferences. The editors would like to thank all contributing authors for their hard work, patience, and willingness to have their work peer reviewed. Presenting at an international conference is one achievement; contributing a paper to a peer-reviewed book is another. We recognise with regret that the process and timelines of compiling this book meant some contributions were left out. Our hope is that the papers in this book connect us with the wider work of IATC contributors and international adventure therapy practitioners.

This book represents an international collaboration, and builds upon the first edition of the book *Emerging Insights*, originally published by European Science and Art Publishing and now out of print. All photographs in this book were taken by Cathryn Carpenter. The editors thank the following people who gave their time to read, review and critique papers: Sandy Allen-Craig, Katie Asmus, Judy Atkins, Almut Beringer, Eric Brymer, Fiona Cameron, Simon Crisp, Michael Gass, Lee Gillis, Tonia Gray, Nevin Harper, Helen Hooper, Sean Hoyer, Christian Itin, Chris Jansen, Jiri Kirchner, Andrea Knepper, Chris Loynes, Denise Mitten, Sandy Newes, Val Nicholls, Barbara Parker-Bell, Luk Peeters, Kaye Richards, Martin Ringer, Stephen Ritchie, Paul Stolz, Anita Tucker, Andy Umbers, Ian Williams, and Allette Willis.

About the Contributors

Kylie Agnew-Pointon is a Provisional Psychologist and Manager for New Directions at Operation Flinders Foundation in Australia. She has special interest in adolescents, behavioural issues, and rehabilitation. Kylie is registered to provide supervised psychological assessment and treatment, and is committed to teaching clients life skills through wilderness and adventure therapy.

Jacqui Akhurst is a Principal Lecturer in Psychology at York St John University. Before her university lecturing career, she taught in primary and secondary schools in South Africa, and following professional psychology training, worked as a School Psychologist. Dr. Akhurst lectured at the University of Natal from 1992 to 2003 (and has recently been appointed as Honorary Professor at its successor, the University of KwaZulu Natal). After moving to the UK in 2004, she worked for two years in the Higher Education Academy Subject Centre for Psychology, then moving to YSJU as a Senior Lecturer. Her research focusses on community-based interventions, often utilizing Action Research and Activity Theory. She is also a Chartered Psychologist with the British Psychological Society (BPS), a Fellow of the Higher Education Academy, and also registered with the Health Professions Council of South Africa (HPCSA) in both Counselling and Educational psychology.

Sandy Allen-Craig is lecturing in Outdoor Education for the school of Exercise Science at the Australian Catholic University. Sandy has developed and implemented a number of units that examine the outdoor experience and therapeutic interventions and the role of mentoring for programs that focus on 'youth at risk'. She was recently awarded an ALTC citation for outstanding contribution to student learning. Her research interests include the use of the outdoors for educational and behavior change and the development of relationships with the natural world. Her passions are her family, her students and being active in the outdoors.

Dene Berman PhD, isa psychologist in practice with Lifespan Counseling Associates in Dayton, Ohio, USA. Part of this practice is the Wilderness Therapy

Program. Dene is also a Clinical Professor at the School of Professional Psychology at Wright State University. He is a former Chair of the AEE Therapeutic Adventure Professional Group (TAPG) and president of the board of the Wilderness Education Association. He has served on the editorial boards of the Journal of Experiential Education and the Journal of Outdoor Research and Experiential Learning, serving as the special editor for two issues of the Journal of Experiential Education on adventure therapy. Dene is the co-author of two books on wilderness therapy, co-author of *The Backcountry Classroom* and has authored numerous journal articles on adventure and wilderness therapy.

Daniel Bowen is a registered psychologist and is currently completing a PhD in Clinical Psychology in the Centre for Applied Psychology at the University of Canberra. Daniels' research focuses on the effectiveness of adventure therapy programs in Australia. For more information, see http://www.danielbowen.com.au/.

Kevin Burrows is a 'Forest School' leader. His first degree was in Fine Art, with Post Graduate training in Teaching, Counselling and Arts Therapies. His work-based M.A. 'Educational Art Therapy' undertook research into how creative group work helped young people with autism to interrelate through their shared creative experiences. He has since gained further experience and qualifications in Ecopsychology, Autism, Groupwork, Expressive Arts Therapy and Person Centred Art Therapy. Kevin has many years' experience working with people who have special needs including autism. He has a small private counselling practice, and teaches at the 'Essential Skills' special needs department of a sixth form college. His PhD research at Anglia Ruskin University is work based within a small woodland in the college campus. Kevin is observing and recording emergent process as part of his PhD where natural, creative experience and sensation enrich his students who have autism's learning experiences. Affiliations include: British Association of Counsellors and Psychotherapists (BACP); Person Centred Art Therapy Association (PCATA); International Expressive Art Therapy Association (IEATA); Counsellors and Psychotherapists Outdoors (CAPO); General Teaching Council (GTC).

Cathryn Carpenter PhD, has implemented outdoor experiential learning programs and courses in commercial, secondary and tertiary settings over the last 30 years. Her PhD examined sociological structures and environments conducive to processes of agency and change in a drug and alcohol adventure therapy program in Australia. Her research interests focus on health and wellbeing through the design and evaluation of therapeutic and developmental programs and via the exploration of human connections to place. Cathryn is a senior lecturer designing curriculum within a youth work degree at Victoria University.

Selena Chandler is an Outdoor Therapist, a UKCP registered Psychotherapist, and an Accredited Practitioner of the Institute for Outdoor Learning, with Summer Mountain Leader qualification. She has over 15 years' experience of integrating outdoor learning and therapy practices in her work. Selena's MA in Development Training from Cumbria University explored the impact of natural outdoor spaces on people experiencing depression. Working both indoors and outdoors, in the voluntary sector and private practice, Selena works with clients including women survivors of sexual violence, youth at risk, adults in recovery from addiction, people in life transitions and individuals seeking personal change. She also teaches Counselling and facilitates Wilderness Therapy retreats for trainee psychotherapists, and workshops for therapists who are beginning to develop an outdoor practice. Selena enjoys walking and canoeing, and maintains respect for nature's abundance and vulnerability through an ongoing dialogue with a wild garden.

Rita Corbiere is a long-standing resident of the Wikwemikong First Nations Reserve. She is retired after spending 40 years in education as a teacher and principal. Aside from her own personal interests, she takes part in community organizations, and she was involved in a research project for the local health centre. Since 2006 she has been working collaboratively with the Waasa Naabin Youth Centre on the Outdoor Adventure Leadership Experience (OALE) program. Currently, she is a member of the Amikook Senior Advisory Committee and the Anishnaabemowin Curriculum Development Advisory Group.

Jennifer Davis-Berman PhD, is a social worker and professor in the department of sociology, anthropology and social work at the University of Dayton in Dayton, Ohio, USA. A regular reviewer for the Journal of Experiential Education, she has published numerous articles on adventure and wilderness therapy over the past 20 years. She has also presented research on various aspects of outdoor adventure at national and international conferences and co-authored two books on wilderness therapy.

Bonnie Dyck MSW, RSW, is a family therapist who for the past six years has been working in the area of youth residential treatment developing and implementing an experiential-based family therapy program. She has over ten years' experience as a therapist focusing on adventure, wilderness, experiential, narrative, motivational interviewing, solution-focused, and family systems approaches. She has over fifteen years' experience working with various adventure and wilderness therapy programs in Canada, the U.S.A., and New Zealand. Bonnie has presented workshops, lectures, and trainings on experiential learning and family-centered practice for various conferences, colleges, and agencies both within Canada and internationally, including at 4IATC and 5IATC. From 2006-2009 she was a Canadian representative on the Adventure Therapy International Committee.

Alan Ewert is a Professor and Chair of Environmental Health, and is the Joel Meier Endowed Chair of Outdoor Leadership at Indiana University. He is the director of the Professional Development Program at Outward Bound and his research examines adventure therapy with veterans, the role of nature in wellness, and outdoor adventure programming outcomes.

Elizabeth Freeman is a Lecturer in Psychology at Sheffield Hallam University in the UK. She completed her BSc (Hons) at the University of Stirling in 2008 and her desire to find effective ways of working with people with mental health issues led to a PhD. In 2013 she was awarded a doctorate by the University of Leeds and her aim is to further examine the effectiveness of walking and solo experiences outdoors with military veterans. Throughout her 8 years of education, she has been a member of voluntary community group committees (e.g. Edible York and York in Transition), volunteered with mental health services (e.g. Open Secret) and completed mental health training (ASSIST, MHFA and counselling skills).

Tonia Gray is an Associate Professor in the Center for Educational Research at the University of Western Sydney. She is a past editor of the Australian Journal of Outdoor Education (AJOE) and a review board member for the Journal of Experiential Education (JEE). Tonia's research interests include: experiential learning in a variety of educational settings; risk taking and risk managements; understanding the motivations and personalities of extreme sports participants; facilitation, leadership and management styles in adventure education and eco-psychology.

Nick Hall lives near Hobart in Tasmania (Australia) with his wife Kathy and their three children. Nick has spent the last fifteen years working and studying in the therapy field, focusing on experiential modalities connected to somatic psychotherapy, shamanism and adventure therapy. For eleven of those years he has worked as an adventure therapy facilitator for The Wilderness Program. Nick has also worked with high needs 'wards of the state' within the Complex Care Program (DHHS Tasmania), and with survivors of torture and trauma at the Phoenix Centre (FASSTT). He works with the Aboriginal Health Service as a counselor; with 'Becoming Men' (a boy to young man rite of passage) in his role with The Wilderness Program; in private counselling and delivering his program called 'A Simple Way To Create A High Functioning Group'. Nick has a degree in fine art from the University of Tasmania, and a graduate certificate in counselling.

Richard Lannowe Hall BEM BA, is founder of Sailaday OK a charity that supports Marine Adventure Therapy. He originally trained as Transactional Analyst psychotherapist; he is the primary therapist and professional skipper with client groups who are recovering from trauma, abuse and addiction. He facilitates residentials on a boat of four days and nights for groups, families and couples. He has developed an integrative models and methodology for the programme with very positive feedback and outcomes. Other activities involve writing and publishing in professional journals.

Sue Parker Hall is a Certified Transactional Analyst (Psychotherapy) (UKCP registered) as well as being a British Association of Counselling and Psychotherapy senior accredited practitioner, a member of the Institute of Transactional Analysis and the Institute of Transactional Analysis in America. She adheres to their ethical frameworks, receives regular supervision and continuously enhances her own personal and professional development.

Nevin J. Harper is a faculty member at the Centre for Sport and Exercise Education, Camosun College, Victoria, British Columbia. Nevin is also the National Research Coordinator for Outward Bound Canada, and an Instructor for the Centre for Sport and Exercise Education at Camosun College, Victoria BC.

Lourens Human PhD, is a registered counseling psychologist with the Health Professions Council of South Africa (HPCSA) and is employed in the Department of Psychology at the University of Pretoria, South Africa. He is primarily responsible for coordinating the MA (Counselling Psychology) program. He lectures in narrative based counseling, adventure based counseling, as well as sports counseling and sport psychology on the program. In general his research interests correspond to his lecturing areas while he has specific interests in the development of professional identity development through adventure in the postgraduate counseling psychology students.

Joe Hinds Following a BA in Social Psychology and a Masters in Psychological Research Methods (MRes) Dr. Hinds gained his D.Phil from the University of Sussex in 2007. Whilst at Sussex, he was employed as a Graduate Teaching Associate in the School of Psychology and as a researcher at the Teaching and Learning Development Unit. Since then, he has been a Visiting Lecturer at the University of East London teaching on their MA in Positive Psychology and at Brighton University teaching Ecopsychology. More recently, between 2010 and 2013 he was at Sheffield Hallam University as a Senior Lecturer in Social Psychology. He is also an Honorary Adjunct Lecturer at University College Dublin, Eire.

Chris Jansen has an extensive range of training and facilitation experience both in New Zealand and also in Singapore, Australia, and the United States. He lectures in outdoor and experiential education at the University of Canterbury, New Zealand and is undertaking a PhD study exploring leadership through appreciative inquiry. He has worked as a counsellor working with adolescent offenders and their families and in substance abuse treatment programmes. He has an M.Ed Counselling and is a registered teacher and member of the New Zealand Association of Counsellors.

Stephen Johnson is a Fellow of the Royal Society of Arts (FRSA) and a health professional with many years' experience as a mindfulness teacher and senior trainer with Breathworks C.I.C. who help therapists and practitioners to deepen their mindfulness practice and become teachers. An Ecotherapist and Humanistic Psychology practitioner, he has a BSc(Hons) in Integrated Therapy and an MSc which examined the role of environment in improving health. He taught at Cambridge, Salford, Lancaster and Manchester Metropolitan Universities, and is researching the role of nature and mindfulness in the Faculty of Health and Well-Being at the University of Cumbria. A mountain leader for over thirty years and former military medic, Steve continues to be involved in pre-hospital care as Casualty Care coordinator of a Lake District mountain rescue team and as a medic on adventure races. He is also a TRiM (trauma risk management) assessor for Mountain Rescue and the Police. He established Tao Mountain to combine these outdoor and health interests through delivering health activities in nature: *www.taomountain.co.uk.* He has worked with young offenders, community groups, environmental and regeneration charities and is currently working with people affected by pain and chronic illness. He was UK delegate to the first Asia Pacific ICHPER (International Congress on Health, Physical Education and Recreation) Conference in Malaysia and is one of two UK delegates to the International Adventure Therapy Committee. He has presented at conferences in Manchester, London, Geneva and Johannesburg, including a keynote presentation at the 3rd Global Change conference.

Peter Kellett has been lecturing in outdoor education at the university of South Australia (Uni SA) in Adelaide, Australia, AustraliWe'a since 2004. He has previously coordinated outdoor programs in South Australian secondary schools, and acted as advisor to outdoor education teachers. In 1981 he established a nature based tour business specialising in walking, cycling and canoe tours in South Australia and Europe, in which he is now working full time.

Carinna Kenigsberg is the Program Manager at Power to Be, an adaptive adventure therapy program in Canada. Combining her love of wilderness and ocean with a passion to support people living with cognitive, emotional, neurological and complex needs, Carinna has embedded her knowledge and years of experience to create profound connection and transformations through nature at Power To Be. Holding a BA in Child and Youth Care from the University of Victoria, Carinna trains staff in behaviour management communication strategies and non-violent crisis intervention. She has been at the helm of the Adaptive Recreation program since 2005, developing, expanding and resourcing Power To Be with staff, students and volunteers to inspire greatness and be stewards of positive change.

Hendrik Sebastiaan (Drikus) Kriek is Director of the Leadership Development Centre and Associate Professor in Human Resource Management and Leadership at Wits Business School. He is a registered Clinical Psychologist and received his MA (Clin Psych) and MBA both cum laude from the Rand Afrikaans University and the University of Stellenbosch respectively. Prof Kriek is a graduate from Yale University in the United States, and received his Doctorate from the University of Pretoria. His research, publications and teaching focus mainly on teams, leadership and change management. He consults in the field of Organisation Development and had been involved in management education projects, leadership development programmes and change initiatives. He regularly conducts local and international teambuilding interventions and is involved in executive education programmes, leadership development and change initiatives to some of South Africa's most well known companies. He has been instrumental in the establishment of the local Adventure Therapy industry and recently completed commissioned research (with a colleague Prof Stella Nkomo) on Sizwe Nxasana, former CEO of Telkom and on African Change Leadership (linking life histories of leaders with change processes). He is a regular speaker on teams, team building and leadership in South Africa and on international forums. In 2006 he was visiting Professor at the Integral Leadership Centre of the Graduate School of Management of the University of Western Australia in Perth. Prof Kriek has lectured, consulted and conducted team interventions in a number of countries including Australia, the Democratic Republic of the Congo, Namibia, Botswana, Zimbabwe and Eretria.

Tarquam McKenna, is a registered art psychotherapist and a Professor within the College of Education at Victoria University Australia. He has been working with arts, psychotherapy, and education using creative processes as psychotherapies and for wellness as a primary focus for all his life. He has taught, supervised and worked with training in education, special education and psychotherapies programs in Australia and New Zealand for more than twenty years. He is past president of the Australian and New Zealand Art Therapies association (ANZATA) and current editor of the journal ANZJAT.

Jamie Mcphie is a Lecturer of Cultural Landscapes and Aesthetics in the Outdoors in the Department of Outdoor Studies, University of Cumbria.

Megan Millar is the Community Development Coordinator at Power to Be. A selfish do-gooder, Megan has spent her life travelling around the world looking for the next opportunity to work with youth and people with diverse needs and connect them with nature. Taking her passion for camping, paddling and adventure, Megan also brings a ton of expertise and education with a BA in social work, extensive wilderness and paddling training, and leadership facilitation to our programs. In her words, "I want my ability to make others laugh, feel cared for and loved to be remembered. I want to accomplish great things through tiny moments. What drives me is my desire to support others. What's the world mean if we don't have one another for support?"

Stephan Natynczuk has over 25 years' experience in adventure therapy and runs the not-for-profit My Big Adventure organization. Stephan draws on a rich experience of being a solution focused adventure therapy practitioner, employer, social-entrepreneur, academic, and chief optimist at My Big Adventure.

James Neill is an Assistant Professor in the Centre for Applied Psychology at the University of Canberra. James' research examines processes and outcomes of outdoor, experiential, and nature-based programs. For more information, see *http://wilderdom.com.*

Aunty Verna Nicholls is a Tasmanian Aboriginal Elder who was born on Cape Barren Island where she spent her early years. She has been teaching traditional and contemporary aboriginal cultural art and craft for much of her adult life and has exhibited her own work in many places including the Tasmanian Museum and Art Gallery. Her work with her own people in connecting to culture, country and community has also occurred during this time. In 2003 she bagan participating and facilitating on Aboriginal Outdoor Recreation Program (AORP) camps significantly helping to develop a style of adventure therapy that would meet the needs of her community, blending cultural elements with the adventure activities. She still continues to be involved with teaching art and craft but has retired from facilitating adventure-based programs.

Val Nicholls has a PhD (Education) from the University of Wollongong; a Bachelor Fine Arts (Hons) University of Tasmania; a Certificate IV Outdoor Leadership, Tasmania; and is a Licentiate of the College of Speech Therapist, University of London. Val lives in Tasmania, Australia and works as an independent educator, consultant and practitioner of nature-based adventure therapy.

Christine Lynn Norton PhD, LCSW, Associate Professor of Social Work at Texas State University San Marcos, received her PhD in Social Work from Loyola University Chicago. She has a Master of Arts in Social Service Administration from the University of Chicago and a Master of Science in Experiential Education from Minnesota State University Mankato. She has over 20 years' experience working with adolescents in a variety of practice settings including therapeutic wilderness programs, juvenile justice, youth and family counseling, schools, and youth mentoring and educational empowerment programs. Her areas of practice and research expertise are in innovative interventions that promote effective treatment in child and adolescent mental health, positive youth development, and youth empowerment. Christine published her edited book Innovative Interventions in Child and Adolescent Mental Health with Routledge. Christine is an appointed research scientist on the Outdoor Behavioral Healthcare Research Council, and is on the Association for Experiential Education's Therapeutic Adventure Professional Group Leadership Council.

Paddy Pawson has worked with young people for the past 25 years in various capacities and across a wide area of needs. For the last 10 years he has worked with and for Waipuna Youth and Community Trust in New Zealand developing and delivering adventure therapy programmes. He is working in a developmental role with adventure therapy in New Zealand to look at ways of expanding practice into more cultural communities and into the fields of education, health, and justice.

Luk Peeters has been working in the experiential outdoors since 1985. He has a Master's degree in Educational Sciences and is a Gestalt-trainer, -supervisor and -therapist with a specialisation in Existential Psychotherapy and Group Psychotherapy. He is responsible for the training department of a challenge course company, coordinates a Gestalt training program, is staff member of a specialisation in Group Psychotherapy and in Emotion Focused Therapy, apart from his private engagements as a psychotherapist and group trainer. He presented at several international conferences and is the author of some articles addressing the use of adventure supporting psychotherapeutic processes.

Duke Peltier set a career goal of enhancing the quality of life for Wikwemikong Unceded Indian Reserve. He is employed as Recreation Coordinator and is studying Native Studies at Laurentian University. Duke was first elected in August 2006 to the Wikwemikong Band Council, and he continues to serve in that capacity with varied responsibilities over the years, such as managing the economic development and education portfolios. He is actively involved in his community and serves on numerous boards and various committees. Some highlights of his work include the development of a 'Better Practices' Manual for Rural, Northern and Aboriginal Communities throughout Canada through his appointment on the Northern Links Expert Committee. He collaborates on research initiatives related to Aboriginal sport programming and positive youth development with Laurentian University.

Scott Polley has been lecturing at the University of South Australia since July 1996. He completed a Registered Nursing Certificate at the Royal Adelaide Hospital in 1986 and a degree in Secondary Physical Education Teaching (Outdoor Pursuits Specialisation) in 1991. He has a Master of Education (Outdoor Education) from La Trobe University, Bendigo. He coordinates the Outdoor Education program (minor, sub-major and major) at the University of South Australia. He holds leadership awards in sea and white-water kayaking, walking, rock climbing and sailing. His interest in adventure therapy stems from working with youth at risk for several months prior to lecturing at UniSA.

Anita Pryor PhD, is an Associate Member of NiCHE (Nature in Community Health and Environment) Research Group of Deakin University School of Health & Social Development; an Associate Member of CFRE (Centre for Family Research and Evaluation); International representative of AABAT (Australian Association of Bush Adventure Therapy); Australian representative of ATIC (Adventure Therapy International Committee); member of the Psychotherapy and Counseling Federation of Australia; member of the Australian Association of Family Therapy; and Director of Adventure Works Pty Ltd. For more information, see: www.adventureworks.com.au

Peter Rae lives in Tasmania and facilitates an alternative education program for youth disengaged from mainstream education that utilizes adventure therapy as a major component. Peter previously worked for Sport and Recreation Tasmania as the Project Officer – Aboriginal Recreation responsible for the planning and implementation of the Aboriginal Outdoor Recreation Program (AORP). He has been involved in the field of adventure therapy since 1999 with the Wilderness Program (formerly Project Hahn), the Dooloomai Youth Project and more recently, Adventure Works.

Brenda Restoule (Waub-Zhe-Kwens – Little Swan Woman) is from Dokis First Nation (Eagle Clan). She is a registered psychologist in Ontario and presently holds dedicated contracts with First Nation communities where she provides direct intervention services, program and community development, and clinical consultation to their mental health programs. She has worked with provincial and federal government departments, and was involved with the Royal Commission on Aboriginal Peoples in Canada (1996). She is the vice chair of the Native Mental Health Association of Canada where she has been an active member since 1995. Her work is dedicated to improving the wellness of Aboriginal people, and she is particularly interested in reducing suicide rates by encouraging a return to traditional practices of caring for each other.

T. Martin Ringer was actively involved in the development of adventure therapy in New Zealand from the early 1970s. He was instigator and convener of the First International Adventure Therapy Conference in Perth in 1997 and actively contributed to many subsequent conferences. From the early 1990's Martin has focused his attention on group dynamics and in particular how systems theory and psychoanalytic theory informs group practice. His book on the subject "Group Action" was published in 2002. From the last ten to fifteen years he has focused on experiential group training of leaders and facilitators as well as applying his skills to teams in corporate settings. Now in his 60's, Martin is drawn more to stone carving, writing and working with those who are passionate about groups and about 'taking the unconscious seriously'. See also www.groupinstitute.com

Stephen D. Ritchie is an Assistant Professor and doctoral candidate at Laurentian University in Canada. He has worked in the outdoor field on and off for more than 25 years as a guide, teacher, facilitator and more recently as professor and program coordinator in outdoor adventure leadership. Stephen has a BPE in Outdoor Pursuits from the University of Calgary and an MBA from Concordia University. Over the past seven years he has taught a variety of under-graduate courses at Laurentian University on topics such as outdoor facilitation and teambuilding; risk management; and adventure therapy. As an instructor trainer, each year Stephen also teaches and certifies students in canoeing and rock climbing. Stephen's research interests are primarily devoted to understanding outdoor and wilderness adventure experiences in the context of achieving personal growth and holistic health.

Lisa Ronalds teaches Outdoor Education and Physical Education. She completed Honours in Exercise Science at the Australian Catholic University in 2005 and completed a Graduate Diploma of Education in Outdoor Education and Physical Education in 2004. Her passion is helping young people to develop to their fullest potential. She is always planning the next adventure in natural places.

Alexander Rose MA, has a professional background related to experiential learning and outdoor skills, focusing his interventions mostly to adolescents, orphans and offenders, coordinating and teaching at the Outdoor School from the Catholic University in Valencia and as lecturer at different universities. Since 2007 his emphasis has been towards Adventure therapy, having presented at several conferences, currently finalizing an introductory manual in Spanish and developing the basis of a Wilderness Therapy program for adolescents. He holds a Master's Degree in Addictive Conducts, and Bachelors Degree in Psychology, Sport Sciences and in Primary School Teaching.

Keith Russell is an Associate Professor in Recreation at Western Washington University, Bellingham, WA, USA. He is the former Director of the Outdoor Behavioral Healthcare Research Cooperative (OBHRC). His research emphasis includes program evaluation, the study of human-nature relationships, the therapeutic value of natural environments, and international protected area management. He teaches courses in statistics, research methods, adventure education and therapy, and human relations. He has been a wilderness educator for more than fifteen years in the US, Mexico, Costa Rica, and New Zealand.

Kim Sacksteder MSW, LISW-S has worked with at-risk youth for over 16 years and has been practicing adventure therapy for 10 years. She supervises the Wilderness Bond Program at Camp Mary Orton in Columbus, Ohio, USA. Kim has been involved in TAPG's efforts to develop best practices since it began. She has chaired the AEE/TAPG Best Practices Steering Committee since 2005. Kim is deeply committed to providing quality service that supports her clients in making the changes they seek and believes strongly in adventure therapy's ability to do just that.

Robert Schinke is a Professor in the School of Human Kinetics and holds a Canada Research Chair, at Laurentian University. Robert is the Editor of Athletic Insight, a peer reviewed journal in sport and exercise psychology, and is the 2008 Canadian Sport Science Research Award recipient for Community Research. Robert's research is funded by the Social Sciences and Humanities Research Council of Canada and the Canadian Foundation of Innovation, and the focus of his work is based upon culturally reflexive motivation and methodology. Robert serves as a motivational consultant to clients from many cultures, and provides applied service mostly in professional sport.

David Segal has been providing adventure therapy for children, youth and families for over 10 years. He is deeply passionate about the natural world and how our inter-being influences our collective and individual well-being. He has given numerous presentations and workshops on cultivating health through contact with nature and adventure and currently works as a clinical counsellor serving youth and families through the Power to Be Adventure Therapy Society and Human-Nature Counselling and Consulting.

David Stacey lives and works in Devon, England. He gained a Postgraduate Certificate in Education (Secondary) the University College of North Wales in Outdoor Education and Science in 1987, and since then has gained a broad range of experience working in the outdoors. Central to this has been his work with the Community of St Antony and St Elias based in Totnes, Devon (England), an organisation specialising in providing care and support towards recovery for adults with severe and enduring mental health problems. For twelve years his main responsibility was that of the Outdoor Activities Manager, developing and running the organisation's Outdoor Activity programme. He has gained a Masters in Philosophy from Exeter University for a research project investigating the ethos and working methods of the Community, which included a broader look at therapeutic communities and related approaches. He is currently part of the senior management team within the Community, and has a broad range of responsibilities including coordinating the overall activity programme. He has made contributions to several conferences both in the UK and abroad based around his experiences of working in the outdoors with adults with mental health problems. David is an Accredited Practitioner of the Institute for Outdoor Learning.

Kaz Stuart has worked in a variety of educational settings (primary and secondary schools and headship of a private school for emotionally and behaviourally difficult young people), as an outdoor instructor for children and adults, and has experience of youth work as a front line worker, consultant and senior manager. She has expertise in experiential learning, and is Cochair of the International Consortium of Experiential Learning. Kaz works for the University of Cumbria, based at Brathay Trust as the Research Leader via a Knowledge Transfer Partnership, she is helping to embed evaluation at Brathay and carries out bespoke research projects for them.

Duncan Taylor has an academic background in the history, politics, and philosophy of the environmental movement in North America. He has worked on forestry issues as part of his more inclusive research on the history and development of environmental thought, and in the larger issue of 'sustainable development' and the question of what it means to meet of human and biophysical needs. His recent work has specialized in the application of integral systems approaches to cultural transformation and environmental changes. He is also involved with the application of complexity theory to ongoing adventure therapy programs for adolescents at risk on Vancouver Island. Duncan's books include: *Off Course: Restoring Balance Between Canadian Society and the Environment* (International Development Research Centre, 1994), *Ecoforestry: The Art and Science of Sustainable Forest Use* (with Alan Drengson, New Society Publishers, *1997),* and most recently the edited anthology *Wild Foresting: Place Based Practices for Diversity and Health* (New Society Publishers, 2009).

Alison Voight is the Coordinator for Therapeutic Outdoor Programs and an Assistant Professor of Recreation, Park, and Tourism Studies at Indiana University. Dr. Voight is a Certified Therapeutic Recreation Specialist, and her research and publications have involved motivation, theory-based processing, and social-psychology of leisure, therapeutic outdoor programs and emotionally disturbed youth, adventure programs and salient benefits, and best practices in accessibility of recreation programs and facilities.

Mary Jo Wabano has worked with Aboriginal youth through program development addressing self-esteem and building confidence since 1985. She is the Health Services Director for the Wikwemikong community. It has been a practice of Mary Jo to work collaboratively on various projects within the community inclusive of other neighbouring First Nations communities. The years of experience that she has gained contribute to her understanding of the life challenges for Aboriginal youth and have helped her realize and acknowledge the potential youth have in terms of striving to become successful young adults. Mary Jo continues to work diligently at providing guidance to a team of Program Managers who are responsible for implementing various programs and services geared towards holistic well-being. She continues to work towards empowering community members to take responsibility for their own health and well-being.

Nancy Young is a Professor at Laurentian University in Canada. She also holds a Canada Research Chair in Rural and Northern Children's Health, funded by the

Canadian Institutes in Health Research. Nancy has a BSc in Physical Therapy, a Masters in Clinical Epidemiology and a PhD in Medical Sciences, all from the University of Toronto. Nancy has been actively engaged in children's health for more than 20 years, both as a clinician and scientist. Her research has underscored the importance of including children's voices in health through their active participation in research.

CONTEXTUALIZING

> Making mental connections is our most crucial learning tool, the essence of human intelligence; to forge links, to go beyond the given; to see patterns, relationships, context.'
>
> -Marilyn Ferguson

Overview of the Fifth International Adventure Therapy Conference

Kaye Richards

Since the inaugural conference in Australia (1997), the Fifth International Adventure Therapy Conference (5IATC) was hosted for the first time in the United Kingdom (2009). Titled 'Adventure therapy as an emerging approach: Towards a profession', this most recent conference pointed towards adventure therapy critically evaluating itself as an approach to psychological therapy, with the longer term goal of enabling greater recognition, deeper understanding, and widening access to adventure therapy interventions across the world.

As adventure therapy practitioners and researchers, our goal is to ensure the reach and positive impact of the work we do. This can only be achieved if (under all its guises) our practice is considered a recognised, validated, effective, and ethical approach, within the broader psychological therapy community. As an international professional group we have to be committed to ensuring that the appropriate knowledge and practice infrastructures are robustly developed and put in place in order to achieve this recognition. This agenda served as a key driver for 5IATC.

Past international adventure therapy conferences have engaged with broader therapeutic, counselling and psychotherapy knowledge and approaches (see Itin,

1998; Richards & Smith, 2003; Bandroff & Newes, 2005; and Mitten & Itin, 2009). As theory, research and practice have developed, the reference to adventure (and outdoor) therapy within mainstream counselling and psychotherapy literature is encouragingly more evident (for example, McLeod, 2009; Brown & Richards, 2005). The ways in which adventure therapy positions itself within mainstream psychological therapies continues to be an important agenda.

Given that the British Association for Counselling and Psychotherapy (BACP) – the leading professional body for counselling and psychotherapy in the UK – hosted 5IATC, this offered a unique platform for the broader recognition of adventure therapy as a legitimate therapeutic approach. BACP's vision 'towards an emotionally healthy society 'and its mission 'to enable access to ethical and effective psychological therapy by setting and monitoring professional standards' – complimented the goals of 5IATC and supported broader engagement with these related professional agendas.

5IATC provided an opportunity for more careful and critical knowledge exchange between adventure therapy and counselling and psychotherapy theory and practice. This was evident particularly in the areas of professionalism, theoretical perspectives, ethical practice, and research. The dynamic interplay between emerging theory and practice across both key strands of outdoor adventure and therapy illustrated the critical discourse required in facilitating future directions, along with the need to re-evaluate theoretical assumptions and perspectives of psychological (transformative) change processes. The documented proceedings of 5IATC demonstrate aspects of adventure therapy theory and practices that underpinned these debates.

Keynote speakers at 5IATC included adventure therapists and outdoor educators from across the world (Dene Berman, Jennifer Davis-Berman, Cathryn Carpenter, Christian Itin, Chris Loynes, Julian Norris, Paddy Pawson and Keith Russell), as well as mainstream counselling and psychotherapist researchers and practitioners (Sally Aldridge, Liz Bondi, John McLeod, Nick Totton, and Alette Willis). Collectively, these speakers identified ways in which adventure therapy is positioned within a history, tradition and profession of outdoor practice, along with the need to embrace the history, traditions, and profession of counselling and psychotherapy. In part, they offered critical theoretical perspectives to a range of approaches of working psychotherapeutically in an outdoor setting, as well as stories of client's individual narratives of change, providing inspiration for recognising the significant impact adventure therapy can and does have.

The workshops and paper presentations reflected diverse international perspectives, and these cultural differences offered innovative examples of practice and perspectives in emerging debates. For example, local political climates, legislation, and cultural needs of therapeutic interventions differ across countries. This diversity brings important understanding to developments as it challenges current knowledge and refreshes perspectives. The papers presented here, therefore, represent different approaches and views from across the globe.

Nevertheless, central questions about the psychological process of change and the benefits of adventure therapy approaches are essential to all international practice. How do we know what kind of adventure therapy intervention works best for what client and when? How can we ensure ethical practice and maintain professional standards? How can we understand the change processes in action and develop theoretical models? How do we build the knowledge and practitioner base of adventure therapy that ensures it is an effective approach? How do we engage policy makers, clients, professionals and the public in this emerging knowledge base? These questions were engaged with during 5IATC and will inevitably continue to underpin the ongoing emergence of adventure therapy as a more widely applied psychological intervention.

Alongside the international adventure therapy community, key organisations supported the success of 5IATC. These included the Adventure Therapy International Committee (ATIC), along with sponsorship from the Association of Experiential of Education (AEE, USA) and the Therapeutic Adventure Professional Group (TAPG, USA); the Institute for Outdoor Learning (IOL, UK), the Routledge/Taylor and Francis Group (UK), Liverpool John Moores University (UK), and the University of Cumbria (UK). It is also essential to acknowledge the presenters and delegates – they all co-created 5IATC itself. Finally, I would like to offer a personal thank you to BACP who embraced my invitation (whilst an employee with them) to host 5IATC. Their willingness to support the conference (and myself in taking the lead role) ensured the success of the event. 5IATC will have a long-standing impact on the endeavours of adventure therapy practices, both in the UK and internationally, and the Adventure Therapy International Committee is grateful to BACP for this support.

In conclusion, as a collective international community we know that adventure therapy has an important part to play in the global endeavour of promoting emotional and psychological health and well-being. The challenge for us all is not only to articulate what our common ground, goals and methods are, but also the more difficult task of finding strategic ways of realising the potential of adventure therapy amongst the complexities of research, policy and therapeutic practice across the world. These challenges will continue to inform, contribute and transform the boundaries of international practices, and an international knowledge base of adventure therapy. These proceedings have captured knowledge, ideas and debates from our shared experiences in Edinburgh (2009), and will help inform and inspire us as we walk along and share the path of adventure therapy with the clients and the professionals we work with across the world.

REFERENCES

Bandoroff, S. & Newes, S. (Eds.). (2005). *Coming of age: The Evolving field of adventure therapy.* Proceedings of the Third International Adventure Therapy Conference. Boulder, Colorado: Association for Experiential Education.

Brown, S. & Richards, K. (Eds.). (2005). Outdoor cure: Therapeutic processes and the natural world. *Therapy Today: The Professional Journal for Counselors and Psychotherapists, Special Issue*, 16(10).

Itin, C. (Ed.). (1998). *Exploring the boundaries of adventure therapy.* Proceedings of the First International Adventure Therapy Conference. Boulder, Colorado: Association for Experiential Education.

McLeod, J. (2009). *An introduction to counseling* (4th ed.). Maidenhead: Open University Press.

Mitten, D. & Itin, C. M. (Eds.). (2009). *Connecting with the essence of adventure therapy.* Proceedings of the Fourth International Adventure Therapy Conference. Boulder, Colorado: Association for Experiential Education.

Richards, K. & Smith, B. (Eds.). (2003). *Therapy within adventure.* Proceedings of the Second International Adventure Therapy Conference. Augsburg, Germany: Zeil Verlag.

Overview of the Sixth International Adventure Therapy Conference

Anita Pryor

The Sixth International Adventure Therapy Conference (6IATC) was hosted in the Czech Republic by ***Dr. Jiří Kirchner*** and ***Associate Professor Běla Hátlová*** along with an organising team from the University of Jan Evangelista Purkyně (UJEP) in Ústí nad Labem. A dedicated team of friendly volunteers provided on-ground support for the conference.

In contrast to the 5IATC hosted by the United Kingdom's professional peak body for counselling and psychotherapy, this conference was supported by a university named after a North Bohemian countryman and scientist called Jan Evangelista Purkyně (1787-1869) whose creative work in the spheres of science, education, social and cultural life was said to be inspired by his relationship with his North Bohemian home, a place of natural and cultural beauty.

The 6IATC was made possible through a European Union Structural Grant for Innovation received by UJEP for the development of a Bachelor program in Outdoor Activities. The conference was considered a foundation for exploring 'the problematics of outdoor activities and their therapeutic utilization'. Conference organisers saw the 6IATC as a good opportunity to bring international adventure therapy practices to the Czech Republic, to share cultural perspectives on uses of outdoor activities for therapy, and to explore possibilities for growing adventure therapy within Eastern Europe. Conference partners included the Faculty of Education, the Institute for Health Studies, the Department of Outdoor Activities, Gymnasion and the Czech Professional Association for Experiential Education.

Cultural practices in the Czech Republic have arguably always included nature-contact, and have long included a particular activity called 'tramping', which began as a means of gaining social and emotional freedom out-of-doors to escape the previously oppressive political regime. Although institutions such as UJEP have researched the physical benefits of physical activity in nature, organisers acknowledged that a focus on the mental health and psychotherapeutic benefits of outdoor activities had not yet gained strong legitimacy in the Czech Republic.

In their proposal to host 6IATC, organisers emphasized the Czech Republic's relative inexperience in the formalised endeavor of using outdoor activities in natural environments for therapeutic purposes. Based on Dr. Kirchner's presentation to the Adventure Therapy International Committee (ATIC) in 2009, members agreed that while the Czech Republic would likely benefit a great deal from an influx of international expertise, that international delegates would also gain inspiration from attending a conference in a cultural setting still in a formative stage of opening up to the possibilities of formsalised adventure therapy.

From the outset, the Czech Republic provided a striking contrast to previous IATCs – environmentally, socially, politically, culturally and professionally. To set the scene: the conference was held in a region called Bohemian Paradise, 100 kilometres northwest of Prague. Conference and accommodation facilities were set within an old castle called Hrubá Skála. The castle sat aloft a sandy mountain-top surrounded by lightly forested gullies, with nearby sand cliffs and caves offering an appeal for tourists and avid sportspeople alike. The conference venue itself was well appointed and charming, and from various towers and turrets, delegates could view nearby hilltops. It didn't take much imagination for foreign delegates to envisage defence fortifications and attacking catapults used by combating medieval armies hunkered down on opposing hilltops in times past. This scene also needs to mention three more Czech elements that helped to shape our 6IATC experience: music, meat, and 'the Czech way'; the significance of these elements will become clearer in delegate descriptions to come.

Keynote speakers at 6IATC included representation from professionals from across the world, including Dr. Michael Ungar, Dr. Alan Ewert, Masego Thamuku and Dr. Christian Itin, as well as local cultural, environmental and heritage specialists who taught all of us about the Czech Way and the history of 'tramping' from which Czech Adventure Therapy emerged (Hubka, 2015). Collectively, these speakers provided a wide perspective on the merits, possibilities and intersections of international adventure therapy. More than ever before, the 'dots were not joined' for delegates at this conference. Arguably, more than at previous IATCs, delegates were invited to draw on their own understandings, meanings and relevancies from the various offerings delivered and received within the cultural smorgasbord of offerings. As guests, delegates were invited to immerse themselves in cultural and historic sensations such as music, feasts of meat, fireside gatherings, outdoor adventures and even in a staged casino experience - as a means of stimulating cross-cultural professional dialogue. As always, some delegates were disappointed at the level or direction of professional stimulation offered by the conference program, whereas other peoples' expeectations were surpassed.

To move from a broad overview to a more focused evaluation of the 6IATC experience, I offer the words of delegates themselves in response to questions posed within a simple evaluation form circulated towards the end of the conference. Their reflections, feedback and advice for future IATC offers insight for those wishing to understand what was experienced in the castle Hrubá Skála in September 2012.

1. What did you appreciate about this conference, what would you like to show gratitude for?

Delegates acknowledged the dedicated team of staff and volunteers who supported the 6IATC: 'thank you to the very hardworking and dedicated organizing team'. The support team was recognised as being willing to change things when necessary, and accommodate the specific needs of delegates: 'the helpers had amazing spirit n' commitment'. The following elements were also highly appreciated:

- The natural features and landscape surrounding the conference venue, the chance to climb and be active
- The diversity of speakers and participants, the quality of keynote speakers
- Networking opportunities, conversations over drinks and meals
- The introduction to Czech culture, the great atmosphere, 'the Czech way' – hospitality, music, tramping, beer, meat, casino.

2. What was your most memorable moment during this conference?

Responses to this question were similar to the previous question: the natural environment (including the climbers memorial); access to outdoor activities (climbing, caving, Frisbee, a good place to go for a walk alone); quality of the keynote speakers and conference presentations (on topics such as existentialism, professional supervision etc.); venue; networking opportunities (including with practitioners from the same country); the inclusiveness and intimacy of the conference (including the social life, the great sense of community); and 'the Czech way' - the fire, the band, tramping songs, playing and singing together.

3. What are 1 or 2 specific things that could be changed or improved?

Delegates provided feedback about the pre-conference information, including the need for more information on the website, such as a clearer registration process, more information about travel and logistics, accomodation and post-conference options, and greater capacity for payment options. Others suggested that more community-building time at the outset would have benefited attendees, and the example given that in future conferences the organising committee could work on creating a welcoming environment for newcomers at the outset. Extra comments made by delegates emphasised some of the points already made, relating to:

- the helpfulness of the organising team
- the inspiring location
- the creativity of workshops, the learning provided by presenters and keynotes
- the overall richness and enjoyment of the 'Czech way' conference experience.

To conclude this overview, I make mention that many previous IATC delegates are looking forward to participating in the Seventh International Adventure Therapy Conference in Denver, Colorado in the United States of America, where we will have the opportunity to receive hospitality from our American colleagues and gain insights into 'the American way' of approaching adventure therapy. This richness of experience that comes from being hosted by international colleagues in their place and way - although accompanied by significant travel and environmental costs - is incredibly valuable. By clarifying what is significant and important about adventure therapy practice in one's own place and way; and to better understand how one's work meets with and diverges from other peoples' ways in distant places; the international adventure therapy arena and three-yearly IATC's are treasured by many.

References

Hubka, P. (2015). *What is Czech tramping? A brief history of Czech tramping in the Czech Republic and former Czechoslovakia*. Retrieved on 1/29/15 from: http://domov-trampu.home.comcast.net/~domov-trampu/Tramping.htm

CONNECTING

'Invisible threads are the strongest ties'

-Friedrich Nietzsche

Cathryn Carpenter

Following on from *Emerging Insights (2012), Adventure Therapy Around the Globe* is a collection of papers developed from presentations, workshops and discussions held during both the 5IATC and 6IATC. Over the years, international adventure therapy practitioners and researchers have considered what adventure therapy might 'look or feel like' if it became more widely recognised as a profession in its own right rather than an adjunct or an alternative process to a number of therapeutic, counselling, health or educational professions. It became clear that becoming a recognised profession could only become an option when a deeper understanding of current practices and practitioner requirements were identified, and the benefits and potential hazards of becoming a 'profession' were clarified. Developing a shared vision for international adventure therapy is still a 'work in progress'.

Vibrant discussions at both the 5IATC generated more questions about the implications of becoming a profession and possible criteria for the inclusion or exclusion of practitioners or programs. Within a smaller community of practitioners and theorists at the 6IATC these conversations focused more practically (and creatively) on expanding adventure therapy as a practice. These debates highlighted the unique approaches to adventure therapy utilised in many countries, by practitioners with diverse qualifications and skills. Whilst future directions were not agreed upon, the shared sense of community and the desire to link ideas and theories indicated a healthy curiosity towards alternative approaches and an individual commitment to professional practices within our own domains.

This collection of papers reflects multiple interpretations of how these developmental, therapeutic, psychotherapeutic and counselling processes are currently being implemented. The contributions of the Adventure Therapy International Committee (ATIC) members from around the world, each author and presenter, every reviewer, and all the conference attendees are what makes these gatherings so valuable. Both conferences and papers included in this book of proceedings offer a myriad of ways to improve and enhance the process and outcomes of adventure therapy experiences.

Connecting

The structure of this book of proceedings reflects our commitment to ensure the multiple voices of practitioners are shared. Some papers have been developed within a theoretical or academic framework that illustrates the author's knowledge and awareness of previous deliberations within this field. Other papers echo the voice of practitioners seeking a deeper understanding of their experiences and provide the lived dimension to adventure therapy practices. All share their unique perspectives and add to our collective knowledge and experience within the adventure therapy community and the broader professions. We encourage you to set aside any critiques on style or rigour, and explore the diverse range of papers offered within these proceedings. We invite you to explore the insights they have to offer you personally, as well as within your practice and profession. We continue the tradition of previous IATC proceedings in respecting the spelling norms of the authors' country of origin, rather than privileging one over another.

The papers in this book are organised according to the nature of their contribution to the field. We have developed the chapters and clustered the papers according to our interpretation of the kind of insights contained within the paper, and how we see their insights enhancing Adventure Therapy: Provoking, Sharing, Reflecting, Adapting, Exploring and Expanding. However, it is important to note that many papers address all aspects, and touch on the multiple dimensions or complexities of articulating Adventure Therapy.

Provoking

This chapter weaves the abstracts from the 5IATC and 6IATC keynote speakers' presentations alongside a series of reflections with the aim to provide an impression of the focus and intent of the session, as well as the nature of the experience and ramifications of ideas and thoughts posed. The selection of keynote speakers for these conferences deliberately attempted to embrace the diversity of theories and practices within our global community. Our collective creativity in constructing so many different and unique ways to combine small groups of people, natural places and adventurous experiences for enhanced health and wellbeing is extraordinary.

SHARING

This initial cluster of papers shares important concepts and frameworks that are developing within international adventure therapy. Chandler's paper begins this section by discussing the role nature has played in the development of key psychotherapists' theoretical frameworks. These frameworks inform practitioners' work today, and Chandler encourages us to ensure current practices also integrate relationships with 'wider nature'. Peeters rationalises the values of taking therapeutic experiences outdoors, provides activities, and discusses a number of pertinent issues within a Gestalt framework. Berman and Davis-Berman have written extensively within the field of wilderness therapy, and in this paper raise questions around the appropriateness of adventure therapy within mental health treatment services for children and adolescents. An Australian research study by Allen-Craig and Ronalds indicates that there is supporting evidence for the use of wilderness therapy as an intervention to help prevent young people prematurely disengaging from school. Pointon also focuses on adolescents demonstrating early signs of 'not conforming', or anti-social behaviour. Discussing the role of self-forgiveness in young people's willingness to change provides another layer of understanding these complex processes. Sacksteder's paper shares the inclusive and consultative processes undertaken by the Therapeutic Adventure Professional Group, in a search for best practices in adventure therapy in the United States.

Jansen and Pawson's paper provides an example of a program that is both philosophically and practically integrated within its community. By including the voice of Ihaka, we share his perceptions of change as he details the lived experience of the program. The final two papers in this section share Indigenous approaches to adventure therapy, and the significance of including country, culture and community. The experiences discussed by Rae and Nichols in Tasmania Australia echo similar experiences shared by Ritchie, Wabano, Schinke, Peltier, Restoule, Russell, Corbiere, and Young. These papers encourage us to respect the deep connections between people and place, and remind us of the rich cultural history and knowledge we are invited to share.

Reflecting

Reflection is one of the key processes we all need to engage with in order to improve practice and outcomes for all involved. All the papers in this section provide either food for reflection for the community of adventure therapy practitioners and theorists, or share the results of reflections discerned through applying a reflective lens to their own practice. The development of the first meta-analysis that focuses specifically on adventure therapy by Bowen and Neil enables us to reflect on short- and long-term effects of programs based on data from over 14,000 participants. This analysis of previous research within adventure therapy programs also provides valuable suggestions for the construction of future research approaches. Voight and Ewert also assist our improvements in future practice by reflecting on the benefits of using social diagnostic theories to understand and anticipate processes and outcomes of programs.

Freeman and Akhurst encourage us to reflect on the role that therapeutic landscapes have in our lives and work and to consider changing relationships people have with natural environments. Hinds takes the role of natural environments in a slightly different direction by clarifying how being immersed in nature is central to our sense of wellbeing. This study by Hinds confirms increased eudemonic wellbeing through identification with nature. Combining many diverse thoughts on what adventure therapy is or could be, Rose shares the diversity of Spanish communities and regulations as he reflects on challenges past and present in the implementation of adventure therapy. The final three papers reflect on what has worked effectively for the authors in their programs or adventure therapy practices. Kenigsberg and Miller outline adaptive recreation practices for all abilities, Lannowe Hall and Parker Hall explain how effective sailing is as a metaphor for life, and Natynczuk reflects on the key aspects of what is important in his adventure therapy programs.

Adapting

The papers in this section challenge us to look more broadly at what is happening in areas aligned with adventure therapy but not necessarily central to our current practice. Dyck's use of motivational interviewing within adventure therapy emphasises an approach in which the overall outcome of the processes are enhanced through borrowing and adapting other theoretical frameworks. Norton provides a theoretical cultural framework that enables us to make sense of personal experiences working across cultures. We are encouraged to apply and test the model further, to increase our sensitivity to people's social and cultural contexts. Stacey's work considers the ways in which the needs of a specific population, in this case people with severe mental health problems, can be met within adventure therapy programs.

Polley within an Australian context and Human and Kriek from a South African context demonstrate that adapting practices from one domain to another can be valuable within the tertiary training sector. Polley outlines the development of an adventure therapy curriculum subject within a University undergraduate outdoor education course in Australia, whilst Human and Kriek describe the inclusion of adventure experiences within a postgraduate counselling psychology course. The creativity of practitioners finding new ways to consolidate and improve the quality of programs and processes is also demonstrated within Gray and Stuart's adaption of storytelling techniques in adventure therapy. Using storytelling to facilitate reflection and personal growth enables us all to understand ourselves, and the world around us, in a different way.

Since presenting their paper at the conference, Taylor, Segal and Harper's work has been published in *Ecopsychology* (June 2010). Their application of integral systems theory to adventure therapy provides theorists and practitioners with a framework for examining practice. Mindfulness is increasingly used as an engagement strategy for a number of educational and therapeutic programs; however in this adaption, Johnson's focus is on enhancing the lived experience within natural locations with an emphasis on mindfulness and sensory recognition. The final paper in this section has Rose outlining the Existentialism paradigm and explaining that it can be utilised as an alternative yet complimentary theoretical framework that focuses on participants grasping a higher purpose for their lives.

EXPLORING

A number of practitioners have been stretching their approaches and understandings of practices within adventure therapy. These papers are pushing us in new directions, inviting us to understand practice through a different lens, or simply explore an idea or issue that is often not discussed. The first paper in this section explores the meaning and implications of 'quiet time' in activity-oriented or challenge-based programs. Nicholls invites us to consider the therapeutic potential of promoting quiet times within programs. Carpenter and McKenna have explored structuring program space through the creation of a reflexive space and discuss how they have been utilising art-focused activities within outdoor programs. Burrows also discusses art in the outdoors, with a focus on the specific needs of autistic students, suggesting that within nature they can develop a free world view and renewed perceptions of self through sensory perceptions. Burrows contrasts this approach to the more typical 'dualistic framework' experienced by neural-typical people.

Human's paper explores the interplay between life and death, raising a number of philosophical questions in relation to our own response to death in the outdoors, and what a subjective grieving process may involve. Within a legal framework, Kellett's paper investigates the ramifications of death in the outdoors by questioning when a serious mistake becomes a criminal act, and what kinds of social constructs shape community expectations.

The final three papers explore contact with nature. Hall provides a brief personal narrative, embodying his personal reflections as practitioner, and proposes that self-perceptions are a valid way of knowing what is, via awareness of synchronicity, immediacy and reciprocity. Harper challenges us to investigate ways of examining the role of contact with nature within therapeutic processes and McPhee explores participants' perspectives on how contact with nature influences their health and wellbeing. The development of an evidence-based research approach that thoroughly investigates the processes, outcomes and impacts of contact with nature is another important step towards adventure therapy coming to be described as a profession.

EXPANDING

The final chapter reflects on the evolution of adventure therapy practice since the first international gathering, and challenges us to consider new ways of understanding the internal and external dynamics within the global community. Pryor's paper from the 5IATC inspires us to broaden our perspectives, and expand our understanding of what international adventure therapy might become when body and soul are more comprehensively integrated as one. In order to expand and encompass our collective expertise into the future, Pryor suggests we need to re-examine our foundations in light of our values. This paper reminds us that all perspectives need to be balanced and retained within AT for the health and integrity of the professional community.

The following papers emphasise key areas of consideration for our professional community: 1) deepen and strengthen facilitator skills, 2) increase nature-embedded AT practices for holistic health and wellbeing, and 3) emphasise community approaches to practice, research and being real in intent, action and evaluation.

Peeters and Ringer's 'hidden adventure' is an opportunity to gain insight into the deeper unconscious processes at work within group dynamics. Facilitators acquiring these skills could further enhance program outcomes. As many AT programs become more explicit about the therapeutic intent of their programs, Schwenk and Natynczuk's paper on the importance of supervision in AT offers strategies to improve professionalism within the field. Ewert draws together a number of central theories confirming the human need for activities in natural environments for the benefit of everyone's health and wellbeing. The final paper by Ritchie, Wabano, Beardy, Curran, Orkin, Vanderburgh, Born and Young demonstrates the benefits of a reflexive team approach to the community-based participatory research that respects shared responsibility in effecting positive approaches to health. Incorporating the whole of community with a realistic emphasis, this approach enables evaluations to be more meaningful and true.

We hope that this collection of papers will challenge, inform, and engage you with ideas, practices and theories that connect us with the diversity of perspectives, skills and 'ways of knowing' within international adventure therapy. We hope that by working through our differences, our shared practices will continue to strengthen and become more innovative, more theoretically and culturally-informed, and more ethically sound. We anticipate that the expansion of knowledge and practice that hopefully emerges as a result of these processes will be felt around the international community of adventure therapy until our next gathering.

PROVOKING

Courage is what it takes to stand up and speak; courage is also what it takes to sit down and listen.

-Winston Churchill

Christine Lynn Norton

A variety of keynote speakers from diverse backgrounds and perspectives were invited to speak at the 5IATC and 6IATC. Speakers were selected because of their practice and research expertise, as well as their cultural worldviews and life experiences. Their addresses to the conference audience as a whole were meant to inspire, challenge, and most of all provoke the international adventure therapy community to think critically about what it is we do, why and how we do it, and in what larger context we practice.

The process of 'provoking' was a call to avoid merely going through the motions of what we already know, and to move past the status quo. We believe that the field of adventure therapy must resist the temptation of complacency, and it is in this spirit, that thought-provoking keynote addresses are provided here.

This chapter presents abstracts and summaries from several of the keynote speeches offered at the Fifth and Sixth IATC, along with a reflective commentary to highlight a selection of insights that emerged from each presentation. Though we were not able to capture all keynote speeches, this chapter provides a broad overview of the expertise and diversity of perspectives that the international adventure therapy community is committed to showcasing. We invite the reader to be provoked, and notice your own emerging insights as you read.

Keynote #1: 5IATC

Thinking about Adventure Therapy as Profession: Issues of Professionalisation

Sally Aldridge

This opening keynote considered the ways in which professions emerge and evolve and the challenges this process may present to adventure therapy in the next few years. One key factor in the development of a profession is that of boundary setting – who is inside the boundary and who is outside. This keynote examined how these decisions are made and how might they be changed.

Looking at the history of the psychological therapies in the UK, two patterns have emerged:

> 1. Exclusive—entry has tight boundaries, for example clinical psychologists whose fixed entry is by a small number of National Health Service (NHS) funded professional doctorates, the British Psychoanalytic Council entry through a limited number of training courses, and the Health Professionals Council (HPC) entry by approved qualifications. A traditional 19th century model of a profession and a professional – entry to people like us – middle class, male, university-educated, in full time work.
>
> 2. Inclusive—entry very open, internal hierarchy of individual accreditation. The second is represented by the caring professions, predominantly female, often part time and often found in workplaces subservient to the professions exemplified in 1 above.

According to Aldridge adventure therapy needs to be aware that wherever and however the process of professionalisation begins there is a tendency for this to become a self-reinforcing dynamic for the future and very difficult to change. A bit like the early decision in a relationship about who puts the rubbish out.

Adventure therapy in particular faces the challenge of bringing together two disciplines and there may be internal divisions of emphasis that will impact on the future. As she understands it, one emphasis is on adventure and the therapeutic gain is implicit, the other emphasis is on the therapy and the therapeutic gain is explicit. The outcome may be the same, but the process of professionalisation will be shaped by where the emphasis rests.

Reflections

Set against the beauty of the green hilltops of Holyrood Park and Arthur's Seat, the 5IATC took place at the University of Edinburgh, Scotland. The 5IATC was generously hosted by the British Association for Counselling and Psychotherapy (BACP) and the theme of the conference was 'Adventure therapy as an emerging approach: Towards a profession.'

Aldridge's keynote address followed on the heels of Kaye Richards of BACP who encouraged the international community of adventure therapy researchers and practitioners to strive together towards the goal of advancing adventure therapy towards becoming a 'recognized psychological therapy'. In doing so, Aldridge urged adventure therapy (AT) practitioners and researchers to build bridges between mainstream psychological therapies and outdoor, adventure practices and to be intentional about how we define ourselves on our journey towards professionalization.

This idea of 'consolidating adventure therapy as a therapeutic approach' (see 'Connecting') followed in the footsteps of four previous international conferences in which 1) an international community was first formed, 2) the therapeutic aspects within adventure were examined, 3) the common and diverse practices from around the world were considered, and 4) the essence of adventure therapy was explored. It is clear that each of these international adventure therapy conferences tell a story and that together, they represent a shared journey in which practitioners and researchers from around the world have come together to find common ground.

Interestingly, Aldridge opened the conference by drawing an important parallel between the processes of professionalization in other fields to what adventure therapy is currently facing. The issues of boundary setting, along with bringing two distinct disciplines together—therapy and adventure—set the tone of the conference in acknowledging the duality that exists in adventure therapy internationally.

Aldridge focused on the importance of intentionally reconciling this duality by making decisions as to which side of the therapy-adventure continuum the international community will lean in moving towards becoming a profession. This challenged many in the audience who were grounded in their own approach to adventure therapy and less aware of the multitude of ways in which adventure therapy is practiced around the world. This keynote also provoked those who wondered if adventure therapy should even be moving towards professionalization in the first place. Left with these important questions, the conference moved forward, entertaining a variety of ideas, while not fully accepting them.

KEYNOTE #2: 5IATC

A Landscape of Re-creation? Aspects of Human Nature Relations in the UK: Reflections on Some Historical Influences from a Therapeutic Perspective

Chris Loynes

Loynes reviewed aspects of the influence of history and culture on the British relationship with nature. Six themes of possible interest to therapeutic concerns were highlighted, these included:

1. The valuing of new places as places of freedom and possibility;
2. The attempts to gain dominion over nature;
3. The rise of the cult of the hero;
4. The emergence of recreation and the recreation movements;
5. The romantics and the idea of transformation; and
6. Power in human and human to nature relations.

The development of outdoor education during the twentieth century suggests that nature became an instrument of education in the pursuit of the social goals of the times. Further themes were identified from this history of outdoor education by Loynes that shed light on the values that can underpin outdoor therapeutic work. These are summarised as:

- What have I got to give to society?
- What can I take from society?
- How do I join in?
- How do I manage the risks of modern life?

The presentation concluded by Loynes expressing concerns about the instrumentalisation of nature in all these social projects. However, it ended on a note of hope with a reference to new trends that can be understood as challenging long held norms of human nature relations in the United Kingdom.

Reflections

As photographs of the natural world flashed over the screen, Loynes' keynote address openly challenged conference attendees to ask ourselves how we relate to nature and how our perceptions of the natural world have been culturally shaped and informed. Is nature a place we go to find the transcendent? Is it a place we go to experience challenge and adventure? Do we compartmentalize the natural world as a commodity that we must use and therefore protect or does nature have intrinsic value in and of itself? As Loynes deconstructed the British (and largely Western) perspective on nature, his talk provoked us to consider how we relate to the outdoor context in which many adventure therapy interventions take place.

As I sat listening, I remembered working for Outward Bound in the Boundary Waters Canoe Area Wilderness (BWCAW) on the border between the United States and Canada. I was working with a group of 7 boys, and I was amazed at how the terrain challenged them to take personal responsibility and not give up. I looked at my co-instructor, and reflected on what a great 'course area' the BWCAW is. He looked back at me smiling, as the sun and the wind hit his face, and said, 'Yeah, and it's a beautiful place too.' The value I gave to the natural world in that moment reflected its therapeutic value in terms of program and treatment goals. However, my co-worker, in his inimitable way, reminded me not to miss the simple beauty of place that existed and had value whether we were there or not. This vignette is my own personal experience of the need to avoid what Loynes referred to as the 'instrumentalisation' of nature.

As practitioners and researchers, this keynote provoked us to understand that various perceptions of the natural world exist and that we need to be self-aware, as well as be aware cross-culturally of how our participants experience the natural world. This is important to the way we practice adventure therapy, as well as the way we develop our programs. If, for example, we think of the natural world as a place in which to challenge ourselves by conquering nature (bagging a peak, tearing up a river, etc.), then the programs and interventions we develop will be skewed towards challenging, adrenalin producing activities. If, however, our view of nature is a haven, a place of quiet reflection, then the opposite is true, and our programs and interventions will be focused on contemplation and connection with the natural world. Loynes' talk was not to say that one perspective was better or worse than the other, but more that we need to be aware of finding a balance and being open to new interpretations of our relationship with nature.

Keynote #3: 5IATC

Exploring an Emergent Dualism in Adventure Therapy Practice

Keith Russell

This presentation argued that the 'body' of adventure therapy (AT) might be in contrast to its 'soul', reflecting an inherent dualism in the field. In North America, the body of AT, manifest in theory, research and current practice, appears to be moving towards validation and acceptance by mainstream behavioural and mental health service delivery systems. Whether this is in reaction to increased public and governmental oversight or due to other causes, the end result seems to be a focus on research, best practices, licensure, and accreditation of AT programs and practitioners. Concurrent with this movement is the growing perception by many that the very essence of AT is being lost in this process, and subsequently that AT is in danger of losing its 'soul'.

This inherent dualism in AT practice seems to be present in discussions heard at conferences, on list serves, and in the literature, and has deep roots embedded in the soil of debate on whether the mountains do indeed speak for themselves. Does movement toward licensure, restrictive accreditation standards, and documented risk management practices move AT farther and farther away from that which makes it special and unique? And consequently, are we losing the opportunity to better understand the core elements of AT that make it truly unique? This presentation examined dualisms in AT and posed questions that guided discourse on the future of potential theory development, research and practice in international adventure therapy. Questions included:

- Do we think AT is currently divided into two competing paradigms?
- Is that a good or bad trend? Can a middle ground be tolerated? Why or why not?

Two areas relevant to AT practice were presented to provide context for the discussion. First, a review of research attempted to address the most fundamental questions of AT practice: Does it work, why, and for whom?

What does the research tell us? Second, current trends in behavioural and mental healthcare delivery systems being practiced in North America were presented in order to begin thinking about how these may impact AT practice. Some of these trends include how organizations are incorporating AT practice in: a) working with First Nation, Aboriginal or Native American peoples, b) treating substance abusing youth and young adults, c) as a prevention tool to promote physical activity and exposure to nature.

Reflections

The process of highlighting dualities apparent in the international adventure therapy community continued with Russell's keynote address in which he spoke about the tension between the structure or form of AT (particularly in the United States) and the magical process of AT that is harder to quantify. However, instead of just stopping there, Russell identified the various aspects of AT, the body (the structure) and the soul (the process), as being like the yin and the yang, complementary and adding to the other.

Bringing these distinct elements together to find common ground seemed especially important at the 5IATC. With over 21 nations represented, the conference emphasized the diversity and pluralism of adventure therapy. This was a part of the richness and beauty of the 5IATC, but also contributed to its challenges. Cultural differences in the practice of adventure therapy as well as cultural differences towards mental health 'treatment' created gaps between AT researchers and practitioners from Western and non-Western parts of the world.

As an American, I came to the 5IATC with the perspective of 'best practices,' professional credentialing, accreditation, and the move towards regulation of adventure therapy as a form of outdoor behavioral healthcare. Given the context of AT in the United States right now, with relevant legislation in Congress and other complicated ethical and legal issues emerging, this structure seems to be an important means of keeping AT alive and well, so to speak.

However, in other less regulated parts of the world, the structure of adventure therapy is less important than the process, and Russell was careful in his talk to also honour the magic and cultural elements of adventure therapy that are so powerful and necessary to preserve. Russell's keynote provoked us to search for this balance of 'body' and 'soul' by dialoguing, debating and searching for common ground.

KEYNOTE #4: 5IATC

Opening Doors in Mainstream Therapy: A Collaborative Pluralistic Perspective on Outdoor Therapy

John McLeod

McLeod discussed the collaborative pluralistic framework for the practice of counselling and psychotherapy as an integrative approach which calls for the therapist and client to work together to develop a shared understanding, and identify therapeutic tasks and methods relevant to the achievement of the client's goals. One of the basic principles of this perspective is that there exist a wide range of activities that may be of therapeutic value in accomplishing therapy tasks. These activities can include not only well-established therapeutic techniques, but also a diversity of cultural resources that open up possibilities for learning and change.

From a pluralistic perspective, outdoor therapies potentially have a major role to play in successful therapy with clients; however, in the community counseling agency where McLeod works, almost none of the clients have any involvement in outdoor activity. Even when it may be apparent to both client and therapist that such involvement would have therapeutic value, McLeod reported that it seems almost impossible to find ways to make it happen.

In this presentation, McLeod explored some of the issues and challenges that confront mainstream office-based counsellors and psychotherapists who are interested in integrating an outdoor dimension into their work with clients in the form of adventure therapy, wilderness therapy, nature therapy, horticultural therapies, or similar approaches, including: a) knowing what is available for clients and developing collaborative referral networks; (b) participating in relevant training to develop an awareness and appreciation of what is involved in different outdoor modalities; (c) being able to access theoretical analysis and research evidence on the processes and outcomes of different types of outdoor therapeutic provision in order to make informed decisions about what types of outdoor activity might be most relevant for each individual client. Suggestions on how these issues might be resolved were discussed, along with a brief discussion of the probable increasing importance of nature-based therapies at a period when the threat and reality of global environmental destruction will inevitably begin to shape the emotional and behaviour change agenda of clients entering therapy.

Reflections

The use of adventure therapy (AT) as an adjunct modality is becoming increasingly well documented as an important best practice (Gillen & Balkan, 2006). McLeod's keynote address gave adventure therapy practitioners an opportunity to consider the opportunities and barriers for bringing AT to mainstream counseling settings. McLeod presented us with a first-hand look at the challenges he faces, and provoked us to consider how to apply AT more effectively as an adjunct modality with other counseling approaches.

This issue is incredibly important if the international adventure therapy community is to provide conventional mental health settings with alternative interventions that do not pathologize clients, but give them new evidence of their strengths experientially. In order to make this happen, we must develop 'collaborative referral networks' in which traditional mental health professionals are informed, trained and open to utilizing AT. Fortunately, research in this area is beginning to occur in which adventure therapy practitioners are beginning to identify 'what every counselor should know about adventure counseling' (Gillen & Balkan, p. 156), which includes the similarities and differences of the two approaches. McLeod's keynote reaffirmed the need for a bridge between practitioners of conventional and adventure therapy approaches.

KEYNOTE #5: 5IATC

Exploring What Makes the Difference in Adventure Therapy Practice

Paddy Pawson

Based on many years as a practitioner in adventure therapy, Pawson examined the processes that seem to make a real difference for those taking part in adventure therapy interventions. Pawson argued that it is not what we do in adventure therapy that is important, but rather it is how we do it that makes the real difference.

Drawing upon the stories of young people who have experienced adventure therapy interventions in New Zealand, this keynote illustrated adventure therapy in action, and in doing so considered practical ways for how to best work in this setting.

Pawson also examined how adventure therapy practices can give meaning to the past, experience 'aroha' in the present, and allow hope into the future. Pawson concluded with an exploration of how we understand dependence, independence and interdependence, and how these understandings translate to processes of change in adventure therapy.

Reflections

Pawson's keynote address brought to us the faces, voices, dances and songs of Indigenous youth in New Zealand who had been profoundly affected by adventure therapy.

Participants shared stories of identity development, connection with nature, and making meaning of their lives. In Pawson's address, we learned of the term 'aroha', which is a Maori term that might be translated as 'unconditional love,' and stands for the utmost respect for fellow human beings (Jarosewitsch, 1997). Clearly, experiencing aroha in the context of an AT program defies quantitative analysis, and exemplified much of the 'soul' of adventure therapy of which Russell spoke earlier. As we listened to the youth who had been impacted by AT, we were invited to connect with the deep 'why' and 'how' of the work that we do.

KEYNOTE #6: 5IATC

Devoured by a Mountain Lion: Original Nature and the Social Ecology of Adventure Therapy

Julian Norris

The nature of our work in supporting transition, healing and development is both deeply personal and inherently systemic. This keynote, inspired by a compelling encounter in the natural world, explored four propositions related to this reality within adventure therapy practice as it pertains to our future development as a field and our relevance in these extraordinary times.

> Proposition One: Our own state of being as practitioners is a critical mediating variable in our field. Who we are is the foundation upon which our practice rests. How might we begin to support the emergence of a generation of practitioners who are both 'professional' and 'awakened'?
>
> Proposition Two: The lasting personal change outcomes sought by adventure therapy practitioners are generally inseparable from the systems within which our 'clients' dwell. Our theoretical and practice models – right the way from diagnosis to follow-up – must shift to reflect this reality.

Proposition Three: The future evolution of adventure therapy lies in being able to go both 'deeper' and 'broader.' Deeper in the sense that we become more effective and sophisticated in supporting individual therapeutic outcomes. Broader in the sense that the best work in our field is likely to emerge in the context of cross-disciplinary, cross-sectional and cross-cultural partnerships.

Proposition Four: Nature remains the greatest healer and teacher. Perhaps our most significant contribution in these times is that we offer an ecologically and experientially grounded approach to human development and wellness. In a sense, our role is to become servants of nature as we weave compelling contexts within which people can connect with and embrace their own creative intelligence and natural resilience.

Reflections

Norris's keynote was predicated on a story in which he was dwelling in a remote cabin in the woods, and that he had to go outside to use the bathroom. His awareness in the moment was that he may encounter, and even by devoured by, a local mountain lion that was roaming those lands. This awareness awoke within him a deep need to consider the context in which we dwell, and also the contexts in which we practice adventure therapy. As he shared this story, I was struck by the deep vulnerability of his situation, and I realized that being aware of our vulnerability is part of the process of knowing who we are something which Norris believes is foundational to our practice. While this idea may seem most connected to the 'soul' of adventure therapy, it is actually supported by the mainstream counseling literature, which argues that self-awareness may be related to counselor effectiveness (Abney, 2002).

Norris also shared his experiences of working with young people in Canada. He had facilitated experiences that incorporated community service, team-building and adventure-based experiences, including program elements that built upon the importance of local context in adventure therapy interventions. In some ways, his community-based model of adventure therapy could be considered a radical approach in which young people could work towards personal growth and change, supported by the community in which they dwell. And yet traditional communities, including Aboriginal and First Nation communities have worked in these ways for millennia. Perhaps some of us have just forgotten about these methods.

The 'community' approach reflects a more collectivist approach to adventure therapy, in contrast to a more commonly conducted 'individual approach, in which the identified client (often a high-risk young person), is removed from his or her community and sent away to a remote location. While adjunctive adventure therapy approaches are emerging, in which young people stay connected to their local communities (OMNI, 2011; CAT, 2011), Norris's keynote provoked us to consider the importance of doing this more often so that our interventions have broad systemic results, while still affecting deep, individual change.

In addition to these ideas, Norris highlighted the central role that nature plays in adventure therapy. These views on the role of nature in adventure therapy provoked us to consider the importance of delivering interventions that are both ecologically and experientially grounded. Some adventure therapy practitioners will caution us that not all adventure therapy occurs outdoors, and resist adventure therapy becoming 'nature therapy'. Yet many adventure therapy interventions do occur outdoors. Perhaps all of us, regardless of the setting or environment in which we work, need to further consider the impact of the actual location as a variable for change. Even more, however, Norris reminded us that the natural world is the primary sustaining context for who we are and what we do, and that perhaps our most valuable role is in reconnecting people to the natural world.

KEYNOTE #7: 5IATC

In Wilderness Therapy Lies the Preservation of the World: Climate Change, Values Change and Consumerism

Kate Rawles

The primary recipients of outdoor and nature-based therapies are people judged to be in need of some kind of 'therapeutic intervention'. In her keynote, Rawles argued that in industrialised 'modern' cultures, therapeutic intervention is also urgently required for the majority of citizens (who would not normally be considered to fall into this category). Industrialised lifestyles require ever-increasing resource consumption, and create ever-increasing levels of pollution on a planet that has ecological limits. Global climate change and catastrophic levels of biodiversity loss are amongst the impacts of these lifestyles, even though these 'privileged' lifestyles are currently only enjoyed by a minority of the global human population. Rawles reaffirmed the idea cited by the World Wildlife Fund, which is that if everyone on earth lived the lifestyle of an average Western

European, we would need three planet earths. She pointed out that modern lifestyles are profoundly unsustainable, and the ecological systems, species and other living beings that make up 'nature' are under severe threat from the 'normal' behaviour of most industrialised citizens including outdoor therapists.

Rawles acknowledged that while there has been some engagement with the role of therapy in helping people deal with the grief and pain caused by climate change and other forms of environmental devastation, we have a potentially much wider role in helping to prevent or at least mitigate these phenomena that has received less attention. Rawles reminded delegates that all of us who attended this conference are consumers; many of us consume more than a sustainable and equitable share of the planet's resources, and almost all find it very hard to consume significantly less even in the light of overwhelming scientific evidence about its consequences. Hence, scientific understanding alone is often not sufficient for action. Rawles stated we need other kinds of engagement and understanding, with particular regard to the links between self-esteem, self-worth, identity, status and material possessions. Her final claim, that nature-based therapies in general, and wilderness therapies in particular, have the potential to be especially potent in this context, provoked us to consider our role as adventure therapists in protecting and preserving the planet.

Reflections

Rawles continued the theme of encouraging us to consider the very broad context in which all of us practice adventure therapy: planet Earth. Rawles provoked us to take ownership of our own role in global climate change, both as individual citizens and as industrialized nations. The ideas presented in Rawles' keynote were further reinforced by a story of her border-to-border bike ride through the United States along the Rocky Mountains, in which she encountered numerous citizens for whom global climate change is at best not a priority, and at worst, a myth. Rawles' story of personal adventure and sacrifice highlighted the need to raise global awareness of this important issue, but also to raise our own internal awareness of our personal roles in relation to global climate change.

Rawles' presentation was emotionally challenging. Some of us felt a strong sense of embarrassment by our countries' conspicuous consumption and denial of the issue. We were also provoked as adventure therapists to consider our professional and ethical obligation to advocate for environmental regulations and protections. Rawles' talk was not meant to be only political but it did move, inspire and provoke all of us to consider the larger macro-level policies that either conserve or destroy the natural environment in which we all both dwell and practice.

KEYNOTE #8: 5IATC

Troubling Adventure Therapy: Constructing and Consuming Wilderness?

Alette Willis and Liz Bondi

Willis and Bondi's keynote was supportive of the goals of adventure therapy to both facilitate the healing of people in 'natural' settings, and to heal human relationships with the 'more-than-human-world'. Their keynote also illustrated the ways in which they are troubled by how concepts and practices may reify some of the western dualisms that underpin contemporary environmental problems. Like adventure therapists and their clients, Willis and Bondi find 'wilderness' environments immensely sustaining and restorative; however, they argued that such experiences are at least partially, expressions of the cultural contexts in which we live.

Without denying the existence and agency of 'non-human others', and the therapeutic potential of being immersed in landscapes that have been altered less by human actions than cities (where most people now live), Willis and Bondi pointed out that 'wilderness' itself is a human concept weighed down with problematic values. They articulated how adventure therapy tends to valorise and propagate a romantic view of wilderness as somehow 'untouched' by humans, a keystone belief in the dualistic separation of nature and culture. They argued that these dualisms are problematic and ultimately counterproductive. The construction of some places as 'wilderness' tends to devalue places that are not considered 'wild' or 'pristine'. These 'non-human' places, which encompass the majority of the globe, thereby become more vulnerable to damage, exploitation and carelessness.

Willis and Bondi also asserted that this radical separation of people's everyday lives from valorised 'nature' also fosters the commodification of nature in practices such as adventure therapy. In its alignment with counselling and other services designed to promote mental health and wellbeing, adventure therapy becomes part and parcel of a consumer society in which individuals attend to their personal needs and wants through the consumption of goods and services. 'Wilderness' and 'nature' are thereby enrolled into the very processes of consumption that its advocates often view as detrimental to the life of human beings and the world they inhabit. Willis and Bondi concluded that if adventure therapy wishes to contribute to positive social change around environmental issues, it needs to take a critical approach to the concept of 'wilderness' and seek ways in which relationships both within and to other types of places might be supported.

Reflections

Whether advertently or inadvertently, 5IATC keynote addresses included a strong theme of the importance of the natural world in adventure therapy. Whether viewed as a healing variable in the treatment process, or as the sustaining context in which all life exists, this conference drew our intentions sharply towards planet Earth. This is no coincidence, given the geopolitical and environmental realities of our time. Even during our time in Scotland, the world was approaching the 2009 United Nations Climate Change Summit in Copenhagen, which sadly turned out to produce nothing more than a weak political statement on the problem, and no real action. With events like this, as well as tell-tale signs of environmental deterioration all around us, we as adventure therapists may be suffering from a collective 'solastalgia', a combination of the Latin word solacium (comfort) and the Greek root – algia (pain)...defined as the pain experienced when there is recognition that the place where one resides and that one loves is under immediate assault' (Smith, 2010, p. 5).

Willis and Bondi's keynote responded to issues of global climate change by critiquing adventure therapy's compartmentalization of wilderness. While most of us who practice in adventure therapy see value in wild places that are less influenced by human intervention, Willis and Bondi's talk further challenged the dualism that both Loynes and Norris had also raised. They took this a step further, by provoking us to consider how this dualistic paradigm may be directly related to the current environmental crisis.

In this context, it is critical to develop a sense of urgency about changing our paradigm to be more inclusive and appreciative of the natural world that is all around us, and perhaps consider more appropriate terminology to describe natural places that have often been carefully tended by Indigenous cultures for millenia (rather than being assumed as 'people-free' places). This may help us to better guard and protect places that have formerly been considered wastelands or not valuable for 'civilized' humans. Not only may this lead to greater environmental protection on a local level, it is also a powerful therapeutic metaphor that reminds us that no place or person should be forgotten.

KEYNOTE #9: 5IATC

Really Wild Therapy: Exploring beyond the Boundaries of the Self

Nick Totton

For Totton, 'wild therapy' refers specifically to two themes: on the one hand, psychotherapy in and through wilderness itself (including adventure therapy), and on the other hand a psychotherapy which sides with the spontaneous as much as the intentional, and with the 'out-of-awareness' as much as the conscious. Totton's presentation linked several highly pertinent topics: the global environmental crisis, the movement of Western culture towards increased regulation and monitoring of many aspects of life (including psychotherapy), new neuroscience research on stress, relaxation, awareness and decision making, and new thinking about the complex relationship between human and 'other-than-human' forms of existence.

Totton focused on the terms 'wild' and 'wilderness', arguing that they identify key areas of contradiction in conventional Western thinking 'wild' means both 'free' and 'dangerous', both 'natural' and 'out of control'. The antithesis of 'wild' is 'domesticated'; and in many ways, civilisation is an ongoing process of human domestication, which in his view has sown the seeds of its own destruction. At the same time, Totton argued that civilisation has plainly multiplied the richness and complexity, as well as the comfort, of human existence. He suggested we don't need to idealise wildness over domestication, but we need to find a way of moving beyond the polarity itself. In this way, Totton encouraged adventure therapists to consider the deeper and wider contexts of their work, including its potential for helping people move away from a domesticated model of power over nature, and towards a positive valuation of self-regulation and spontaneity.

Reflections

Totton's address continued the important theme of reframing how we conceptualize the natural world. This continuous message of moving beyond the duality of wildness versus domestication may seem redundant; however to a largely Western audience, it was an important message to reiterate. For so long, the wilderness component of adventure therapy has been described as separate and remote, and while profound individual changes can and do occur in these remote environments (Norton, 2011; Russell, 2000), the transfer of learning may be greater if we did not construct and emphasize such a strong dichotomy between the urban and natural environments, humans and nature. Totton's keynote gave us reason to consider that what is truly 'wild' may include spontaneous gestures of courage and shared adventure, in both remote and local settings.

The prospect of dissolving traditional power relationships between people and the natural world poses a number of interesting possibilities. An exploration of the theories of biophilia, and the need for humans to be seen as an evolutionary element of nature emphasizes yet again, the value of adventure therapy processes that enable people to gain a deeper understanding of, and connection with, the natural world. 'Wild therapy' provoked us to look beyond current limitations, and embrace and adapt alternative understandings of our potential impact on clients or participants, theories underpinning practice, and the morphing of therapeutic approaches.

KEYNOTE #10: 5IATC

Controversial and Critical Debates in Adventure Therapy: An Interactive Process

Cathryn Carpenter and Christian Itin

As adventure therapy continues to grow and evolve across the world many controversial debates are posed in its international development. The first critical question centers on whether the adventure therapy community wants to be considered an international field of endeavour. If so, there may be a need to develop and consolidate the field of adventure therapy, building a shared sense of identity, purpose, ethics and perhaps regulation, training and accreditation.

Yet, adventure therapy is understood and practiced differently in each region of the world. Each culture has developed diverse ways of working with people within their landscape and country, to promote enhanced health and wellbeing. As each international region evolves their unique approach to using adventure as a part of this work, adventure therapy appears to be defined differently.

The second critical question centres on the possibility and or role of an international definition of adventure therapy. Can an understanding of this practice be universally shared? Is adventure therapy a unifying theme or construct, and is this really what draws the profession together? This keynote involved an interactive debate, highlighting a range of perspectives from practitioners and academics from around the world, and challenged our understandings of what adventure therapy means now. The hope was that the shared insights might help us in developing a framework for where the profession may head in the future.

Reflections

This debate depended upon the active participation of the entire conference community. Rather than have 'expert' panels discussing these questions, the aim was to hear the voices of the broader 'expert community'. The structure of the debate required people to physically locate themselves along a continuum, depending on how strongly they agreed with a series of statements. After placing themselves along a continuum, conference attendees were offered a short time to discuss their rationale with the people around them. Carpenter and Itin wandered along the line interviewing people with a microphone in order in order to gather and share different perspectives and viewpoints. The following questions formed the basis of movement along the continuum:

- *'Adventure therapy is what we are centrally organised around' versus 'Some other factor is what we organise around'.*
- *'We should work towards one shared international definition of adventure therapy' versus 'We should accept the richness of diverse definitions from regional and national perspectives'.*
- *'Specific clinical qualifications lead to best practice' versus 'Diverse perspectives reflecting many pathways lead to best practice'.*
- *'Outdoor/Nature is an effective part of adventure' versus 'Adventure need not include outdoor/nature'.*

Whilst this debate (across the conference floor) clarified the diversity of opinions and the spectrum of practice, values and beliefs within the international adventure therapy community, it left many of us realising the enormity of the task to find common ground. This session did not necessarily move us closer to defining international adventure therapy as a cohesive profession.

Nevertheless, from the range of meaningful dialogue, cross-cultural exchange, provoking keynotes, and practical and inspiring workshops, and out of this interactive debate emerged various insights, including

1. *Defining what is and what is not adventure therapy may not be as important as critically examining how adventure therapy is practiced, ethically and effectively in all its many cross-cultural forms.*

2. *Cultural differences can frustrate and enlighten, but the cultural bridging that can occur through mutual empathy and dialogue can create new wisdom in the field of adventure therapy, and beyond.*
3. *Regardless of how it is practiced, adventure therapy must avoid the paternalism of mental health 'treatment' in the West, which can imply treatment 'done to' the client by experts. The locus of control must be with the client, and the process of adventure therapy must be one of collaboration.*
4. *Adventure therapy must value the inherent wisdom found in the individual and in the community. It must involve multiple systems and domains of a client's life, including professional helpers, as well as the wisdom of elders and Indigenous peoples and cultures.*
5. *Sustainability is critical to the survival of the wild lands in which we often practice adventure therapy. Our ecological resources are key to our health and sanity, and all communities need to take ownership of their role in global climate change.*

And finally ...

6. *The 'body' of adventure therapy does not need to threaten the 'soul' of adventure therapy nor vice versa. It is imperative to remember that both are predicated on the ideas of protecting client wellbeing, promoting healing and growth, and maintaining our ability to continue to practice adventure therapy around the world.*

General Public Lecture (5IATC)

Meeting the Mental Health Needs of Children and Adolescents: The Role of Adventure Therapy

Dene Berman and Jennifer Davis-Berman

Berman and Davis-Berman presented a public speech during the 5IATC, which they translated into a paper entitled 'Finding a place for adventure therapy and therapeutic adventure on the continuum of care'. Their speech is not included in this chapter, as it is included as a full paper within Chapter 4 (Sharing).

Reflections

The Bermans' talk provided a complex mix of theory, research and practice ideas that merited an entire paper in this book. We have included mention of the presentation here because as well as being a key presentation, their address was also noted as one of the more provoking talks given. It presented a distinctly Western perspective on adventure therapy. The presentation sought to distinguish between adventure therapy and therapeutic adventure and, much like Aldridge's keynote, reminded us that if we take steps to specifically define adventure therapy, we have to decide who is in and who is out.

While the Bermans' keynote utilized the 'continuum of care' model to make space for both adventure therapy and therapeutic adventure as viable interventions, they encouraged us to define adventure therapy as a 'clinical' mental health treatment intervention administered by 'licensed professionals'. While speaking to an international audience, these ideas provoked audience members to engage in meaningful dialogue about these complex issues. (See 'Sharing' for a full copy of their paper).

KEYNOTE #11: 6IATC

Too Safe for Their Own Good: How the Right Amount of Risk and Responsibility Helps Children and Teens Become Resilient

Michael Ungar

Dr. Michael Ungar, well known for his research on the topic of resilience, presented a keynote speech at 6IATC. A summary of what he presented is included here. Dr. Ungar is the founder and co-director of the Resilience Research Centre that coordinates millions of dollars in research in more than a dozen countries looking at building resilience in individuals and communities. Though he does not have a background in adventure therapy, he has written about the role that camps can play in fostering resilience and positive youth development (2012). Ungar defines resilience as the capacity to **navigate** the world (and having what is needed made available and accessible) as well as having the capacity to **negotiate** the world (and influence what is provided). In his keynote address, Ungar discussed the dangers of overprotecting young people and the actual risks children and youth face, compared to the positive risks inherent in adventure therapy. According to Ungar (2012), 'Too much exposure to risk (adventure and responsibility) endangers children. Too little exposure to risk (adventure and responsibility) fails to provide a child opportunity to grow up healthy.' In order to develop the seven tensions of resilience (see Table 1), youth need positive risk taking experiences, like the kind that are often found in adventure therapy programs.

Table 1: Seven Tensions Related to Resilience

Tension	Explanation
1. Access to supportive relationships	• Relationships with significant others, peers and adults within one's family and community
2. Development of a desirable personal identity	• Desirable sense of one's self as having a personal and collective sense of purpose, ability for self-appraisal of strengths and weaknesses, aspirations, beliefs and values, including spiritual and religious identification
3. Experiences of power and control	• Experiences of caring for one's self and others, the ability to affect change in one's social and physical environment in order to access health resources
4. Experiences of social justice	• Experiences related to finding a meaningful role in one's community that brings with it acceptance and social equality
5. Access to material resources	• Availability of financial, educational, medical and employment assistance and/or opportunities, as well as access to food, clothing and shelter
6. Experiences of a sense of cohesion with others	• Balancing one's personal interests with a sense of responsibility to the greater good; feeling a part of something larger than one's self socially and spiritually
7. Adherence to cultural traditions	• Adherence to, or knowledge of, one's local and/or global cultural practices, values and beliefs

(Adapted from: Ungar, M., Brown, M., Liebenberg, L., Othman, R., Kwong, W.M., Armstrong, M. & Gilgun, J. [2007]. Unique pathways to resilience across cultures. Adolescence, 42(166), 287-310)

Reflections

The main focus of Ungar's keynote address was pointing out how adventure therapy may serve as a much-needed context for positive risk-taking that can facilitate components necessary for developing resilience. Current adventure therapy research shows that outdoor adventure programs provide asset-building experiences that contribute to positive youth development (Norton, Watt, & Penn, 2013). Though no research has been done to measure the impact of adventure therapy on resilience, specifically, Ungar's resilience framework fits well with the goals of adventure therapy, and could be widely applied and empirically tested in the future.

KEYNOTE #12: 6IATC

Adventure Therapy and Natural Environments

Alan Ewert

Ewert presented a keynote during the 6IATC, which discussed the influence that natural environments can play in the field of Adventure Therapy. Various theories and concepts were discussed that highlighted the potential ways that natural environments can be effective in both therapy and overall human health. More specifically, Ewert asked the question 'is there a connection between adventure-based therapeutic programs that occur in natural environments and human health?' This presentation argued that the answer to this question is unequivocally "yes." The extant literature and personal experience suggests that adventure therapeutic programming is positively associated with issues related to human health, and this connection is greatly strengthened when these programs occur in natural and outdoor environments. Moreover, Ewert presented three reasons why adventure therapeutic programming can be effective in promoting health and wellness: (1) the environment in which most adventure activities take place, (2) the activities themselves that typically require physical activity and movement, and (3) participation in adventure activities often help develop social networks and support, that is conducive to personal health. His full paper on the topic of adventure therapy and natural environments can be found within Chapter 8 (Expanding).

Reflections

Ewert's keynote encouraged us to consider the healing role that nature plays in adventure therapy. However, instead of focusing solely on adventure therapy from a mental health perspective, Ewert looked at the intervention more holistically, coming from a health and wellness perspective. As such, he was able to invite the audience to consider various aspects of the intervention that contribute to wellness, including the actual environment, but also exercise, social support, etc. Too often we view adventure therapy solely as a clinical intervention in mental health, but Ewert's keynote framed adventure therapy within a broader framework of human health. In this vein, time spent pursuing outdoor adventure can be seen as 'personal medicine' that all humans can utilize on their path to wellness and recovery.

KEYNOTE #13: 6IATC

Adventure Therapy with HIV/ AIDS Orphans

Masego Thamuku

Thamuku is the Director of Ark 'n Mark Trust, which runs wilderness retreats as part of a larger psychosocial support program for HIV/AIDS orphans in Botswana. During her talk, Thamuku highlighted the theoretical approach used in her program. Per her keynote and highlighted specifically on the Ark 'n Mark Trust website (2015):

The wilderness retreats are done using a child strengthening therapeutic approach called EARTH. It is a wilderness based therapeutic technique that carefully and creatively combines the Setswana and the Western psychology to child strengthening and psychotherapy. It was developed for adolescent orphans of Botswana to help them confront and mitigate the psychosocial effects of grief and trauma as a group. This is done using the wilderness as a foundation, utilizing its healing properties. EARTH is an acronym that stands for the various qualities of the intervention:

E - Empathy Based
A - Action Oriented
R - Relationship Building
T - Transformative
H - Healing Therapy

EARTH therapy uses a combination of the following approaches to ensure a thorough, well rounded and successful rehabilitation:

- Psychoanalysis
- Group Therapy
- Therapeutic Play
- Rites of Passage

- Individual Focused therapy

These intensive therapeutic techniques are done in the beginning of the day and are partnered with nature education and outdoor challenge activities, in the afternoon. The education sessions vary widely from game drives to crafts allowing for ongoing self-exploration and reflection of therapy.

After completion of these retreats follow-up support is done to complete the methodology. Home-based networks that are formed during retreats are strengthened and monitored by local volunteers (Bommabana) and Social Workers. Follow-up support strengthens the foundation that was given during the retreat resulting in the following outcomes:

- Build social skills
- Decrease a sense of isolation and build a sense of belonging
- Decrease self-blame
- Negotiate rather than confront
- Help children make their own connections between feelings and actions
- Help children reframe how they interpret situations
- Support children in taking action when appropriate

In sharing about the EARTH methodology employed in the wilderness retreats, Thamuku also discussed how this intervention creates a much-needed space for young people to grieve the loss of family members due to HIV/AIDS. According to Thamuku, this is not a commonly accepted practice, and provides the young people with nature-based rituals and rites of passage to help them move forward both in their grief journey and in their own development.

Reflections

Anyone who had the privilege of hearing Thamuku speak will remember how she moved the 6IATC audience to tears. Not only did Thamuku bring to life the EARTH methodology to life via case studies and powerful anectdotes about the flora and fauna in Botswana, she also led us in song. She began singing "Will the Circle Be Unbroken" as an example of something she does in the field to process grief with the youth in her program, and many of us sang along with her. This powerful moment illuminated how the culturally relevant spiritual underpinnings of the intervention are a key part of the healing process. However, the magic that happens in the field does not stand alone. This program goes a step further and provides psychosocial support and follow up for two years post-wilderness retreat. To me, this intervention is a wonderful example of a hybrid model of adventure therapy, which combines the backcountry expedition with community-based social work follow up. I think there is room to replicate a program like this in other parts of the world to help young people cope with trauma and loss.

KEYNOTE #14: 6IATC

Rethinking the Use of Metaphor in Adventure Therapy

Christian Itin

Building on his work looking at the seven generations of adventure therapy (Itin, 1998) (see Table 2 below), Itin reviewed the various paradigms of the use of metaphor in adventure therapy and engaged the audience in drawing up on our own figurative, 'hypnotic' language to develop metaphors that were kinesthetic, generative and isomorphic all at once.

Table 2: The Seven Generations of Adventure Therapy

1st Generation	*2nd Generation*	*3rd Generation*	*4th Generation*	*5th Generation*	*6th Generation*	*7th Generation*
Letting the experience speak for itself	*Speaking for the experience*	*Debriefing the experience*	*Frontloadin g the experience (direct)*	*Framing the experience (metaphor)*	*Frontloading the experience (Indirect/Para-doxical)*	*Flagging the experience*

Rather than taking an 'either/or' approach to the issue of the use of metaphor, Itin helped practitioners understand the need to intentionally engage the client to co-create metaphors in a variety of different ways.

Reflections

During his keynote, Itin broke us into small groups in order to discuss a dilemma that one person in the group was facing. Once one person's dilemma was identified, we were instructed to ask open-ended questions and listen with empathic attunement to the language the person was using to describe his/her dilemma. The other group members took notes identifying figurative, 'hypnotic' language that the person was using to describe his/her situation. Group members then read back these statements to the person sharing, in order to see what emotions or images these phrases elicited. From here, group members discussed experiential, adventure-based activities that might provide an isomorphic experience matching the person's figurative language and kinesthetic activity. This process was a wonderful training opportunity for the practitioners in the audience, and was a reminder that our 'elicitation of responses or the suggestion of possible actions enables the practitioner to support the client in drawing upon and developing those unconscious resources for change that are neede' (Itin, 1998, p. 125).

REFERENCES

Ark 'n Mark Trust. (2010). *EARTH methodology.* Retrieved on 1/29/15 from: http://www.arknmark.org/earth_methodology.php

Abney, P.C. (2002). *A study of the relationship between the levels of self-awareness within students enrolled in counselling practicum and the measurements of their counselling effectiveness.* (Doctoral dissertation). University of North Texas. Retrieved on 9/20/2011 from http://www.worldcat.org/.

Chicago Adventure Therapy. (2011). *Programming.* Retrieved on 9/20/2011 from www.chicagoadventuretherapy.org/.

Gillen, M. C. & Balkin, R. S. (2006). Adventure counselling as an adjunct to group counselling in hospital and clinical settings. *Journal for Specialists in Group Work*, 31(2), 153-164.

Itin, C. (1998). The seventh generation in adventure therapy. In C. Itin (Ed.), *Exploring the boundaries of adventure therapy*, pp. 12-130. Boulder, CO: The Association for Experiential Education.

Jarosewitsch, R. (1997). *Aroha or what constitutes healing in psychotherapy*? Retrieved on 9/20/2011 from: http://www.g-gej.org/1-3/aroah.html.

Norton, C.L. (2011). Wilderness therapy: Creating a context of hope. In C. Norton (Ed.), *Innovative interventions in child and adolescent mental health.* New York: Routledge.

Norton, C.L., Watt, T., & Penn, A. (2013). Exploring the impact of a wilderness-based positive youth development program for urban youth. *Journal of Experiential Education.* DOI: 10.1177/1053825913503113

Omni Youth Services. (2011). *Journey: Skills for life.* Retrieved on 9/20/2011 from: http://www.omniyouth. org/programs-services/journey-skills-for-life.

Russell, K.C. (2000). Exploring how the wilderness therapy process relates to outcomes. *Journal of Experiential Education,* 23(3), 170-176.

Smith, D.B. (2010, January 27). Is there an ecological unconscious? *New York Times Sunday Magazine*, p. 36.

Ungar, M. (2012). Camps help make children resilient. Camping Magazine, Sept/Oct 2012. Martinsville, IN: American Camping Association. Retrieved on 1/29/2015 from: http://www.acacamps.org/campmag/1209/camps-help-make-children-resilient

SHARING

I chose to risk my significance, to live so that which came to me as seed goes to the next as blossom, and that which comes to me as blosom, goes on as fruit.

-Living Wide Open

The Aboriginal Youth Resilience Study: A Look at Promoting Resilience and Wellbeing through Outdoor Adventure Leadership Experience
Steven Ritchie, Mary Jo Wabano, Robert Schinke, Duke Peltier, Brenda Restoule, Keith Russell, Rita Corbiere and **Nancy L. Young**

CHAPTER 1

Counselling and Psychotherapy Outdoors: Grounding Our Practice in our Theoretical Roots

Selena Chandler

ABSTRACT

In the United Kingdom (UK), therapy training predominantly prepares counsellors and psychotherapists to work with individuals in indoor settings. Increasingly therapists are responding to the challenges of our times, such as the impact of lack of contact with nature on childhood development and the relationship of our psyche to environmental destruction and climate change. Therapists are seeking to expand the therapeutic alliance, to make space for wider nature in the therapy room, as well as creating therapy spaces in the outdoors.

This paper aims to support this broadening of therapy practice by seeking to discover what part wider nature played in the childhoods and adult lives of key therapists, and whether awareness of wider nature is present in their theory and practice. Towards this aim, the lives and ideas of Freud, Jung, Rogers, Perls and Milton are considered, as they have informed much counselling training and practice in the UK. These explorations have highlighted that seeds of outdoor therapy and elements of ecopsychological understandings were present in the theories and practice of these early founders of counselling and psychotherapy. Fertile ground exists for contemporary therapists to acknowledge their own theoretical roots, and to grow practices that integrate relationship with our wider nature.

Introduction

The explorations recorded here arose from a curiosity following conversations with colleagues about practising therapy outdoors, and the personal and planetary benefits that might exist when we include acknowledgment of relationships with wider nature in the psychotherapy process. In the UK, counsellors and psychotherapists are increasingly interested in the possibilities of undertaking the adventurous journey of therapy in the outdoors. However as yet, it seems that an awareness of relationships with wider nature plays little, if any, part in counselling training in the UK.

As a therapist, I work with people to explore their hidden stories, to give voice to less familiar aspects of themselves, and to discover new elements of their taken for granted ways of being. I have wondered whether our place in the web of life featured in any theories of psychological development, and also whether there are any recent traditions in models of Western psychotherapy for conducting therapy outdoors. Has wider nature been completely written out, or is it present but not yet visible?

To begin with, and to give a context to what follows, some forms of working outdoors based on a therapeutic intent are briefly outlined. Many of these practices underpin our work, with models and ideas from experiential education and development training which may warrant further investigation by counsellors and psychotherapists (Gass, 1993; Schoel & Maizell, 2002). However, for the purposes of this paper, it is contributions from some of the more prominent theorists and practitioners in Western models of psychotherapy, such as Rogers, Freud, Jung, Perls and Erickson that are explored, in order to discover how they might inform counselling and psychotherapy outdoors.

Therapeutic Outdoor Practices

Adventure therapy draws on principles from experiential education. People take part in adventurous activities such as high ropes courses, kayaking or abseiling, usually in a group setting, where these novel experiences and group interactions can act as a therapeutic catalyst. Adventure therapy can take place either indoors or outdoors. Wilderness therapy often takes the form of expeditions, allowing significant time away from the home environment, allowing a period of immersion in simple, self-sufficient living, again often as part of a group. Wilderness therapy also usual seeks remote locations, where evidence of human activity in the landscape is limited, and where in learning new skills and building a community people can generate new experiences of themselves.

There have been critiques of both adventure therapy and wilderness therapy, such as by Beringer (2003), suggesting that often the natural worlds in which the therapy is embedded is invisible, and the pivotal contribution of the natural setting to therapeutic success is unacknowledged. Eco-therapy, as with most of these terms, is a broad ranging category of practices, which do aim to specifically recognise the outdoors as a therapeutic setting. Use of the label eco-therapy is becoming more widespread with, for example the publication in the UK of a report on the benefits of green exercise for mental health by the national mental health charity (MIND, 2007). In this context, it is time in green space and social interaction that are seen to be the primary elements that promote improved wellbeing.

Eco-psychology is a practice concerned with exploring and deepening our relationship with the earth, utilising psychotherapeutic processes for the benefit of human and planetary wellbeing (Roszak, 1995). Therapists work both indoors and outdoors to address alienation from aspects of self, from our bodies, and from human relationships. They also work to address alienation from nature, both from our own 'wildness', and from an organic bonding with the wider world. Outdoor therapy practices may include elements of all of these, whilst also specifically including the developing field of counsellors and psychotherapists who are working outdoors with individuals, within the conventions of a therapeutic hour.

NATURE AND THE THERAPISTS

Nature played an interesting part in the lives of Rogers, Freud and Jung. For example, at the age of twelve, Carl Roger's family moved to a farm, on which the young Carl managed chickens and reared livestock. He also developed an interest in breeding moths. According to Thorne, Rogers:

> became totally fascinated by the great night-flying moths which inhabited the woods around the farm (and) began himself, to breed the moths in captivity, reared the caterpillars and watched over the cocoons during the long winter months, learning what it means to wait patiently for nature to reveal her secrets. (Thorne, 2003, p.2)

Rogers later went to university, undertaking agricultural studies for a short time with the intent of becoming a farmer. For a while he had a job in a lumberyard where stacks of tree trunks were being seasoned: life stories recorded in their growth rings; the smell of sawdust and the texture of the wood.

Sigmund Freud was also a country child. He was born in a small market town near a river and surrounded by meadows and mountains. Reportedly, he resented his family's move to Vienna when he was three years old because he lost his rural paradise. According to Burke:

> All his life, Freud reveled in nature, taking summer holidays in spectacular mountain regions of Austria and the South Tyrol where he enjoyed hiking and swimming, as well as leading his six children on long rambles through the forest. (Burke, 2006, p.3)

We also know that he took a daily constitutional walk around the Ringstrasse in Vienna; a daily walk of four to six kilometres along a grand, tree-lined boulevard which passed through green parks and along the river, a walk that Freud usually undertook at quite a brisk pace.

Carl Jung was born near Lake Constance in Switzerland, and he continued to live on the shores of lakes throughout his life. Although he grew up alongside country girls and boys, his childhood was not a happy one. He wasn't keen on school, and was absent for a significant period of time. He spent as much time in the woods as he could, responding to his passion for solitude and nature.

Jung often talked of his experiences using descriptions of nature or in terms of his relationship with nature. He recorded one of his earliest memories where he was lying in a pram, in the shadow of a tree with the warmth of the sun, the blue sky and golden sunlight darting through the green leaves. Descriptions such as this draw attention to the ability of nature to engage our senses and the importance of our preverbal knowing. Jung stated:

> I have just awakened to the glorious beauty of the day, and have a sense of indescribable well-being. (Jung, 1962, p.6)

In his late thirties Jung had what is known as his 'creative illness'. He had a period of about five years when he felt an uncertainty and disorientation; a feeling that he had not yet found his own footing. During this time, Jung returned to playing childhood games, building houses and villages from stones. He found that time outdoors in contact with the land helped him to connect to his fantasies and creativity.

Jung also recognised the risk of romanticising nature, and he drew attention to its dark side, 'earthworms tormented to death by ants, insects that tear each other apart piece by piece', saying 'I knew myself well enough to know that I was only gradually, as it were, distinguishing myself from an animal' (Jung, 1962, p.69).

From such explorations it seems that Freud's response to moving to a city was a sense of loss of relationship with rural nature. Rogers was engaged in intimate, patient, observing relations with insects and animals until at least his late teens, and Jung felt himself merged with, and an integral part of nature throughout his life.

As these examples illustrate, in contrast to the current daily experiences of many urbanised people, for these developers of psychotherapy practice, easy access to and regular time in natural outdoor spaces were commonplace. As therapists, we can be aware that the usual patterns of someone's life, the taken for granted things' that may not be subject to critical reflection, and their impact on psychological development and functioning may pass unnoticed until they are highlighted and held in attention in a therapeutic exchange.

Having looked at the place of nature in the personal lives of Rogers, Freud and Jung, we can consider nature's presence and influence in their theories and concepts.

The Person-centred Concepts of Rogers

Rogers proposed the idea of self-actualisation, an inherent tendency for the human organism to maintain itself and to move towards the constructive accomplishment of its potential. In his explanation of this tendency, Thorne suggests it is likely that Rogers drew on his background in agricultural science to propose a simple principle that is present and observable 'throughout the natural order' (Thorne, 2003, p.26). It is not hard to imagine how observation of the life cycle of caterpillar to cocoon to moth would suggest an innate capacity for healthy growth.

Rogers suggested that the only constraints to this arise from the conditions of the environment. Just as a cabbage is unlikely to thrive in poor soil without proper care, watering and the regular removal of slugs, similarly the growth of the human being will be compromised if conditions are unfavourable. In developing his ideas Rogers focussed on the conditions of the human environment and identified the core conditions in human relationships of congruence, unconditional positive regard and empathy (Mearns & Thorne, 2000) as being the environment in which the 'seed' of human potential can grow.

The concept of unconditional positive regard may in some ways be familiar to adventure and wilderness therapists, in terms of nature's fair and equal consequences. Whilst individuals will have their own ideas and feelings about how nature has treated them, in many ways nature simply is. If it's raining on me, it's raining on you too; it's just raining and we are accepted as we are.

Whilst warmth, honesty, openness, and acceptance are elements in human relating that facilitate growth and development, it can be interesting to extend consideration of the optimal conditions for wellbeing to our wider environment. For example the regard in which we hold land, air and water, our impact on nature of which we are an integral part, and our recognition that what we do to the Earth we do to ourselves. What are the core conditions for relating that facilitate the mutual thriving of both humans and wider nature, and how can counsellors encourage greater awareness of this web of connections?

Psychodynamic Concepts and Practice

With his concept of the 'boundaried ego', Freud was focussed on internal processes and was specific in his reservations about a sense of relationship with animals, plants and the land. He regarded the 'oceanic feeling', with its sensation of eternity, of feeling limitless and unbounded, and of being in connection with the wider world as strange. And despite spending much time in nature himself, he says the sense of connection was not something he felt. In contrast, Freud did acknowledge strengths of connection felt with people:

> towards the outside… the ego seems to maintain clear and sharp lines of demarcation, there is one state when this is not the case. At the height of being in love the boundary between ego and object threatens to melt away. Against all the evidence of his senses, a man who is in love declares that 'I' and 'you' are one, and is prepared to behave as if it were a fact. (Freud, 1991, p.253)

For Freud such feelings only relate to human relationships, and he cautions that this normal function can become distorted and pathological. Similarly, and to illustrate his ideas about the separate self, Freud drew on anthropological descriptions of Native American and Aboriginal beliefs. He regarded their ecological interactions with their natural environments, descriptions of totem animals, and beliefs about being connected to nature as evidence of primitive and childlike thinking and a lack of psychological maturity (Freud, 1913).

For Roszak (1995), along with other ecopsychologists, this determined boundary between the ego and the external world, the idea that psychological maturity is evidenced in separate, self-contained individuals, has had detrimental consequences for the wellbeing of humans and of the Earth. Deep ecologists such as Macy (2007) have proposed that love for the world (where 'world' includes humans as an integrated element rather than somehow separate and apart), is a necessary and healthy response for life.

One of the developments in psychodynamic thinking was 'object relations theory' (Hinshelwood, 1989), which put simply, describes how as babies our personality and identity are formed and developed as we internalise our positive and negative experiences of our most significant human caregivers. Clinebell (1996), an eco-therapist, extends this idea to propose that we internalise both our human and our natural environment. He suggests that the forming of our identity is influenced at a deep, preverbal level by our early experiences in and of nature. We are influenced by our experiences of direct contact with nature and also by our family and culture's views of the natural world, which we experience both directly and through our parents' feelings, attitudes and ways of relating with nature. Clinebell argues that the quality of our continuing relationship with nature is a major dynamic in our sense of being firmly grounded or feeling 'up in the air' and unrooted.

More recently Randal (2005) has identified how psychoanalytic concepts can be utilised to give us some ways to understand our individual and communal responses to environmental crisis and climate change. Self-protective defence mechanisms and seeking to reduce our sense of anxiety can be observed in many of our responses. People may engage in 'splitting' and 'denial', processes by which we can prevent ourselves from fully knowing our experiences. For example we can watch television coverage of human behaviours that are damaging nature, and then because of the pain that this generates within us we can separate and distance ourselves from knowing what we've just seen, or deny that it's true. Similarly, regression to childish responses of instant gratification such as 'I need more / the latest / bigger', or 'why should I change my behaviour when no one else is', and 'it's okay because parents /scientists / technology will sort it out', allow us to continually consume to compensate for a lost sense of connection.

The senses of guilt, anger, conflict, fatigue, helplessness, illusion and powerlessness that these processes of distancing and trying to separate and disconnect from relationship with wider nature can generate may be presented by people seeking therapy support. Eco-psychologists are increasingly aware that these responses and human behaviours towards wider nature may be representations of intrapsychic or interpersonal conflicts and they may also be the direct responses of our nature-selves.

To return to Freud's therapy practice for a moment, there are records describing how he was willing to extend the boundaries of his work by meeting with his clients outdoors. In an early example of outdoor therapy, he conducted a 'walking analysis' of Max Eitingon, which included Freud and Eitingon meeting for sessions twice a week for five weeks, whilst walking in a park in Vienna.

JUNGIAN CONCEPTS AND ANCIENT MEMORIES

Whereas Freud found the idea, if not the practice, of connecting to nature difficult, Jung describes his sense of interconnectedness in the following way:

> At times I feel as if I am spread out over the landscape and inside things, and am myself living in every tree, in the splashing of the waves, in the woods and the animals that come and go, in the procession of the seasons. There is nothing … with which I am not linked. (Jung, 1962, p.225)

While object relations concepts can be expanded to consider the influence of our own direct nature experiences (as well as those filtered to us by our immediate parents and culture), Jung extends this even further. He introduces the concept of the collective unconscious, through which our relationship with wider nature can be influenced by our shared ancient memories. 'All those factors, that were essential to our near and remote ancestors will also be essential to us, because they are embedded in our inherited organic system' (cited in Stevens, 1994. p.51).

Stevens (1994) highlighted that this was similar to findings in behavioural biology, the study of animals in their natural habitats. Every animal species has a repertoire of behaviours which is dependent on structures that evolution has built into the central nervous system of that particular species. These structures, known as 'innate releasing mechanisms' are primed to become active when an appropriate stimulus is encountered in the environment. When the stimulus appears, the animal responds with a characteristic pattern of behaviour, which has been adapted through evolution, to the situation. So for example, a mallard duck becomes amorous at the sight of the green head of a mallard drake; the green head is the 'sign stimulus', which releases in the duck's central nervous system the innate mechanism responsible for the characteristic patterns of behaviour associated with duck courtship.

In Jung's 'collective unconscious', as humans we share archetypes, nueropsychic centres, that if activated give access to our common myths, feelings, images and ways of being human. Given that for much of our history our ancestors were actively engaged with the land in which they lived, it is useful to consider what the impact on both our physical and psychological wellbeing might be when, due to lack of contact with appropriate experiences and stimuli, these well adapted patterns for being do not receive stimulation.

The biologist E. O. Wilson (1984) conducted studies focussed on the importance of biodiversity and suggested a similar idea. With his 'biophilia hypothesis', the idea that we have an inherent need to affiliate deeply and closely with the natural environment, is part of our evolutionary inheritance. This theory suggests that at a deep body-mind level we know, however dimly, that if we continue to reject this inheritance and do not establish a respectful interaction with wider nature, we will lose a vital dimension of our humanness.

We live in times where the rational, scientific and technological tend to be given prominence. Jung suggested that we give too much attention to our consciousness and leave the unconscious behind. By focussing on the outer physical world, we have neglected our own inner nature. Practical advice that Jung gave for remedying our loss of contact with nature, both within and without, includes: to work shorter hours, to make the sparest use of TV/radio/ and technological gadgets, and to have a plot of land to cultivate with the intent of letting nature affect us, so that our instincts come back to life (Sabini, 2002).

People often cite gardening as being necessary for their psychological wellbeing (Sempi, Aldridge & Becker, 2002). Practices of digging, weeding, sowing and watering have been introduced into psychotherapy work with people who have experienced trauma or dislocation from their homeland (Linden & Grut, 2002). There is also an increasing range of research evidence from the field of environmental psychology that supports such outdoor therapy practice (Natural England, 2007). The evidence suggests that engagement with wider nature beneficially impacts our psychological wellbeing, with trees and vegetation lessening aggression, resting in a garden improving concentration, views of landscapes assisting recovery from mental fatigue, green exercise enhancing self-esteem, and sounds and views of nature facilitating quicker healing, reducing stress and reducing anxiety.

In the development of their theories of psychological processes, both Rogers and Freud saw themselves as engaged in the adventure of therapy. Rogers said he was 'an adventurer who thirsts for new terrain to conquer and problems to overcome' (Thorne, 2003, p.16). Freud described himself as 'an adventurer exploring the unknown hinterlands of the mind' (Stevens, 2008, p.141). They tended to focus their attention on the mind and internal processes, on individualism and the immediate client-therapist relationship rather than on wider connections. In the ideas of Fritz Perls and Gestalt therapy, there is a more explicit recognition of our body-mind connection.

Perls and Gestalt Therapy

> It makes no sense to speak, for instance, of an animal that breathes without considering air and oxygen as part of its definition... there is no single function of any animal that completes itself without objects and environment. (Perls, Hefferline & Goodman, 1951, p.228)

Perls puts emphasis on present-centeredness, body awareness and sensory experience; the contact between the self and its environment. He understood that body and mind function as a totality and that the boundary of the self is not fixed:

> The very moment that we breathe, is the air that comes in still part of the outside world, or is it already our own?... where is the place where the self begins, and the otherness of the environment ends? (Perls, cited in Clinebell, 1996, p.47)

Cahalan (1998) is a Gestalt therapist who works outdoors. He suggests that our mechanistic, dualistic worldview has allowed us to become alienated from Earth, and that we adopt an armoured stance to maintain this alienation. We blunt our senses, tense against the weather, distract our thinking and talking. In armouring, sensory, muscular-emotional and verbal dimensions are interwoven, and we separate ourselves from the world in which we are embedded. Cahalan has found that by working outdoors, often during a conventional therapy session, the quality and energy of therapeutic exploration is enhanced by the immediate multisensory presence of the natural community.

Erickson's Therapeutic Nature Tasks

Multisensory engagement is also foregrounded in the therapy practice of Milton Erickson. 'I've sent more than one depressed man to go and dig, and plant a flower garden for someone' (cited in Burns, 1998, p.19). Like Rogers, Erickson grew up on a farm where, following a serious episode of polio, which left him virtually paralysed, he spent a lot of time observing and listening to the natural world around him. Erickson gradually recovered some mobility and shortly before going to university, still unable to walk well he set off on his own adventure therapy, a long distance solo canoe trip.

These experiences found their way into Erickson's psychotherapy practice and he often suggested activities in nature, such as visits to lonesome places, giving attention to particular plants at the botanical gardens, mountain walks and gardening, for clients to engage in between sessions. Erickson believed that the metaphorical richness and physical engagement of these nature tasks, along with the relaxed states of consciousness induced by such activities, could allow people to access wider ways of knowing themselves and their place in the world (Hayley, 1985).

Rossi, a student of Erickson, explained the usefulness of the altered, relaxed states induced by activities such as walking and gardening, suggesting that these states are necessary for the processing of the integration of change, for 'bringing the learning home' in adventure therapy terms. Rossi highlighted that neurons respond to exercise just as muscles do, and that exposure to enriched environments can influence growth in the brain. 'Novelty, exercise, training, and the voluntary focussing of attention can facilitate the growth and re-organization of neural networks of the brain' (Rossi & Rossi, 2008, p.8).

Periods of rest and relaxation are necessary in order to consolidate new life experiences, so when a client has been engaging in emotional experiences, therapeutic dialogue, exploring different perspectives or new possibilities, the opportunity for rhythmic walking and quiet time in nature facilitates the effective embodiment of a new sense of self.

Conclusion

This exploration has revealed that within the theoretical models of counselling traditionally taught, there is evidence of the significant influence of nature in the childhoods and in the adult lives of key therapists such as Freud, Rogers, Jung and Erickson. In the development of their therapeutic theories, it is possible to find the seeds of awareness of the mutually beneficial effect of acknowledging our relationships with wider nature as relevant to the therapy process.

Counselling is an evolving practice, responding to the needs of our times, and informed by a new awareness of factors that affect psychological development and wellbeing. Similarly, the broadening of counselling and therapy practice to respond more effectively to multicultural and diverse communities has been informed by critiques that question some of the familiar ideas of counselling.

In considering therapy as a process that includes awareness of relationships between humans, as well as wider nature relationships, many authors have questioned traditional western ideas of psychological normality and have highlighted models of wellbeing that integrate mind-body-spirit-Earth.

As therapists we spend much time listening to our fellow humans, yet as Starhawk (2004) reminds us 'everything around us is always speaking'. There are clear grounds for counselling outdoors and indoors with wider nature in mind. If we and our clients spend more time listening, what will we hear?

Reference

Beringer, A. (2003). Toward an ecotherapy framework in adventure therapy. In B. Humberstone, H. Brown,& K. Richards (Eds.), *Whose journeys? The outdoors and adventure as social and cultural phenomena.* United Kingdom: Institute for Outdoor Learning.

Burke, J. (2006). *Freud's Vienna.* Retrieved on 10/14/2008 from www.smh.com.au/news/europe/freuds-vienna

Burns, G. (1998). *Nature-guided therapy.* USA: Taylor & Francis.

Cahalan, B. (1998). Remembering Earth: From armored spectator to sensuous participant. *British Gestalt Journal*, 7(2), 99-105.

Clinebell, H. (1996). *Ecotherapy.* USA: Fortress Press. Freud, S. (1991). Civilization and its discontent. In *The Penguin Freud Library Volume 12, Civilization, Society and Religion*. UK: Penguin.

Freud, S. (1913). *Totem & taboo: Some points of agreement between the mental lives of savages and neurotics.* UK: Routledge Classics 2001.

Gass, M. (1993). *Adventure therapy: Therapeutic applications of adventure programming*. Boulder, CO: Association for Experiential Education.

Hayley, J. (Ed). (1985). Conversations with Milton Erickson. In *Volume 1, Changing Individuals.* USA: Triangle Press.

Hinshelwood, R. (1989). *A dictionary of Kleinian thought.* UK: Free Association Books.

Jung, C. & Jaffe, A. (1962). *Memories, dreams and reflections*. UK: Collins.

Linden, S. & Grut, J. (2002). *The healing fields: Working with psychotherapy and nature to rebuild shattered lives.* UK: Francis Lincoln, Ltd.

Louv, R. (2006). *Last child in the woods: Saving our children from nature-deficit disorder*. USA: Algonquin Books.

Macy, J. (2007). *World as lover, world as self.* USA: Parallax Press.

Mearns, D. & Thorne, B. (2000) *Person-centered therapy today: New frontiers in theory & practice.* UK: Sage.

MIND. (2007). *Ecotherapy report.* Retrieved on 1/25/2010 from www.mind.org.uk

Natural England. (2007). *Mental health and the natural environment.* Retrieved on 1/25/2010 from www.naturalengland.org.uk/ourwork/enjoying/health.

Perls, F., Hefferline, R.F. & Goodman, P. (1951). *Gestalt therapy: Excitement and growth in the human personality.* USA: Souvenir Press.

Randall, R. (2005). *A new climate for psychotherapy.* Retrieved on 1/25/2010 from www.cambridgecarbonfootprint.org.

Rossi, E.L. & Rossi, K.L. (2008). *The new neuroscience of psychotherapy, therapeutic hypnosis & rehabilitation: A creative dialogue with our genes.* Retrieved on 1/25/2010 from www.ErnestRossi.com.

Roszak, T. (Ed.). (1995). *Ecopsychology: Restoring the Earth, healing the mind.* USA: Sierra Club Books. Sabini, M. (Ed.). (2002). *The Earth has a soul: The nature writings of C.G. Jung.* USA: North Atlantic Books.

Schoel, J. & Maizell, R. (2002). *Exploring Islands of Healing: New perspectives on adventure based counselling.* USA: Project Adventure.

Sempik, J., Aldridge, J. & Becker, S. (2002). *Social and therapeutic horticulture: Evidence and messages from research.* UK: Thrive Reading.

StarHawk. (2004). *The Earth path.* USA: Harper Collins. Stevens, A. (1994). *Jung: A very short introduction.* UK: Oxford University Press.

Stevens, R. (2008). *Sigmund Freud: Shaper of the unconscious mind.* UK: Palgrave Macmillan.

Thorne, B. (2003). *Carl Rogers* (2nd ed.). UK: Sage. Wilson, E.O. (1984). *Biophilia.* Cambridge, MA: Harvard University Press.

CHAPTER 2

Taking Therapy into the Outdoors: Why and When and How to Do So

Luk Peeters

ABSTRACT

This paper presents arguments for taking therapeutic pursuits into the outdoors and using adventurous activities to help the therapeutic process. The author describes and illustrates characteristics of suitable activities, and looks at specific issues regarding implementation in a therapeutic process. A Gestalt perspective provides the framework for this discussion.

INTRODUCTION[1]

This paper attempts to look at different aspects of using outdoor or adventurous activities, or a wilderness environment, as a means for therapeutic growth or healing. Gestalt-experiential and existential therapeutic perspectives form the framework for this discussion, which are also influenced by the psychodynamic approach.

WHEN DO THE BENEFITS OF THIS THERAPEUTIC APPROACH OUTWEIGH THE COSTS?

Taking people outdoors often entails a significant financial cost, heightens certain risks, is time-consuming and might even endanger fragile natural ecosystems. So it might be interesting to start this article by looking at some of the advantages of this approach.

---

[1] Note: the author alternates the use of 'he' or 'she' in the text when referring to patients in order to keep the reader attentive and ensure non-discrimination towards gender.

When the Individual or Group Processes Stagnate within a Classical Approach

The adventure therapy approach can serve as a kind of catalyst for individual, inter-relational or group-processes when the more classical indoor or 'talking' approach stagnates within an individual or a partner-relation therapy, or when a group seems to be stuck at a certain level of its development. The adventure therapy methodology seems to possess a certain set of strong characteristics which can provide a renewed dynamic within the person and the group, who are then able to visualise and 'unfreeze' the present.

When Rationalisations and Intellectualisations are Hard to Overcome

Helping a group or client avoid the pitfalls of rational escape routes or intellectualising a possible solution could be another motivation to take them into the outdoors. Words by themselves offer few solutions in an outdoor environment, where action is necessary and where action also becomes very visible. When words do not touch the essence, solutions must inevitably be active. Zinker (1977) stated:

> The experiment is the cornerstone of experiential learning. It transforms talking about into doing, stale reminiscing and theorizing into being fully here with all one's imagination, energy and excitement. (p.42)

The Invitation to Act

The initial hesitation to act is often lower in an adventure setting and the presented activities are often experienced as being less artificial than the 'exercises' or 'experiments' being presented in classical therapeutic settings. The task seems to be more functional and useful. In this respect, the approach heightens the attractiveness to engage for a number of target groups. I suspect this to be one of the reasons why an adventure or outdoor setting is often used in work with adolescents. A participant after a youth at risk program reflected:

> I think it has been the very first time in my life that I really felt useful. That my presence, my existence, my life made a difference. That it mattered that I was there. That I was really needed. That I made a difference. (Participant #1)

Sometimes the need to act is more urgently present. To stall or to postpone has more visible and immediately unpleasant consequences. Being 'stuck' is bodily felt. As a participant, you may find yourselves hesitating between two alternatives. As another participant stated:

> You feel stuck. You want to ask for help but the words don't come. You stay put, with your mouth open, hands reaching out. The long abseil attracts you but frightens you at the same time. You stand up, sit down and stand up again. You feel your hesitation taking you from the one position back to the other: standing, sitting, standing... You can't stay here forever either. You'll have to choose. Yes or no. (Participant #2)

In less urgent situations we can postpone the decision more easily by waiting, by looking for distraction, by arguing, by buying more time for a decision: 'But this water is so damn cold, or you are getting tired, and the therapist just sits there; without moving, waiting patiently. It's up to you to do something' (Participant # 3).

Especially participants who hardly ever make choices, who seldom actively take decisions, are urged by a particular situation to leave their old and well-known patterns and engage themselves in the new and unknown; to feel how the new experience of actively taking a stance and acting can help them. As Clarkson (1989) stated: 'for the client who tends to be stuck most of the time in an indecisive and non-committed way, the greatest learning may be gained from learning to make this final contact' (p.113).

Accelerating a Diagnosis

Counsellors and therapists often witness how this approach rapidly makes the existing dysfunctional personal or group mechanisms visible, thus bringing these mechanisms more quickly to the fore and accelerating the search for behavioural alternatives. The most important reasons for using the active adventurous approach are found in some specific characteristics of this working methodology.

WHAT IS SO TYPICAL?

A Comparison between Activities in the Outdoors and a Classical Therapeutic Set-up

If we want to explore the specifics of the outdoor approach we are drawn towards the similarities with therapeutic approaches such as Gestalt and Emotional Focused Therapy (EFT) where experimentation has a central role in the therapeutic practice. The way in which clients engage themselves in various outdoor activities can be considered as a series of enlarged and linked 'therapeutic experiments'. While this is similar to a classical therapeutic session, a significant difference is the explicit distinction made in a classical approach between what happens 'within' versus 'outside' of the session. This contrasts sharply with, for example, a multi-day hike where the entire event is part of the 'session'. The therapeutic contract is extended and also includes the more daily habitual activities of our functioning (Ray, 2005). Do we take part in the cooking and with whom? Do we insist on the privacy of a tent? Do we help carry someone else's gear? How do we want to appear in the pictures that are taken?

An illustration of the latter is provided: During a wilderness therapy program a participant's harsh self-criticism was one of her central themes. The way she tried to avoid being photographed was unexpected by the other participants, and became a clear illustration of this theme.

We explored in depth the link between this avoidance and her self-image and sense of self-worth. Later on in the same program, we experimented with her explicitly posing for a picture while reflecting how she would like to be pictured in that environment.

Our Total Existence is Condensed to 'Me-in-this-Situation'

Wilderness therapy gains further strength from another source. Due to the simplicity of the challenge, the isolation and the interdependency of the group members and the duration of the experience, our whole existence is condensed to what I term the 'me-in-this-situation.' Or, as a participant described it:

> It's inevitable. It becomes impossible to not look at oneself and see how you present yourself in the everyday tasks. How much weight do I carry for the group? How much of the meal do I serve myself? Why don't I get involved in the map and compass route-finding?. (Participant #4)

The Strength of Nature as a Surrounding and Healing Frame

The immersion in natural surroundings during a hike, or having nature as the background in which the adventurous activities take place, has always been very appealing for most human beings. Nature can be a reflection of a lost 'home' with possibly lost ideals, childhood dreams, longings and desires. This immersion can be supported with poetry, stories and myths and presented as a place for rest, withdrawal, contemplation and renewal. Literature speaks of the restorative function of a natural environment, a place in which people can not only learn and grow but also restore mental and physical wellbeing (Muir, in Miles, 1993).

The strong metaphysical impact of the natural setting has an immediate effect on the meaning-making process of people, especially when the immersion is complete (we don't just step out of the van to look at the landscape, but become part of the landscape itself). The use of a natural setting together with physical activity is often offered as 'common sense' advice in how to deal with mental health problems. Depressed people are advised to regularly go for a hike or practice a sport. Clients themselves have provided testimony as to how a daily walk outdoors or practicing an intensive sport helped them through a psychologically difficult period. These are examples of physical activity that was disconnected and not integrated in the actual 'official' therapy, but were effective nonetheless.

Natural and Spontaneous Movements and Exertion

Outdoor activities often require natural body movements and effort, and the situation itself guides us how to proceed. We 'know' how to act if we listen attentively to our body. Look at how a child climbs: fluently, spontaneous, and sensitive to his own balance or equilibrium, sensitive to his own being-in-the-world. Technical mountaineering handbooks emphasize this in their own way. Eric Langmuir, in Mountaincraft and Leadership stated:

> It is one of the great joys of climbing that it is such a spontaneous and uncomplicated activity. Of course, there are techniques to learn and some modern climbing involves the use of a lot of highly specialised hardware, but in spite of this, at its roots, it is very much a matter of doing what comes naturally. (Langmuir, 1984, p.137)

Given enough awareness of myself in-this-situation, these movements present themselves, almost naturally to me. As a result of this, it also becomes very clear when we choose to take another, less natural action, or where we choose another, a more preferred style of interacting.

The Vitalising Effect on the Person

In a natural environment people often feel a desire to become more active. They feel they are gaining control of the situation. They again become the driving force of their life, their authentic choices, and their own decisions. This is in contrast with the dependency and the lack of impact that one experiences in our high-tech, complex world. The promise that we would become more able to master and control our environment proves to be an illusion in contemporary urban society. As a result, frustration, impotence and dependency are steadily growing.

In nature everything is more simple and straightforward. Behaviour in this realm has clearly visible consequences, no arbitrary rewards or punishments. The areas where we can be in control and where we have no control at all are clearly separated. Where we have no control we can anticipate or adapt ourselves. Kaplan and Talbot (1983) stated:

> Yet the assertion of individual control is incompatible with much of what wilderness offers and demands; rather than struggling to dominate a hostile environment, the participants come to perceive their surroundings as quite safe as long as one responds appropriately to environmental demands. Thus there is tendency to abandon the implicit purpose of control because it is both unnecessary and impossible. (p.54)

Or, as the participants put it themselves:

> If it continues to rain like this we know that we'll not be able to cross the river until the water level drops again. We can't control the water level. But we can make the choice to stay on this side of the river for the rest of this day. It's not easy walking, but we'll find a good camping spot here. (Participant # 5)

> We're not sure if this beautiful weather is going to hold or change suddenly into thick mist or a downpour. Weather forecasts are not very reliable in the mountains. But we have our waterproofs and warm clothing and a tent in our backpack. We can anticipate what might happen. (Participant # 6)

The Central Role of Awareness

The concept of awareness deserves a special mention in this paper. Often, it is heightened awareness that provides the key, which unlocks the door of change. Our senses, the instruments that guide our awareness, are not completely suited for their task anymore. Dullness is caused by an overload of sensory stimulus, and impressions that each in themselves cry out for our attention in a cascade of images, sounds, colours and tastes. We encounter difficulties at the level of sensing, but all too quickly we move on to the level of interpretation.

Lambrechts (2001) stated that we have great problems to see, hear, feel, without judging. All too often we have to focus our attention for a longer period on something that does not attract our attention by itself. This brings us back to the distinction that James (1899) made between two types of attention, depending on the amount of energy needed to focus and stay focussed on an object or a thought: involuntary attention is effortless; and voluntary attention demands energy to focus and ignore other distracting stimuli.

Within Gestalt Therapy, we try to reclaim a larger space for the direct experience, and put thinking and knowing on hold for a while. Activities in natural surroundings can help to foster this process by means of their simplicity, tranquillity and harmony. We can become more sensitive to the small differences and changes so that our senses become sharpened again. Through this process we learn to look more accurately, feel more subtly, hear better, smell more distinctively and taste more delicately.

The unknown and new aspects of the activities themselves also have their effect. On the one hand they attract our attention effortlessly and they awaken our interest and fascination. But on the other hand, in their contrast with triviality, they point out where we act out of routine or habit and where we do not genuinely contact what is 'obvious'.

Perls (1973) stated that routine and habits are established functions, and any need to change them requires that they should be brought into the focus of awareness afresh.

Removed from our predictable, daily routine this is easier. We touch the environment, and the environment touches us. We experience, and at the same time co-create the paddling, the climbing, the hiking, all in interaction with the surrounding nature. Lambrechts (2001) stated that we experience ourselves as a living whole and we experience the surrounding world by means of seeing, hearing, smelling, tasting, feeling, by breathing, by moving. At the same time we experience the world that shapes us and we experience ourselves shaping the world.

Archetypes Come Alive

Other authors have already mentioned the connection between adventure therapy and the notion of the archetype. Miles cited Stephen Bacon when he described the 'Sacred Space' as a collective age-old pattern that is passed down unconsciously over generations and transcends culture (Miles in Gass, 1993). Wilderness environments possess all of the characteristics to bring that archetype alive and can thus become a place pervaded by a sense of power, mystery and awe that facilitates positive empowerment and transformation for the one who enters it.

In the author's experience, archetypes are strongly activated during outdoor programs and work along with other therapeutic factors. I have witnessed the rise of heroes and outcasts, and of families, with new-found brothers and sisters, fathers, mothers, sons and daughters.

Something which may not be real in everyday-life, may become a powerfully felt reality on a wilderness therapy program, along with its therapeutic effects. This experience may transcend the individual meaning-giving process. I have observed how family roles spread through a group and are recognised by most of its members when asked (e.g. there is significant consensus about who is being seen as the father, the mother, the teenage child etc.).

The adventurous activities that we undertake in a wilderness context often draw on age-old patterns and archetypes. For example all of a sudden, participants find themselves in a situation where they are able to experience an archetype. For a moment, they might become a real hero, making the difference for another living being making a difference between life and death! Or, they might become the caring big sister that they may have unconsciously always wanted to have been for a younger sister. The process seems to crystallise something that has perhaps long been present only as loose particles, of whose presence they weren't even aware.

> Due to the experience of sitting by myself on that solo-activity I realised for the first time how strong my need is to be alone and by myself. Because I was invited by outsiders (the therapists) to take the challenge and sit for 36 hours on the same spot, with nothing to do, as a hermit, I could finally give that permission to myself as well and feel fully how good that felt for me. Just being there, by myself. (Participant # 7)

Since my whole being is reduced (in a condensed way) to 'myself-in-this-situation', the actions that I undertake gain an almost symbolic meaning for the way I deal with the same theme in other situations. Two examples are provided:

Example 1

Heather had already communicated a few times how the dependency that she felt during the multi-day hike reminded her of what she wanted to flee from: the submissive way she related to her colleagues at work, a pattern she recognised in her own family relations as well; a pattern which she had started to dislike, but had not yet managed to change. That morning she was invited to guide the group on the day's hike. The role involved scheduling the route and deciding on the breaks, speed and place to set up camp in the evening. At first she refused, then she carefully started to try, and after a couple of hours she was fully immersed in her new role. She had a deliberate look, a straighter posture and a backpack that didn't feel as heavy any more. She even had difficulty stopping when the group found a suitable campsite late afternoon; she herself could have kept on walking for hours.

Example 2

Because she felt inferior in relation to Helen, another participant, Marian choose to do an activity with her where equality was needed to succeed. Helen agreed to work with Marian on the activity. Once they got up on the beam and looked at the gap in the middle of the crossing, however, there was no sense of equality any more. Completely unexpected, Helen became very frightened and unsure, while with each step Marian's confidence grew. Although she was not sports-like at all, she felt balance and stability and trust in herself and was able to use all of this while relating to Helen to successfully help her cross the gap to the other side.

The Generating of Metaphors

The activities presented during an outdoor therapeutic adventure seem to possess intrinsic qualities, which generate strong metaphors. Almost spontaneously, they give birth to images and meaning (Peeters, 1997). Meaning-giving and metaphors cannot be sought or invented, they present themselves and emerge from the interplay between participant and activity. An example is provided:

> Mark during a rock-climbing session, became stuck. Mumbling to himself, shouting and cursing, tears were running down his cheeks. He was refusing to give up and be lowered down.
>
> Leave me, I have to finish something off here'. The rock-climb took him almost an hour, but gave him a lot of relief and satisfaction when he eventually succeeded in getting to the top (as well as pain and sadness).

> Later, Mark described how when he was climbing, he wasn't on the rock-face any more. He was fighting against his father's judgment, his father who always undervalued him, underestimated his achievements and judged that he would not succeed in the challenges he chose or the studies he wanted to undertake. His own father predicted him to fail, and saw him as a loser.

Phrases and expressions from our different native languages regain their authentic, physically tangible meaning. For example, we 'can't see the forest for the trees, ''get off track, ''loose ones' bearing', 'feel safe', 'reach out for someone', 'feel stuck...' During such activities there is a direct and essential experience of theme's which are normally only expressed or felt symbolically. As a result of this direct and bodily-felt connection, this lived-experience can be brought back to behaviour or challenges in daily lives by means of the same expression or metaphor. An example to illustrate this is provided:

> The group members are surprised by Danny's courage. He climbs to the very top of that pole. Then he stands on top of it, turns around and jumps off while being belayed by the other directors of the hospital where he works as a manager. Back in the hospital he is known as being very careful and even hesitant in the decisions he has to take there. Reflecting on his contrasting behaviour there versus here on the ropes course he concludes:
>
> Here I feel safe. And when I feel safe (and he points to his team members holding the belaying ropes) I dare to take risks. At work I don't have such a safety system to protect me when taking risks. (And after another thoughtful moment). Perhaps I should ask the board members more to hold the ropes if I want to make a potentially risky jump at the hospital. (Participant # 8)

This described process is a very idiosyncratic one to me the author. It is my firm belief that one cannot prescribe or dictate metaphors to make them emerge. Neither does a specific activity lead to a specific and generalised metaphor that is meaningful for any group of participants, as is suggested by some authors such as Gass (1995) or Bacon (1983). As opposed to a superficial easy to handle 'cookbook', I believe there is no pre-set recipe for cooking up a metaphor. The presence of a respectfully close and skilled therapist, empathically attuned to the language, the non-verbal communication and the meaning-giving process of the clients might be a more honest but less easy-to-use approach to the facilitation of true-felt metaphors, be it on an individual or a group level.

Some Specific Issues Regarding the Implementation

How to Choose and Shape the Activities

In my opinion, the most suitable activities for this kind of work are the ones which require only a short learning period before one masters it enough to immerse oneself into the activity and live the experience ('non-technical' activities so to speak). For me, activities such as downhill skiing, vertical caving, diving and the like require too long a training period to be used effectively for this purpose. So the activities that require almost no technical guidance or training, where participants can easily rely on their everyday mental and bodily knowledge to act, seem to be best suited.

In trying to make them therapeutically workable, Gestalt therapy theory about the use of 'active therapeutic experiments' offer us some guidance. As Wollants (1997) stated:

> The experiment is open-ended and its sole purpose is the creation of an opportunity to 'experience', to help the client examine what exists, to bring this into awareness and to give it meaning. (p.22)

When working therapeutically with outdoor activities, it is very tempting to choose activities, which might evoke a so-called catharsis, or to be led by predictions regarding the chances of success and the possible effect that this might have on the wellbeing of the client. So, it is important to remain sufficiently open-ended, with the attitude of a novice, in our choice of activities or in the way we observe clients in the activities.

The chosen 'intervention' is a co-creation between the participant and the therapist. This is an interesting issue, given that activities and challenges are often chosen and presented by the therapist or the program organizer and can often no longer be altered. However, we can easily overcome this possible contradiction. The practical design of the chosen activities and the filling-in of the different parameters can still be created together. If the high ropes course is on the program for that day, there are still numerous ways to shape and create that activity together with the group and with the different individual participants involved.

Closely linked to the previous point, an appropriate activity must always be presented at the client's level of readiness. Zinker (1977) described this process as 'grading'. Sonia Nevis spoke of 'grading up' and 'grading down' to describe the process of shaping an activity so that it is suitable and do-able on the one hand, and challenging enough with learning opportunities on the other hand. Other aspects have to be taken into account as well (cited in Peeters, 2003, p.136):

Thus, grading should be done, not only at the level of readiness of the participant, but also taking into account surrounding circumstances, such as the length of the program or group dynamic mechanisms. In this way, participants can take part in standard adventure activities which have nonetheless been personalized for them.

Risk of Physical Injury

The explicit involvement of the client's body in the therapeutic process heightens the risk of getting injured. Even more so, the 'bodily' presenting of major life-themes can become an extra element of risk as well. The non-verbal signals that accompany certain psychological issues can then necessitate assistance, treatment, follow-up or even urgent intervention. The therapist must realise that he can find himself (medically-speaking), in a 'wilderness' situation (i.e. external medical care is more than 2 hours away). In addition, work with special target groups (for example individuals with traumatic brain injury) may require medical assistance during the program. For example:

> I remember a client who had developed a personal coping style of fighting himself mentally through difficult situations he got involved in. Changing his mind or giving up had never been an option for him. It even seemed that the possibility of looking back and choosing to step out never occurred to him. Sadly, he only told us this after the cave exploration that we had chosen to do.
>
> When he got stuck and jammed in a difficult and narrow passage that he had actively chosen to try, his medical history of two heart attacks came frighteningly close. In that narrow passage he once again did not see the option of retreating and moving backwards; physically trying to force his way through was for him the only way to continue. During the debrief afterwards, he told how painfully clearly he had experienced that his coping style (not only physically but also mentally) blocked him and added to his heart problems as well. Perhaps his 'heart-attacks' were the only 'solution' his entire being could come up with to stop him.

Building in the Necessary Reflection Time

Especially in wilderness programmes or hiking expeditions in remote areas, it is important to take precautionary care and put those practical things into place which make it possible to reflect back on the lived experiences from a certain position of comfort. Dry clothes, warm drinks, a hut with fireplace can provide the necessary distance to look back and integrate what has taken place. For example:

> During a therapeutic program in New Zealand it rained almost continuously during the first three days of the hike. Luckily, a mountain cabin had been booked for a night somewhere halfway along the six-day route. Up until that moment, refection time had been brief, squeezed together under a small tarp, facing away from the smoke of a campfire that constantly needed the group's attention, while at the same time trying to dry clothes and grasp some of the warmth of the flames. The shelter and the comfort of the hut provided the group with the opportunity to explore the lived experiences, and to process them further with enough space and time.

The Temptation of Accomplishment and Success

The underlying temptation to focus too much on performance and on task achievement during activities is ever-present. The activity itself often seems to dictate the moment or place of success. For example, the top of the rock-climb, the exit of the cave, or the end of the trail on the map. There is also the achievement of other participants as a point of comparison and measure of personal success. Hovelynck (1999) argued that we need to make a shift from a task-success orientation to a frame-orientation. The frame will then decide what can be called successful. In this regard, the 'quitting' of the participant with a history of heart attacks could be looked upon as a success. 'Failing' within a task-orientation can be a real victory if viewed from a frame orientation. Or, in Wollants (1997) words, 'an experiment cannot fail'. Even an experiment which is rejected or aborted by the client, is in itself already a success. Once again, an experiment has by definition an open and uncertain end. Thus, I would also add that the rejection itself must then be explored as a part of raising consciousness of oneself in-that-situation. An example is provided:

> John tried hard to get on top of the high pole and then jump off. His goal in the activity was to experiment with his desire to trust others more. However he didn't make it to the top of the pole. He was visibly disappointed, and asked the therapist for a second chance. The therapist told him that he should discuss it with his belayers. The belayers were already putting the gear away and seemed rather relieved that they could finally take off their harnesses and helmets. John hesitated for a long time and finally dared to interrupt the clean-up process and personally ask everyone if they would be willing to belay him a second time. After everyone agreed and replaced the harness and helmets, John was ready to give it another try. He looked up to the top of the pole, and then to his obliging and patient belayers. He then told everyone:
>
> My second attempt can stop here. I feel like I've already completely succeeded in my objective. By taking the huge risk to be rejected when asking you to belay me while everyone seemed to be glad that the activity was finally over, I placed a large amount of trust in you. This is the most daring jump I could make. (Participant # 9)

The Group Context

Group context could be the content of a full article in itself. The fact that this kind of therapy is most often undertaken in a group, be it an existing group or as co-participants in an open enrolment program, has huge consequences for the meaning-making process for different individuals. It is the author's belief that any leader of such a program must be trained in group-dynamic phenomena, so that they can understand and work with the effect of a group on individual behaviour, and can also understand the meaning and function of individual behaviour for the group-as-a-whole. Emerging roles, phenomena such as projective identification (Ringer, 2002), the group focal conflict, or basic-assumptions of group behaviour are just some examples of theoretical concepts, which can help to shape our understanding and practice of working within a group context.

The Therapist as Active Partner in the Venture

Much more explicitly than in a classical therapeutic setting, the adventure therapist is a partner in the therapeutic journey of the client or the client-group. The therapist has his own wishes, desires and needs, which of course have their right to exist but must not become the dominant issue. It could become problematic, for instance, if it is always the therapist who is slow and who needs to be waited for when leaving camp in the morning, or when he is the least physically fit person. Or if she herself is too exhausted, too hungry or too cold to leave the group members with the necessary space to decide for themselves when they want to take a break or decide on the route of their hike.

Hindrances in the Creation of an Emotionally Safe Therapeutic Environment

When offering outdoor activities as a therapeutic instrument, it is of the great importance to ensure an emotionally safe working and experimental context. In adventure therapy the sessions do not take place in the safe and enclosed bubble of a therapy room, but in the public space of the natural environment. As a result, in certain locations there is a risk of exposure to by-passers or spectators or fellow outdoor-lovers. Those people might react in a very specific way, or even intervene in the processes the therapist carefully tries to establish. In spite of best intentions, such interventions often do not fit the therapeutic goals or methods of working, as illustrated by the following story:

> Two cavers decided to help the woman who was very clearly having difficulty trying to find the exit of the cave. Her difficulties were apparently compounded by the 'negligence' of her guide, who was seemingly unaware of her needs (so they thought). Furthermore, the woman was clearly pleased with the pushing and pulling and helping hands the cavers provided. All of this made the cavers feel quite justified in the 'help' they provided. Later on, reflecting on her 'caving-session' the woman told her guide and therapist (who himself was an experienced caver as well) how sorry she felt about not having managed to do it completely on her own and how she was disappointed in how she had given away her independence too easily to others.

Such 'interventions' might also take place in situations where technical staff are hired to provide help or provide the necessary qualifications to undertake an activity. It is of the greatest importance that support staff are briefed ahead of time about how the therapist wants to run the activity. Technical support staff can also be evaluated on their affinity for the therapeutic facilitation of these activities. Often, it is best to stay away from spectacular or well-known natural sites. Participants do not need a dramatic location in order to explore and develop awareness for what is and what might be.

Conclusions

As author of this paper, I had the objective of sharing some of the passion I feel towards working with groups therapeutically in the outdoors. I wanted to explore together with the reader, the kaleidoscope of richness that lies within a use of nature and adventure as an instrument for growth, discovery and healing. I hope I realized part of this aim, and that the paper stimulates other therapists and counsellors to take their client system on a wonderful inward adventure, outdoors and into nature.

Acknowledgements

Many thanks to Nick Ray and to Jen Nold for her stimulating help with the English writing.

References

Bandoroff, S. (2003). Family therapy with a twist and a shake and a shout: Adventure family therapy in practice. In K. Richards & B. Smith (Eds.), *Therapy within Adventure*. Augsburg: Ziel.

Bacon, S.B. (1983). *The conscious use of metaphor in outward Bound*. Denver: Colorado Outward Bound School.

Davis-Berman, J., & Berman, D. (1994). *Wilderness therapy: Foundations, theory and research.* Dubuque: Kendall/Hunt.

Clarkson, P. (1989). *Gestalt counselling in action.* London: Sage Publications.

Gass, M. (1993). *Adventure therapy: Therapeutic applications of adventure programming.* Dubuque: Kendall/Hunt.

Gass, M. (1995). *Book of metaphors, Volume II.* Dubuque, IA: Kendall/Hunt.

Gillis, H.L. & Ringer, T.M. (1999). Therapeutic adventure programs. In S. Priest & J. Miles (Eds.), *Adventure programming.* USA: Venture Publications.

Gilsdorf, R. (1998). Gestalt and adventure therapy: Parallels and perspectives. In C. Itin (Ed.), *Exploring the boundaries of adventure therapy: International Perspectives*. Boulder, CO: Association for Experiential Education.

Gilsdorf, R. (2004). *Von der erlebnispädagogik zur erlebnistherapie.* Bergisch Gladbach: EHP.

Hovelynck, J. (1999). Facilitating the development of generative metaphors: reemphasizing participants' guiding images. *Australian Journal of Outdoor Education,* 4(1), 12-24.

James, W. (1899). *Talks to teachers on Psychology: And to students on some of life's ideals.* New York: Henry Holt.

Kaplan, S., & Talbot, J.F. (1983). Psychological benefits of wilderness experience. In I. Altman & J.F. Wohwill (Eds.), *Behaviour and the environment.* New York: Plenum Press.

Lambrechts, G. (2001). *De Gestalttherapie tussen toen en straks.* Berchem: EPO.

Langmuir, E. (1984). *Mountaincraft and leadership.* Leicester: Cordee.

Miles, J.C. (1993). Wilderness keeping by wilderness educators. *The Outdoor Educator*, June, 9-13.

Peeters, L. (1977). 'De Paal' als werkinstrument binnen een experiëntiele Gestaltpsychotherapiebenadering. In *Kwestie van techniek: Gestalt, tijdschrift voor gestalttherapie* (4th ed.), p. 5. Turnhout: Bureau Gestalt.

Peeters, L. (2003). From adventure to therapy: Some necessary conditions to enhance the therapeutic outcomes of adventure programming. In K. Richards & B. Smith (Eds.), *Therapy within adventure.* Augsburg: Ziel.

Peeters, L. (2009). Hooofdstuk 18: Over het inzetten van avontuurlijke werkvormen. In P.derkinderen, E. Knijff, & S. Meijer (Eds.), *Praktijkboek Gestalt,* (271-286). Utrecht, De Tijdstroom.

Penner, C. (1997) A Gestalt approach to experience. In R. Nadler & J. Luckner (Eds.), *Processing the experience.* Dubuque, IA: Kendall/Hunt.

Perls, F. (1973). *The Gestalt approach and eye witness to therapy.* USA: Science and Behaviour Books.

Ray, N. (2005). Transactions on the rock face. In *Therapy Today: The Professional Journal for Counselors and Psychotherapist*, Special Issue, 16(10),15.

Ringer, T.M. (2002). Group action: *The dynamics of groups in therapeutic, educational and corporate settings.* London: Jessica Kingsley Publishers.

Wollants, G. (1997). Gestalt als symmorfoseproces. In *Kwestie van techniek: Gestalt, tijdschrift voor gestalttherapie* (4th ed.), p. 5. Turnhout: Bureau gestalt.

Zinker, J. (1977) *Creative process in Gestalt therapy.* New York: Random House.

CHAPTER 3

Finding a Place for Adventure Therapy and Therapeutic Adventure on the Continuum of Care

Dene Berman and Jennifer Davis-Berman

ABSTRACT

This paper was delivered as a public presentation as part of the 5IATC, at a special session open to conference delegates and the general public. From a mental health perspective, the authors discuss the appropriateness and applicability of adventure therapy to mental health services for children and adolescents. Particular attention is paid to developing strategies to gain acceptance from the mainstream mental health community. The mental health systems in the United States and the United Kingdom are used as examples. Finally, recommendations for an evidence-based approach, and use of the GRADE system for evaluating research are presented. The authors suggest that in order to operate within the mental health treatment system, adventure therapy programs must go to greater lengths to document effectiveness.

INTRODUCTION

This paper represents a public lecture delivered as part of the larger 5IATC. As such, it is geared toward professionals in the field, as well as those who might be completely unfamiliar with adventure therapy and its applications. Although a difficult task to reach such diverse audiences, the authors are excited about the possibility that their words might generate some thought and discussion among a wide variety of people. Thus, this paper speaks to those who have done the research and writing in the field of adventure therapy, and those who have developed and run some of the most widely respected programs in the world. We are also writing for parents or other family members who are curious about an adventure therapy program for a loved one, or who have had a loved one participate in such a program. Some of the readers may have participated in outdoor adventures and have directly experienced the ways in which adventure and the outdoors can combine to create transformative experiences that shape who we are and who we will be. Most likely, the readers are young people trying to determine the direction of their profession and their practice. Like the presentation upon which it is based, this paper offers an opportunity to continue to join together in the discussion and generation of ideas.

The authors come to the field of adventure therapy as people with a passionate interest in these programs and their effectiveness. Being mental health therapists, we are keenly interested in the place of adventure therapy in mental health treatment both in North America and throughout the world. Our experience in the field includes running wilderness therapy trips, training wilderness therapists, and functioning in both academic and practice settings. We've also conducted a great deal of research, and have written about adventure therapy rather extensively. We have argued that from a mental health perspective, therapists must have the same credentials on wilderness therapy trips as they do in office settings (Davis-Berman & Berman, 1994; 2008).

This presentation explores the application of wilderness therapy to mental health treatment, using the United States and the United Kingdom as examples. An argument is made for the need for increased professionalization of the field. Of course, this is a biased perspective, reflecting the mental health laws and regulations in both the United States and the United Kingdom, and may not be applicable in other parts of the world. The following case study gives the reader a taste of some of the issues that can arise when dealing with serious mental health issues while on a wilderness therapy trip in the United States:

Kelly was referred from the community mental health clinic where she had been seen for depression. She was quiet and somewhat isolated during base camp, and hung back for the first few days on the backpacking trail in a National Forest. We knew more was at stake than depression when Kelly approached the staff after three or four days of not seeing anyone on the trail, talking about how we were being followed by the mafia, who were intent on murdering her. The next evening after we set up camp but before it was time to start dinner, Kelly approached me with a trowel and toilet paper in hand to say she was headed off into the woods. She was wearing her compass and whistle, and pointed in the direction she was headed. As I was nodding off, leaning against a tree, I heard a blood curdling scream and then someone crashing through the brush. We executed our emergency plan, gathering the remaining participants into a circle as Dave, our outdoor leader, went into the woods to find Kelly. Kelly came back by herself, with Dave entering the camp from another direction. I approached Kelly, who was staring off in space with a faraway stare, asking what happened. Kelly replied, 'My name is KC. Kelly was murdered by the mafia man.' Kelly then became catatonic, sitting up all night. Over the next two days we worked on evacuating Kelly and getting her to a small community hospital, where some of her many personalities emerged, others to be revealed to us in the months and even years when I continued to see her in therapy.

The point to be made here is that high levels of both outdoor leadership and therapy skills are needed to work with troubled adolescents in adventure activities, especially in more remote settings where support services are not readily available. This is a radically different venture than taking at-risk youth out on an adventure, and equally different than providing psychotherapy in an office, clinic, or hospital setting.

PUBLIC PERCEPTIONS OF WILDERNESS THERAPY

Some readers may remember the Brat Camp television series, which was airing at the time of the Fourth International Adventure Therapy Conference. Viewers in the United States, the United Kingdom, and even Australia were avidly glued to their TV sets to watch troubled kids in the wilderness. The first season was developed and filmed in the United States, but participants were selected in London. The major stated goal of the project was to expose parents in the United Kingdom to wilderness therapy as an alternative to traditional approaches to working with troubled teens.

These television shows have certainly exposed the public to the process of wilderness therapy as conducted by some programs. People seem more interested in this field, and might even be more open to considering it as an option for one of their family members. In fact, RedCliff Ascent, the site of the first series, reported that since their Brat Camp exposure the number of website visits per month doubled (Jones, 2005).

Clearly, exposure and publicity work. People are now better informed about adventure therapy as a treatment option. But, is this Brat Camp type of exposure the kind of public relations effort that is good for this field? Does this promote our field in ways that enhance the promise of wilderness therapy? The airing of this series led to a debate among professionals in the outdoor adventure field. Concerns were raised about the derogatory labels being placed on participants like 'angry punk', 'drug addict', and 'compulsive liar'. Some raised concerns about the use of Native American names for staff and participants. The issues of privacy and confidentiality were also extensively debated, as was the issue of deprivation. Even if the parents had consented to the television cameras, did this mean that the adolescents wanted this exposure? Did the adolescents feel pressured to participate, due to the high cost of the program being covered? Even if they did want to participate, is it clinically and professionally ethical for them to? These are just some of the questions being debated since the airing of the program.

Brat Camp is not the only public view of wilderness therapy in the United States and the United Kingdom. Particularly in the United States, adventure and wilderness therapy are identified with boot camps where participants are treated punitively, with an attempt to break them down in order to build them back up again. Deprivation, verbal abuse, the withholding of basic sustenance, inadequate shelter, and failure to provide for basics are characteristic of these kinds of programs. A cursory glance at American daytime television reveals situations where teens are identified as being 'troubled', forcibly taken to boot camps, filmed, and then interviewed on talk shows. Often, these teens were brought back for encore or follow up appearances, as American audiences seem so fascinated with the boot camp experiences.

A third way in which the public gets a view of wilderness therapy programs is via reports of tragedies in wilderness therapy trips. Unfortunately, deaths on trips, with resulting lawsuits, often garner a great deal of media coverage and attention, tainting the image of the good work done. A recent study by the United States Government Accountability Office exposed abuse and neglect in wilderness programs, grouping wilderness therapy programs with more punitive boot camp programs (Government Accountability Office, 2007). As an example of how the image of adventure therapy has been corrupted, the authors undertook a simple Google search of the words *Death and Wilderness Therapy*, and the first item to pop up was about a teen death due to a staph infection in a juvenile corrections boot camp facility.

This year, a story was told in the United States about two judges who pled they were guilty of taking bribes for sentencing thousands of adolescents to private detention programs. The picture that accompanied a nationally published editorial of this story showed a picture of a young woman who was sentenced to a wilderness camp 'for building a spook MySpace page that lampooned her assistant principal'. This same editorial went on to cite a National Associated Press survey that revealed 13,000 claims of abuse, including rape, by juvenile correction staff (Associated Press, 2009). Stories like this one, and the report of the United States Government Accountability Office erroneously and harmfully lumped therapy programs that involve adventure and wilderness into the same category as correctional facilities, boot camps, and the like.

The authors make the plea to distance adventure therapy programs from other programs by calling for high standards that include: increased attention to safety, both physical and emotional; lack of coercion in programs; the accreditation of programs; and proper credentialing or commissioning of individuals. Some of our forthright positions have created controversy in the field, and we've had our share of disagreements over this idea of standards. However, given the climate of misperception about adventure therapy in the United States in particular, we believe this is essential. Furthermore, this kind of dialogue is what keeps the field alive, and it should be encouraged and welcomed.

We have talked for decades about the challenges of wilderness therapy programs to be recognized by the mainstream mental health community (Davis-Berman & Berman, 1994; 2008). Since the recent near collapse of the American and world economies, this acceptance has become even more difficult. Also, the aforementioned investigation of residential treatment of youth by the United States Government Accountability Office sent shock waves through the adventure therapy and traditional mental health communities.

In this paper, we present some of the obstacles that adolescents face, both in the United States and in the United Kingdom. For example, adolescents face obstacles to therapy, and more specifically wilderness therapy. In the United States obstacles include the unemployment crisis, where even basic needs such as housing and food are in jeopardy for many. Currently, the healthcare system in the United States is being debated, and there are about 50 million uninsured people. As an example in the United Kingdom, we will touch on debates about the provision of psychotherapy within the health care system.

Rather than restricting ourselves to adventure therapy programs that can be conceptualized to be psychotherapy, we want to consider (and thus promote), thought and discussion about a continuum of care in child and adolescent mental health that exists both in the United States and in the United Kingdom. Based on this continuum, we can begin to figure out what kinds of programs are appropriate. We introduce an evidence-based model to help place programs on the continuum of care.

For our purposes, we make a distinction between adventure therapy and therapeutic adventure. For us, adventure therapy programs are based on identified or diagnosed disorders, by individuals trained and credentialed in mental health, with the systematic application of assessments and treatments. Such an approach is inherent in the mental health treatment field. On the other hand, therapeutic adventure programs are those that may promote positive change, but in a less formal way, or by non-professionals, or with a less systematic approach, often without the goal of alleviating the symptoms of a disorder (Davis-Berman & Berman, 1994). The questions to be addressed in this paper concern the extent to which therapeutic adventure programs can function within the field of organized mental health treatment, to help alleviate some of the psychological problems confronting young people. Again, these perspectives and ideas are based on an analysis and understanding of the mental health treatment systems in the United States and in the United Kingdom.

The Mental Health Needs of Youth

Around the world, the rates of psychiatric disorders among youth vary from 8 percent in the Netherlands to a high of 57 percent in areas surrounding San Diego in the United States. Australian rates for the 18 to 24 year old group are somewhere in the middle at 27 percent. When looking at the 13-to-15 age group, the rate in the United States drops to about 12 percent. Studies of youth between the ages of 13 to 15 in the United Kingdom report this same 12 percent, and estimates suggest that worldwide, one in every 4 to 5 young people has a mental health disorder in any given year (Patel, et al., 2007).

A large study in the United Kingdom looked at the mental health of children and youth between the ages of 5 and 16 (Green, McGinnity, Meltzer, Ford & Goodman, 2005). It was reported that, in general, 10 percent of the young people had a clinically diagnosed mental health disorder, with a 4 percent rate of anxiety or depression, a 6 percent rate of conduct disorder, a 2 percent rate of attention deficit hyperactivity disorder, and a 1 percent rate of autism and eating disorders. There was also a 2 percent rate of co-occurring multiple disorders. More than one in four children and youth had attempted to harm or kill themselves. According to this study, the rates of mental health disorders among youth in the United Kingdom had remained essentially unchanged since 1999 (Green, McGinnity, Meltzer, Ford & Goodman, 2005).

Estimates of mental health problems in American youth also vary widely from 5 to 20 percent. When substance abuse problems are included, it has been suggested that 21 percent of children and adolescents in the United States have a diagnosable mental health disorder, with 11 percent of those having disorders that are described as significantly impairing (United States Department of Health & Human Services, 2001). Similar to the data reported from the United Kingdom, anxiety disorders were found to be most common.

The different health care systems in the United States and the United Kingdom will be addressed later in this paper. However, it is interesting to note at this point that, in both countries, there is a gap between the mental health needs of adolescents and the services available to them. Some researchers in the United Kingdom have claimed that help for adolescents is often not available or not effective. Others have pointed out that many of the major mental health disorders begin in adolescence, and noted that this is where service provision is weakest. In the United States, there is a similarly recognized lack of mental health treatment for youth and adolescents. Recent estimates confirm that 70 percent of adolescents who need care are not getting it (Chandra & Minkovitz, 2006).

A current United States Government report revealed that 7 million United States young adults meet the diagnostic criteria for a substance abuse disorder but 93% of them – 6.3 million people – are not getting the specialty care they need (SAMHSA, 2006). This apparent service gap opens the door for adventure therapy and other creative approaches to fill the gap between the needs of youth and the services available to them.

ORIGINS OF OUTDOOR THERAPY IN NORTH AMERICA

There is a history in North America of attempts to use the outdoors and adventure to address mental health needs. One of the earliest examples, although not with youth, is a use of tent therapy that can be traced back to the United States when in 1901, nature played a role in the treatment of mental illness. During that summer, psychiatric patients with tuberculosis were housed in tents on the grounds of the Manhattan State Hospital East in New York. Not only did the physical health of these patients improve as a result of this program, their mental health did as well (Wright & Haviland, 1903). Tenting programs arose in other places in the United States around that same time (American Journal of Insanity, 1910; 1916).

Another source of outdoor programming to meet mental health needs comes from the *therapeutic camping* movement. Camp Ahmek, in Ontario, Canada, represents the first recorded use of a camp to try to effect social change in youth. It was founded in 1921, with a girls' camp established in 1927. Based on the founder's experience of the Young Men's Christian Association (YMCA), there was an emphasis on the development of their intellectual, social, and physical lives, within a religious framework (Dimock & Hendry, 1939). Other early camps included the Dallas Salesmanship Camp, which closed in 2004 after a 60 year history of focusing on the emotional growth of youth (Loughmiller, 1965). The Fresh Air Camp at the University of Michigan operated from 1944 until its decline in the 1970s. It was the first camp to specifically target youth with mental health problems, and use psychotherapy. This camp used students from the fields of social work, education, psychology, nursing, and sociology under the supervision of trained mental health professionals (Morse, 1957). Perhaps the most famous outdoor program in the United States that has focused on growth and development has been *Outward Bound.* Founded in the United Kingdom in 1941, its influence has been wide reaching (Miner & Boldt, 1981). Early Outward Bound programs deserve comment not only because of their work with youth, but also because of their attempts to collect data and show the effectiveness of their programs. These early programs cleared the way for adventure and outdoor therapeutic programming for youth in the United States.

There are numerous types of programs that utilize the out-of-doors to work with youth. Many of these programs do wonderful jobs of working with at-risk adolescents, addressing personal growth and self-esteem. Our discussion about therapy and the need for treatment based in evidence is in no way meant to take away from the impact of these therapeutic programs. They are quite powerful.

Many adventure programs, such as those offered to facilitate adjustment in college, have been aimed at education and growth. The use of the outdoors has also been extended to programs that cater to people with certain health conditions, while others focus on leadership training and can be connected to universities. Regardless of the program type, the outdoor environment often helps facilitate personal growth and awareness. The range of adventure programs can be compared to a continuum of care in mental health.

Continuum of Care

A model that we have discussed related to outdoor programs is one that includes a range of services, listed below with an increasing level of intervention, with more intensive levels of care, and more specialized models of delivery of that care (Berman & Davis-Berman, 2009):

- Recreation
- Growth and enrichment
- Self-esteem
- Adjunct to Therapy
- Outpatient
- Day Treatment
- Partial Hospital
- Residential
- Inpatient Hospital

Complicating one's ability to gain a clear picture of the mental health delivery system in the United States is the fact that individuals who are covered by third-party payers (e.g. insurance companies, or government programs such as Medicare or Medicaid) are limited in the types of services they are eligible to receive. Services must often be pre-certified as necessary, usually requiring that patients fail in less restrictive levels of care.

In the United Kingdom, where there is one health care system, a continuum of care is incorporated into the Department of Health framework for child mental health. This 4-Tier model is outlined here (Department of Health, 2007):

- Tier 1. Child and adolescent mental health services are aimed at providing early screening and referral, as well as general advice and treatment for 'less severe' problems. Providers at this level include teachers, social workers, volunteers, and primary care physicians.
- Tier 2. Early assessment and intervention are provided by mental health professionals.
- Tier 3. Provides for children and adolescents with 'severe, complex and persistent mental health disorders' using a multi-disciplinary model for such serious problems as psychosis, and for individuals who may be at risk for hospitalization.
- Tier 4. For those needing inpatient care for assessment or treatment.

The irony of the situation is that while we can all think of adventurous ways of helping youth, at the same time, there is no obvious, ready-made place for adventure therapy in the mental health continuum of care for children and adolescents. Adventure therapists without specialist training in mental health and without a role in a mental health system, are not easily conceptualized to fit within these practice models. If we want funding for adventure therapy in the United States and the United Kingdom, we must fit into the mental health or health care system. In order to fit in, we must have evidence of effectiveness.

Evidence-Based Practice

Fifteen years ago an American Psychological Association Task Force on Promotion and Dissemination of Psychological Procedures called for well designed, randomized controlled studies that showed superiority to a placebo or equivalence to established treatments, with a treatment manual and homogeneous treatment population (APA Presidential Task Force on Evidence-Based Practice, 2006).

The importance of this initiative is that it established a precedent for the evidence-based practice of psychology in the United States. It is now expected that psychologists in the United States will practice in a manner consistent with Evidence-Based Practice of Psychology. What that means is that psychologists will utilize the best available research in their assessments, treatment planning, and interventions. This is consistent with the Institute of Medicine's call for evidence-based practice as 'the integration of best research evidence with clinical expertise and patient values' (Task Force on Promotion and Dissemination of Psychological Procedures, 1995, p. 4). Social work has also supported evidence-based practice for a number of years (Gilgun, 2005).

Evidence-based practice in mental health treatment is not limited to psychology the United States Government has a website with links to evidence-based substance abuse practices around the world.

In the United Kingdom, health care standards are promulgated by the National Health Service (NHS). An independent organization within the NHS, the National Institute for Health and Clinical Excellence (NICE) has within its purview a responsibility for providing guidance on health and illness. NICE currently has 15 published guidelines on psychiatric disorders (Khele, 2008).

NICE and more than 20 international organizations (including the World Health Organization), utilize a system for evaluating the quality of research called 'Grades of Recommendation, Assessment, Development and Evaluation' (GRADE) (Higgins & Green, 2008). This system has four levels of evidence quality: high, moderate, low, and very low. Highlights of high quality evidence within the GRADE system include: a clear research question with relevance to patients; randomised trials; and large effect size. This approach, and the conclusions drawn from it when applied to mental health have been the subject of recent controversy with allegations of flawed strategies for searching and interpreting the evidence. Lesser levels have increasing limitations on research evidence. Randomized Controlled Trials research methods are preferred, but weaker designs can be upgraded if there are big treatment effects.

It is notable that adventure therapy research, while ongoing and with some promise, lies outside of the research reviewed or recommended by APA, NICE, or any of the organizations utilizing the GRADE system. This puts the field of adventure therapy outside of the mainstream of the evidence-based realm of healthcare, social programming, or psychotherapy. Our challenge as a field is to identify what we do best, determine which populations we are effective in serving, and then to design, staff and execute those programs.

IS THERE A SEAT AT THE TABLE?

Adventure Therapy

Is there a seat at this table for adventure therapy? There are wonderfully creative, curative, and transformative programs that use adventure and the outdoors. However, for those who aspire to change personalities, remediate psychological problems, augment or supplant traditional therapies, or receive healthcare funding, thereby aspiring to be adventure therapy, continued work needs to be done. In other words, if we want a seat at the table that includes healthcare, mental health treatment, and social programs, we will need to speak the language of the mental health treatment system.

Research

Based on the current emphasis on evidence-based approaches in both the United Kingdom and the United States, if adventure or wilderness therapy programs want to be recognized and respected by mainstream mental health, research evidence must support their effectiveness. We extensively reviewed the literature in the field of wilderness therapy, and have concluded that while excellent studies have been done, the field has not met the standards set forth to qualify as an evidence-based approach.

Continuum of Care

If wilderness therapy programs are to be accepted into mainstream mental health, they must fit into the continuum of mental health treatment care. We have discussed these levels of care in the United Kingdom and the United States. The field of adventure therapy must take stock of what services it can and cannot provide, and must position itself at the level of care for which it is qualified. Implicit in these levels of care, are different types of credentials for practitioners.

For example, growth-oriented groups often work with adolescents who are basically highly functioning, with no major mental health or addiction problems. In these types of programs, no mental health credential may be needed to provide effective and safe care. This would be similar to Tier 1 in the system in the United Kingdom where volunteers, teachers or social workers might be delivering the service. As the level of complexity of problems increases, so does the need for mental health training and credentials. For example, in outpatient mental health in the United States there is an obvious need for appropriate credentialing. Only licensed mental health professionals can provide psychotherapy services. This resembles the commissioning of programs and practitioners for Tiers 2, 3 and 4 in the United Kingdom system. There will soon be a push for the credentialing of mental health professionals in the United Kingdom. Credentialing and cross-training of adventure professionals and therapists is an issue that continues to cause contention in the United States and internationally. We have said that we feel that the future of wilderness therapy, especially in the United States and the United Kingdom, rests on licensure and credentialing if movement into mainstream mental health treatment or health care is possible.

Beyond Research and Training

For an intervention to be successful, it is not enough to have research, a range of services, and well-trained staff. One model that holds promise for the field (in that it sheds light on issues to be considered) is the RE-AIM model. RE-AIM goes beyond efficacy data to look at variables that determine the impact of programs, in order to bridge the gap from research to practice. It does so by considering five variables (Zweben, 2007, p. 25):

- Reach into the target population
- Efficacy or effectiveness
- Adoption by target settings or institutions
- Implementation—consistency of delivery of intervention
- Maintenance of intervention effects in individuals and populations over time.

The RE-AIM website (www.re-aim.org) suggests ways in which each of these factors can be addressed. A framework such as RE-AIM goes beyond the narrow focus of some evidence-based research to include important issues such as reaching the intended audience, being concerned about the adoption of the approach, and factors such as cost (Glasgow et al., 2006).

Therapeutic Adventure

The critique presented in this paper does not mean that therapeutic adventure programs that address growth or Tier 1 type of populations are unimportant. In fact, they are critically important and may actually serve as excellent prevention programs. For those in this field who run therapeutic programs, there may be little that needs to be done, except to continue to share their programs with the public.

Enhancing and facilitating personal growth might be a way to limit the development of future mental health problems in adolescents.

CONCLUSIONS

Some adventure therapy programs do cater specifically to adolescents with mental health problems. These programs in the United States are regulated, often accredited and use credentialed staff. These efforts should continue. Those who are not able to meet that level of care are best to focus on prevention, early intervention, education, and growth. These programs are no less important, they just don't meet the standards to which mental health professionals must adhere. In this way, both adventure therapy and therapeutic adventure can become a part of the continuum of care in child and adolescent mental health.

While all of this may appear to be a daunting task, there are clear steps to be taken. Let us take up the challenge to put together an international task force to analyze the research on adventure therapy by using the same system, GRADE (www.gradeworkinggroup.org), used by so many of the major health organizations in the world (including the World Health Organization). We need to promote what we can do effectively and safely, and set an agenda to overcome what we find is lacking. From there, looking at the steps involved in RE-AIM will also help us to implement programs that are effective and sustainable.

REFERENCES

American Journal of Insanity. (1910), 67.

American Journal of Insanity. (1916), 73.

American Psychological Association Presidential Task Force on Evidence-Based Practice. (2006). Evidence-based practice in psychology. *American Psychologist*, 61, 271-285.

Berman, D. & Davis-Berman, J. (2009). *Wilderness therapy in the desert*. Keynote address presented at Lotan's Way: The First Israeli Wilderness Therapy Conference, Hatzeva, Israel.

Chandra, A. & Minkovitz, C. S. (2006). Stigma starts early: Gender differences in teen willingness to use mental health services. *Journal of Adolescent Health,* 38, 754-758.

Davis-Berman, J., & Berman, D. (1994). *Wilderness therapy: Foundations, theory & research*. Dubuque, IA: Kendall/Hunt.

Davis-Berman, J. & Berman, D. (2008). *The promise of wilderness therapy.* Boulder, CO: Association for Experiential Education.

Department of Health. (2007). *National service framework for children young people and maternity services: The mental health and psychological well-being of children and young people: Standard 9.* Retrieved from: http://www.dh.gov.uk/en/Publicationsandstatistics/Publications/PublicationPolicy AndGuidance/ Browsable/DH_4868712.

Dimock, H., & Hendry, C. (1939). *Camping and character: A camp experiment in character education.* New York: Association Press.

Gilgun, J. (2005). The four cornerstones of evidence-based practice in social work. *Research on Social Work Practice,* 15, 52-61.

Glasgow, R., Nelson, C., Strycker, L., & King, D. (2006). Using RE-AIM metrics to evaluate diabetes self-management support interventions. *American Journal of Preventive Medicine*, 30, 67-73.

Government Accountability Office. (2007). Residential treatment programs: Concern regarding abuse and death in certain programs for troubled youth. Retrieved on October 10, 2007 from: www.gao.gov.

Grade Working Group. (2009). Retrieved from: www. gradeworkinggroup.org.

Green, H., McGinnity, A., Meltzer, H., Ford, T., & Goodman, R. (2005). *Mental health of children and young people in Great Britain*, 2004. Retrieved from http:// www.statistics.gov.uk.

Higgins, J. P. & Green, S. (2008). *Cochrane handbook for systematic reviews of interventions (Version 5.0.1).* The Cochrane Collaboration. Retrieved from: www. cochrane-handbook.org.

Jones, J. (2005). *Wilderness therapy and the white-hot glare of publicity.* Woodbury Reports. Retrieved on 12/28/2005 from http://www.strugglingteens.com.

Juvenile Law Center. (2008). Retrieved from: http://www.jlc.org/files/luzernecounty/charging.pdf

Khele, S. (2008). NICE guidelines for mental health. *Therapy Today*, 19(10), 40-41.

Loughmiller, C. (1965). *Wilderness road.* Austin, TX: Hogg Foundation for Mental Health.

Miner, J., & Boldt, J. (1981). *Outward Bound USA: Learning through experience in adventure based education.* New York: William Morrow & Co.

Morse, W. (1957). An interdisciplinary therapeutic camp. *Journal of Social Issues, 13* (1), 15-22.

National Cancer Institute. (2009). Retrieved from: www.re-aim.org.

Patel, V., Flisher, A., Hetrick, S., & McGarry, P. (2007). Mental health of young people: A global public health challenge. *Lancet, 369,* 1302-1313.

SAMHSA. (2006). *OAS Reports: A day in the life of American adolescents: Substance use facts*. Retrieved on 11/05/2007 from http://www.oas.samhsa.gov

Task Force on Promotion and Dissemination of Psychological Procedures. (1995). Training in and dissemination of empirically validated psychological treatments: Report and recommendations. *The Clinical Psychologist, 48*, 3-23.

United States Department of Health and Human Services (2001). *Youth violence: A report of the surgeon general.* Rockville, MD.

Wright, A., & Haviland, C. (1903). Additional notes upon tent treatment for the insane at Manhattan State Hospital East. *American Journal of Insanity, 60,* 53-59.

Zweben, J. (2007). *Evidence-based practices and treatment interventions: A clinician's perspective.* Retrieved on 7/14/2009 from: http://www.coce.samhsa.gov/ cod_resources/PDF/EBP%27s-Clinician%27sPerspective-COCE-COSIG6-21-07.pdf.

CHAPTER 4

A Wilderness Based Therapeutic Intervention for Young People at Risk of Homelessness and Educational Disconnection

Sandy Allen-Craig and Lisa Ronalds

ABSTRACT

The research upon which this paper is based aimed to evaluate the life effectiveness of participants involved in a wilderness therapy program, in order to determine its value as an early treatment intervention for youth 'at risk' of homelessness and educational disconnection. The study focused on participants from five Australian Regional Extended Family Services (REFS) wilderness programs. The programs were designed as an early intervention for young people at risk of homelessness, to help prevent educational and family disengagement. The study investigated the effectiveness of the program in promoting change in program participants. The study examined outcomes of the program associated with the risk factors of homelessness as measured by the Life Effectiveness Questionnaire (LEQ). The LEQ was used in three of its forms in order to determine the changes that took place.

The results of the research show that there was change between the pre and post program responses across the overall LEQ-I and YARPET scores, with small to moderate effect sizes of 0.31 and 0.22 respectively. Greatest improvements are seen in time management ($d = 0.43$), task leadership ($d = 0.45$), social competence ($d = 0.35$) and achievement motivation ($d = 0.32$). The observer results consistently support those of the participants. An effect size of 0.2 represents an 8% increase in student perceptions of their skills. These results give preliminary support for the use of wilderness therapy as an intervention to help prevent young people prematurely disengaging from family and the education system.

INTRODUCTION

Youth homelessness is a serious social issue within the Australian community. On Census night 2001, a total of 99,900 people were estimated to be homeless (ABS, 2002). Close to half of the 99,900 homeless people were less than 25 years of age (46%), with those aged 12-18 years a prominent group (26% of all homeless people), and those under the age of 12 years making up ten percent.

Ninety percent of homeless young people presenting at Salvation Army Youth Care centers are not currently involved in any formal education (HREOC, 1989). This may be due to inadequate living conditions, instability regarding location, a lack of privacy and space, or difficulty being motivated. However, leaving the education system greatly limits future career opportunities (Smith, 1995). Research conducted by the Council to Homeless Persons in Victoria supported these findings, revealing that the majority of young homeless people do not participate in education at any level. Of young homeless people aged 15-19, 69% were not in education (CHP, 1998).

The combination of past trauma, lack of supports, and managing a precarious life with a poor view of the future, often results in these young people being depressed and angry, or demonstrating a range of other emotions. Previous negative experiences (either with adults or with support services), combined with poor communication skills, often result in young people appearing hostile or aggressive when seeking support (Australian Institute of Health and Wellbeing, 2003). In order to address the issue of youth homelessness in Australia, the Liberal-National Party Government in 1996 established the Reconnect Program, which places great emphasis on early intervention strategies for youth ‘at risk’ of homelessness.

Regional Extended Family Services (REFS) is one of many services involved in delivering the Reconnect Program, and currently provides early intervention wilderness-based therapeutic strategies for targeted young people at school, or those disengaging from the education system in local communities. This study evaluated the outcomes of one REFS program by examining factors associated closely with the risk factors of homelessness as measured by the Life Effectiveness Questionnaire (LEQ) in order to determine its value as an early treatment intervention for youth ‘at risk’ of homelessness and educational disconnection.

Risk and Protective Factors for Youth

Young people grow and develop in the context of their social, physical and natural environments. In these environments, they experience both risk and protective factors, which may either inhibit or enhance the developmental process. When young people have a preponderance of risk factors, they are often considered 'youth at risk'.

Youth At Risk The commonly used phrase 'youth at risk' generally refers to children and teenagers who display problem behaviours, difficulty in school, use of drugs, are in trouble or have conflicted relationships with their parents (Conner, 2004). Being 'at risk' is not a problem relegated solely to lower socioeconomic groups or to ethnic minorities. 'At risk youth' is a term used to describe youth who live in a negative environment and/or lack the skills and values that help them become responsible members of society (Kallusky, 1997). By labelling a young person as 'at risk', it implies that this person has a greater chance of negative life outcomes, such as depression, suicide and homelessness.

Young people who are deemed to be 'at risk' often share many similar personal characteristics such as low self-esteem (Beautrais, Joyce & Mulder, 1999; Fergusson et al., 2000; Groholt et al., 2000; Kienhorst, at el., 1992), limited educational achievement (Andrews & Lewinshohn, 1992; Beautrais, 1998; Groholt, et al., 2000), high external locus of control (Beautrais et al., 1999; Kienhorst et al., 1992; Pearce & Martin, 1993), high scores on measures of hopelessness (Beautrais et al., 1999; Benjaminsen et al., 1990; Shaffer et al., 1996), and high scores on measures of impulsivity, recklessness, and risk taking (Beautrais et al., 1999; Fergusson, Beautrais, & Horwood, 2003; Shaffer et al., 1996). Many of these risk factors are in line with the identified risk factors for homelessness.

Homelessness

Homelessness is a state in which people have no access to safe and secure shelter of a standard that does not damage their health, threaten their personal safety, or further marginalise (Neil & Fopp, 1992). The Human Rights and Equal Opportunity Commission (1989) suggested that this insecurity of shelter and detachment from family leads to an individual becoming vulnerable to dangers from which they would normally be protected. According to Kids Help Line (2003) some of the more common factors that may contribute to homelessness are poverty, family breakdown, mental illness, drugs, alcohol, learning difficulties and abuse (emotional, physical and sexual). There are many reasons why a child or young person might find themselves homeless, and there is no one thing that can be identified as a cause of homelessness (Neill & Fopp, 1992).

Youth Homelessness and Family Relationships

Most homeless children leave home because they feel there is no alternative. They are faced with issues such as serious abuse, sustained family conflict or family breakdown, poverty, social isolation, and a sense of hopelessness that places near intolerable stresses on families (CHPA, 2003). A study conducted by Dangar (1999) found that the greatest cause of unhappiness for Australian kids is conflict within their family. The study suggested that good relationships between parents and children assist children to be socially and emotionally competent, resilient, and able to cope with adversity. Good relationships also facilitate a sense of optimism, positive self-image and high self-esteem (Dangar, 1999).

Resilient Youth

Research focusing on resilience suggested that children are able to overcome adversity more effectively when they possess certain internal resources (Werner & Smith, 1992). If these resources can be developed, the child's level of resilience may subsequently increase and thus reduce the risk factors associated with youth homelessness.

Protective factors of the individual, or 'internal resources' (Werner & Smith, 1992) include level of intelligence, self-efficacy, self-esteem, internal locus of control, positive temperament, self-confidence; communication skills and social skills, competence and realistic goal setting (Garmezy, 1985; Rutter, 1987; Luthar, 1991; Werner & Smith, 1992; Masten & Powell, 2003; Bolger & Patterson, 2003; Fergusson & Horwood, 2003). Many of the factors considered as being relevant to homelessness may be addressed during a wilderness therapy experience, especially the factors that are considered 'internal resources' to the individual, (for example self-esteem, self-efficacy, and internal locus of control). The results of a number of studies suggests that wilderness therapy may be a successful intervention program for increasing an 'at risk' adolescent's 'internal resources' (Bolger & Patterson, 2003; Werner & Smith, 1992; Fergusson & Horwood, 2003; Masten & Powell, 2003).

The REFS wilderness program aims to enhance these factors and thus reduce the likelihood that the participants involved in the programs will enter the homelessness cycle. Using a combination of wilderness therapy, narrative therapy, experiential learning, family mediation and counselling, and development of community interconnectedness, REFS seeks to prevent students from disengaging with their family and education systems prematurely, and from entering the homelessness cycle.

Wilderness Therapy

Wilderness therapy is an emerging intervention in mental health practice to help adolescents overcome emotional, adjustment, addiction, and psychological problems (Norton, 2011). Wilderness therapy often involves participant immersion in an unfamiliar environment, group-living with peers, individual and group therapy sessions, educational curricula and the application of skills such as fire-making and back country travel. Programs are designed to address problem behaviours by fostering personal and social responsibility and emotional growth of clients (Russell, 1999). Research on the therapeutic effects of wilderness therapy has suggested that the holistic nature of the experience facilitates changes to the physical, psychological, social, emotional and spiritual self (Davis-Berman, Berman, & Capone 1994; Norton, 2011; Russell, Hendee, & Phillips-Miller, 2000; Russell, 1999; Russell, 2000).

Russell (2000) stated that research shows wilderness therapy can improve self-perceptions, increase social adjustment, and reduce recidivism of adolescent participants. Such outcomes would appear to address several of the issues related to youth homelessness, thus suggesting the possible benefits of wilderness therapy as a strategy to prevent youth homelessness.

Although the REFS program uses multiple interventions, this study aimed to explore the outcomes of the extended wilderness journey component of the REFS program.

Methodology

Participants

The criteria for inclusion in the present study were that participants were aged above thirteen years of age, that they were considered 'at risk' by the referral agency, and were believed to be able to monitor personal and others' levels of safety during the activities, as determined by the program observers.

Initial referral to the program was made through private and public education, justice and welfare agencies. The observers participating in the research were workers from each of the referring agencies who were involved in the entire process of the wilderness therapy program.

The initial pre-test sample was twenty-four participants, which was the total number of participants to go through the program during the research period. The post-test was also twenty-four participants, and the follow-up was nine participants. There were sixteen male participants and eight female participants. The age range of the participants was between thirteen and twenty-three years, with the average being fifteen. Participant data decreased from post-test (n = 24) to follow-up (n = 9), as transitory participants became less contactable or were involved in a different program during the final stages of data collection.

PROCEDURE

Ethical approval was obtained from the Australian Catholic University Human Research Ethics committee. Upon receiving informed consent from parents/guardian, the participants involved in the research were asked to complete two questionnaires during their one-hour participant interview. The participants were informed of the nature of the study in general terms and were under constant supervision by the test administrator. The observers were given the same instructions as the participants, and completed their questionnaires at the same time as the participants.

Instrumentation

The measure chosen was the 'Life Effectiveness Questionnaire' (LEQ) as it measures many of the protective factors relating to youth homelessness. For the purposes of this study it was used in three forms:

1. The Life Effectiveness Questionnaire (LEQ-I) Participant Version;
2. The Life Effectiveness Questionnaire (LEQ-I) Observer Version; and
3. The Life Effectiveness Questionnaire (YARPET) Youth at risk Version.

The Life Effectiveness Questionnaire

The Life Effectiveness Questionnaire (LEQ-I) is a twenty-nine item, nine factor self-report instrument specifically designed for the purpose of measuring the impact of educational, psychological, and training interventions which aim to enhance the personal development of participants (Neill, 2003). Developed by Neill, Marsh and Richards in 1997, the LEQ-I assesses multiple dimensions of personal effectiveness, which are typically changed through experiential education programs. The LEQ was developed and tested in a wide variety of outdoor education programs. It is particularly relevant to personal development aims, which are typical of these programs. The LEQ was developed within the context of adventure programs, however the instrument is also intended for broader use with experiential education and personal development intervention programs (Neill, 2003).

The authors (Neill et al., 1997) claimed that this is an adequate, short, easy-to-administer, self-report instrument for evaluating the outcomes of programs which aim to enhance multiple areas of personal effectiveness, and is psychometrically appropriate for a variety of ages and gender. This was determined by a three-step procedure, from congeneric analyses, to multifactorial analyses, then to invariance testing, representing a particularly powerful statistical process. The authors caution that ideally, further testing of the test-retest stability of the instrument should be conducted (Neill et al., 1997). The LEQ has developed into an instrument with identifiable factors, with good internal consistency, and with a stable factorial structure for both males and females, adolescents and adults (Neill, 2003).

The nine dimensions of the LEQ include: achievement, motivation, active initiative, emotional control, intellectual flexibility, self-confidence, social competence, task leadership, time management, and locus of control (Neill et al., 1997). A number of these dimensions are related to those factors that have been identified as risk factors for homelessness.

The observer version of the LEQ-I was used in order to compare the self-reported results to those of an onlooker who has had significant personal contact with the participant. It was felt that it would be beneficial to assess the responses of an adult observer who was able to draw on previous interactions and experiences with the participants as this could serve to validate the responses of the participants. The questionnaire includes the same questions as those in the LEQ-I, however they are worded appropriately to an onlooker.

Although the original LEQ has been used successfully for evaluating and researching some ‘youth at risk’ programs, the developer had concerns that the scales didn’t address many of the common goals of ‘youth at risk’ programs. In order to address this, the YARPET was developed from the original LEQ by Neill (2003). It was designed to assess typical youth objectives for youth at risk adventure-based or experiential intervention programs. Seventeen youth developmental objectives were designed through consulting with a range of youth at risk programs and outdoor education organisations (Neill, 2005). Neill (2005) recommended that users select from the 17 objectives in order to reduce the overall items, and to customise the instrument to be relevant to the program and research goals. Neill suggested evaluators too often use full instruments, for fear of undermining the overall validity of the questionnaire when only part of the instrument is relevant to program objectives.

Through consultation with REFS facilitators, the researcher customised the questionnaire according to program aims and subsequently created a thirteen dimension, thirty-eight item questionnaire. The thirteen dimensions include:

- Personal Objectives: self-esteem, self-confidence, locus of control, effective problem solving, goal setting, creative self-expression and healthy risk-taking.
- Social Objectives: respect/understand personal boundaries, conflict resolution, communication skills, cooperative teamwork and effective leadership.

Data Analysis

Initially this study examined significance levels. However, program evaluation studies with less than approximately 50 participants are understood to lack sufficient statistical power for detecting small, medium or possibly large effects and therefore it was decided that it would be more appropriate for this study to report effect size (Neill, 2008). Rather than simply answering the question of whether or not a program was effective, effect sizes indicate the quantified amount of change between two times, i.e. before and after the program.

Researchers have offered suggestions about the meaning of different effect sizes. For example, it has been suggested that an effect size of 0.50 is a change of practical significance while 0.25 is educationally significant (Wolf, 1986). Cohen (1977) suggested that 0.2 was small, 0.5 moderate, and 0.8 large. Other authors have warned against global guides to interpreting effect sizes since who and what is being measured needs to be identified before a genuine assessment about the value of a particular effect size is made (Neill, 2008).

In practice, a small effect size can be very impressive if, for example, the outcome is difficult to change (e.g., a personality construct) or if the outcome is very valuable (e.g., an increase in life expectancy). On the other hand, a large effect size does not necessarily mean that there is any practical value in the change, particularly if it isn't related to the aims of the intervention (Neill, 2008). A benchmark for Outdoor Education programs with school students was set at an effect size of 0.2 and represents an 8% increase in student's perceptions of their skills (Neill, 2008). This study had a small sample size, therefore we are mindful that it is inappropriate to generalise results to a wider population or to other wilderness therapy programs.

RESULTS

Changes in Total Life Effectiveness (YARPET *and LEQ-I)*

In order to determine the overall change from pre-test to post test for both the LEQ-1 and the YARPET effect sizes were calculated (see Figure 1).

Figure 1 shows that that there was a small to moderate effect size (d = 0.31) from pre-test to post test the LEQ-1. From pre-test to post test the YARPET showed a small effect size (d = 0.22).

Effect sizes for LEQ-I components

To examine the changes in each individual component of life effectiveness from pre-test to post test, effect sizes were calculated for each factor of LEQ-1 (see Figure 2).

Task leadership (d = 0.45), time management (d = 0.43), social competence (d = 0.35) and achievement motivation (d = 0.32) all showed a small-moderate change. Locus of control (d = 0.29), self-confidence (d = 0.29) and emotional control (d = 0.23) also showed a small-moderate change. Active initiative (d = 0.13) and intellectual flexibility (d = 0.17) fell into the range of no effect from pre-test to post test.

Effect sizes for YARPET components

To examine the changes in each individual component of life effectiveness from pre-test to post test, effect sizes was calculated for each factor of YARPET (see Figure 3).

A moderate change was seen in effective leadership (d = 0.5). A small-moderate change was reported for respect personal boundaries (d = 0.34), self-esteem (d = 0.29), communication skills (d = 0.29), conflict resolution (d = 0.29) and self-confidence (d = 0.24). The remaining factors showed no change.

Participant versus Observer Responses to Life Effectiveness Questionnaire

To determine if the participants and the observers observed similar change, effect sizes for both the Pre and Post LEQ-I observer and participant were compared (see Figure 4).

Both the participants and the observers showed a small to moderate effect, participant pre to post (d = 0.31) and observer pre to post (d = 0.23). This suggests that the observers did in fact have an accurate perception of the participants. The smaller change results of the participant compared with the observer may reflect that the participants gained a greater understanding of the different aspects of life effectiveness and therefore were able to reassess themselves with greater insight.

Changes in LEQ-I and YARPET Life Effectiveness from Pretest to Follow-up

Due to the small number of follow-up data obtained (n = 9) no analysis was undertaken on this data.

Discussion

Change in Overall Life Effectiveness

The results showed that there was change between the pre and post program responses across the overall LEQ-I and YARPET scores, with small to moderate effect sizes of 0.31 and 0.22 respectively. An effect size of 0.2, which is the suggested benchmark for outdoor education programs with school students, represents an 8% increase in student perceptions of their skills. Thus, while the overall effect size may be described as small, an 8% increase in personal, social and environmental skills through a relatively short intervention, particularly if sustained, may be considered a strong outcome (Neill, 2008).

Small to moderate changes in participants' life effectiveness for both questionnaires gives preliminary support that the REFS program provided an appropriate mechanism for enhancing the life effectiveness skills of participants.

Changes in Individual Components of Life Effectiveness

Active initiative and intellectual flexibility showed no effect from pre to post test. It may have been that participants became more aware of their lack of flexibility through participation in the wilderness experience. This is supported by Owen, et al., (2001) who reported participants' self-perceived behaviour changes remained unchanged or lowered from pre-test to post test. They believed the participants' experiences gave them awareness and an understanding of themselves and the impact of their behaviour, and that with this extended awareness, an individual's motivation for change could be influenced. (For example a pupils' reporting of 'change for the worst' might mask an increased motivation to 'change for the better').

The largest changes were seen in effective leadership (d = 0.5), time management (d=0.43), and task leadership (d = 0.45). Time management in particular consistently reported large changes (Neill, 1999; McLeod, & Allen-Craig 2005), this could be contributed to the nature of these programs, with an expectation of having to reach certain destinations before dark, be 'ready to go' in the mornings, and other organisational aspects of the program. If the participants do not learn to manage themselves well there are very real consequences in terms of their enjoyment and wellbeing during the program.

Figure 1: Effect Sizes for YARPET and LEQ-1, Pre to Post Test

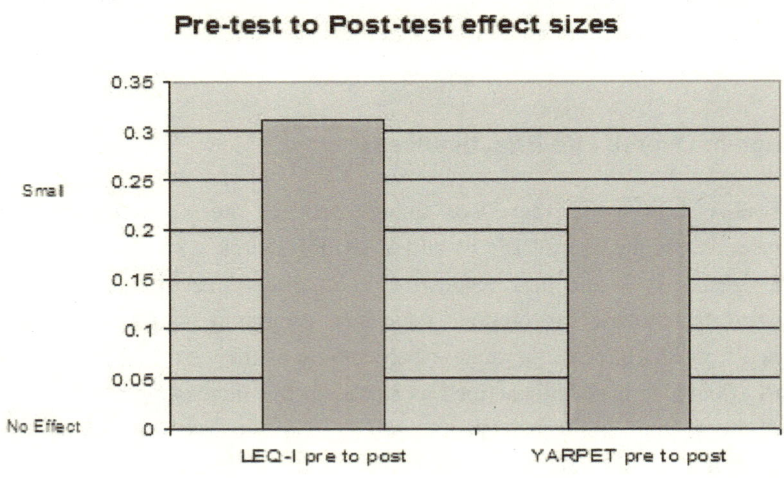

Respect of personal boundaries (d = 0.34), social competence (d = 0.35), achievement motivation (d = 0.32), locus of control (d 0.29), self-confidence (d = 0.29), self-esteem (d = 0.29), conflict resolution (d = 0.29), communication skills (d=0.29) and emotional control (d = 0.23) all showed a small-moderate change. These results are supported by other studies of wilderness intervention programs found in the literature (Neill & Flory, 2000a; Neill & Flory, 2000b; Neill, 1999; Russell, 1999).

The small to moderate change in measures of internal locus of control is an important change to note as a high level of internal locus of control is suggested to increase resiliency and subsequently decrease the risk factors associated with suicidal behaviours (Borowsky et al., 1999; Frederico & Davis, 1996; Quinn, 1999; Resnick, 2000). Improvement in this component is therefore very important with respect to youth at risk.

Effective problem solving, goal setting, cooperative team work, creative self-expression, healthy risk taking, community engagement, active initiative and intellectual flexibility showed no effect from pre to post test.

RATIONALE

Wilderness therapy places people in the position where they must make decisions which could have a dramatic impact on their experience, requiring people to work together, respect the needs and interests of others and take charge of the group or themselves where necessary. It is therefore important to consider why some of these components showed no change. Previous studies have also shown that intellectual flexibility is more difficult to enhance through outdoor education programs (Neill, 1999; Neill & Flory, 2000a; Neill & Flory, 2000b). It is certainly possible that the participants gained a greater understanding of the different aspects of life effectiveness as the program progressed and therefore were able to reassess themselves with greater insight.

Discussions during the wilderness experience are often focused on being in control of one's life, being confident in ones abilities, taking on leadership roles within the group, and setting goals, which are challenging yet achievable. With this in mind it is not surprising that the participants' understanding of these concepts is possibly heightened, and their responses following the experience may reflect this.

Figure 2: Effect sizes for LEQ-1 components

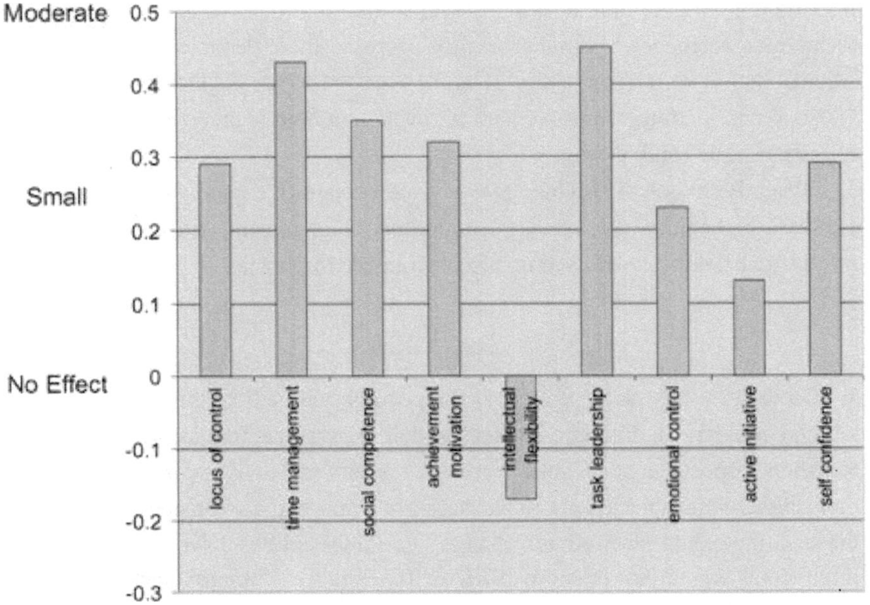

Figure 3: Effect sizes for YARPET components

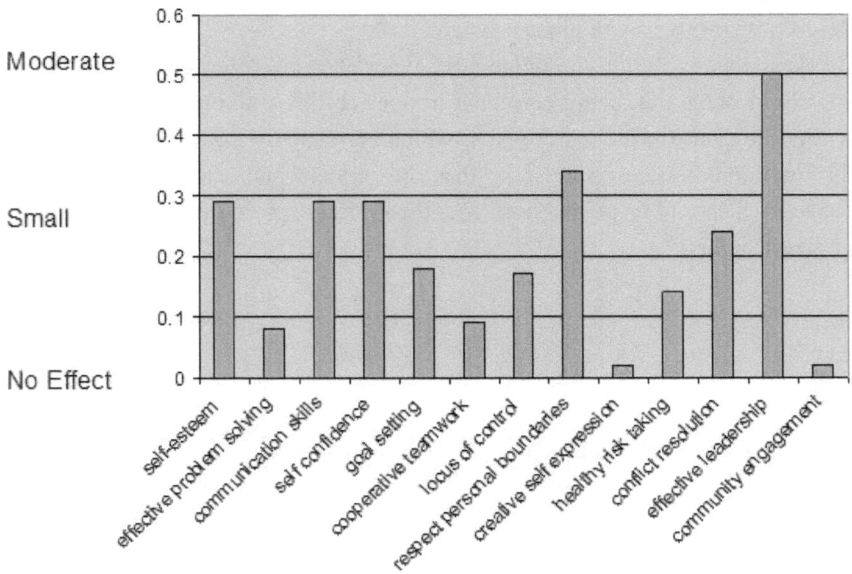

LIMITATIONS

There are many problems encountered when young people are expected to complete self-assessment reports. Truthfulness and accuracy may be compromised by both cognitive and situational factors (Brener, et al., 2003; Shrauger & Osberg, 1981; Sudman, 1987; Wallendorf & Brucks, 1993). Adding to this was the fact that the young people involved in the study were considered 'youth at risk' and more likely to display literacy problems, lack of motivation, and possible mental health issues. These factors may impact the way in which participants comprehend and respond to questions. There is potential for bias within these results, as the observer's role within the referring agency may influence their responses. Although the intention is for the observer to note possible changes in behaviour of the participants, they may also wish the program to be seen to be achieving program outcomes.

All participants involved in the REFS wilderness program over the research period were involved in the research; however, the sample size of the study (N = 24) is small. There was a high attrition rate of participants. Some participants were unavailable or unwilling to either complete the self-report questionnaires or did not complete the questionnaires adequately. This resulted in difficulties in data collection and analysis. This problem was particularly apparent for the follow up data, with only nine of the twenty-four participants completing this component of the research. Due to the REFS program being only offered biannually, and the time constraints on this study, there was no other opportunity for the researcher to collect additional data. This, combined with the risk of high attrition rates meant that the possibility of small sample sizes was high, with no foreseeable opportunity to address this in the design of the study.

Figure 4: Participant and observer responses

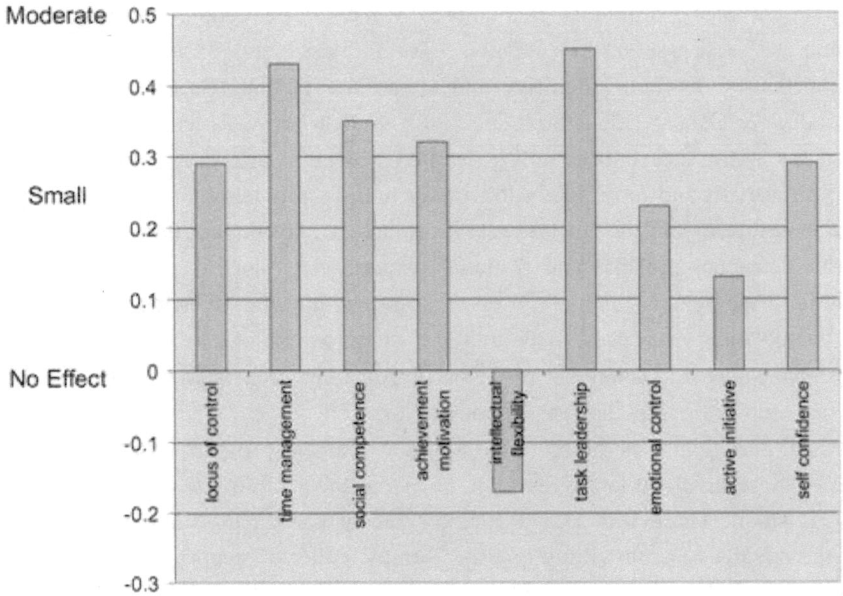

The REFS program is a multidimensional intervention and although considerable effort was made to time the testing in such a way as to isolate the extended journey component of the program, it is possible that additional variables such as client selection or pre trip preparation may have impacted the findings.

Other limiting factors include a lack of a control group, participants' varying degrees of 'risk', external distractions during questionnaire completion and the fact that not all groups took part in the same wilderness activities.

Considering that the aims of the program relate to long-term changes in life circumstances, this longer term follow up information is invaluable in understanding the benefits of the program. This is a difficult challenge due to the chaotic nature of the participants' lives.

Conclusion

As a pilot study of Regional Extended Family Services wilderness program, this research offered a reasonable 'initial' validation of the quality and appropriateness of the REFS approach to the development of a number of life effectiveness skills for youth at risk of homelessness. The REFS wilderness program was found to have a positive impact on a number of the Life

Effectiveness skills of participants, suggesting that the program provides participants with the opportunity to change their perceptions of themselves.

Positive change was seen in eight of the nine LEQ-I components and ten of the thirteen PET-A components. The positive improvements in these areas of life effectiveness are encouraging; however the lack of change of other factors is worthy of further investigation, and perhaps warrants some programmatic or facilitation changes for more effective enhancement of these areas.

The results of students' self-evaluations were supported by the results of the observer evaluations, thus suggesting that the participants' self-evaluations responses were an accurate and honest assessment of themselves. There is also preliminary support that the REFS programs had positive short-term effects on participants' overall self-perceived life effectiveness.

The results of this preliminary study provide encouraging empirical support for the use of wilderness therapy as an intervention to create change and increase protective factors in youth 'at risk' of homelessness and disconnection with families and education, with more investigation required.

Implications for Future Research

REFS wilderness program seeks to prevent the premature disengagement of 'at risk' youth from their family and the education systems, and subsequently decrease the likelihood of young people entering the homelessness cycle. It would be advisable then that future research should consider participants' school attendance rates over the course of the research, in order to determine the outcome of this specific aim. Long-term studies with good follow-up data are essential to understand the long-term effects of these types of interventions.

Various program designs and activities are utilised during wilderness therapy programs. There is a need for research to focus not only on whether outcomes are being achieved, but how the outcomes may be achieved.

It is imperative that wilderness therapy programs, such as REFS, continue to conduct research relating to program outcomes in order to further develop our understanding of the impacts of these programs on the lives of young people.

References

Andrews, J. A., & Lewinshohn, P. M. (1992). Suicidal attempts among older adolescents: Prevalence and co-occurrence with psychiatric disorders. *Journal of the American Academy of Child & Adolescent Psychiatry, 31*, 655-662.

Beautrais, A .L. (1998). Risk factors for serious suicide attempts among young people: A case control study. In R. J. Kosky, H. S. Eshkevari, R. D. Goldney, & R. Hassan (Eds.), *Suicide prevention: The global context* (pp. 167-181). New York: Plenum.

Beautrais, A. L., Joyce, P. R., & Mulder, R. T. (1999). Personality traits and cognitive styles as risk factors for serious suicide attempts among young people. *Suicide and Life-Threatening Behaviour, 29*, 37-47.

Benjaminsen, S., Krarup, G., & Lauritsen, R. (1990). Personality, parental rearing behaviour and parental loss in attempted suicide: A comparative study. *Acta Psychiatrica Scandinavica, 82,* 389-397.

Bolger, K. E., & Patterson, C. J. (2003). Sequelue of child maltreatment: vulnerability and Resilience. In S. S. Luthar (Ed.), *Resilience and vulnerability: Adaptation in the context of childhood adversities.* New York: Cambridge.

Borowsky, I. W., Resnick, M .D, Ireland, M., & Blum, R .W. (1999). Suicide attempts among American Indian and Alaska Native youth: Risk and protective factors. *Archives of Paediatric and Adolescence Medicine*, 153, 573-580.

Brener, N. D., Billy, J. O. G., & Grady, M. A. (2003). Assessment of factors affection the validity of self-reported health-risk behaviour among adolescents: evidence from the scientific literature. *Journal of Adolescent Health, 33*, 436-457.

Conner, M .G. (2004). What are 'Special Needs' and "Youth At Risk"? Retrieved on 2/27/2003 from: www.Wilderness-Therapy.Org

Council for Homeless Persons Australia. (2003). *Youth homelessness*. Retrieved from: www.chpa. org.au/youth.html.

Dangar Research Group. (1999). *Kids-on-Kids: Growing up in Australia.* Sydney.

Davis-Berman, J., Berman, C. S., & Capone, L. (1994). Therapeutic wilderness programs: A national survey. *Journal of Experiential Education, 17*(2), 49-53.

Fergusson, D. M., Beautrais, A. L., & Horwood, L. J. (2003). Vulnerability and resiliency to suicidal behaviours in young people. *Psychological Medicine, 33*, 61-73.

Fergusson, D. M., Woodward, L. J., & Horwood, L. J. (2000). Risk factors and life processes associated with the onset of suicidal behaviour during adolescence and early adulthood. *Psychological Medicine, 30*, 23-39.

Fergusson, D. M., & Horwood, J. (2003). Resilience to childhood adversity: Results of a 21 Year Study. In S. S. Luthar (Ed.), *Resilience and vulnerability: Adaption in the context of childhood adversities.* New York: Cambridge.

Frederico, M., & Davis, C. (1996). *Gatekeeper training and youth suicide prevention.* Canberra: Department of Health and Family Services.

Garmezy, N. (1985). Stress resistant children: the search for protective factors. In J. E. Stevenson (Ed.), Recent Research in Developmental Psychology, *Journal of Child Psychology and Psychiatry.*

Groholt, B., Ekeberg, Wichstrom, L., & Haldorsen, T. (2000). Young suicide attempters: A comparison between a clinical and an epidemiological sample. *Journal of the American Academy of Child & Adolescent Psychiatry, 39*, 868875.

Human Rights and Equal Opportunity Commission (1989). *A guide to our homeless children.* Report of the National Inquiry into Homeless Children by the Human Rights and Equal Opportunity Commission. Canberra, AGPS.

Kallusky, J. (1997). *Constructing an urban sanctuary for at-risk youth in physical education: An artistically crafted action research project in an inner-city high school.* Greeley, CO: University of Northern Colorado.

Kienhorst, I. C. W. M., De Wilde, E. J., Diekstra, R. F. W., & Wolters, W. H. G. (1992). Differences between adolescent suicide attempters and depressed adolescents. *Acta Psychiatrica Scandinavica, 85*, 222-228.

Kids Help Line. (2003). Infosheet 3: Family Relationships. Retrieved on 2/27/2003 from: www.kidshelplince.com.au/research/INFOSHEETS/03 Familyrelationships

Luthar, S. S. (1991). Vulnerability and resilience: a study of high-risk adolescents. *Child Development, 62*, 60-616.

Masten, A. S., & Powell, J. L. (2003). A resilience framework for research, policy, and practice. In S. S. Luthar (Ed.), *Resilience and vulnerability: aptation in the context of childhood adversities.* New York: Cambridge.

McLeod, B., & Allen-Craig, S. (2007). What outcomes are we trying to achieve in our outdoor education programs? *Australian Journal of Outdoor Education, 11*(2), 41-49.

Neill, C., & Fopp, R. (1992). *Homelessness in Australia.* Melbourne: CSIRO Australian Housing and Urban Research Institute.

Neill, J. T., & Flory, M. (2000a). *Brief report on the effects of a Colorado Outward Bound school program on the life effectiveness of adult gay and lesbian participants.* Unpublished. Retrieved on 2/27/2003 from: www.unh.edu/outdoor-education/leq.html

Neill, J. T., & Flory, M. (2000b). *A pilot study of the short-term and long-term effects of the Women's Wilderness Institute "Girlz in the Woods" courses on adolescents' personal effectiveness and self-esteem.* Unpublished. Retrieved 2/27/2003 from: www. unh.edu/outdoor-education/leq.html.

Neill, J. T. (2003). *Selecting tools, instruments, & questionnaires for outdoor education research and evaluatio*n. Australia: Outdoor Education Research & Evaluation Centre.

Neill, J. T., Marsh, H. W., & Richards, G. E. (1997). *Development and psychometrics of the Life Effectiveness Questionnaire.* Sydney, Australia: University of Western Sydney.

Neill, J. T. (2008). *Meta-analytic research on the outcomes of outdoor education.* Paper presented to the 6th Biennial Coalition for Education in the Outdoors Research Symposium, Bradford Woods, IN, 11-13 January, 2002.

Norton, C.L. (2011). Wilderness therapy: Creating a context of hope. In C. Norton (Ed.), *Innovative interventions in child and adolescent mental health*, pp. 36-74. New York: Routledge.

Pearce, C. M., & Martin, G. (1993). Locus of control as an indicator of risk for suicidal behaviour among adolescents. *Acta Psychiatrica Scandinavica, 88*, 409-414.

Quinn, J. (1999). Where need meets opportunity: Youth development programs for early teens. *Future of Children, 9*, 96-116.

Owen, J., Fletcher, C., & Richards, K. (2001). Firm foundations? Evaluation of a school based experiential personal development course. *Horizons, 16* (Winter), 27-31.

Resnick, M. D. (2000). Protective factors, resiliency, and healthy youth development. *Adolescent Medicine: State of the Art Reviews, 11*, 157-164.

Russell, K. C. (1999). *Theoretical basis, process, and reported outcomes of wilderness therapy as an intervention and treatment for problem behaviour in adolescents.* Unpublished doctoral dissertation, University of Idaho, Moscow, ID.

Russell, K. C. (2000). Exploring how the wilderness therapy process relates to outcomes. *Journal of Experiential Education, 23*(3), 170-176.

Russell, K. C., Hendee, J. C., & Phillips-Miller, D. (2000). How wilderness therapy works: The wilderness therapy process for adolescents with behavioural problems and addictions. In D. N. Cole, & S. F. McCool (Eds.), *Proceedings from wilderness science in a time of change conference.* Fort Collins, CO: USA.

Rutter, M. (1987). Psychological resilience and protective mechanisms. *American Journal of Orthopsychiatrics, 57*(3), 316-330.

Shaffer, D., Gould, M.S., Fisher, P., Trautman, P., Mareau, D., Kleinman, M., & Flory, M. (1996). Psychiatric diagnosis in child and adolescent suicide. *Archives of General Psychiatry, 53*, 339-348.

Shrauger, J. S., & Osberg, T. M. (1981). The relative accuracy of self-predictions and judgments by others in psychological assessment. *Psychological Bulletin, 90*(2), 322-351.

Sudman, S. (1987). Perspectives for future development. In H. Hippler, N. Schwarz, & S. Sudman (Eds.), *Social information processing and survey methodology* (pp. 212-219). New York: Springer-Verlag.

Wallendorf, M., & Brucks, M. (1993). Introspection in consumer research. *Journal of Consumer Research, 20*, 339-359.

Werner, E. E., & Smith, R. S. (1992). *Vulnerable but invincible: A study of resilient children.* New York: McGraw-Hill.

Wolf, F. M. (1986). *Meta-analysis: Quantitative methods for research synthesis.* Beverly Hills, CA: Sage.

CHAPTER 5

Prevention of Anti-social Behaviour: Genuine Self-forgiveness and Willingness to Change

Kylie Agnew Pointon

ABSTRACT

An exploration of the mechanisms behind how a wilderness-based intervention program, designed to improve anti-social behaviour for young people at risk, can positively impact on an individual's willingness to change was undertaken. A pretest-posttest control group design compared participants (n = 39) and controls (n = 16) on measures of genuine self-forgiveness, value affirmation, self-affirmation and willingness to change. Results suggest that genuinely forgiving oneself for a transgression assists in improving willingness to change negative behaviour. Furthermore, if a person desires to genuinely forgive themselves, results suggest that affirming values acts as a mediator in this process.

INTRODUCTION

Young people are over-represented in the justice system with statistics indicating almost 50% of apprehensions by police in Australia involve people aged 10-24 years (Smart, Vassallo, Sanson & Dussuyer, 2004). Anti-social behaviour, which is defined as actions and words that have a negative impact, can be a significant issue during an individual's school years and can set in motion a path of long-term deviant behaviour and associated problems (Farrington & Ttofi, 2011). This anti-social behaviour during adolescence has been linked to future criminal behaviour, violence and incarceration. This issue has varied and far-reaching consequences which impacts on the whole community, including families, schools, social services, police and government (MacKenzie, 2000; Rutter, Giller & Hagell, 1998). Anti-social behaviour in schools can negatively affect both academic achievement levels (Smith, 1998) and retainment in education (DETYA,

2001). This behaviour can also be an indicator for future involvement in criminal activity (Berridge, Brodie, Pitts, Porteous & Tarling, 2001).

In the interest of the young person and potentially their community, it is therefore considered important to intervene early and assist in returning the individual to a greater level of adjustment. Early intervention aimed at achieving positive behaviour change has been shown to relate to lower rates of criminal activity and better health and economic outcomes (Greenberg, 2006; Moffitt, Caspi, Harrington & Milne, 2010). However, in order for the intervention to be effective it must be carefully designed to maximise the chance of success for young people. Research has demonstrated that poorly implemented programs are less likely to be effective in encouraging positive change (Abbot, 1991).

Considering the mechanisms that may lead to changes in cognitions and behaviour, the present study will focus on young individuals' awareness and coming to terms with their previous wrongdoing through the process of self-forgiveness. Self-forgiveness is defined as *"a positive attitudinal shift in the feelings, actions, and beliefs about the self following a self-perceived transgression or wrongdoing committed by the self"* (Wohl, De Shea & Wakhinney, 2008, p. 3). It is one proposed mechanism for explaining how a person moves on from a transgression. Fisher (2006) argues that individuals who acknowledge their transgressions and do not 'play down' their wrongdoing, genuinely forgive themselves and will subsequently show a greater willingness to change (Fisher & Exline, 2006).

This research will investigate the role of self-forgiveness in the effects of an intervention (an 8-day wilderness adventure program conducted by Operation Flinders Foundation) for young people identified by their school or community agency, as being at risk of developing deviant behaviours. More specifically, this research aims to identify the significant mediating mechanisms behind a positive shift in "willingness to change" following an intervention program for youth at risk of anti-social behaviour.

Crime Prevention

The link between anti-social behaviour in early adolescence and a range of problems later in life has been well established. Vassallo et al. (2002) conducted a longitudinal study to analyse anti-social behaviour patterns and found that school based anti-social behaviour in younger adolescence was a precursor to engaging in criminal activities in later adolescence and early adulthood. Other longitudinal studies by Moffitt et al. (2002) focused on school-based antisocial behaviour, and found that engaging in bullying-type behaviour correlated with long term antisocial behaviour (Moffitt et al., 2002). It is therefore recommended that interventions must be focussed on the early stages of adolescence to be most effective (Loeber & Farrington, 1998; Bender & Losel, 2011), but careful consideration must be given to their design and presumed mechanisms in order to provide the most effective intervention possible to benefit young people (Wilson & Lispey, 2001).

Crime prevention in Australia takes many forms and various programs have been devised in order to encourage young people to modify antisocial behaviour (MacKenzie, 2001). One type of intervention program involves at-risk youth participating in wilderness adventure experiences over an extended period of time (e.g. 8-30 days). These programs are designed to allow young people the chance to challenge themselves and gain subsequent self-esteem improvements (Raymond, 2003). Wilderness adventure programs are ultimately designed to promote pro-social behaviour changes for young people at risk of breaking the law who are engaged in anti-social school-based behaviour (Barrett, 1993).

There are over 25 wilderness-based intervention programs in Australia competing for funding in the area of crime prevention and school retention (Pryor, 2009). Research indicates that early intervention is vital, effective and can save government money compared to incarceration and rehabilitation (Berridge et al., 2001). Research into such programs indicates that they are effective in helping young people feel that they can achieve positive outcomes, as there is an increase in self-confidence gained from overcoming challenges (Cason & Gillis, 1994; Raymond, 2003).

Wilderness adventure programs have both high levels of public support and research to support outcomes (Crisp, 1996). However, there is a need for these programs to be as effective as possible and regular evaluation, modification and research is crucial to ongoing success. The outcome-focussed research on these programs evaluates positive results which may lead to a reduction in future criminal activity (Mohr et al., 2001; Raymond, 2003). It is valuable to measure more than the positive outcomes, and instead to delve into the psychological processes behind them. This research is important in order to better understand how and why pro-social change is actually achieved through intervention programs (Newes, 2001; Armstrong & Francis, 2003).

Intervention programs aim at increasing the participants' intrinsic motivation and self-perceived capacity to turn their lives around, rather than using deterrence or other forms of social control (Berman & Davis-Berman, 2001). Willingness to change is therefore one key outcome that has been highlighted as a potential explanation for the positive behaviour changes observed in young people following wilderness adventure intervention programs (Brand, 2001). By analysing the mechanisms behind willingness to change and how people move on from transgressions (to choosing to engage in pro-social behaviour), it allows for possible improvements in program design.

The focus of this study will be on fostering willingness to change and identifying barriers for young people, which prevent them from engaging in changing their behaviour.

Willingness to Change

A key aim of interventions, such as wilderness adventure programs, is to increase or enhance the participants' willingness to change. Willingness to change is described as a conscious shift in cognitions regarding behaviour; from fixed and unwilling to change to open and motivated to change (Lispey, 2009). In order for young people to be willing to modify their antisocial behaviour, they need to accept that their behaviour is problematic and see themselves as capable of changing their behaviour or learning new ways. Furthermore, willingness to change indicates that the young person is ready to engage in novel cognitions regarding change and potential alternative pro-social behaviour (Raymond, 2010).

One proposed model for explaining willingness to change is the Trans-theoretical Model of Behaviour Change. This is a model of behaviour change that is described as occurring in stages and involves conscious decision-making, and both intrinsic and extrinsic motivation (Prochaska & Velicer, 1997). The model starts with 'pre-contemplation', moving through to 'contemplation', 'preparation', 'action', and finally the 'maintenance' stage is reached. The first stage is 'pre-contemplation', when there is no recognition of a behaviour problem and no consideration of a need to change. A person who is in this stage would not see a need for change and would be content for their behaviour to stay the same. Once a person begins to recognise that there is a problem with their behaviour and they are considering a need for change, they enter the 'contemplation stage' proposed in the Trans-theoretical Model of Change. When a person has entered this stage they may be searching for support or methods, which can help them with behaviour change (Gottfredson, Wilson & Skroban-Najaka, 2002).

If a person acknowledges that there is a problem and makes a conscious decision to change then they are entering the 'preparation stage' of change and begin establishing the best way to put the desired change into action. The support and methods to assist them to achieve change need to be enlisted for them to move into the 'action stage'. The 'action stage' is characterised by conscious actions to bring about the change. Once change has occurred through actions the person moves into the final 'maintenance stage' and will need to engage in conscious actions to maintain the changes in behaviour (Hemphill & Howell, 2000).

To illustrate the Trans-theoretical Model of Change, we may imagine a young person who is constantly disrupting class in school. If they are in the pre-contemplation stage they will not see this as an issue and have no motivation to stop disrupting the class. It is when they have entered the contemplation stage, they will start to see that their behaviour is problematic, but they may not be sure what they can do to change this behaviour. Once the young person starts to realise what needs to be done to elicit the necessary behaviour changes, they have entered the preparation phase. During the preparation stage they will need support from teachers and some strategies to put this behaviour change into action. During the action stage the actual behaviour change is visible to outsiders and teachers can see that the young person is making an effort not to disrupt the class. Finally, the last stage of behaviour change is maintenance stage, the young person must make a continual and conscious effort to not disrupt the class to ensure that the positive behaviour change is maintained.

If a young person engaging in anti-social behaviour can move from the pre-contemplation stage through to the preparation and action stages of change, and ideally to the maintenance stage, then subsequent pro-social behaviour change is more likely to occur. Research has found that this is the case in school based anti-bullying programs and other crime prevention programs (Gottfredson et al., 2002). However, there is limited research into the internal mechanisms that encourage an individual to move from the pre-contemplation stage of change through to the action stage.

Involvement in a wilderness adventure program may increase a young persons' willingness to change but there is still a need to identify and analyse the key mechanisms behind this shift in thinking and subsequent behaviour change. This study will investigate what will assist a young person to engage in the process of change and what can eliminate barriers preventing young people from changing. It is important to acknowledge that a wilderness program alone may not successfully transform an individual from the pre-contemplation stage through to the maintenance stage (Prochaska & Velicer, 1997). It is reasonable to suggest that the intervention program can encourage a young person to move from pre contemplation to contemplation or preparation stages as a direct result of the program (Russell, 2000). However, it is likely to take additional follow-up support and guidance to move through the action and maintenance stages after the individual has returned to the school environment (Hemphill & Howell, 2000; Ttofi & Farrington, 2010).

To help understand how wilderness adventure programs might foster willingness to change and to explain the intrinsic motivation underlying change, the psychological concept of self-forgiveness may shed light. Willingness to change arguably requires that individuals accept that they have done wrong, but learn to see this as not too self-threatening to the extent that they become paralysed or defensive in their management of their shame (Ahmed, Harris, Braithwaite, & Braithwaite, 2001). They can take responsibility for their wrongdoing yet be accepting of and trusting in their self. This is what we argue the process of genuine self-forgiveness entails. If a young person is able to self-forgive there will be motivation towards willingness to change. This is because self-forgiveness can foster positive thoughts and direct attention away from self-destructive behaviour that is likely to compound the problems they are facing (Woodyatt, 2010).

SELF-FORGIVENESS

Self-forgiveness is the facing of one's transgression while abandoning negative thoughts and behaviors directed at the self and replacing them with positive cognitions (Maltby, Macaskill & Day, 2001). It is achieved through a process of motivational changes, involving a reduction in avoidance of thinking about the transgression. This is accompanied by a reduction in motivation to act in a self-punitive way or engage in self-destructive behaviour (Wohl et al, 2008). At the same time, an individual who self-forgives becomes more motivated to have positive thoughts about themselves and to envisage themselves as distinct from their negative behaviours (Hall & Fincham, 2005). When a person realises they have "done wrong" but also acknowledges that they are still a good person and can change then this is referred to as genuine self-forgiveness (Holmgren, 1998).

The benefits of achieving a state of genuine self-forgiveness include lower levels of depression, anxiety and higher levels of life satisfaction and general health scores (Maltby et al, 2001; Thompson et al., 2005). This genuine self-forgiveness is the desired form of self-forgiveness as studies have shown that it is a strong indicator for willingness to change and positive behaviour change (Woodyatt, 2010). It is suggested that genuine self-forgiveness involves a severing of the link between responsibility acceptance and the negative cognitions and emotions about the self which prevents a person from wanting to change their behaviour (Wenzel, Woodyatt & Hendrick, 2011). Genuine self-forgiveness will imply that individuals will be willing to change, demonstrate this in their future behaviour and will more likely to achieve and maintain the positive behaviour change.

Based on these arguments, genuine self-forgiveness might be an important mechanism through which an intervention program supports willingness to change.

However, self-forgiveness research is a relatively new area of psychology and research has been conducted in criminal groups engaged in rehabilitation programs and in university student samples with scenario-based research (Woodyatt, 2010). This research can be applied to the problem of antisocial behaviour in youth, but only to a limited extent. Preliminary research into offender samples has shown that achieving a higher level of genuine self-forgiveness following interpersonal offences is associated with better restorative outcomes for the offender (Woodyatt & Wenzel, 2010). This research also highlights different types of self-forgiveness and the impact on change related cognitions. However, further research investigating the mechanisms behind self-forgiveness and subsequent willingness for change in young people at risk will encourage development of effective intervention programs and therefore warrants further research.

Self-affirmation and Value Affirmation

Since genuine self-forgiveness is the desired outcome of an intervention program (in order to achieve a positive shift in willingness to change), it is important to analyse how this state of genuine self-forgiveness can best be achieved. Genuine self-forgiveness, and the acceptance of wrongdoing it implies, requires the young person to be self-critical and these thoughts can be threatening to the individual's sense of self. It has been found that individuals are more willing to accept criticism or negative information about themselves when they were first allowed to affirm themselves as a "good" person (Dillon, 2001).

Self-affirmation is a process of maintaining self-integrity, which allows an individual to perceive herself as efficacious and capable (Sherman et al., 2009). If a person is self-affirmed they should have the self-confidence to acknowledge transgressions and are more likely to forgive themselves without threatening their perception of being a worthwhile person (Sherman et al., 2009). Hence, on the one hand it can be argued that self-affirmation should enable genuine self-forgiveness. A wilderness adventure program is designed to build young people's self-esteem by overcoming challenges and helping establishing themselves as capable individuals (Brand, 2001).

This study seeks to examine more specifically how the wilderness program impacts on self-affirmation. These programs aim to provide young people with an opportunity to encourage positive experiences regarding their ability, efficacy, endurance and/or courage. It is through these experiences that they can see themselves more positively (Raymond, 2003). Realising these alternative positive dimensions (self-affirmation) then makes them less defensive to threats to their integrity deriving from acknowledging their wrongdoing. Self-affirmation is thus predicted as a mechanism behind genuine self-forgiveness. Overcoming the threat to self enables a young person to affirm himself and to feel empowered to move past a transgression.

On the other hand, the affirmation of values has been proposed to be an alternative, mediating pathway towards genuine self-forgiveness. Value affirmation means that an individual is more likely to have a strong sense of who they are and where they stand in relation to values that have been violated, rather than just feeling good or better about themselves. Furthermore, value-affirmation involves a process of strengthening an individual's belief that a particular value is true, important and is worth upholding (Woodyatt & Wenzel, 2010). This process allows acceptance of responsibility without having deleterious effects on one's self-esteem, thus allowing individuals to accept shame and trust in their capacity improve behaviour.

Essentially, value affirmation assists an individual in clarifying their personal values (in contrast or in alignment) regarding community behaviour expectations. Wenzel et al. (2011) demonstrated that the affirmation of values (violated by the transgressor), and a recommitment to those values, limits the negative self-implication of responsibility acceptance (Wenzel et al. 2011). In simple language; acknowledging that anti-social behaviour violates community values, and that these values are meaningful, helps a person take responsibility for their actions. Furthermore, value affirmation encourages a young person to fully acknowledge the impact of the transgression on the community, which is an important step in genuine self-forgiveness (Holmgren, 1998; Fisher & Exline, 2006).

Wilderness adventure programs are also designed to have pro-social values reinforced, with the concepts of trust and respect for others in the wilderness adventure context, highlighted through modelling, role play or structured activities and discussions (value affirmation) (Brand, 2001). Therefore, an intervention program that is aiming to increase willingness to change should work towards achieving higher levels of genuine self-forgiveness along with self-affirmation and/or value affirmation.

In summary, an intervention program designed to change anti-social behaviour in young people at risk aims to move individuals from the pre-contemplative stage to the action stage of change proposed in the Trans-theoretical Model of Behaviour Change. This positive behaviour change is predicted to involve aspects of genuine self-forgiveness. Genuine self-forgiveness is one proposed way for an individual to meaningfully address the transgression(s) and values that have been violated and move on to positive behaviour change.

HYPOTHESES

This study compared the effects of a wilderness therapy program on willingness to change and measures of the highlighted aspects of self-forgiveness with a wait list control sample. To the extent that the program achieves positive changes in self-affirmation and value affirmation, participants are more likely to gain genuine self-forgiveness. This self-forgiveness, in turn, will be associated with a greater willingness to change. Based on these arguments the following hypotheses are put forward:

> H1. The program (relative to control group) will lead to an increase in genuine self-forgiveness and, mediated by this, in willingness to change.
>
> H2. (a) The program (relative to control group) will lead to an increase in value affirmation, and this will partially mediate the program's effect on change in genuine self-forgiveness. (b) The program (relative to control group) will lead to an increase in self-affirmation, and this will partially mediate the program's effect on change in genuine self-forgiveness.

METHOD

Design

A 2 (Program, Control) by 2 (Pre-test, Post-test), quasi-experiential design was used in this study. The program group (41 participants) completed a questionnaire two weeks prior to attending the Operation Flinders program (pre-test) and one week after attending the program (post-test). The 45 item questionnaire asked participants to respond in relation to a self-identified school based issue or problem. The control group (49 participants) completed the same questionnaire during the same time frame but did not attend the intervention program until later in the year.

Participants

The participants (N = 90) were 63 male and 27 female students aged 14-18 years (M = 14.8, SD = 2.1) from secondary schools in South Australia; 52% from metropolitan areas and the remainder from regional areas, 9% identified as Indigenous. They were selected (by their school or a welfare agency) to attend a South Australian based wilderness adventure program (Operation Flinders) in either June or August 2011. Participants were nominated by their school or community agency to attend the program, as they were at risk of criminal behaviour or engaging in antisocial school based behaviour. This selection was made independent to the research and schools could choose up to 10 young people to attend the program each year. The majority of the schools had a history of participating in the program; only 4 of the 18 schools were participating for the first time. Young people were encouraged to voluntarily attend the program and they were able to obtain educational points (towards the South Australian Certificate of Education) for attending.

Allocation of participants to the program group (June program) or wait-list control group (August program) was (semi) random for the purpose of research. The allocation was done without considering the design of this research and not based on any systematic factors. The schools nominated to attend the program based on convenience (e.g., the time of year that best suited the school) and the program provider randomly allocated schools to a particular program time.

Fifty-two secondary schools, behaviour centres or community groups from across South Australia nominated to attend the Operation Flinders program in 2011. From these 52 schools 9 attended the June program and 9 attended the August program. At the end of 2010 the schools nominated to send a team of 5 or 10 young people on the program in 2011. The allocation of schools to either the June or August program was made by Operation Flinders the previous year, independent of the present research and can therefore be used as a random allocation to conditions (although, since there was no true randomization as part of the research design, it should correctly be characterised as quasi-experimental). That is, the allocation to either June (Program group) or August (Control group) was based on the schools' request to attend the program and then Operation Flinders (more or less) randomly choosing the month that a school would attend.

In order to analyse the change in pre and post-test scores, only participants who had completed both the Time 1 and Time 2 questionnaires were utilised.

Unfortunately, some participants failed to return their pre-test and/or post-test questionnaires. This meant the number of usable cases reduced to 50, with 29 males and 21 females. In the program group (N = 41), 34 participants completed both pre and post-test questionnaires, representing a response rate of 83%. In the control group (N = 49), only 16 participants completed both questionnaires, representing a response rate of 32.7%.

Gender

The valid longitudinal sample showed an unintended gender difference between groups. The attended program group (N = 34), gender division was 61.8% females and 38.2% males compared to the control group (N = 16), which reported 100% males. To check the role of gender on the independent variables, gender was analysed using the hierarchical multiple regression framework. No significant gender effects were found and gender was excluded from the analyses reported here so as not to further limit statistical power refer to Tables B.1 and B.2 (Appendix B).

Measures

All psychological measures used 7-point Likert-type scales (1 = *strongly disagree*, 7 = *strongly agree*); higher scores on this scale indicated greater levels on each construct. The full list of measures used in this study is shown in Appendix A.

Self-forgiveness

Self-forgiveness was measured with the 15-item *Differentiated Self-forgiveness Process Scale* (Woodyatt & Wenzel, 2010) that measures 3 sub-types of self-forgiveness: genuine self-forgiveness, pseudo self-forgiveness and self-punitiveness. Past studies by Woodyatt & Wenzel (2010) found this scale to have adequate internal consistency with the individual measurements of genuine self-forgiveness α =.60, pseudo self-forgiveness α =.70 and self punitiveness α =.85.

Genuine self-forgiveness refers to the process of coming to terms with one's guilt, maintaining a positive sense of self while acknowledging one's responsibility. This construct was measured by five items, such as "I am trying to learn from my behavior." Internal consistency for this scale was high (Pre α =.76, Post α =.82). Pseudo self-forgiveness refers to engaging only in positive self-affirmation without addressing values that their transgression has violated. It was measured by 5 items; for example, "I wasn't the only one to blame for what happened" (Pre α =.72, Post α =.62). Self punitiveness measured with 5 items, refers to focussing on the values that their transgression has violated and holding onto a negative self-concept, for example, "I can't seem to get over what I have done" (Pre α =.76, Post α =.71).

Value Affirmation and Self-affirmation

Value affirmation is the belief in the importance of the values violated by one's negative behaviour. The value affirmation 5-item measure was derived from the measures by Woodyatt (2010) and Wenzel et al (2011). Value affirmation focussed on reconfirming one's own values in line with the schools values; for example, "I share with the school an understanding of what is important". Internal consistency for this scale was adequate (Pre α = .79, Post α = .71). Self-affirmation means having conviction in oneself as a capable and worthwhile person. The self-affirmation 5-item measure focussed on reconfirming one's own sense of self-worth, based on the *Self Integrity Scale* by Sherman et al (2009); for example, "I am comfortable with who I am". Sherman et al. (2009) found the consistency to be high (α = .84). Internal consistency for the scale was also adequate in the present study (Pre α = .81, Post α = .88).

Willingness to Change

Willingness to change was measured using a 15-item scale developed for evaluating the success of Northern Territory wilderness programs to bring about increase in willingness to change (Raymond, 2010). The measurement tapped into participants' self-identified willingness to change their behaviour (e.g. "I am ready to start making changes to improve my life") and related aspects of willingness to change, such as self-efficacy (e.g. "I can succeed at almost anything I set my mind on"), problem awareness (e.g. "There are things in my life I could do better") and seeking helping relationships (e.g. "I am happy for others to help me improve my life"). The measurement had been used on smaller sample groups that did not allow for internal consistency to be established, but when used in this study the measurement had high consistency (Pre α =.82, Post α =.88).

Procedure

Permission letters and information about the study were sent to all school principals, parents and students participating in the June (Group 1program) and August (Group 2control) Operation Flinders programs. Questionnaires and administration instructions were forwarded to the teachers, who were coordinating each school's involvement in the Operation Flinders program. They were instructed to administer the first questionnaire in the two weeks prior to the June program. Questionnaires could be done either on paper or online; only one school chose the online version.

As a crucial part of the administration process, the participants were invited to identify a school based behaviour problem or issue they were experiencing. This behaviour was used as a consistent reference point for both pre and post-test questionnaires. To create a memory prompt for the post-test questionnaire the participants were instructed to briefly note the problem or issue on a separate sheet of paper. After completing the first questionnaire, the memory prompt was kept by the administering teacher in a sealed envelope ready for the post program questionnaire.

The most common behaviours that were identified included fighting with other students (N = 13), arguing with teachers (N = 11), disrupting classes (N = 9), truanting ("wagging") school (N = 9) and general disrespectful behaviour (N = 7). Participants were instructed to answer the questionnaire focussing their attention on the identified behaviour problem or issue. Participants also reported their age, gender and the school that had referred them to the program.

The program group attended the June Operation Flinders program and the wait list control group was undertaking regular school based activities during this time. After the program group returned from the June Operation Flinders program, the second questionnaire was sent to schools involved in the research project. Before answering the second questionnaire all the participants were given their sealed memory prompt, which encouraged participants to think about the same issue identified earlier.

RESULTS

Preliminary Analyses

In an initial step of the analyses, the mean levels of pre and post-test scores were inspected (see Table 1). First, the mean scores on all dependent variables were compared between program group and control group. Independent samples t-tests revealed no significant differences between groups for all pre-test measures. Independent samples t-tests revealed also no significant differences between groups for the post-test measures of genuine self-forgiveness and willingness to change. However, compared to the control group the program group had significantly higher post-program scores for value affirmation, $t(48) = 2.19$, p

=.019, with a medium effect size, d = .57 and self-affirmation, t (48) = 2.48, p =.048, with a small effect size of d = .29.

Second, pair-wise t-tests were used to test for change from pre to post-test scores within groups. For the program group, the paired comparisons revealed a significant increase in genuine self-forgiveness $t(33) = 2.51$, $p = .017$, $d = .41$, value affirmation, $t(33) = 2.51$, $p = .017$, $d = .60$, and willingness to change $t(33) = 1.96$, $p = .050$, $d = .27$, with medium to small effect sizes. This was in contrast to a significant decrease in value affirmation $t(15)$ 3.70= , $p = .002$, $d = .56$, self-affirmation, $t(15) = 2.47$, $p = .026$, $d = .52$, and willingness to change $t(14) = 3.55$, $p = .003$, $d = .75$, from pre to post-test in the control group, with moderate to large effect sizes.

Table 1: Mean differences between groups (standard deviation)

	Program Group		Control Group	
	Pre	Post	Pre	Post
Genuine Self-forgiveness	3.56 (1.36)	4.15 (1.30)	3.88 (1.22)	4.06 (1.22)
Self-affirmation	4.86 (1.43)	5.27 (0.99)*	5.31 (1.35)	4.90 (1.61)*
Value Affirmation	3.38 (1.06)	4.14 (0.96)*	4.15 (0.94)	3.60 (0.71)*
Willingness to change	3.92 (0.78)	4.36 (0.84)	4.30 (0.89)	4.22 (0.74)

* p < .05

Effects on Willingness to Change via Genuine Self-forgiveness

The program (relative to control group) was predicted to lead to an increase in genuine self-forgiveness and, mediated by this, in willingness to change. In order to test the mediation hypothesis a series of regression analyses were undertaken, allowing the statistical control of baseline levels while testing the mediation process. After the effect of the program on willingness to change was established in the preliminary analyses (see Table 1.), the effect of the program on the mediator genuine self-forgiveness was examined. Attendance on the program had a significant effect on genuine self-forgiveness (β -.30) $p = .018$, with higher genuine self-forgiveness associated with higher willingness to change.

Table 2: Summary of Hierarchical Regression Analysis for Variables Predicting Willingness to Change (N = 49)

Variable	B	SE B	β
Step 1			
Program	-.64	.20	-.37**
Pre-program Genuine Self-forgiveness	.08	.07	.13
Pre-program Willingness to Change	.61	.12	.63**
Step 2			
Program	-.43	.19	-.24
Pre-program Genuine Self-forgiveness	.01	.07	.01
Pre-program Willingness to Change	.47	.12	.49**
Post-program Genuine Self-forgiveness	.24	.08	.38*

Note: R2 = .474 for step 1; ΔR2 = .090 for step 2 (ps < .05) * p < .05

** p < .001

The mediation effect of genuine self-forgiveness was then further tested through a hierarchical regression of post-test scores of willingness to change on the factor group, controlling for base levels of genuine self-forgiveness and willingness to change at the first step and post-test genuine self-forgiveness at the second step. The results are shown in Table 2. Attendance on the program explained a significant positive change in reported willingness to change (β = -.37) p = .002. When post-test genuine self-forgiveness was entered in Step 2 it was significantly associated with willingness to change (β = .38) p = .004, while the effect of the program was no longer significant (β = -.24), suggesting a mediation effect of genuine self-forgiveness. This mediation is shown in Figure 3. Sobel's tests revealed that the indirect effect via genuine self-forgiveness was marginally significant (Z = 1.90, p = .057). The prediction that genuine self-forgiveness would mediate the effect of the program on willingness to change was supported.

Effects on Genuine Self-forgiveness via Value Affirmation and Self-affirmation

The second hypothesis predicted that A) self-affirmation and/or B) value affirmation would mediate the effect of the program on genuine self-forgiveness.

The program (relative to control group) was predicted to lead to an increase in both value affirmation and self-affirmation then, mediated by this, in genuine self-forgiveness. In order to test the mediation hypothesis a series of regression analyses were undertaken. The effect of the program on the first mediator value affirmation was examined while controlling for all relevant base-line measures. Attendance on the program had a significant effect on value affirmation (β -.47) p = .012. The effect of the program on the second mediator self-affirmation was examined. Attendance on the program also had a significant effect on reported self-affirmation (β -.33) p = .009.

The mediation effect of value affirmation and self-affirmation was then further tested through a hierarchical regression of post-test scores of genuine self-forgiveness on the factor group, controlling for base levels of value affirmation, self-affirmation, genuine self-forgiveness and willingness to change at the first step and post-test value affirmation and self-affirmation at the second step. The results are shown in Table 3.

The attendance of the program was significantly related to higher levels of reported genuine self-forgiveness (β = -.27) p = .039. When post-test value affirmation and self-affirmation were entered in Step 2 only value affirmation was significantly associated with genuine self-forgiveness (β = .43). While the effect of the program was no longer significant (β = -.11), suggesting a mediation effect of value affirmation but not self-affirmation. This mediation is shown in Figure 4. Sobel's tests revealed that the indirect effect via value affirmation was significant (Z = 2.18, p = .029). The prediction value affirmation that would mediate the effect of the program on genuine self-forgiveness was supported. In contrast, the prediction self-affirmation that would mediate the effect of the program on genuine self-forgiveness was not supported.

In summary, it was verified that young people who attended the program had reported a significant positive change in willingness to change and this was mediated by genuine self-forgiveness. The effect of the program on genuine self-forgiveness was mediated by value affirmation but not by self-affirmation.

Table 3: Summary of Hierarchical Regression Analysis for Variables Predicting Genuine Self-forgiveness
(N = 49)

Variable	*B*	*SE B*	*β*
Step 1			
Program	-.73	.34	-.27*
Pre-program genuine self-forgiveness	.32	.14	.33*
Pre-program willingness to change	.37	.24	.34
Pre-program value affirmation	-.04	.19	-.03
Pre-program self-affirmation	.20	.14	.22
Step 2			
Program	-.30	.33	-.11
Pre-program genuine self-forgiveness	.25	.13	.26
Pre-program Willingness to Change	.40	.21	.26
Pre-program value affirmation	-.11	.17	-.09
Pre-program self-affirmation	.15	.15	.16
Post-program value affirmation	.60	.17	.43**
Post-program self-affirmation	.02	.15	.02

Note: R^2 = .392 for step 1; ΔR^2 = .157 for step 2 (ps < .05)

* p < .05 **p < .001

Discussion

The aim of the study was to gain an in-depth understanding of the mechanisms behind the effect of the intervention program on young people who were identified as having behaviour problems in the school context. Specifically, it aimed to examine the relationships between reported willingness to change, self-forgiveness, self-affirmation and value affirmation following attendance on the Operation Flinders program. Analysis between a group of 39 young people attending the 8-day wilderness based intervention program and a control group of 16, found that genuine self-forgiveness significantly mediated the effect of the program on willingness to change. The positive change in self-forgiveness was mediated by higher levels of value affirmation but not significantly mediated by self-affirmation. These results give interesting insight into the theories of self-forgiveness and behaviour change. However, the conclusions must be sensibly limited by sampling constraints and reflective of the small number of participants who responded to both pre and post questionnaires.

Willingness to Change and Genuine Self-forgiveness

Overall, the results support the first proposition that the effect of the Operation Flinders intervention program on willingness to change was mediated by genuine self-forgiveness. Willingness to change was measured as the desire to modify anti-social school-based behaviour. In this study, these behaviours included fighting with other students, arguing with teachers, disrupting classes and truancy. The results show that the participants who went on the program (and responded to both questionnaires) had a significant positive change in reported levels of genuine self-forgiveness and willingness to change. The results suggest that, on average, young people who attended the program reported that they had higher self-reported levels of self-forgiveness related to the identified school based behaviour. It is important to note that the effect of the program on willingness to change this behaviour is at least partially mediated by levels of self-forgiveness.

Interestingly, one of the key theoretical implications of this finding is that because genuine self-forgiveness was shown to mediate the effect of the program, we can contribute to knowledge of the benefits of genuinely forgiving oneself. Theoretically, genuine self-forgiveness involves accepting that the transgression was their fault but also removing the associated negative emotions, which prevent a person engaging in the change process (Wenzel, Woodyatt & Hendrick, 2011). To enhance a program's effect on willingness to change anti-social behaviour it is reasonable to suggest that the program targets genuine self-forgiveness.

Genuine Self-forgiveness, Value Affirmation and Self-affirmation

This study also found support for mediating effects behind the program's relationship with improvements in genuine self-forgiveness. The results support the proposition that the effect of the Operation Flinders intervention program on genuine self-forgiveness was mediated by value affirmation. However there was no support for the prediction that the effect of the intervention program on genuine self-forgiveness was mediated by self-affirmation.

Value-affirmation is a process of strengthening an individual's belief that a particular value is true, important and is worth upholding (Woodyatt & Wenzel, 2010). This indicates that genuine self-forgiveness involves truly acknowledging that a value has been violated. Moreover, if a particular value has to have been perceived as personally important to a young person (indicated by higher levels of reported value affirmation) then they are more likely to acknowledge this transgression and genuinely forgive themselves rather than downplaying or blaming others for their behaviour (Dillon, 2001). However, some caution regarding the direct effects attributed to value affirmation needs to be exercised, as there may be alternative causal variables that were unmeasured in this study impacting on genuine self-forgiveness. The relationship between value affirmation and self-forgiveness suggested in the results would need to be tested further in order to empirically show that those who affirm values are more likely to self-forgive.

When compared with past studies focussed on self-forgiveness these findings are in line with Wenzel and Woodyatt's proposition (2010) that failing to genuinely self forgive assists in severance of responsibility acceptance and self-regard (Woodyatt & Wenzel, 2010). This study was also adding weight to Woodyatt experiential study, which found that only value affirmation had an effect on genuine self-forgiveness (Woodyatt, 2010). As the mediating effect of value affirmation was supported by the results, it can be suggested that the program has a positive effect on self-forgiveness through changes in value affirmation. Therefore, an important component to include in an effective intervention program targeting anti-social behaviour is reinforcing values. To assist in the analysis of the role of value affirmation in the process of genuine self-forgiveness further exploration into the effects of value affirmation on the different types of self-forgiveness (and self-punitiveness) would be beneficial (Presser & Van Voorhis, 2002).

In contrast to the mediation effect of value affirmation on genuine self-forgiveness, self-affirmation was not a mediating factor. According to the predicted model, this indicates that self-affirmation does not impact on genuine self-forgiveness and subsequent willingness to change. It implies that an intervention program may want to target value affirmation whilst trying to encourage willingness to change. However, this result does not mean that increasing self-affirmation should be completely disregarded as a goal of an intervention program designed to improve anti-social behaviour. Self-affirmation may have other additional benefits for young people that were not captured in the measurements used in this study, such as building resilience (Gillespie & Allen-Craig, 2009) and personal confidence to overcome future challenges (Ungar, Dumond & McDonald, 2005).

Theoretical Implications

This study fills in the gaps in self-forgiveness literature by extending the previous findings with offender adult groups in an interpersonal transgression setting (Woodyatt, 2009) to a youth sample with anti-social behaviour that can be a precursor to criminal activities. Positive changes in genuine self-forgiveness and responsiveness and willingness to change are outcomes of the program, but in order to understand how the Operation Flinders program relate to the findings to historical Operation Flinders evaluation work, plus relate the findings to the wilderness therapy literature in general. In addition as value affirmation was identified as a mediating factor, it is imperative to reflect on the sort of values Operation Flinders aims to reinforce.

Limitations

This study could be improved by having additional follow up measures. A longitudinal study to follow up the effect of the intervention on life outcomes for young people at risk would be optimal (Wilson & Lipsey, 2000). This would need to look at relationship between self-reported willingness to change and objective indicators such as behaviour measurements including 3rd party observations or school behaviour reports.

An important limitation to acknowledge is the lack of true randomisation. This is linked to an existing sampling bias as whole schools rather than individuals were randomly allocated to conditions. As the study is quasi-experimental, any conclusions regarding causation need to be viewed with caution as the correlational nature of the design means that certain variables may have been missed. In addition, the allocation to conditions by schools rather than individuals may have contributed to the un-equal response rate. Although a total of 90 participants were involved in the study only 49 completed both the pre and post measures. One reason for the low response rate of participants on the program was that many of the participants may have struggled to complete the QA's due to literacy. The literacy, self-awareness and self-reflection skills required to complete a number of the questions may have been problematic for some young people (Humber & Snow, 2001) and may have contributed to the low response rate. The control sample had a lower response rate which gives the results a more conservative measure of differences, which is a strength, but this also meant that there was a smaller than planned sample size for the analyses.

Implications for Wilderness Adventure Intervention Programs

There are important implications for wilderness intervention programs trying to target behaviour change. Study results point to the program being valuable and effective in improving value affirmation, self-forgiveness and willingness to change. Genuine self-forgiveness will imply that they will be willing to change and demonstrate this in their future behaviour and will more likely be related to the change and maintain the positive behaviour change. The program affected genuine self-forgiveness through its effects on value affirmation. As value affirmation was a significant mediator of change, programs should enhance this aspect of the program and make explicit the importance of values.

Future Research Directions

Further studies into the elements of the intervention program with bigger groups of participants would assist in understanding the emphasis that can be placed on genuine self-forgiveness and value affirmation. In addition to testing other elements of the program, future research should consider other measurable behavioural outcomes. This will assist in examining the link between self-forgiveness, willingness to change and observable positive changes in school-based behaviour following attendance on the program. The changes also need to be examined both short term and over an extended period of time to further understand the full impact of attending the program (Newes, 2001). Another possible research direction is to identify the individual characteristics that make young people receptive to wilderness-based intervention programs (Howells & Day, 2003). This information will assist schools and agencies in selecting the young people who will most benefit from attending the program and who are ready to instigate change (Raviv, Sills, Raviv & Wilansky, 2000).

Conclusion

In summary, the analyses demonstrate that the wilderness adventure program had significant effects on self-affirmation, value affirmation and willingness to change compared to not attending the program. The results of this study are significant because intervention programs such as Operation Flinders can be further developed to enhance goals in improving behaviour in young people, especially when the mechanisms behind how the program works are better understood. Knowing that value affirmation is important in fostering self-forgiveness in young people with school behaviour problems can improve program development. However, further research into self-forgiveness and the relationship between positive behaviour changes will strengthen the impact the program can have with young people. A focus on this area will assist in improving the current and future social behaviour of young people and communities, which is the ultimate and most significant aim of any intervention program.

References

Abbott, C. (1991). The Outdoor Experience program: what it does and how it works. In Cianchi, J. (ed.). *Proceedings of the First National Symposium on Outdoor/Wilderness Programs for Offenders*. Canberra, ACT, Australia: Adult Corrective Services. 171-174.

Ahmed, E., & Braithwaite, V. (2006). Forgiveness, reconciliation and shame: Three key variables in reducing school bullying. *Journal of Social Issues*, 62(2), 347-370.

Ahmed, E., Harris, N., Braithwaite, J., & Braithwaite, V. (2001). *Shame management through integration.* Cambridge, UK: Cambridge University Press.

Armstrong, A. & Francis, R. (2003). Difficulties in evaluating crime prevention programs: What are some lessons for evaluators of community-based programs? *Paper presented at the Evaluation in Crime and Justice: Trends and Methods Conference convened by the Australian Institute of Criminology in conjunction with the Australian Bureau of Statistics and held in Canberra,* 24-25 March 2003

Barrett, J. (1993). Survey of outdoor activity provision for young offenders and young people at risk. *The Journal of Adventure Education and Outdoor Leadership*, 10(4), 24-27.

Bende, D., & Losel, F. (2011). Bullying at school as a predictor of delinquency, violence and other anti-social behaviour in adulthood. *Criminal Behaviour and Mental Health.* 21, 99-106.

Berman, D.S., & Davis-Berman, J. (2001). Critical and emerging issues for therapeutic adventure. *The Journal of Experimental Education*, 24, 68-69.

Berridge, D., Brodie, I., Pitts, J., Porteous D, & Tarling, R. (2001). The independent effects of permanent exclusion from school on the offending careers of young people. *RDS Occasional Paper,* 71, London: Home Office

Brand, D. (2001). A longitudinal study of the effects of a wilderness-enhanced program on behaviour-disordered adolescents. *Australian Journal of Outdoor Education* 6(1): 40-54.

Cason, D. & Gillis, H.L. (1994). A meta-analysis of outdoor adventure programming with adolescents. *The Journal of Experiential Education*, 17(1): 40-47.

Crisp, S. (1996). When does wilderness adventure become therapeutic? The need for broader frameworks: Experiential reconstruction of developmental foundations. *Australian Journal of Outdoor Education,* 2(1): 9-18.

DETYA (2001). *Innovation and best practice in schools: Review of literature and practice.* Canberra: Department of Education, Training and Youth Affairs. Dillon, R.S. (2001). Self-forgiveness and self-respect. *Ethics*, 112(1), 53-83

Farrington, D.P, & Ttofi, M.M. (2011) Bullying as a predictor of offending, violence, and later life outcomes. *Criminal Behaviour and Mental Health,* 21, 90–98.

Fisher, M. L. & Exline, J. J. (2006). Self-forgiveness versus excusing: The roles of remorse, effort and acceptance of responsibility. *Self and Identity,* 5(2) 127-146.

Fisher, M. L. and Exline, J. J. (2010), Moving Toward Self-Forgiveness: Removing Barriers Related to Shame, Guilt, and Regret. *Social and Personality Psychology Compass*, 4, 548–558.

Gillespie, E. & Allen-Craig, S. (2009). The enhancement of resilience via a wilderness therapy program: A preliminary investigation. *Australian Journal of Outdoor Education.* 13(1), 39-49.

Gottfredson, D.C, Wilson, D.B. & Skroban-Najaka, S.(2002). "School based Crime Prevention". In Sherman, Lawrence W. et al. (Eds.) *Evidence-based crime prevention.* New York: Routledge, pp. 56-164.

Hans, T. (2000). A meta-analysis of the effects of adventure programming on locus of control. *Journal of Contemporary Psychology*, 30(1) 33-60.

Hall, J.H & Fincham, F.D. (2005). Self-forgiveness: The stepchild of forgiveness research. *Journal of Social and Clinical Psychology*, 24(5), 621-637.

Hemphill, J.F., & Howell, A.J. (2000). Adolescent offenders and stages of change. *Psychological Assessment*, 12, 371-381.

Holmgren, M. (1998). Self-forgiveness and responsible moral agency. *The Journal of Value Inquiry*. 32, 75-91.

Howells, K., & Day, A. (2003). Readiness for anger management: Clinical and theoretical issues. *Clinical Psychology Review*, 23, 319-337. Humber, E., & Snow, P.C. (2001). The oral language skills of young offenders: A pilot study. *Psychiatry, Psychology and Law*, 8, 1-11.

Lispey, M.W. (2009). The primary factors that characterise effective intervention with juvenile offenders: a meta-analytic overview. *Victims and Offenders*, 4(2), 124-147

Loeber, R. & Farrington, D.P. (1998). Never too early, never too late: risk factors and successful interventions for serious and violent juvenile offenders. *Studies on Crime and Crime prevention*, 7, 7–30

MacKenzie, D.L. (2000). Evidence based corrections: Identifying what works. *Crime and Delinquency*, 46, 457-471.

Maltby, J., Macaskill, A. & Day, L. (2001). Failure to forgive self and others: A replication and extension of the relationship between forgiveness, personality, social desirability and general health. *Personality and Individual Differences*, 30, 881-885

Moffitt, T.E., Caspi, A., Harrington, H.L. & Milne, B.J. (2002). Males on the life-course persistent and adolescence limited antisocial pathways: follow-up at 26 years. *Development and Psychopathology*, 14, 179– 207

Mohr, P., Heseltine, K., Howells, K., Badenoch, D., Williamson, P., & Parker, A. (2001). *Evaluation of Operation Flinders wilderness-adventure program for youth at risk.* Report to Attorney-General's Department. Adelaide: FAPRG, University of South Australia.

Newes, S.L. (2001). Future directions in adventure-based therapy research: Methodological considerations and design suggestions. *The Journal of Experiential Education*, 24, 92, 99.

O'Brennan, L. L., Bradshaw, C. P & Sawyer, A. L. (2009). Examining developmental differences in the social-emotional problems among frequent bullies, victims, and bully/victims. *Psychology in the Schools*, 46(2), 100-115.

Presser, L., & Van Voorhis, P. (2002). Values and evaluation: Assessing processes and outcomes of restorative justice programs. *Crime and Delinquency*, 48(1), 162-188.

Prochaska, J.O. & Velicer, W.F. (1997). The transtheoretical model of behaviour change. *American Journal of Health Promotion*, 12, 38-48.

Pryor, A. (2009). Australian outdoor adventure interventions: Existing empirical evidence. *Unpublished report*. Burwood, Victoria: NiCHE Research Group, Deakin University School of Health and Social Development.

Raviv, A., Sills, R., Raviv, A., & Wilansky, P. (2000). Adolescents' help seeking behaviour: The difference between self and other referral. *Journal of Adolescence,* 23, 721-740.

Raymond, I. (2003). Risk, crimonogenic need, responsivity: An evaluative framework applied to the Operation Flinders wilderness therapy program for youth at risk. *Unpublished Thesis*. Adelaide, South Australia: University of South Australia.

Russell, K.C. (2000). Exploring how the wilderness therapy process relates to outcomes. *The Journal of Experiential Education*, 23, 170-176.

Rutter, M., Giller, H. & Hagell, A. (1998) *Antisocial Behaviour By Young People.* Cambridge: Cambridge University Press.

Sherman, D.K., Cohen, G.L., Nelson, L.D., Nussbaum, A.D., Bunyan, D.P, & Garcia, J. (2009). Affirmed yet unaware: Exploring the role of awareness in the process of self-affirmation. *Journal of Personality and Social Psychology,* 97(5), 745-764.

Shrout, P.E. & Bolger, N. (2002). Mediation in experiential and non-experiential studies: New procedures and recommendations. *Psychological Method,* 7(4), 422-445.

Smart, D., Vassallo, S., Sanson, A. & Dussuyer, I. (2004). Patterns of antisocial behaviour from early to late adolescence. *Trends and Issues in Crime and Criminal Justice.* Vol 290, Dec 2004.

Smith, R. (1998). *No Lessons Learnt: A Survey of School Exclusions*. London: The Children's Society.

Stuckey, M.E. & Stukas, A.A. (2009). Overcoming self-defeating behaviour in areas of contingent self-worth; The effects of self-affirmation on self-handicapping. *Presented at the annual meeting of the Society of Australasian Social Psychologists,* Melbourne, Australia.

Tangney, J., Boone, A.L., & Dearing, R. (2005). Forgiveness of the self: Conceptual issues and empirical findings. In E.L. Worthington (Ed.). *Handbook of Forgiveness*. Hoboken, Brunner-Routledge.

Thompson, L.Y., Snyder, C.R., Hoffman, L., Michael, S.T., Rasmusen, H.N., Billings, L.S. et al. (2005). Dispositional forgiveness of self, others and situations. *Journal of Personality*, 73(2), 313-358.

Ttofi, M.M., & Farrington D.P. (2010). School bullying: Risk factors, theories and interventions. In Brookman F, Maguire M, Pierpoint H, Bennett TH (eds.) *Handbook of Crime.* Cullompton, Devon: Willan pp. 427–457.

Ungar, M., Dumond, C., & McDonald, W. (2005). Risk, resilience and outdoor programs for at-risk children. *Journal of Social Work*, 5(3), 319-338.

Vassallo, S., Smart, D., Sanson, A., Dussuyer, I., McKendry, W., Toumbourou, J.T, Prior, M., & Oberklaid, F. (2002). *Patterns and precursors of adolescent antisocial behaviour, the first report.* Melbourne: Crime Prevention Victoria.

Wenzel, M., Turner, J.K., & Okimoto, T.G. (2010). Is forgiveness an outcome or initiator of sociocognitive processes: Rumination, empathy, and cognitive appraisals following a transgression. *Social Psychological and Personality Science*, 1(4), 369-377.

Wenzel, M., Woodyatt, L. & Hedrick, K. (2011). *Confessing one's wrongdoing: Genuine self-forgiveness as the severance of the negative link between responsibility acceptance and positive self-regard.* Manuscript submitted for publication.

Wilson, S.J., & Lipsey, M.W. (2000). Wilderness challenge programs for delinquent youth: A meta-analysis of outcome evaluations. *Evaluation and Program Planning*, 23, 1-12.

Wohl, M.J.A, DeShea, L. & Wahkinney, R.L. (2008). Looking within: Measuring state self-forgiveness and its relationship to psychological well-being. *Canadian Journal of Behavioural Science* 40(1), 1-10.

Woodyatt, L. & Wenzel, M. (2010). Self-forgiveness and the restoration of offenders following an interpersonal transgression. Paper presented at the 13th Biennial Conference of the International Society of Justice Researchers (ISJR), Banff, Canada.

Woodyatt, L. & Wenzel, M. (2011). Encouraging genuine self-forgiveness. *41st Annual Conference for the Society of Australasian Social Psychologists, Manly, Australia.*

Woodyatt, L. & Wenzel, M. (2010). Is self-forgiveness associated with restoration of a transgressor? *13th Conference of the International Society for Justice Research.*

Woodyatt, L. & Wenzel, M. (2010). Self-forgiveness and restoration after an interpersonal transgression. *40th Annual Conference of the Society of Australasian Social Psychologists.*

CHAPTER 6

Development of Best Practices for Adventure Therapy

Kim Sacksteder

ABSTRACT

The field of adventure therapy has experienced a growing need to demonstrate efficacy and establish standards as the professional environment demands increased accountability. The Therapeutic Adventure Professionals Group (TAPG) of the Association for Experiential Education (AEE) has been working toward the development of best practices for adventure therapy in order to address this need. This paper outlines the emergence and rationale behind ethical standards, best practices, and evidence-based practice as they relate to adventure therapy, and describes the history and process utilized by TAPG to address these needs. The implications for international adventure therapy are also explored.

INTRODUCTION

Over the last decade, the demand to identify best practices has emerged as a priority within the mental health field, as 'managed care' has influenced programs to demonstrate their effectiveness. At the First International Adventure Therapy Conference in 1997, Crisp clearly identified the importance of developing best practices for adventure therapy (Crisp, 1998). Additionally, media reports, public pressure and high-visibility deaths in programs have highlighted a need for standards in the practice of adventure therapy. The Therapeutic Adventure Professionals Group (TAPG) of the Association for Experiential Education (AEE) has sought to create a set of best practices for adventure therapy that could begin to unite the field behind standards regarding the practices of quality programs and practitioners. This paper represents the efforts of TAPG in creating a set of best practices for adventure therapy, explores the history and process used to accomplish this task, discusses the potential impact upon programs, and offers areas of potential impact to the international community.

TAPG is a professional organization committed to the development and promotion of adventure-based programming and the principles of experiential education in therapeutic settings. TAPG is also committed to the professional development of our members and the profession as a whole. AEE members within this group typically work within the fields of health, mental health, corrections, education, and other human service fields. Our primary purpose is to facilitate networking for professionals within our various fields and to share information, techniques, and concerns regarding the therapeutic use of adventure. We represent the interests of our membership to the Board and larger professional communities through workshops, conference and pre-conference activities, and best practices development (TAPG, 2010). It is important to note that, although TAPG has international membership, the majority of members are from the United States, and the resulting best practices reflect a predominantly American perspective.

THE NEED FOR A STANDARD

Media trends and public perceptions related to adventure therapy and in particular, wilderness therapy, have fluctuated over the last decade. Television programs in the Unites States, such as 'Man vs. Wild' and 'Survivorman' have glorified the ideal of survival in nature. The popularity and public awareness of wilderness therapy grew when it entered the television spotlight with Brat Camp, a reality TV program that premiered in the United Kingdom and drew a wide audience in the United States that featured a wilderness therapy program (Russell, 2006). Louv's (2005) book entitled 'Last Child in the Woods', and the subsequent No Child Left Inside movement have renewed the idea that children being in nature is not only healthy, but an integral part of their development. This has resulted in some government legislation mandating environmental education programs in school curriculums in the United States (Govtrack, 2009).

However, these positive trends have been countered by reports of abuse, neglect, and even deaths in residential programs, including wilderness programs. There has been confusion in public perceptions about the distinction between therapeutic programs and boot-camp style programs, which operate with fundamental philosophical differences (Russell, 2006). This, in turn, has launched the regulation of wilderness programs into the political spotlight as the General Accountability Office (GAO) completed its 'Report on Abuse' (Kutz & O'Connell, 2007). In this report, the GAO indicated there was a lack of internal regulation and standards related to wilderness treatment programs and cited numerous cases of abuse, neglect and death occurring in residential programs.

Following this report, Representative George Miller presented the 'Stop Child Abuse and Neglect in Residential Programs for Teens Act of 2009' to Congress that proposed legislation and governmental oversight of these and other residential programs. To date, this bill has not been enacted into law (Govtrack, 2009).

The 2007 GAO Report also commented on the lack of 'definition' in our field, and proposed its own definition of wilderness therapy in lieu of finding agreement among professionals or even professional organizations about who we are and what we do (Kutz & O'Connell, 2007). Our field has been plagued by lack of definition and unclear boundaries identifying who we are, what we do, and conversely, who we are not and what we don't do (Newes, 2000; Newes & Bandoroff, 2004). Part of this issue arises from an ethic of respect for diverse perspectives and a desire to be inclusive of all who engage in the process. Additionally, many practitioners and programs view governmental oversight or regulation as a hindrance to operating an effective program rather than as a safeguard of an effective industry. As a field, we have struggled to balance this ethic with the need to define boundaries, establish standards for practice, and explore what is 'best practice'.

Another criticism of adventure therapy arising from some in the mental health community is that we have not demonstrated the efficacy of our interventions through research (Newes, 2000). In order to establish research evidence, we must first seek clarity regarding what we are testing. We need to create definition and begin to collect data under a banner of common language (Crisp, 1998; Newes, 2000). Developing best practices assists in addressing this issue and supports operationalizing our work.

TAPG opted to address these concerns by establishing best practices for adventure therapy that create a standard for practice, establish boundaries, and are supported by endorsement from the field. Ultimately, ethical practice demands we provide quality care that relies on the best available evidence (Stuart & Lilienfield, 2007; Hagemoser, 2009). TAPG is committed to the ethical principle that we should strive to provide the best possible care, to focus on the continuing development of best practices, and to implement best practices as they emerge.

The Evolution of Best Practices

The concept of 'best practices' arose out of the corporate sector in response to an increasingly competitive international business environment (Horton, 2000). This focus on attending to evolving strategies for increased efficiency and effectiveness extended into the world of healthcare and medicine with the advent of 'managed care' (Kramer & Glazer, 2001). Glazer (1998) asserted that if the mental health field had clearly demonstrated the value of our treatments early in the managed care era, we would never have been subjected to the current level of intrusion from forces purchased by payers. The concept of best practices has infiltrated almost all professions with a call to identify, develop and implement practices within each profession that promote continuous quality improvement (Glazer, 1998; Manela & Moxley, 2002; Kramer & Glazer, 2001). Although there are varying reactions to this movement and how it has been applied and translated, the primary concept is intrinsically consistent with the values and ethics of mental health practice – be aware of what works and use it to provide the best possible care for your clients.

Within international adventure therapy, the publications from each International Adventure Therapy Conference have consistently articulated a need for identification of best practices (Crisp, 1998; Gillis & Priest, 2003; Crisp, 2004). Crisp (2004) discussed this to greater extent in the proceedings from the 3IATC, providing a framework for key elements of best practices and exploring the barriers impacting on the achievement of his vision of a unified paradigm in which adventure therapy emerges as an evidence-based practice with clearly outlined ethics and best practice standards.

Definitions of best practice are numerous and vary somewhat, but most definitions include the following concepts:

- Best practices are methods, actions, elements of planning or design, etc. that lead to superior outcomes and are more effective and efficient than others.
- Best practices rely on the best knowledge or evidence available.
- Sources of evidence may include research, historical precedent, expert opinion and experience.
- Best practices are dynamic and must be updated as new knowledge and superior ways of doing things emerge.
- Best practices are recognized by peer organizations within an industry as 'best' (Manela & Moxley, 2002; Kramer & Glazer, 2001; Wikipedia, 2009).

This standard of 'best practices' is the dominant paradigm within which most TAPG member organizations operate. Although the majority of TAPG members practice within the United States, members from other countries such as Canada exist in a similar climate of accountability (Public Health Agency of Canada,

2002). Kramer & Glazer (2001) stated that the ability to identify and implement best practices has differentiated the successful organization from the unsuccessful organization. They describe collaborative partnerships among professional organizations and governmental initiatives pushing for the development and implementation of best practices throughout the healthcare and mental health industries. This highlights the importance of the need for best practice standards throughout the international adventure therapy community, particularly if we desire to emerge as a recognized and respected profession (Crisp, 2004).

THE RISE OF EVIDENCE-BASED PRACTICE

Many events of the late 1990's and early 2000's have led to the rise of evidence-based practice (EBP) as the paradigm in which mental health services are evaluated. In the early 1990's, the healthcare industry became dominated by the value of funding and providing EBP (Parker, Ritchie, & Kirchner, 2009). As part of the healthcare system in the United States, this focus quickly moved into the mental health care continuum.

In 1999, the U.S. Surgeon General published a report on the state of mental health in the United States, which recommended fundamental changes to the mental health treatment system (U.S. Department of Health and Human Services, 2009). Although this report indicated that the efficacy of mental health treatments was well-documented, the recommendations included a call for evidence-based interventions and continued research in order to deliver the most state-of-the-art treatment to people coping with mental health issues. This report was followed up by the President's 'New Freedom Commission on Mental Health' (2003), which stated that consistent use of evidence-based treatments and best practices will become standard practice in the United States. This has indeed become the state of mental health treatment in the United States and Canada, and it is currently well accepted that practice is to be based on the best evidence available (Manela & Moxley, 2002; Hagemoser, 2009; The President's New Freedom Commission on Mental Health, 2003).

The American Psychological Association Presidential Task Force on Evidence-Based Practice (2006) provided the following definition of EBP:

> Evidence-based practice in psychology is the integration of the best available research with clinical expertise in the context of patient characteristics, culture, and preferences. The purpose of EBPP is to promote effective psychological practice and enhance public health by

> applying empirically supported principles of psychological assessment, case formulation, therapeutic relationship and intervention. *(p.1)*

This task force acknowledged that EBP had become a key feature of policy-making, funding, and health care systems. In fact, the current funding priority is most often providing funding for empirically supported treatments (EST's), which are treatment approaches shown to be efficacious in clinical controlled trials. EST's often have a manualized approach to training and treatment, in which a manual is provided that outlines the steps practitioners are to take in providing treatment. Where EST's require rigorous research methodology and evidence, EBPP is a more comprehensive approach that incorporates multiple sources of evidence and acknowledges the integration of research and clinical expertise to establish an evidence base (APA Presidential Task Force on Evidence-Based Practice, 2006).

Regardless of one's beliefs about EBP or how it is implemented, the context of the TAPG membership is one in which practitioners are expected to provide evidence to demonstrate the efficacy of their work, from both ethical and business perspectives. Adventure therapy practitioners and programs operating within this context must demonstrate effectiveness; if not, the results are often job loss and program closure.

Best Practices versus Evidence-based Practices

The process TAPG engaged in is not designed to establish adventure therapy as an evidence-based practice, although that may be the ultimate goal of this project and the adventure therapy field. Rather, our goal is to establish what we believe to be best practices for adventure therapy in the United States based on the best available evidence. This includes drawing upon research, relevant literature, and expert opinion. Even in the EBP paradigm, there is room for more than research as a source of evidence (Hagemoser, 2009; Messer & Wampold, 2002; APA Task Force on Evidence-Based Practice, 2006). The APA Presidential Task Force on Evidence-Based Practice (2006) state that where data is sparse, practitioners are to use their best clinical judgment. The report asserts that research related to EBP indicates that sensitivity, flexibility and response to client characteristics are more effective than rigid compliance with a manualized EST (APA Task Force on Evidence-Based Practice, 2006).

Efforts to establish adventure therapy as an evidence-based practice will require more coordinated efforts to conduct quality research, such as those being organized within the Association for Experiential Education. Establishing adventure therapy as an evidence-based practice has several benefits for the field. These include an increased understanding of how adventure therapy works, what aspects of our practice are effective, and better quality care for our clients. Additionally, demonstrating the effectiveness of our work improves our ability to market and fund our services and gain credibility with-in the mental health field (Crisp, 2004). Part of our solution is to join debates occurring in the mental health field, to represent ourselves through publication in peer-reviewed journals, and to present at professional conferences outside of our 'own' professional organizations.

History of TAPG Efforts

TAPG members have been strongly influenced by the developments in behavioral healthcare in the United States as well as the ongoing discussions in the international adventure therapy community. These influences contributed to a motivation to act, and TAPG made a decision to move forward on developing best practices.

Initial Steps

TAPG holds a pre-conference yearly in conjunction with AEE's Annual International Conference. In 2000, the assembled membership identified three areas of focus for future membership development: accreditation/ certification; development and delivery of professional development curriculum; and best practices. Based upon the political and practice climate of the time, best Practices was identified as the most vital and feasible. Between 2000 and 2005, these pre-conferences engaged attendees in identifying key components of effective practice, developing definitions, drawing boundaries, creating categories and outlining a set of standards and best practices to help clarify issues such as:

- What is an adventure therapy program or an adventure therapist?
- What is adventure therapy?
- What program philosophies are therapeutic versus. punitive?

Initial best practice discussions centered on educating attendees on current trends in mental health policy, funding, and ethics in order to establish the motivation to engage in the process. Attendees expressed concerns related to potential 'manualization' or prescribed treatments as a threat to the creativity, diversity, and 'magic' of adventure therapy. These disparate perspectives presented challenges for attendees to negotiate. How do you balance the need to establish a standard and demonstrate efficacy with the need to maintain flexibility and responsiveness in client care? These struggles and more were addressed in the early development of this project, just as they were in the mental health field as a whole. Often, we tended to think of ourselves as 'outside the mainstream' of the mental health field, whilst the same discussions were being held in the mental health profession (Parker, Ritchie, & Kirchner, 2009; Weinberger & Rasco, 2007). In recent years, there has been encouragement to rid ourselves of this separation from 'conventional' practice due to its detrimental impact on our ability to be an accepted and respected approach to treatment. At times, concerns were expressed about stagnation as the discussion continued. This discussion, and the initial buy-in from the membership, was critical to the success of the project, but there remained a concern of 'all talk and no action'. Also, differences of opinion remained as people managed reactions to the changing climate and rise of the evidence-based paradigm.

The leadership supported continued progress by calling for attendees to seek the intersection of ideas; to find the places where people could agree. Members were invited to think about the place where common ground was reached. Pre-conference leaders solicited attendees in identifying themes, components, and aspects of adventure therapy that they believed should be included in best practices. These components were organized into thematic clusters that would eventually produce an outline for the best practices document. The focus of these efforts was to ensure the membership was engaged in the process in a meaningful way, rather than to produce a set of standards 'for' them. A tone was set from the beginning that placed value on respecting the diversity of our members and our practices.

In February 2005, TAPG hosted the first Adventure Therapy Best Practices Conference in Buffalo Grove, Illinois at OMNI Youth Services. This conference brought together top practitioners to focus on the experiential and practical application of adventure therapy, even utilizing volunteer 'clients' to make presentations as experiential as possible. Gillis presented on the 'State of the Field' and Russell presented on the 'State of Research'. This gathering led to a serious push to move forward in the development of best practices; to move past the discussion and brainstorming into focused action.

TAPG committed to hosting Adventure Therapy Best Practices conferences every 2 years in order to maintain our momentum in this important process. In 2007, the conference was held at the University of New Hampshire, (New Hampshire, USA) and in 2010 at Camp Mary Orton (in Columbus, Ohio, USA). In 2007, AEE also began the process of incorporating standards for therapeutic programs into the Accreditation Standards, which have been successfully implemented into the AEE Accreditation program.

At the AEE International Conference in October 2005, a committee was tasked with taking the next steps by coordinating efforts to develop adventure therapy best practices, and transition to acting outside of the limitations of an annual TAPG pre-conference, which was where the bulk of the work was done in the past.

TAPG focused on gathering a diverse and representative group of people to engage in the process. From 2005 to 2010, this committee, along with over 60 practitioners, educators, and researchers worked to develop and implement a process to create a best practices statement. Teams developed a structured outline and completed literature reviews related to each established outline area. The outline drew upon work from the previous pre-conferences.

Through this process, the group found that of the three essential elements of best practice (historic precedent, research, and expert opinion/experience), it was necessary to rely heavily on expert opinion and practitioner experience to complete the project. The literature and research could be summarized, but this expert opinion was critical to providing the most current evidence to establish best practices.

Challenges and Limitations

There were numerous challenges related to this process, as well as limitations associated with the evolution and state of the field. Some of the primary issues encountered are described below.

Website versus Publication

TAPG debated producing a published text or a website. A published text provides a differing level of credibility in mainstream channels, while a website has the needed flexibility to be updated as the field develops. Additionally, the electronic medium provides accessibility to the most current information by varied audiences including the potential client, current or developing practitioner, academician, researcher, and governmental entity. At the onset, TAPG decided to create a website with the intent that it may lead to publication at a later point.

Another concern related to the product was authorship. While it was important to recognize contributors, it was also critical that this work emerge from a diverse group of professionals in the field and not 'belong' to certain people. Thus, it was decided to pursue a product that credited contributors but lacked authorship, as it was produced from the efforts, review and endorsement of a wide range of professionals and organizations.

Components of Best Practice

As discussed earlier, the primary components of best practices are research, historic precedent, published literature, and expert opinion. Although there are significant numbers of studies related to adventure therapy, there are challenges associated with compiling, organizing, and analyzing this research. Also, while there is quality and relevant research, it is not enough at this time to establish a solid evidence base for most aspects of adventure therapy. Much of the published literature reflects practitioner experience and opinion rather than solid research evidence. Therefore, our process relied heavily on practitioner experience and was informed by research evidence where it was available.

Definition of Adventure Therapy

Many questions emerged related to definition. This issue was identified by Crisp (1998) early on in the international discussion related to best practice, and continues to be a factor today. What is adventure therapy? Who is our population? Do these practices address therapeutic programs or treatment programs specifically? Establishing the definition of 'what' we are producing best practices for was a critical step in this process.

We had to stay focused on what was particular to adventure therapy so that we did not engage in reinventing mental health treatment standards, while simultaneously addressing a need to establish that for adventure therapy to be an accepted practice modality, accepted aspects of mental health treatment must be incorporated into any adventure therapy practice.

Diversity of the Adventure Therapy Field

The field of adventure therapy incorporates many diverse areas, with practitioners who work in office-based settings, community mental health agencies, and in wilderness environments on extended expeditions. Finding the intersections of these areas presents challenges in being specific enough to be useful, while being general enough to be inclusive of our diverse approaches. This issue was also identified by Crisp (2004).

In the beginning, it was decided to include a diverse range of practitioners and there was a focus on gaining endorsement from the adventure therapy field, rather than attempting to create a single document from a single organization. If the field is to come together and address our issues of public perception and lack of clarity, we must find agreement about what we feel is the best way to practice our profession.

The Process

The results of the work from the pre-conferences were organized into an outline for the project. This outline included seven major sections. These sections included:

- Historical foundations
- Theory
- Ethics
- Treatment applications
- Clinical decisions
- Practitioners
- Research

Initially, over 40 professionals were identified and divided into seven teams, one for each outline section. These teams were responsible for reviewing the outline and completing a literature review.

Next, a process was developed that utilized 'writer's weekends' to overcome barriers that had slowed earlier attempts to produce results. This process hinged on utilizing the strengths of face-to-face meetings (for gaining depth and clarity), combined with the breadth of multiple perspectives accessed through scheduled participation of professionals at a distance.

For a writer's weekend, three to five professionals gathered in a central location for the purpose of developing content for their assigned outline section. Up to ten additional professionals who could not be present, were scheduled to support at various times throughout the weekend. Three roles were identified for a writer's weekend. These included:

- *Content Team:* This team develops the structure and content for each section. These were people who were present at the writer's weekend.
- *Review Team:* This team reviewed the work of the content team and made recommendations for clarification, restructuring, missing or inaccurate information, and re-wording of key descriptions. This team worked at a distance at scheduled times. Work from the content team was typically reviewed twice during a writer's weekend.

- *Writer:* One writer was selected to take the work of the content team and structure it into written form. A single writer was designated to support consistency in the 'voice' of the writing.

The following steps were utilized to develop the statement of best practice for a given outline section:

1. *Add content to the outline headings.* This was accomplished through discussion and agreement on which content points should be included. Content teams were asked to avoid negotiating over wording, which stopped progress and were asked to focus on the content message instead. However, they were required to balance this with the need for clarity in their content message.
2. *Initial content sections sent to reviewers.* Reviewers were scheduled to look at content at designated times. Content teams would continue working through their section, but send what they had completed to reviewers. This initial review allowed reviewers to provide an outside perspective to the structure 100 and direction that a content team was taking and provide feedback.
3. *Content revision.* Once reviewer comments were reviewed, content teams would revise content accordingly, taking into account the feedback provided. At times, this feedback was contradictory and content teams were asked to consider diverse perspectives. If agreement could not be found, this was noted in the document.
4. *Drafting.* At this point, the designated writer would move forward with organizing the content into a draft document.
5. *Final review.* At the end of each writer's weekend, the drafted best practices were sent out to a wide range of reviewers. These reviewers were asked to think of themselves as 'co-authors', meaning that rather than just sending out critiques, they were asked to send suggested rewordings, alternate definitions, and their own perspectives on complex issues.
6. *Attach literature.* Literature citations are finalized that reflect support for the stances taken in the best practices document. Throughout the process, various literature and published research may be utilized to develop content, but this step ties the work to an important piece of the best practices process, published literature and historic precedent.

At the time of 5IATC, we are in the drafting stage of the process. The website has been created, with a URL of tapg.aee.org/tapg/ bestpractices. The content and writer's weekends have been completed and much of the content is posted and available for review and feedback. Some literature has been attached to the available content. As a continually evolving document, all readers are encouraged to provide feedback and support the development of the site. It is the significant contributions of the adventure therapy community that will contribute to the eventual impact of best practices for our field.

Following completion of these steps, the plan is to circulate the final 'Best Practices' document to professionals and organizations in the field for feedback and endorsement. Once established, a system for updating and maintaining these practices must be established in order to keep them current. As this develops and our evidence base is strengthened, this document will hopefully become published.

International Implications

In presenting this process and the history behind it to the international adventure therapy community, it has been important from the outset that we were clear that the best practices produced and identified were context-specific and relevant to TAPG members and organizations who were in vital need of such a product. We maintain that adventure therapy, as defined and practiced in our context, requires this type of definition and boundary-setting in order to emerge as a profession that is accountable to the clients we serve.

The rise of the EBP paradigm is not applicable to the entire international context, but is certainly relevant in many areas of the globe and to many practitioners in the international adventure therapy community (particularly in mental health treatment, for example Crisp, 2004). It is apparent that in an international context, definitions of adventure therapy vary considerably and there are few agreed-upon lines drawn (Crisp, 2004).

The best practices developed as a result of our process are relevant in the context of our member organizations and should not be assumed to be automatically transferable to other contexts. Alternately, when something is asserted as 'best practice' in one environment, there is an inevitable comparison that will impact practitioners in other environments. Therefore, it is expected that establishing best practices in the TAPG context will have unexpected positive and negative effects in other areas of the world.

Although this process is context-specific, it may be utilized effectively in other countries seeking to develop structures required by governmental agencies or by other adventure therapy communities in order to establish standards for effective practice. Also, articulating best practice standards allows practitioners from different environments to learn from one another. The benefit of having an international community of practitioners is based on the idea that, though we come from many different perspectives, we have much to offer one another to enhance our practice.

It seems the international adventure therapy community is experiencing a parallel process to what TAPG experienced in 2000-2005, in which there is a tension between the need to establish standards, research aspects of practice and draw boundaries, and the need to preserve the diversity, freedom, and flexibility of our practice. During the 5IATC, the international adventure therapy community exhibited a split in perspectives and questioned how to move forward. Some issues brought up included:

- How do we define ourselves? Do we have to?
- Do we strive to become a profession and draw boundaries or continue as a loose association of people who do similar things and learn from one another's experience?
- Do we have a professional responsibility to establish standards?
- How do we do this in a way that incorporates diverse perspectives and contexts?

A major implication of this TAPG process for the international community lies in looking at the same barrier TAPG experienced – how to move past our differences in order to continue developing as a field. The answer for TAPG was to focus on the areas where we agreed in order to move forward. For example, what are the things that bring us together as an international community? This process suggests that if we are able to seek the intersection of our ideas, the aspects of practice that bring us together, it will support us in developing as a field rather than being stalled in debate. The debate has intrinsic value in the process, but that value is undermined when it continues without forward movement. The aspects of adventure therapy that connect us are the source of our strength as a community and may be utilized to propel us to reaching our greatest potential.

REFERENCES

Albright, A. & Salmanowitz, M. (2009). From Committee on Education and Labor: *House overwhelmingly approves legislation to stop child abuse in residential treatment programs*. Retrieved from: http://edlabor.house.gov/newsroom/2009/02/house -over whelmingly-approves.shtml.

American Psychological Association Task Force on Evidence-Based Practice for Children and Adolescents. (2008). *Disseminating evidence-based practice for children and adolescents: A systems approach to enhancing care*. Washington, DC: American Psychological Association.

APA Presidential Task Force on Evidence-Based Practice. (2006). Evidence-based practice in psychology. *American Psychologist* 61(4) 271-285.

BusinessDictionary.com. (2009). *Definition of best practice*. Retrieved from: http://www.businessdictionary.com/definition/best-practice. html.

Crisp, S. (1998). International models of best practice in wilderness and adventure therapy. In C. Itin (Ed.), *Exploring the Boundaries of Adventure Therapy: International Perspectives*. Boulder, CO: Association of Experiential Education.

Crisp, S. (2004). Envisioning the birth of a profession. In S. Newes & S. Bandoroff (Eds.), *Coming of age: The evolving field of adventure therapy*. Boulder, CO: Association of Experiential Education.

Gillis, H. L. & Priest, S. (2003). Adventure therapy: Past, present and future. In K. Richards & B. Smith (Eds.), *Therapy within adventure*. Augsburg, Germany: ZIEL.

Glazer, W. (1998). Best practices: Defining best practices: A prescription for greater autonomy. *Psychiatric Services*. 49(8), 1013-1016.

Govtrack. Bill Sponsor Reed, J. (2009). *No Child Left Inside Act of 2009*. Retrieved from: http://www.govtrack.us/congress/bill.xpd?bill=s111-866.

Hagemoser, S. (2009). Breaking the bandwagon: Scrutinizing the science and politics of empirically supported therapies. *The Journal of Psychology*, 143(6), 601-614.

Horton, S. (2000). Introduction to the competency movement: Its origins and impact on the public sector. *The International Journal of Public Sector Management*. 13(4), 306-318.

Louv, R. (2005). *Last child in the woods: Saving our children from nature-deficit disorder*. Chapel Hill, NC: Algonquin Books of Chapel Hill.

Kramer, T. and Glazer, W. (2001). Best practices: Our quest for excellence in behavioural health care. *Psychiatric Services*. 52(2), 157-159.

Kutz, G., & O'Connell, A. (2007). *Residential Treatment Programs: Concerns regarding abuse and death in certain programs for troubled youth*. Report of the U.S. Government Accountability Office.

Manela, R. W. and Moxley, D. P. (2002). Best practices as agency-based knowledge in social welfare. *Administration in Social Work*, 26(4), 1-24.

Messer, S., & Wampold, B. (2002). Let's face facts: Common factors are more potent than specific therapy ingredients. *American Psychological Association* (9)1, 21 25.

Newes, S. (2000). *Adventure-based therapy: Theory, characteristics, ethics, and research*. A paper written to fulfil the comprehensive examination requirement in Psychotherapy, Ethics, Methodology. State College, PA: Pennsylvania State University.

Newes, S. & Bandoroff (2004). What is adventure therapy? In S. Newes & S. Bandoroff (Eds.), *Coming of age: The evolving fleld of adventure therapy*. Boulder, CO: Association of Experiential Education.

Parker, L., Ritchie, M., Kirchner, J. (2009). Balancing health care evidence and art to meet clinical needs: policymakers' perspectives, *Journal of Evaluation in Clinical Practice,* 15, 970-975.

The President's New Freedom Commission on Mental Health. (2003). *Achieving the Promise: Transforming mental health care in America.* Retrieved from: http://www.mentalhealthcommission.gov/reports/Finalreport/toc_exec.html.

Public Health Agency of Canada. (2002). *Review of best practices in mental health reform.* Retrieved from: www.phac-aspc.gc.ca/mh-sm/pubs/bp_review/reves-eng.php.

Russell, K. C. (2006). Brat camps, boot camps, or....? Exploring wilderness therapy program theory. *Journal of Adventure Education and Outdoor Learning,* 6,(1), 5167.

Stuart, R., & Lilienfeld, S. (2007). The evidence missing from evidence-based practice. *American Psychologist*, p. 615-616.

U.S. Department of Health and Human Services. (1999). *Mental health: A report of the Surgeon General—Executive summary*. Rockville, MD: U.S. Department of Health and Human Services, Substance Abuse and Mental Health Services Administration, Center for Mental Health Services, National Institutes of Health, National Institute of Mental Health.

Visitask. (2009). *Project management training and resources*: Definition of best practices. Retrieved from http://www.visitask.com/ best-practice-g.asp.

Weinberger, J., & Rasco, C. (2007). Empirically supported common factors. In S. Hoffman & J. Weinberger (Eds.), *The art and science of psychotherapy* (pp. 103-129). New York: Routledge/Taylor & Francis Group.

Wikipedia. (2009). Definition of best practice. Retrieved from: http://en.wikipedia.org/wiki/ Best_practices.

CHAPTER 7

Developing 'Challenging' Young People: Honouring their Authentic Story

Chris Jansen and Paddy Pawson

ABSTRACT

Worldwide, a multitude of adventure-based outdoor programmes exist that are designed to develop 'challenging' young people. Recently, Aotearoa/New Zealand has seen a resurgence of interest from central government in implementing programmes for such young people that draw on military models of practice. The philosophy and format of adventure therapy programmes implemented by St John of God Waipuna in Otautahi/ Christchurch Aotearoa/New Zealand present a strong contrast to these military-style programmes. Evaluation of these programmes suggests that if adventure-based programmes are to be effective in developing young people and sustaining change, they must focus on developing all aspects of the young person.

This approach is grounded in building respectful and meaningful relationships among everyone involved with the programme, and that approach, in turn, is predicated on power sharing and taking responsibility for oneself. The over-arching aim is to give young people a sense of ownership. This is achieved by an intentional shift throughout the programme from dependence, through independence and on to interdependence. This descriptive paper interweaves consideration of these aspects, especially in terms of how they have informed the design and delivery of the Waipuna programmes, with various models of personal development and leadership, along with the self-reported narrative of a young person involved in one of these programmes.

INTRODUCTION

What we do is important, but how we do it is what makes the difference. Young people are required to participate in a world that has been created by preceding generations, often without input from their generation. We maintain that any setting, whether school, church, community, family, workplace or outdoor programmes, which give young people little opportunity to 'map and walk their journey' into adult life limits their ability to make a meaningful and satisfying life for themselves, let alone make a meaningful contribution to this planet we inhabit together. Conversely, situations that help young people gain respect for themselves and their abilities will help them to feel their contribution is important, give them resiliency, and provide them with hope and aroh. These situations, we believe arise out of settings, both formal and informal, where young people are able to form respectful, robust relationships with more experienced others (usually adults) who are prepared to walk with them as they transition through a state of dependence through independence and on to interdependence. Adventure therapy programmes offer one such setting.

The majority of adventure therapy programmes are implemented by adults for adolescents, many of whom are designated as 'at risk', or to use the term we prefer to use, 'challenging' in terms of their behaviour, learning, and life skills. How do those of us delivering these programmes balance our philosophical beliefs with the needs of the young people? How do we support them to make reasoned choices, take responsibility for their actions, and build respect for themselves and others? How do we honour, respect and do justice to their journey to develop their own philosophy of understanding? Why should they invest in us and our philosophy when after all, in their view, it is we who 'stuffed' the world. How do we create therapeutic enhancing environments for young people who consider themselves 'bombproof and bulletproof'?

These are questions that the Waipuna Trust in Otautahi/Christchurch, Aotearoa/New Zealand, has kept in mind since first implementing its adventure therapy programmes for 'challenging' young people. These questions inform the account we give in this paper of Waipuna and the principles and practice underpinning its programmes. We begin this account with a brief overview of the characteristics of adventure therapy programmes, followed by an outline of Waipuna's adventure therapy programmes. This is followed by a summary of an evaluation of these programmes undertaken in 2007, outlining the success factors and themes that emerged from that evaluation. We then discuss these themes in more detail, drawing in particular on the models that underpin the programmes' principles and practice. During this section of the paper, we draw on the experiences of Ihaka, a young man who recently participated in the programme.

ADVENTURE THERAPY: HISTORY AND CHARACTERISTICS

In 1997, Hattie, Marsh, Neill, and Richards undertook a meta-analysis examining 'the effects [for young people] of adventure programmes on a diverse array of outcomes such as self-concept, locus of control and leadership' (p. 43). The authors concluded from their analysis, which focused on 96 studies featuring over 12,000 participants, that 'adventure therapy programmes can obtain notable outcomes and have particularly strong, lasting effects' (p. 77).

Jansen (2004) outlined both the nature and the strengths of adventure therapy approaches and presented a similar picture. Such programmes, Jansen explained, are characterised by an engaging and action-orientated setting within an unfamiliar environment, which serves as a catalyst for change. The programmes typically focus on finding solutions, on gaining immediate understanding of the consequences of actions, and on success. Staff facilitate supportive peer groups, opportunities to process intense emotions, and opportunities to create new stories about one's life. The programmes offer approachable professionals and role-modelling, and an overall approach underpinned the principle of developing young people holistically. The literature also cautions that not all adventure therapy programmes are inherently good, in particular that some may have very limited long term outcomes (Hattie et al., 1997; Jansen, 2004).

THE WAIPUNA PROGRAMMES

The St John of God Waipuna (Waipuna) is a service of St John of God Hauora Trust. It has, for over 25 years, operated a range of services and programmes that supports young people and their families who encounter risk from poverty, abuse, neglect, violence, low self-esteem, addiction to alcohol and drugs, and/or other addictive behaviours. Adventure therapy at Waipuna integrates Maori (NZ indigenous people) concepts and understanding into its programme as part of honouring its commitment and belief in Te Tiriti O Waitangi (treaty between Maori NZ indigenous people, and Pakeha visitor settlers, signed in 1840).

The adventure therapy (AT) programme featured in this paper has evolved over 11yrs. Its initial philosophy achieved specifically targeted behavioural change outcomes in young people, and has evolved to having an overt focus on meeting the developmental needs of each person within the family and community that surround them. Young people are referred by self, agencies or schools, and the interview process identifies a match between the young person and the programme. The age range is 13-19 years and groups are single gender, with 80% of total participants being male. Each programme differs according to the needs of participants but includes:

- Interview with participant and family (within first 3 weeks of day programme)
- 12-16 weeks – one full day per week with AT experiences
- Family AT day
- 4 hrs per week meeting one on one with young person (2 seen each week)
- Participant and parent/guardian evenings (four evening 2 hour sessions)
- Natural world journey of 6 days in area of participants' ancestors
- Family natural world weekend
- Celebration

Selection on to a programme involves the young person being informed about all aspects of the programme and given time to think about it. If the young person is still interested in the programme, Waipuna staff set up an interview with the young person's whānau (family), followed by an extended period of time to ensure that the young person makes a fully informed decision to engage in the programme. During this time they and a Waipuna staff member sit down together to talk about the programme, the nature of the young person's involvement in it, and what outcomes they hope and want for the young person a 'you chose, we chose' consensual approach is taken. The interview may also clarify that the timing is not right or there is not a match with the programme and the family. Once admitted to the programme, the young person spends the first four days (over four weeks) experiencing the 'medium' outdoor experiences and processes. Following this a further interview takes place where the young person can now make an informed choice for further involvement.

The natural world journey is scheduled after the day programme component and the parent/young person evenings. The young people receive a letter from the facilitators inviting them to participate. Further interviews follow with all young people, thus maintaining the approach of focussing on the development of each young person regardless of their choices made. Despite most young people in week two of the day programme component indicate they are not interested in the journey component, by week twelve, 80% write a letter applying to participate in a natural world experience. The weeks leading up to this opportunity allow each young person to make an informed choice about whether to apply to go on the natural world journey.

Originally these programmes have tended to be imposed on the young people, but they have now evolved to have the needs of young people as the reference point. The natural world journey is now theirs, which means that the facilitators within the programmes must have a sufficiently flexible approach to ensure a progression of experiences that meet the developmental needs of individual programme participants. Over this time of change we have developed and trialled, in collaboration with the young people, various tools and models that we consider helped us address the questions raised above. We emphasise that the tools are simply guidelines because individual facilitators take those tools and use and shape them in ways that suit their own ways of working *with* and *alongside* young people.

Journal Writing

An important component of the natural world journey is journal writing. According to West and Crompton (2001), journal writing enables young people to understand the relevance of their experiences. This is because journal writing requires self-reflection, both individually and in group contexts. Journal writing thus helps young people to make sense of and to learn from their experiences in ways that benefit their skills acquisition and social interactions with others. These gains, say West and Crompton, tend to be transferred to the home environment. Cassidy (2001) makes the important point that the value of journal-based reflection is not determined by programme staff and facilitators; rather the value lies in what the experience means for the individual participants and how they use that learning to advance and inform their own understandings of their lives, past, present, and future. Invariably, the ability for the young person to experience, reflect and then write, and finally 'speak their truth' is a part of the value of narrative approaches with young people. The ability to transfer new knowledge to various other circumstances in their lives is significantly enhanced. Because this unconditional supported writing allows young people to tell authentic (their truth) stories, those stories begins to merge with their bigger life stories, helping them gain new understanding, and engendering hope within their lives.

During the natural world journey, reflective journaling starts on Day one. Each evening participants answer questions and then move to sentences, and on to stories. They do not have to write for long, but they must write something. It does not matter if their writing is not well formed; their 'unpolluted' writing is what has meaning within the world of their truth. This comment from one young person on Day four of the wilderness journey is typical: 'My confidence is getting deeper and deeper and my thoughts more usable'. On Day five of the wilderness journey, the programme facilitators interview each participant with a focus on the young person's inner journey (as opposed to his or her outer journey). Each person then spends the rest of the day writing his or her story of both the inner and the outer journey. Typical questions used to spark this writing include 'what have you noticed about yourself in this time away? What thoughts have been your friend along the way? What has excited you and who has known about it? What would your friends/ family be saying if they observed you over the last 6 days?

SUCCESS FACTORS EMERGING FROM THE EVALUATION PROCESS

In 2007, Waipuna commissioned an extensive evaluation of the impacts of the adventure therapy programmes on the young people involved in them. The researchers opted to use qualitative research methods to gather and analyse data because they considered this approach the best one for encouraging the participants to readily discuss relevant matters with them. Interviews were conducted with four focus groups, comprised of the different people associated with the programmes, 80% of all invited accepted this invitation. The groups were the young people, their parents or care givers, key community representatives, and the programme facilitators.

The interviews were conducted with one researcher interviewing, one writing, and each session was recorded for transcribing and analysis. These interviews typically took 1-2 hours and involved groups of between 6 12 people. The researchers used thematic analysis (Boyatzis, 1998) to explore the data and determine major themes and success factors.

One of the major positive impacts of the programmes that the researchers identified was the development of healthy personal and social skills among the young people involved. The researchers noted improved school work, higher school attendance rates, and improved relationships with peers, family and adults. They also noted that the skills the young people developed expanded to influence other sectors of their lives, such as school and the wider community.

The researchers attributed much of the success of the programmes to the facilitators' skill and ability to form effective relationships with the young people. Every focus group gave examples of how facilitators used adventure therapy experiences to develop strong relationships with the young people, and from there, help instil positive change in their behaviours and life skills. The facilitators also identified these relationships as the particular strength of the programme, and said that the aspect of the relationship most crucial to success was trust. Trust, they said, enabled the programmes' facilitators to challenge (especially through the adventure therapy experiences) the young people with the idea that the power to change resided within them. This process, the facilitators explained, helped young people develop a sense of ownership and responsibility for their own journey and outcomes.

The young people's parents and caregivers also acknowledged the broader impact the programme had on their parenting skills and the relationships within their families and their family support networks. They reported growing in confidence as a result of the changes they saw in their children, the support they received from facilitators, the skills they learned at the GAIN (family) programme, and the informal support networks they developed with other parents and caregivers on programme courses.

In summary, three key themes emerged from the evaluation which are considered embedded as core principles in the Waipuna programmes: (1) development of the whole person; (2) respectful and meaningful relationships; and (3) building ownership through the sharing of power. These principles are discussed in the following sections, drawing on models of personal development and leadership from the literature, and the community perspectives gathered in the research. Throughout our discussion, we interweave a journal narrative from a young man, Ihaka, who participated in one of Waipuna's adventure therapy programmes, and make explicit how these principles are practically applied in programmes.

Ihaka's Story

Ihaka was a 14-year-old young man who came to Waipuna because he was experiencing some major challenges in his life, both at home and at school. He wrote his journal account over many days while involved in a Waipuna programme called Te Tira Horomaka. (Te – the / Tira – travelling party / Horomaka – geographical area of Banks Peninsula). Ihaka has given his consent to use his writing and story within the context of this paper; his writing as it appears in this paper is his own authentic authorship. As Ihaka's story unfolds, we make links between it and the key success factors/ themes. Italics are occasionally added to Ihaka's writing to emphasise these links.

Theme 1: Development of the Whole Person

My Journey Writings: Ihaka Moody

> *Today I woke up with a pit in my stomach. I was dreading the week ahead and didn't want to leave my stable position at home. I knew that I*

would get homesick and was a little bit scared. I wasn't sure how I would fit into the group.

When we arrived at the beach I was sort of hoping that I was in the wrong place or missed them but as soon as I saw them I knew that my journey had begun.

The work was tiring and I was getting frustrated and in a way wished I had of either slept in or just not come, but I knew that was selfish because so many people wanted to come on the trip and I was chosen. It felt great when I reached the top of the hill and I felt happy when we were standing on the rocks with the names in them. It made me feel like I was standing on top of the world.

I started to wonder where we were going now because I couldn't see any route down. Then came the dreaded gorse bush, it hurt and it was everywhere. The campsite was ok and I was feeling a lot of emotions when we started writing the pages. Then when I showed my paper to Bevan [facilitator] and we started talking and I shared a lot of them with him.

One of them was how I get angry a lot when I am at home/school. And how instead of taking control of my own problems, I take out a lot of that anger on other people. Another way I let go of anger is by swearing which I think is wrong. I feel a lot happier now and I think that from now on at home, school or wherever I am I will be nicer and more considerate of other people.

How do you develop a person? Answers to these questions have been explored in the various models of development that underpin the Waipuna programmes; we consider three here. The main principle informing the first two models is that development of the whole person must be holistic if we are to have healthy communities and societies. The third model considers how the developmental journey of young people from dependence to independence might be best expedited.

In Aotearoa/New Zealand, Dr Mason Durie (1994) developed a Māori philosophy toward health that is based on a holistic health and wellness model called Te Whare Tapa Wha the house with 4 walls (see Figure 1). For Durie, health is underpinned by four dimensions representing the basic beliefs of life: te taha tinana (physical health); te taha hinengaro (psychological or mental health); te taha wairua (spiritual health); and te taha whānau (family health). These four dimensions are represented by the four walls of a house. Each wall is necessary to ensure the strength and symmetry of the building. Thus, if a troubled young person is to gain wellbeing and resilience, his or her needs in all of these areas must be met. Durie's model also suggests that the various cultures we come from express holistic development from their own perspectives.

Taha tinana describes our capacity for sound physical growth and development. Good physical health is required for optimal development; our physical 'being' supports our essence and shelters us from the external environment. For Māori, the physical dimension is just one aspect of health and wellbeing and cannot be separated from the aspect of mind, spirit, and family. Taha hinengaro (mental health) describes our capacity to communicate, to think and to feel. Thoughts, feelings and emotions are integral components of the body and the soul.

Taha wairua (spiritual health) describes our capacity for faith and wider communication. Our physical and mental health is related to unseen and unspoken energies; the spiritual essence of a person is his or her life force. Spiritual health determines us as individuals and as a collective; it 'tells' us who and what we are, where we have come from, and where we are going. Taha whānau (family health) relates to our capacity to belong, to care and to share; individuals are part of wider social systems. Whānau or family provides us with the strength to be who we are. Whānau is also the link to our ancestors, our ties with the past, the present, and the future. Understanding the importance of whānau and how it contributes to illness and how it assists in curing illness is fundamental to understanding health issues, especially for Māori.

Figure 1. A Mãori conception of holistic development model developed by Durie (1994).

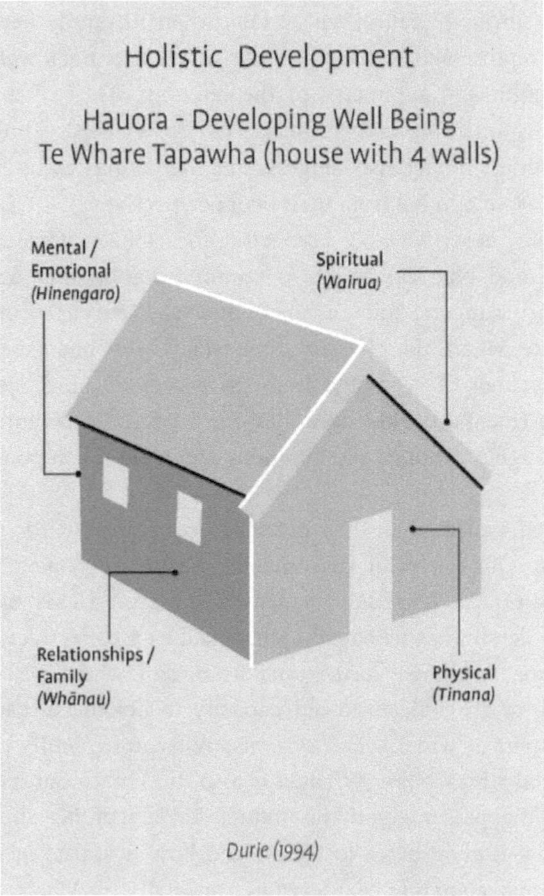

Another model of youth development underpinning the Waipuna programmes is the Circle of Courage (see Figure 2), which grew out of North American Indigenous philosophy and resilience research, and focuses on the development goals of generosity, belonging, mastery, and independence (Brendtro, Brokenleg & Van Bockern, 2002). The Circle of Courage is a philosophy that integrates what Brendtro et al. consider to be the best of Western educational thought with the wisdom of Indigenous cultures and emerging research on positive youth development. The model has four core values: belonging, mastery, independence, and generosity.

Figure 2. The circle of courage – model developed by Brendtro, Brokenieg, and Van Bockern (2002)

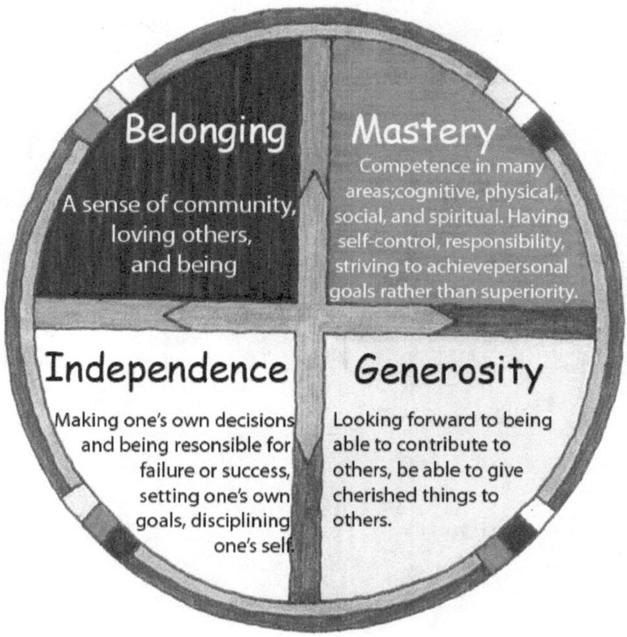
Belonging
A sense of community, loving others, and being
Mastery
Competence in many areas;cognitive, physical, social, and spiritual. Having self-control, responsibility, striving to achievepersonal goals rather than superiority.
Independence
Making one's own decisions and being resonsible for failure or success, setting one's own goals, disciplining one's self.
Generosity
Looking forward to being able to contribute to others, be able to give cherished things to others.

As is evident from the figure, the model is represented by a circle (the medicine wheel) divided into quadrants. The circle is sacred and suggests the interconnectedness of life. It also expresses the sacredness of the number four: the four directions (East, West, North, South), the four elements (wind, water, fire, earth) of the universe, and the four races (red, white, black, yellow). Each quadrant of the circle of courage stands for a central value belonging, mastery, independence, and generosity.

The third model outlined in Figure 3 describes the changes in our relationships that we encounter as we grow from being a child, to an adolescent, and finally to an adult. This process is biologically mandated it is a natural and necessary part of our lives. It suggests that part of this process is to move through the stages of dependence, independence and eventually interdependence. The circles in the diagram represent the growth and separation of a young person from his or her parents and caregivers. The descriptions on the right denote some of the characteristics likely to occur during each stage of our developing relationships.

Figure 3. Growing in our relationships - model developed by Pawson (2004)

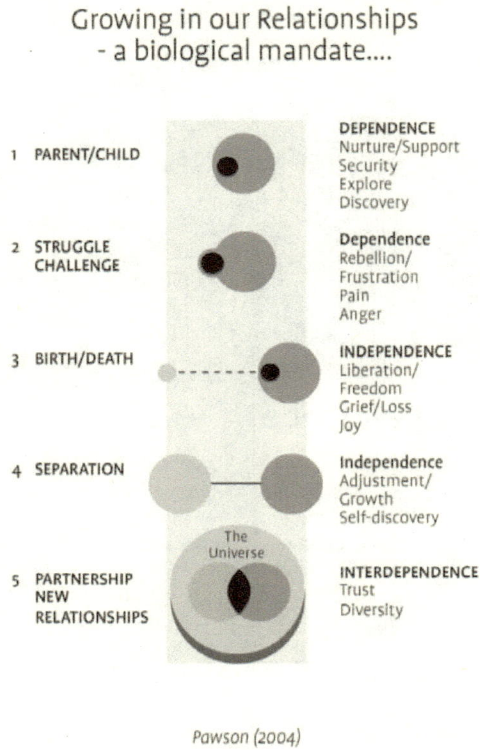

The essence of the process outlined in Figure 3 is that, as we grow, we seek to gain more say over our lives (locus of control), a stance that can create conflict with those who have previously supported us. The Waipuna programme maintains that the sole purpose of any developmental experience with young people should be to give voice to their life story; once they and we hear it, we are all in a better position to avoid this conflict.

Programme Example: Needs-focused Flexible Programme Design

The underpinning theories contained in the three models are seen in the structure of Waipuna programmes, which are built around meeting the developmental needs (emotional, physical, intellectual, social and spiritual) of young people. Each young person, with facilitator guidance, selects programme activities that accord with where the young person is 'at' and which then allows him or her to progress through various experiences, which again are primarily of the young person's choosing. Choice is important because Waipuna does not want its programmes to provide environments of situational change in which young people are put under so much stress and pressure that they have to change without necessarily 'buying into' the change. Imposed change, we believe, equates with short-term, non-lasting situational change in the young person. Positive developmental change, brought about by the individual being able to choose the growth and change trajectory, equates with long-term, lifelong change. Waipuna programmes focus on meeting the needs of the whole person inclusive of the wider relationships that surround a young person's life. For example in Aotearoa/New Zealand the Indigenous Maori people have concepts of spirituality that are important in forming their world view, which without makes it difficult for them to fully develop.

Theme 2: Respectful and Meaningful Relationship

My Journey Writings: Ihaka Moody

> *Today was completely different to yesterday. Somehow I woke up feeling a little bit happy. I felt a bit nervous when we put the kayaks out in the water. It was so hard at the start and even turning was a problem. It was scary when we got caught on the rocks and I started to get angry when we couldn't turn to get out of the waves. As soon as we swapped over it was all good until our boat flipped over, I was afraid that I might drown. If I couldn't undo my skirt so I just panicked, and pushed off the boat. In a way I was glad that I was in a double hull because me and Karape were a good team and we always had someone beside us for support.*
>
> *I was actually disappointed when I found out we weren't riding the bikes but that all went away when I saw my Nana and Granddad. I was so pleased to see them and it was great to be able to have a laugh and some kai with them as well. It was sad when I left but I know I would see them again soon. I think that I handled my swearing well today. And I kept my anger to a minimum.*
>
> *When I was at the front of the group it made me feel like I belonged somewhere because I had to control the pace of the entire group. With this also came a lot of responsibility. The bike ride was awesome I had so much fun.*

> *I have great respect for my Nana and Granddad. They have been so good to me and even though sometimes I admit that I am a nuisance, they have always been good to me and brought me up with good morals. It makes me feel happy when I see all of the things I have in life and see the way I could have turned out.*
>
> *I never really knew my father ... one day I might want to meet him but I'm still not sure because I might be disappointed.*
>
> *The reasons that I like my dad are because he brought me into this beautiful earth and because he chose to bring me into this earth through my mother.*
>
> *And I love my mum, she's awesome. Even though she wasn't able to bring me up herself, she still stood by me and put me in the best care she could.*
>
> *I think if my dad saw me now he would be happy with the way I turned out and the hands that care for me now...*

What type of relationship best fits the need of the developing adolescent who has the innate desire to be the author of their own life? What relationships enhance the journey through independence to interdependence and thus grow people into contributing young adults who can have relationships that are healthy for themselves and all around them? Counselling literature is unanimous in stating that the strength of the 'therapeutic relationship' is the most significant factor in the development of healthy outcomes for a client. Rogers (1960), the founder of person-centred counselling, coined the phrase 'unconditional positive regard' as a prerequisite for any effective therapy.

In 2003, an extensive educational research project titled Te Kōtahitanga, conducted by researchers at Waikato University in Aotearoa/ New Zealand, sought to investigate how to improve the educational achievement of disengaged Māori students in mainstream secondary school classrooms (Bishop, Berryman, Tiakiwai & Richardson, 2003). One of the main approaches of the research was to talk extensively with Māori about their educational experiences. The Māori students, those parenting these students, their principals and some of their teachers saw that the most important influence on Māori students' educational achievement was the quality of the in-class face-to-face relationships and interactions between the teachers and Māori students. In contrast, the majority of teachers suggested that the major influence on Māori students' educational achievement was the children themselves and/or their family/ whānau circumstances, or systemic/structural issues (p. 1).

The researchers concluded that deficit theorising (emphasising reasons that undermine a young person's development) by teachers is the major impediment to Māori students' educational achievement because it results in teachers having low expectations of Māori students. This, in turn, creates a downward spiralling, self-fulfilling prophecy of Māori student underachievement and failure. Bishop et al.'s research has had a strong impact across educational provision in Aotearoa/New Zealand, particularly with respect to highlighting the importance of a reciprocal trusting relationship between teacher and student.

Figure 4 outlines two types of relationship that young people encounter in our society as they consciously and unconsciously seek to have their developmental needs met. The relationship on the left fits within a dependence framework and is characterised by power/weakness. The person on the receiving end of power typically feels a sense of weakness, which leads him or her to want to have power over others. The process becomes one of a vicious cycle because both parties seek not to feel weak. Ultimately, the downward spiral ends in the destruction of the relationship. Also, because the relationship is a very dependent one, it does not allow growth or development. This kind of relationship produces temporary situational change at best, and perpetuates power relations at worst.

Figure 4. Characteristics of dependent and independent relationships - model developed by Pawson (2009)

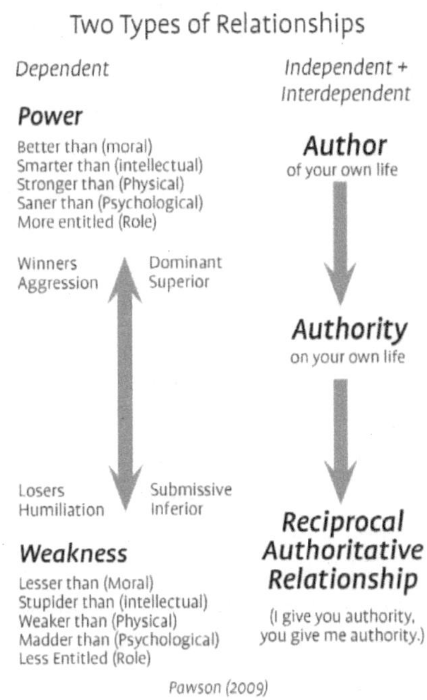

In contrast, the relationship on the right is characterised by independence and interdependence. With the onset of puberty, the relationships that characterised the early stage of young people's lives tend to become less central as the desire to be the 'authors' of their own lives takes over. At this point, young people generally want adults to relate to them in ways that allow these youngsters to have some authority over what happens to them. We all have a biological mandate to become responsible for our lives; this mandate gives each of us the impetus and drive to be the authority on our own life. But the mandate will only be realised if the relationships that surround young people are reciprocal in nature, that is, each person in the relationship gives the other (or others) permission to be the authority on his or her own life.

A respectful and meaningful relationship is also one that is characterised by the twin imperatives of high challenge and high support. Figure 5 depicts four quadrants that blend combinations of low and high challenge and support. The Waipuna programme have found that environments of high challenge and high support are more conducive to effecting long term positive development. The black quadrants tend to lead to situational change. Wachtel and McCold (2001) in restorative justice literature refer to a similar diagram as the Social Discipline Window, which describes four similar environments: neglectful, punitive, permissive and restorative.

Figure 5. Characteristics of robust relationships - model developed by Pawson (2008)

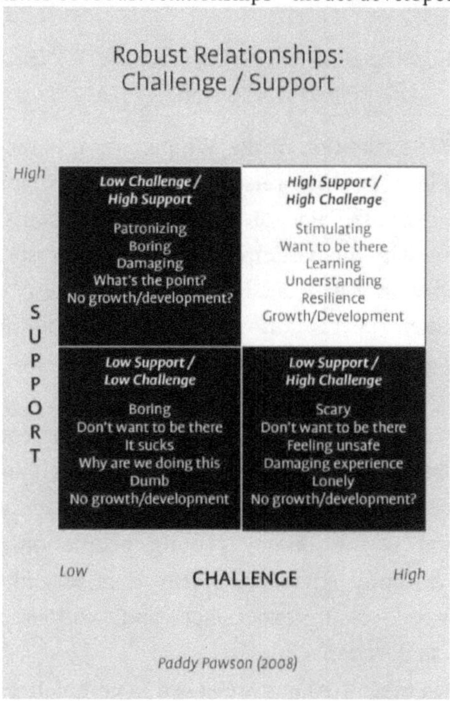

We consider that the staff of many programmes and organisations that claim to be focused on 'youth development' use the right language but offer programmes through relationships between programme staff and young people that are punitive or coercive in nature. The need to control young people through reward and coercion is often at the heart of these 'relationships'. There is a public perception that coercion works ('a bit of discipline never hurt me'); unfortunately, we consider that schools and educational settings are often the worst for using coercive methods to 'control' young people.

We need to ask ourselves if the change we hope to see in young people is being brought about by power-based relationships, in which the adult is the one providing the intrinsic or extrinsic motivators. We maintain that genuine change for young people happens only when they experience environments, situations, and relationships that are meaningful to them within the context of their respective developmental journeys. Change does not become meaningful or long-term for individuals until it becomes one that they have internalised and not had imposed on them. We note here that sometimes young people do need extrinsic motivators to instigate change, but these motivators should be gradually removed in accordance with the goal of supporting intrinsic motivators.

Programme Example: Positive Relationships between Participants and Whanau

McKay et al.'s (2007) evaluation of the Waipuna programmes showed that with respect to the building of positive relationships between participants, facilitators and others in their lives, the line of positive impact starts with a facilitators' respectful relationship with the participant. This then sets the scene for the culture of relationships both within and outside the programme (transfer), followed by their family, then their peers, followed by the school and then the wider community. The programmes' resources and energy follow the above sequence, with family receiving the following interventions:

After the interview process, the young person, parent(s)/caregiver(s) and other supporters commit to four evening sessions, each two hours long, of a facilitated, interactive engagement on the issues that impact on their home lives.

After the natural world journey (young people only), the participant's families gather for a family adventure weekend in a wilderness location. This opportunity offers two adventure experiences and two therapeutic sessions, each one and a half hours in duration.

All participants in these sessions are asked to complete evaluations at the end of them. This comment from a parent is of a kind we often see:

> The relationship the boys have with adults has changed. They are more confldent with adults. I have had comments from others in the community that have been very impressed with the way the boys communicate and their confidence. This course has bridged the gap between parents and teenagers. (Parent of participant, 2010)

Theme Three: Building Ownership through Sharing of Power

My Journey Writings: Ihaka Moody

- *Ko Aoraki te maunga*
- *Ko Waitaki te awa*

- *Ko Takitimu te waka*
- *Ko Ngai Tahu te iwi*
- *Ko Ihaka toku ingoa*

Aoraki (Mount Cook) is my mountain
Waitaki is my river
Takitimu is the canoe on which my ancestors arrived (into Aotearoa)
Ngai Tahu is my tribe
Isaac is my name

To me this means the places and tools my ancestors used to use a long long time ago. I feel happy when I see or say this because it makes me feel like I really belong in the tribe. And I can see where my ancestors grew up. I guess in a way this is to me like a family tree. This tells me where I came from.

Before I came on Te Tira Horomaka I never thought I would truly be able to express my feelings. But as I have found on this journey it's ok to express yourself to others. And there is nothing wrong with speaking the real truth. It feels good to be able to let off some steam. And instead of keeping everything bottled up inside, actually express yourself and let it all out.

On Te Tira Horomaka, I have discovered that you don't always have to do things for yourself. Sometimes you can do things for others without wanting anything in return but a simple thank you. I have found that thank you is a beautiful word and can mean so much to a person who is happy to help.

There is some ways that I have found to express myself throughout this journey.

At the start of this journey I was feeling UNSURE about the road ahead and how I would handle the challenges that would come my way, and whether I would handle those challenges well or breakdown under pressure.

> *Not all of the road was HARD, but it just depends whether you just push on and put up with it or you take your anger out on your fellow peers, or whether you realise that they have to go through everything that you are going through, and help them out with their problems.*

Covey (2004) identified human growth as a sequence of three stages: dependence, independence, and interdependence (see Figure 6). As we noted in Theme 1, the natural development process is that of moving from dependence as a child, through to a growing independence as a person during adolescence and on into adulthood and a growing interdependence.

What role do we, as programme leaders have in this development process, and what options does this role give us? How do we create opportunities for healthy development to happen? The top half of Figure 6 illustrates the development process we have outlined. The bottom half of the figure is based on the theory of situational leadership, developed by Hersey and Blanchard (1982). This theory holds that there is no single 'best' style of leadership but that the particular leadership style chosen at any stage in a programme is based on the developmental level of the individuals being led.

The leadership style depicted in the bottom left-hand side of Figure 6 is that of a leader who is directive and who sets boundaries and parameters that are not negotiable. This means, within the context of the Waipuna programmes, that the young people involved in them have no input into them. On the right-hand side of the continuum, we see a leader who has become much less directive, whose role is that of facilitating the decisions being made by the individual and/or the group. This role involves aspects of power-sharing of providing choices, allowing for negotiation, and building responsibility. This is the style of leadership/facilitation that Waipuna ultimately promotes.

In reality, it is seldom that leaders will give total responsibility to a group, however, from the young person's perspective, even a small amount of choice can feel considerably different from having no choice at all, which is often their experience. This consideration presents a challenge for those of us leading and facilitating the Waipuna programmes. The challenge is that of providing a programme of activities and opportunities that have structure and boundaries, yet offer young people room to move within those boundaries so that they can exercise choice as they progress along their developmental pathway. We will return to this matter shortly.

Figure 6. Individual and group development through situational leadership - model developed by Jansen (2008)

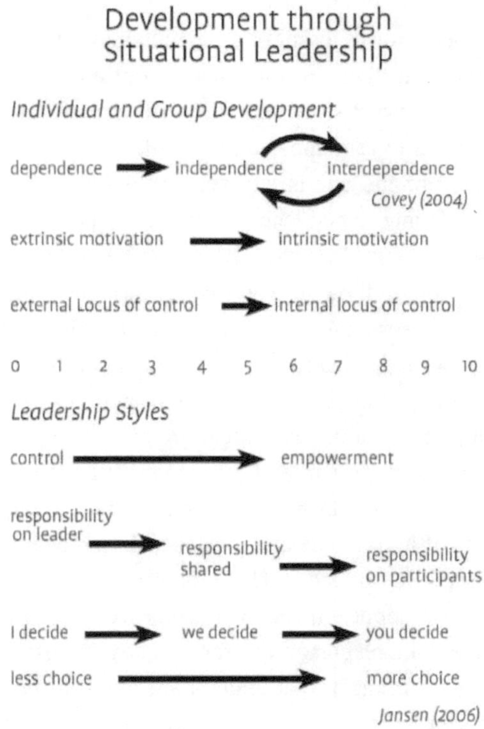

Programmes that have adolescent development as a primary objective thus need to focus on an intentional shift throughout the programme from dependence through independence and on to interdependence, and from a more directive to a less directive style of leadership. Schusser (2005) describes how he sees this process occurring with the young people he teaches:

> *My students are highly at risk when they enter the programme. Most students are dependent on me to guide them down the bumpy road. ... In the second and third term a change starts to occur ... our relationship deepens and they experience a class feeling that they like and want more of ... a feeling of respect, dignity and trust. In this setting independence grows, skills grow and students are challenged on their selfishness... In the third and fourth term magic occurs; challenges to behaviour are met with consideration rather than cursing, acceptance and apologies rather than violence. People are feeling more empowered and interdependent.*

> *They help each other and some of this is transferring into other areas of life* (p. 107-108).

This implies that if we choose to adopt a development model for the individuals and groups we work with, then we must also adopt a situational or contingency leadership model, so that our style and role can vary as the individual and the group develop. We need to remember that not all individuals and groups start on the less cohesive side of the continuum set out in Figure 6; some may already have a strong degree of interdependence and maturity in place, so leaders may not always have to begin their leadership style on the directive side. Among the factors that influence the individual's and the group's development, and that can act as indicators of current developmental needs, are the participants' ages, the size of group, how well the leader knows each individual and the nature and composition of the group, the setting and type of activity on offer, and the prior experience and competence of the individual/group.

The models of development and of situational leadership that we have considered here, and the relationships between the two, require leaders who are tuned in to the needs of individuals and groups and who adapt their style and role to suit the current needs of each. The models also require leaders who are continually looking for opportunities to share power with the individual or the group by having them take responsibility for as many as possible of the choices in the programme. We are mindful that leaders are likely to have a preferred style and that tensions can exist when the leadership style required to match a participant's or a group's developmental stage does not accord with this 'natural' style. However, unless these challenges are met, it is possible (probable even), that the leader will impede the healthy development of both individuals and groups.

Programme Example: Intentional Focus on Developing Choice and Responsibility

This focus within the Waipuna programmes starts with the referral process and increases as the programmes continue. Programme staff make clear to participants from the outset that if participants are to develop healthily within their own worlds, they need to make intentional choices a practice that fosters personal responsibility and accountability for one's decisions and actions. This approach makes the journey wholly that of the participants, and one that they can celebrate as an achievement of their own (development). A family member provided this account of the process in her evaluation of the programme:

> *It takes a while, the shakedown period, when they are first in the group, you know, about how the leaders are not going to be telling them what they should be doing ... [there are] really clear processes. So building a raft like they did ... that's all got to be them pushing that thing ... it's not all going to come along on the back of a trailer ... they've got to build it, they have got to work out what they've got to do. ... [It's] their responsibility* (Family member of participant, 2010).

Pearce and Boyes's (2004) findings are consistent with those of Mossman (2005) and Russell (2005), both suggesting that a young person's readiness to make changes is an important element of the therapeutic change process. Mossman argues that consideration of young people's motivation to attend adventure therapy programmes is overlooked. Often, she says, the young people who enter such programmes do so on the recommendation (or direction) of adults, such as parents, teachers and counsellors, and they may not have the desire to make changes in their lives. An individual who self-refers into a programme usually has a degree of insight into their personal circumstances, abilities and behaviours. However, the young people who do enter adventure therapy programmes generally have been referred by others, partly because they do not have the degree of self-reflection/insight to take this step themselves. Such tends to be the case with the Waipuna programmes. While we do encounter young people who are very keen to participate (just as Mossman found), many have been pressured (or required) to attend the programme and, as a result, are not highly motivated to engage in processes focused on change processes. Working with these young people to establish goals can be a particularly complex and challenging situation. Interestingly, Mossman reported higher levels of motivation amongst young people who had been referred by peers. Peer referral is an approach that Waipuna promotes and supports.

My Journey Writings: Ihaka Moody

> *Sometimes when people make mistakes you automatically get ANGRY at them. But all you can do is remember that everyone makes mistakes and it's better for everyone if you just forgive and forget rather than just hold a grudge.*
>
> *I have improved a lot of things on this journey as well as I have had a lot to think about. I haven't got as angry because I have learnt to control my anger. As a result of that I haven't cursed as much either. Another thing*

> *that I haven't yet had a chance to practise is helping out my Nana, Granddad, Mum and even my brother.*
>
> *I'm sure that when I arrive back home they will all see a difference in the way I act towards them. I won't be as selfish and I will never backchat about doing a job when a job needs to be done.*
>
> *This journey has been cool but I still can't wait to be back in my own bed again!*
>
> *Bevan and Paul [facilitators] have been awesome to us. They have led the way and put so much into this journey. I sort of see them as role models. If I grew up to be like them that would be all good. If I had anything else to say it would be thank you Paul and Bevan and ... TE TIRA HOROMAKA Rules!!!!!!!!*
>
> *But last and definitely not least is HAPPY.*
>
> *This journey has really opened my eyes to the better things in life. Not everything is life has to do with technology. Sometimes it makes you feel good about yourself to just get outside, have some time to think, and really get into the idea of MANA.*

Ihaka's writings are sprinkled with unconscious reference to the programmes' success factors/themes identified by the evaluation undertaken by McKay and colleagues (2007) and confirmed by us, through our engagement with the Waipuna and its programmes during its eleven years of operation. Opportunity to share power and engage in mutual authoritative relationships along with the appropriate holistic approaches that honoured the 'whole of Ihaka' are the 'sunshine moments' in his writing, for they express life, growth and hope. Ihaka arrived at Waipuna with some significant challenges. He finished the programme having encountered critical experiences that allowed him to view his world through a different lens. By respecting and meeting Ihaka's developmental needs, Waipuna and its staff helped Ihaka confront, reflect on, and address the challenges and concerns that had long confronted him.

Ihaka's new discovery of who he is (identity, belonging) made for a cloak of many people hanging over his shoulders; he now felt he belonged. His ability to understand himself gave him more understanding of his whānau and of his taha whānau (reality) understanding that flowed on to a sense of growing mana within his whānau structure. When the opportunities (developmental experiences) arose, he grabbed them with a desire that was both intuitive and innate (biological mandate). Each progression added a piece to the jigsaw making up Ihaka's present life. The natural world (journey with ancestors) gave him reflective (and writing) space to encounter a new narrative. Paramount to his success was the relationships that walked with him; the trust he gathered through them meant he had a supportive reference point as he took more risk with his feelings, actions, peer relationships and the challenges associated with discovering himself. Ihaka expressed through his writing, qualities that were already inherent in him. The programme did not give him something he did not have but rather gave him relationships and experiences that allowed him to discover what was already there. All of this is embodied in Ihaka's comment that 'This journey has really opened my eyes to the better things in life.'

Conclusion

What we take from Ihaka's story and our consideration of the facets of the Waipuna trust programmes that he and many other 'challenged' young people have been part of is that a change of mind-set is needed if we are to truly address and honour the developmental needs of 'challenging' young people and their families. Young people need to be viewed as having wisdom. Because they generally do not know they are wise, they need experiences and supportive relationships that give them the ability to discover what is already inherent. Older wise people do not give these younger people wisdom but rather facilitate their ability to recognise their inherent wisdom. This wisdom then becomes their wisdom, their story, their contribution, and the ongoing ownership of that wisdom and of the decisions and actions it engenders logically follows. This positioning is very different from that in which young people are viewed as empty vessels that need filling up with everyone else's wisdom something young people encounter regularly, even in well-meaning adventure therapy programmes. We strongly believe that 'seeing young people as inherently wise' will make a significant difference to how we respect our young, across not only our programmes but indeed our whole society.

Authentic development programmes understand that young people are the biggest stakeholder, they form relationships based on mutual respect and honour the unique journey each individual must make and create within their diverse world views. This consideration needs to be reflected in decisions relating to the structure and delivery of the programmes; honouring every person with a respectful relationship, developing the whole person, power sharing, developing choice and responsibility, and creating a safe environment so each authentic story is honoured. Our role, as facilitators and leaders within these programmes, is to ensure we remain focussed on meeting the holistic needs of the participants, ensuring our structures from governance to management through to practice reflect a culture that is committed to fully developing every person as we choose to walk together.

REFERENCES

Bishop, R., Berryman, M., Tiakiwai, S., & Richardson, C. (2003). *Te Kōtahitanga: The experiences of Year 9 and 10 Māori students in mainstream classrooms*. Report to the Ministry of Education. Wellington, New Zealand: Ministry of Education.

Boyatzis, R. E. (1998). *Transforming qualitative information: Thematic analysis and code development.* Thousand Oaks, CA: Sage Publications.

Brendtro, L., Brokenleg, M., & Van Bockern, S. (2002). *Reclaiming youth at risk: The hope for our future.* Bloomington, IN: Solution Tree Press.

Cassidy, K. (2001). Enhancing your experiential programme with narrative theory. *Journal of Experiential Education, 24*(1), 22-27.

Covey, S. R. (2004). *The seven habits of highly effective people.* New York: Free Press.

Durie, M. (1994). *Whaiaora: Māori health development*. Auckland, New Zealand: Oxford University Press.

Hattie, J., Marsh, H., Neill, J., & Richards, G. (1997). Adventure education and Outward Bound: Out-of class experiences that make a lasting difference. *Review of Educational Research, 67*(1), 43-87.

Hersey, P., & Blanchard, K. (1982). *Management of organizational behaviour: Utilizing human resources* (4th ed.). Englewood Cliffs, NJ: Prentice-Hall.

Jansen, C. (2004). Adventure approaches with challenging adolescents: Ko Tane Mahuta Pupuke. *New Zealand Journal of Outdoor Education, 1*(3), 10-20.

Mckay, S., Donaldson, K. & Schroeder, R. (2007). *Project evaluation, adventure therapy: Pumanawa atawhai with young people and their families programme, St John of God Waipuna Trust*. The Collaborative for Research and Training in Youth Health and Development.

Mossman, E. (2005). *What works with youth? An evaluation of the Adventure Development Counselling programme.* Unpublished doctoral thesis. University of Canterbury, Christchurch, New Zealand.

Pearce, K., & Boyes, M. (2003). Determining readiness for therapeutic adventure programmes: The Transtheoretical Model. *Australian Journal of Outdoor Education, 7*(1), 37-45.

Rogers, C. (1960). *On becoming a person: A therapist's view of psychotherapy.* New York: Houghton Mi'in.

Russell, K. (2005). Two years later: A qualitative assessment of youth well-being and the role of aftercare in outdoor behavioural healthcare treatment. *Child and Youth Care Forum, 34*(3) 209-244.

Schusser, E. (2005). Making a difference. In T. Dickson, T. Gray, & B. Hayllar (Eds.), *Outdoor and experiential Learning: Views from the top* (104-108). Dunedin, New Zealand: Otago University Press.

Watchel, T., & McCold, P. (2001). Restorative justice and everyday life. In J.Braithwaite & H. Strang (Eds.),*Restorative justice in civil society* (pp. 117-125). New York: Cambridge University Press.

West, S. & Crompton, J. (2001). A Review of the impact of adventure programmes on at risk youth. *Journal of Park and Recreation Administration, 19*(2), 113-140.

Glossary of Maori Terms

Aotearoa New Zealand, land of the long white cloud

Aroha to love, feel concern for, feel compassion and empathy

Haka dance, to perform

Hinengaro mind, thought, intellect, consciousness, awareness

Kai food

Kawa protocols; customs related to greeting and the like

Mana prestige, authority, status, spiritual power

Rangatiratanga sovereignty, chieftainship, right to exercise authority

Te tira Horomaka tiraa®travelling party; Horomaka-Ngai Tahu geographical area

Tikanga correct procedure, custom, practice, convention

Tinana the main part of anything person, self, reality

Wairua spirit, soul of a person that exists beyond death

Whānau family group, extended family

Ihaka's self-narrated story has been shared with audiences throughout New Zealand, Australia, and Scotland. Each time the audience has been invited to write brief notes telling him how his story has affected them. He now has over 600 pieces of feedback and he continues to be humbled and moved that people think his story has added meaning to other people's lives. The ongoing therapeutic value continues well after the programme has finished its delivery.

CHAPTER 8

The Aboriginal Outdoor Recreation Program: Connection with Country, Culture, Family and Community

Peter Rae and Aunty Verna Nichols, Aboriginal Elder

ABSTRACT

The journeys of the Tasmanian Aboriginal people from European invasion to contemporary culture provides a unique opportunity to explore the impact of an adventure therapy approach in reconnecting people to country and family. This paper explores the impact the Aboriginal Outdoor Recreation Program (AORP) has on Aboriginal people in Tasmania and their communities.

The AORP provides participants opportunities for personal growth in an environment of cultural practices, both historical and contemporary, supported by outdoor recreation activities. One of the key factors is supporting participants to spend time on country of cultural significance to them. This has proven to have powerful impacts on individual behaviour and the community-building process.

Family is an important aspect of this community, and there are often strong family connections between participants, cultural facilitators and Elders on a program. Personal growth outcomes for younger members of the community in this environment are increased by the presence of senior family members or community Elders. They are witnesses to positive behavioural change and can later reinforce these in the family or community setting. Thus, old patterns of behaviour are no longer supported by either family or community. The transfer of positive attitudinal and behavioural change witnessed in the program is enhanced by the ongoing support of senior family members or community Elders participating in the program.

> One of the most significant observations from this program is the power of the country (bush/natural environment) to allow a safe and respectful space for communities and individuals to gain strength. People connect with each other at a deep level uninhibited by modern distractions in the urban environment.

INTRODUCTION

> *'Time spent on Aboriginal land is so important and can do more than anything else in helping our people and community reconnect to their culture and heritage'* (Nichols 2009)

As a facilitator and project officer for the AORP, and based on the author's experience of over ten years in the field of bush and adventure therapy, I believe we can do no better than to listen to the voices and ancient wisdom of the Indigenous Elders of our country, in order to use the bush/wilderness/outdoor environment in ways that support people to heal and grow. This wisdom comes from a culture based on practices that are connected with the landscape and country, and from the understanding that 'we belong to the land' rather than the land belongs to us (Sveiby & Skuthorpe, 2006; West, 1987). These practices have been disrupted over the last two hundred years in Tasmania, since European invasion and settlement. In Tasmania, the contemporary Aboriginal community are actively reawakening this wisdom of culture and country, to help heal and strengthen a community and people that are suffering from trauma since this invasion (Atkinson, 2002; West,1987).

A populist view of adventure therapy as a recently-evolved form of 'treatment' is possibly only relevant to contemporary cultures that have long forgotten their Indigenous roots. For some Australian Aborigines, the therapeutic benefits of the bush are still part of a living history, even in Tasmania where near genocide removed almost all trace of an Aboriginal people that were an integral part of the landscape and environment (Reynolds, 1995; Smith, 1965; Sveiby & Skuthorpe, 2006). A small number of Aboriginal people in Tasmania survived, and continued to practice elements of traditional culture; this knowledge is now helping to reawaken other aspects of their culture.

This is being supported in part through the AORP (a wilderness therapy program), and other 'Back on Country' programs delivered in Tasmania, such as melythina tiakana warrana (Heart of Country) (Matson-Green, 2009).

The experiences and perspectives of the Elders, the middle mob, the youth and children connecting to their country, the culture, family and community define the essence of the AORP.

This paper tells the story of the AORP through the voices of Tasmanian Aboriginal participants. Observations for how and why this program impacts participants are discussed under the following sections:

- AORP description
- Author's perspective
- An Elder's story
- The Aboriginal community's journey of healing through connection to country, culture, family and community
- Wilderness therapy within the context of a contemporary program
- Now and for the future the continuing journey.

Program Description

The AORP is a State Government program delivered through Sport and Recreation Tasmania (part of the Department of Economic Development, Tourism and the Arts).

The AORP program has been running for ten years, and has evolved as part of a much larger journey towards healing for the Aboriginal people in Tasmania. Individual people in the Aboriginal community began the process of reconnecting to country for healing and wellbeing. This process then progressed to include families, which prompted the Tasmanian Aboriginal Centre to deliver several 'Back to country' and 'Health and wellbeing for women' programs (Langford, R. personal communication, August 2009).

In 2000, the Project Hahn program (now the Wilderness Program a mainstream community adventure therapy program service provider, also delivered through Sport and Recreation Tasmania) began implementing the AORP. This program has since developed through feedback from participants, community leaders, facilitators and Elders to its present status within the Tasmanian State Government. The AORP will continue to evolve and grow to meet the changing needs and priorities of the Aboriginal People in Tasmania.

Within AORP, one full time employed position is allocated to manage relationships with community organisations and individuals, develop program proposals and implement the delivery. Wilderness therapy facilitators, cultural leaders and community mentors are employed on a part time basis to meet the unique needs of each program's activities. The Wilderness Program assists the

AORP (as a sister organization) through program delivery. The AORP delivers programs to meet community needs using cultural, adventure and wilderness therapy activities that include:

- A range of cultural/bush/adventure camps
- Residential (on country) 'Wilderness therapy' and 'Community Mentor' training programs
- Day activities as part of the pre and post camp program
- Single day activities

DEFINITIONS USED IN THIS PAPER

WiT Wilderness therapy, as underpinned by the bush counselling processes used by the Wilderness Program (formerly Project Hahn) (Adams & Sveen, 2000).

AORP Aboriginal Outdoor Recreation Program delivered by Sport and Recreation Tasmania through the Department of Economic Development, Tourism and the Arts Tasmania, Australia.

WiP Wilderness Program delivered by Sport and Recreation Tasmania through the Department of Economic Development, Tourism and the Arts Tasmania, Australia.

Black fella an Aboriginal person of Australia.

White fella a person of European descent or non – Aboriginal heritage.

Middle mob members of the Tasmanian Aboriginal community from young to middle aged adults.

Full Value Agreement a contract of social norms that is formed at the beginning of each program or activity by the participants and facilitators. The words and descriptions will vary but will always cover at least: physical and emotional safety, positive/constructive feedback, no putdowns, respect of each other and environment, no drugs/alcohol, no sexual/intimate relationships or other exclusive behaviour and goal setting (Adams & Sveen, 2000; Priest & Gass, 2005; Schoel, Prouty & Radcliffe, 1988).

AUTHOR'S PERSPECTIVE: PETER RAE

The Aboriginal story of the last 200 years cannot be separated from the European story in this country. For me it is a real honour and a privilege to be a part of telling this story of the Aboriginal people of Tasmania. My story is from the perspective of a facilitator, program coordinator and white fella. It is about observations on country with participants, and through conversations following time spent on country. It is not based on a quantitative scientific study or review of the program (which is often the white man's way). However, qualitative evaluations are completed by participants after programs, and these have been used to inform the process of program evolution. My intent here is to keep closer in essence to the way the Aboriginal people in Tasmania would tell their story; I am also a participant in this story.

For me it has been an interesting journey to be involved with an Aboriginal program and community in Tasmania. In the beginning it was about understanding their journey, where they have come from, where they are, and now where they are heading. I observed early on many of the strengths and values that the Aboriginal people and their community held, and how these had shaped and maintained the present community. These must also have been integral to this community over thousands of generations. From my perspective as an outsider to the Aboriginal community, I could observe the great value that these may have for all communities.

Slowly over time I have built trusting relationships with participants, community leaders and Elders, through which deeper issues could be discussed. I have witnessed and been involved in the increasing acceptance of cultural values and differences from both Aboriginal and non-Aboriginal people in this program over the last seven to eight years. It has been recognised by both black fellas and white fellas that this is a journey that we are taking together.

Why is this increasing acceptance occurring? I believe that through a connection to land/ country, culture and community/family some healing of past trauma is occurring. Pain and grief are being released through this process and people have the space or capacity in themselves for acceptance and reconciliation. This is reflected in the feedback from participants, community mentors and Elders. The journey of black and white fellas together is significant in this process to allow healing across the whole community. It cannot happen fully for one without the other.

An Elder's Story: Aunty Verna Nichols

This story may be best described through the voice of an Elder of the Aboriginal people of Tasmania. In the following paragraphs, Aunty Verna Nichols tells a part of her story as an Aborigine from Tasmania, her connection to the country, and how the AORP is supporting many of her community to reconnect with country and their Aboriginal heritage:

> *'To me an Aboriginal person is one with their country. By this I mean that we have a connection to the earth; the earth is our mother, our heart, which in turn ties us together to the rest of our country. We have had this connection for over 30 thousand years in Tasmania.*
>
> *For a long period in our Aboriginal history the invasion of Europeans made life hard as our land was taken over and killing of my people became common practice. The Government of the day paid soldiers and European settlers money for capture or killing of Tasmanian Aboriginal people. Many were rounded up and sent to a reserve on Cape Barren Island, in Tasmania. My mother was born on this reserve and I was 4 years old when this reserve was closed. Our land, heritage, some cultural practices, some traditions, language were denied my ancestors and it was thought that through assimilation Tasmanian Aboriginal people would be gone forever. I speak to you now from what I call a living history, this living history is not only my story but of Aboriginal people back home. We are a very proud, strong race of people and I believe that our cultural practices, traditions, have only been asleep in us, not lost forever. We have been awakened by the spirits of our ancestors. Secret women's business and secret men's business is practiced once again by my people.*
>
> *The AORP allows participants to reconnect with family old and new, make new friends and strengthen connections between ourselves and the wider community.*
>
> *Some of the youth and young adults of my community know they are Aboriginal but for many different reasons have never been out in the bush, out into their country, not experienced the land and what it can offer them; not been able to find their heart, their connectedness to mother earth. This program enables all participants to learn country and*

for some to travel ancestral land. Important lessons are learnt on the way, spiritual connections, survival skills. Long, long walks enable people to talk, laugh and learn together, sometimes it is all too much for some. At the end of the day participants are feeling different about themselves, they are glad that they made it to the end. Other activities that look too hard are completed by some; others don't try, but this is ok. This continues for the length of the camp and towards the end my heart is flt to burst as I watch them go from strength to strength.

Sometime, somehow, somewhere on their journey they found that they do belong, have found their connectedness to mother earth. Finding out about their ancestors, speaking up for the first time in front of others, asking questions and finding answers. This program is so very important for participants' self-esteem, confidence, well-being, trust, faith and respect for themselves and each other. This program brings the best out in people, enables some to reach out to others for the first time, realising that they are not the only one with problems, speaking about them, knowing people are really listening and are prepared to help if they can.

The Aboriginal Outdoor Recreation Program run by Sport and Recreation Tasmania is offered to the Aboriginal community to strengthen individuals and community through culture and adventure. Dedicated people from this department and Aboriginal community have not only planned this program but more importantly have put it into action' (Nichols, 2009).

The Aboriginal Community Journey: Healing through Connection to Country, Culture, Family and Community

Since the invasion by Europeans of their country in the early 1800's and the following destruction of their culture and heritage, the Aboriginal people in Tasmania have been on a journey to reconnect with each other, their country and culture (Reynolds, 1995; Smith, 1965).

Through the voices of participants of the AORP, their closer connection to country, culture and community through its activities are described. Observations as to why and how this is occurring are offered, along with some conclusions as to the impact on the contemporary Aboriginal community in Tasmania. The strengthening and healing begins through listening to the voices of the Elders.

Connection/Reconnection to Culture

> It is important that we pass on our knowledge now, to our youngster, because if we don't when we are gone it will go with us. (AORP Elder, Gathering at Murrayfield, Bruny Island Tasmania, April 2009)

The traditional culture of the Tasmanian Aboriginals was one strongly connected to the country and the natural environment in which they lived, where large family groups were the basis of their small communities. In recent times the Aboriginal people in Tasmania, as a people, have begun the conscious process of reconnecting with the land and culture. They are doing this through the knowledge and understanding of traditional culture, with the Elders, and reawakening cultural understanding by participating in and creating contemporary cultural practices which strengthen this connection. The concepts that are used in adventure therapy programs today were once an integral part of traditional culture. The AORP is one contemporary avenue where this process has been reinvigorated. The program is continually being strengthened as the community leadership and sense of ownership of it grows and evolves.

From recorded conversations before, during and post programs, and written comments on evaluation forms from participants, community leaders and Elders, it has become apparent that the community is in a phase of strengthening identity and healing, and that the AORP can have a significant role in supporting this.

In Tasmanian Aboriginal people, the anger and pain of past trauma is carried in the current generation, and needs to be 'heard' to allow the healing to begin. After participating in an educational/cultural activity called 'Gum Nuts to Buttons', a young man on the program provided his response to the European/Aboriginal conflict over the last two hundred years:

> It makes me really angry to learn and understand how my people and culture have been treated. (personal communication, November, 2006)

When this pain and hurt is expressed physically and emotionally, what is done with it? Time spent on country with family or community Elders, reconnecting to the land and practicing traditional and contemporary cultural activities helps healing. Listening to the voices of the Elders (their own stories of trauma and healing) may help guide the anger to some positive outcomes in identifying as an Aboriginal, understanding the culture and connecting to non-Aboriginal people. The connection of Elders to the younger generations is absolutely vital for the health and wellbeing of individuals, families and community. It is essential that opportunities for this to occur are created and then supported by the Aboriginal community, broader society and the government.

As highlighted below, the health and wellbeing of Aboriginal and non-Aboriginal people cannot occur in isolation from one another. One twelve-year-old participant wrote about what part of the cultural and heritage program was most meaningful to him in a post program evaluation questionnaire:

> Realising that some Europeans are not bad!' (AORP participant questionnaire, 2008). Belonging/connection to country 'I realise I need to continually connect with country even as simply as spending an evening around a fire yarning with a group of fellas. (personal communication with King during a Wilderness Therapy course for AORP community mentors, September 2008)

The importance of connection to country cannot be overstated. In Tasmania the Indigenous people and culture have been relatively recently removed from their land. This physical removal has not been enough to sever the emotional and spiritual connection to country, and these links are strongly felt and described when the opportunity to spend time on significant country is available. Although this physical connection was taken away, their emotional and spiritual connection to the land remains, and allows people to reconnect to country. This seems to be highlighted when Aboriginal groups go out on country in the context of a family or community setting. While a sense of belonging for individuals is immediately apparent in this bush environment, the practical understanding is sometimes lacking and needs to be learned. It is clear that Aboriginal participants feel comfortable and at home in the bush, it is a safe place for them. This is highlighted in the following comment by an AORP facilitator in a post program letter to a participant:

> Another incident that stuck in my mind was when we got lost on the way back from the cave. You managed to work with the group to find your way back to track. Excellent work! You are obviously really comfortable walking around the bush. (Facilitator, Tasmanian Government, 2009)

This reflects positive risk-taking in terms of behaviours and actions, despite the group heading in the wrong direction. In this supportive and safe environment, where mistakes can be made and lessons learned without fear of negative peer pressure or punishment, participants are encouraged to make decisions even if their choices are poor. The consequences for their choices and actions are held in place by being on country in a community setting that includes an agreement made on social norms (or full value agreement).

What is essential in maximising the level of healing and wellbeing from the AORP, is the opportunity for participants to spend time on culturally significant land. The therapeutic and healing benefits are evident from the comments of participants during and following opportunities to spend time on country. During a multiday walking program to a remote culturally significant Aboriginal site a participant stated:

> This has helped give me an understanding why I have been carrying this anger with me, what I can do to help others in similar situations so they don't have to go through all that I have. I can see how this (AORP) can benefit so many of our fellas who don't even realise why they are angry and keep getting into trouble. (personal communication, January 2009)

Traditional/Contemporary Culture

> I feel so relaxed out here with no stress, more comfortable in the bush. I'd like to go back to the islands (Bass strait Islands) to go birding (mutton birding, a traditional/contemporary cultural practice) after I get out. (personal communication with a 16-year-old male participant in the middle of the southwest world heritage area of Tasmania, January 2009)

What can happen in this environment when people are feeling safe and comfortable is a reconnection to culture through participation in contemporary cultural activities based on traditional practices. This occurs in the context of the landscape where the participants are asked to consider the traditional practices of their ancestors. The following types of questions guide cultural facilitators: Why and how would our ancestors have lived here? Where are the food, water and shelter? Spending time on country is about connecting on an emotional/spiritual level with the land. The transfer of knowledge and understanding that occurs from Elders to youngsters through these questions and stories is about connection and healing at physical, mental, emotional and spiritual levels. All these elements are vital in strengthening culture and community so that the pain and suffering of the past can begin to be addressed. Community mentor Ruth Langford surmises this succinctly:

> In the urban environment the intergenerational post-traumatic stress is numbed through alcohol and other drugs and may be vented through

> anger and violence which does not allow any real healing to occur. (personal communication with Langford, August 2009)

Family and Community

> I am amazed how well they have got along, no arguing or whining and it has been easier to hold my tongue. It has been fantastic to watch them really give things a go that they struggled with and achieved, not do it for them! (personal communication with a father after observing his son's actions and behaviours during a community camp, Dickson, June 2008)

The community-building process may occur more easily when a group undertakes a journey together. For participants attending the AORP, it is significant that this journey is out on country that is either of cultural significance, or owned and managed by the Aboriginal community. The community-building is further strengthened when family relationships, mentor roles and Elder connections are considered in the participant selection. This deeper community structure mirrors the past and taps into the traditional practice of traveling across the landscape in family groups or tribes.

What has been observed when the processes described above are put into place? There is often a strong level of respect between Elders and younger participants that is evident from the beginning of the AORP experience, which helps to create a safe and supportive environment. This encourages positive risk taking when opportunities for participants to try new behaviours or attitudes present themselves. This is evident by the group working cooperatively to prepare a meal, when they are facing the challenge of an abseil or caving activity, or involvement for the first time in a cultural practice. For example a week out in the bush on culturally significant country practicing traditional and contemporary culture supported by adventure activities allowed two young boys to shine in a strong family and community setting without the distractions of the urban environment. On the journey back to town at the end of the program, the negative behaviours exhibited by these two young boys in the back of the vehicle as we approached city limits strongly contrasted with the positive strengthening behaviours of the past week in the bush. This was brought to their attention before they left later in the day, and again with Elders, uncles and aunties during post program debriefs and discussions.

This type of experience is often observed when aunties, uncles and Elders relate to the younger participants on program, spend time together on country.

The impact for the youngsters is that positive behavioural change is observed and supported by significant older people in their lives. This allows strengthening of follow-up opportunities after programs where continuing positive behaviours can be supported and relapses into old patterns of behaviour are highlighted. The impact on the Elders in witnessing this behavioural change can be an increased understanding of the youngster's abilities, and an understanding about how to support this in the future.

It is through these program experiences that strategies for future programs have been informed and developed to strengthen community involvement and support for positive behavioural changes. This can create change at a community level and not just be isolated to a behavioural shift at the individual level.

Wilderness Therapy (WiT)

WiT, as outlined by the bush-counselling model, is adapted in various ways to support the cultural and adventure based program activities (Adams et al., 2000). WiT practice is based on theories and practices such as lifespan development, behaviourist theory, Gestalt therapies, person centred therapy, existential therapy and brief therapies, and uses tools that include edgework and disequilibrium, experiential and heuristic learning, social norm setting, non-directive group work, group developmental dynamics, natural consequence, individual goal setting, mastery and journey (Adams et al., 2000).

At the beginning of each program, the main emphasis is on building trust, support and a safe physical, emotional and spiritual environment. When this occurs, issues of depth or stories of healing are allowed to come from the participants as they spend more time on country with families and Elders learning their culture. In contrast to some mainstream wilderness therapy processes, the wisdom of the Elders precludes the use of direct methods of questioning and formal counselling in the early formative part of programs. Instead, facilitators, mentors and Elders use storytelling and allow time for participants to gain the understanding and confidence so that they can begin to tell their own stories.

Now and for the Future

The AORP will continue to allow a safe and respected space for community and individuals to gain strength, healing and wellbeing through connection to country, culture, community and family. It will continue to be a place for contemporary culture to grow and evolve, and for connection with existing and reawakened elements of traditional culture and heritage. And it will continue to support a community and a people who have survived past traumas and who can gain strength and a sense of purpose from this awareness to continue their journey of healing and wellbeing.

This program has provided opportunities for Aboriginal and non-Aboriginal people to work together towards healing, as individuals and communities, and to share knowledge within the sphere of wilderness therapy.

The AORP will endeavour to inform mainstream practices in adventure therapy and wilderness therapy in ways of 'being and doing' that come from the wisdom of the Aboriginal culture and its Elders. These wisdoms hold significance and relevance for all people who find themselves on a journey of healing and wellbeing.

REFERENCES

Adams, A. & Sveen, R. (2000). An holistic model of bush counselling: Cornerstones of practice. *Australian Journal of Outdoor Education, 5*(1) pp. 28-38.

Atkinson, J. (2002). *Trauma trails: Recreating song lines, The transgenerational effects of trauma in indigenous communities*. North Melbourne: Spinifex Press.

Matson-Green, V. (2009 November 11). *Melythina tiakana warrana (Heart of Country) program*. Speech presented for the Tasmanian Aboriginal Healing Project community workshop, Hobart & Launceston, Tasmania, Australia.

Nichols, V. (2009). *AORP-connection to country, culture and family.* Speech presented at the 5IATC, Edinburgh University, Edinburgh, Scotland.

Priest, S. & Gass, M.A. (2005). *Effective leadership in adventure programming* (2nd ed.). Illinois: Human Kinetics Publishers.

Reynolds, H. (1995). *Fate of a free people*. Australia: Penguin Group Australia.

Schoel, J., Prouty, D. & Radcliffe, P. (1988). *Islands of healing*: *A guide to adventure based counselling.* Hamilton, MA: Project Adventure.

Smith, P. A. (1965). *Moonbird people.* Adelaide: Rigby Limited.

Sveiby, K-E., & Skuthorpe, T. (2006). *Treading lightly.* Sydney: Allen and Unwin.

Tasmanian Government Internal Reports. (2008). *AORP annual report, June 2008.* Hobart, Tasmania: Rae, P.

Tasmanian Government internal reports. (2009). *AORP participant report, January 2009.* Hobart, Tasmania: Fairlie, R.

West, I. (1987). *Pride against prejudice*. Canberra: Montpelier Press.

CHAPTER 9

The Aboriginal Youth Resilience Study: Promoting Resilience and Well-being through Outdoor Adventure Leadership Experience

Stephen Ritchie, Mary Jo Wabano, Robert Schinke, Duke Peltier, Brenda Restoule, Keith Russell, Rita Corbiere, and Nancy Young

ABSTRACT

It is imperative that we improve the mental health of Aboriginal youth in Canada. From an Aboriginal worldview, mental health must be approached in concert with the promotion of spiritual, physical, and emotional health. This holistic approach is concordant with the processes implicit in programs using outdoor adventure and experiential education (OAEE). Programs using OAEE have proven effective in improving the mental health of youth at risk in mainstream populations; yet there is little evidence of their effectiveness on the resilience and well-being of Aboriginal youth.

We used a 3-phase study design that began with a community-based participatory approach to develop an outdoor adventure leadership experience within one Aboriginal community in Canada (Phase 1). We then applied culturally reflexive strategies in the context of a mixed method research design to evaluate the program's effect on the resilience and well-being of youth using both quantitative methods (Phase 2), and qualitative methods (Phase 3). This paper describes the methods, description of the sample, and initial findings from the qualitative analysis. The qualitative results suggest that the outdoor adventure leadership experience had a positive effect on resilience. These initial findings are encouraging, since the program has been fully accepted and endorsed by the community.

Introduction

The promotion of mental health is a well-documented priority for Aboriginal Canadians (Dumont-Smith, 2005; Government of Canada, 2006, chap. 12), especially among youth (First Nations Inuit and Aboriginal Health [FNIAH], 2003). Since Aboriginal people live throughout Canada, and their youth are the most rapidly growing segment of the Canadian population, their well-being should be a critical national concern. In 2008 a group of Aboriginal leaders and university researchers collaborated to refine, implement, and evaluate a novel intervention using principles of outdoor adventure and experiential education (OAEE). The intervention was designed to promote the resilience and well-being of Aboriginal youth from one Canadian reserve. This paper describes the research design phases, and presents early results from the study. Additional papers will follow that will provide more detail on a broader array of outcomes.

Background

The term Aboriginal, in the Canadian context, usually refers to indigenous populations and includes status and non-status Indians, Métis, and Inuit (Indian and Northern Affairs Canada, 2004). The term First Nations refers primarily to North American Indian communities (or status and non-status Indians living on and off reserves throughout the country). However, the terms Aboriginal and First Nations are sometimes used interchangeably because First Nations are the largest group within the Canadian Aboriginal community. Oppressive colonial policies over the years, such as the residential school system, and the centuries long legacy of imperialism, have left a dramatic negative impact on Aboriginal health and mental health status (for a review see Royal Commission on Aboriginal Peoples in Canada, 1996). The Aboriginal population in Canada has been marginalized and has suffered from poor socio-economic conditions comparable to those in developing nations (Canadian UNICEF Committee, 2009; Dumont-Smith, 2005).

The rapidly growing First Nations (FN) population has poorer health status than the rest of the Canadian population with higher rates of many chronic and infectious diseases, higher hospitalization rates, and lower life expectancy (Adelson, 2005; Dumont-Smith, 2005; Government of Canada, 2006). Mental health is critically low among FN people, as seen in higher rates of anxiety and depression (Government of Canada, 2006), and suicide rates that are twice the Canadian rate (Health Canada, 2005). Suicide rates among FN youth (15-24 years of age) are five to seven times higher than national rates for males and females respectively (Canadian Institute of Child Health, 2000). The aforementioned is not a problem unique to Canada, as these suicide rates are similar to those reported for indigenous people in other colonial countries such as the United States and Australia (Hunter & Harvey, 2002).

In 2001, a federal task force met to discuss youth suicide in Canada (FNIAH, 2003). Their report, entitled 'Acting On What We Know: Preventing Youth Suicide in First Nations', underscored the need to develop strategies to address youth suicide in a holistic way, emphasizing culture (FNIAH, 2003). In particular, two of the main themes were: (a) supporting a community-driven approach; and (b) creating strategies for building youth identity, resilience and culture (FNIAH, 2003). Concurrently, Kirmayer and colleagues concluded that 'mental health promotion that emphasizes youth and community empowerment is likely to have broad effects on mental health and well-being of Aboriginal communities' (Kirmayer, Simpson, & Cargo, 2003, p. S15). This study takes a look at how these recommendations were incorporated into a strategy to address the compelling need for mental health promotion among children and youth within one Aboriginal community.

An Aboriginal approach to mental health promotion encompasses the concept of well-being, which is holistic (spiritual, mental, physical, and emotional), relational (self, others, and nature), and integrated (individual, community, and culture) (Hart, 1998; Hill, 2006). Aboriginal well-being and healing philosophies do not separate mental health from other aspects of health, and include a more comprehensive and inter-connected view of a state of balance and harmony within the individual as well as within the family, the community, and the larger environment (Hunter, Logan, Goulet, & Barton, 2006; Wilson, 2003).

Resilience is an important mental health construct for this study since it was identified as a priority for Aboriginal youth suicide prevention (FNIAH, 2003), and it is considered a protective factor for community and youth development (Brennan, 2008). Wright and Masten (2006) stated that 'resilience typically refers to a pattern of positive adaptation in the context of past or present adversity' (p. 18). Wagnild and Young (1993) described the moderating effect of resilience on the negative effects of stress and suggested that it promotes adaptation. Others have defined resilience similarly, suggesting that the concept is characterized by the development or promotion of positive factors in the face of adversity, risk, and negative experiences (Ahern, 2006; Fergus & Zimmerman, 2005). Beyond the individual, the concept of resilience can also include family, interpersonal, community and social/cultural characteristics that function as assets or protective factors that are not necessarily linked directly to risk and adversity (Wright & Masten, 2006).

The holistic approach in Aboriginal health and resilience is concordant with the holistic processes that are implicit in outdoor adventure (Berger & McLeod, 2006; Beringer & Martin, 2003; Martin, 2002) and experiential education contexts (Foster & Linney, 2007; Quay, 2003). Outdoor adventure contexts involving groups of people can be holistic in developing a sense of community through physical, mental, emotional, and often spiritual experiences that occur collaboratively in natural environments (Foster & Linney, 2007; Martin, 2002). Pryor, Carpenter, and Townsend (2005) referred to this holistic process as a spectrum of outdoor experiences and interventions that they described as a socio-ecological approach to promoting health and well-being.

Many OAEE-type programs follow an expeditionary model, where a program is delivered to a small group of participants during a wilderness excursion. The excursion is planned to include multiple natural challenges requiring teamwork and individual effort to overcome. Hence, these challenges could represent a proxy natural intervention for the risk experiences and adversity characteristic of resilience in life. Ungar (2005) described this connection further, suggesting that there is a 'remarkable similarity between the anticipated outcomes from outdoor adventure programming and characteristics of resilient individuals' (p. 325). Thus, we hypothesized that an OAEE-type experience may provide an intervention well-suited to Aboriginal youth.

In the past few decades, there has been mounting evidence of therapeutic benefits of OAEE in a variety of populations (Neill & Richards, 1998). In particular, a meta-analysis of 96 studies using adventure education indicated that well designed OAEE-type programs are effective (Hattie, Marsh, Neill, & Richards, 1997). Russell (2003) demonstrated the efficacy of targeted wilderness therapy programs for youth at risk through improved behavioral functioning, and Clark, Marmol, Cooley, and Gathercoal (2004) demonstrated significant behavioral change, and also positive chacterological changes (personality) for troubled adolescents in wilderness therapy. Additionally, Neill and Dias (2001), Ewert and Yoshino (2008), and Shellman (2009) conducted independent studies with experimental designs and concluded that resilience was enhanced via outdoor adventure education.

Despite the accumulating evidence from outcome studies, there is a dearth of evidence on the efficacy of OAEE-type programs with respect to resilience and well-being among Aboriginal youth. Hence, our research team used a collaborative approach to develop, implement and evaluate an intervention program entitled the Outdoor Adventure Leadership Experience (OALE). The OALE targeted Aboriginal youth who live on reserve, a cohort identified as a high-risk age group within an at-risk population (FNIAH, 2003; Health Canada, 2005).

METHODS

The methods reflected a collaborative approach between community leaders from Wikwemikong Unceded Indian Reserve (WUIR) and researchers from Laurentian University (LU). Both WUIR and LU are located in northern Ontario, Canada, the study setting. This region of northern Ontario is in a Boreal forest, and the topography includes many lakes, rivers and rocky outcroppings, and rolling terrain typical of the Canadian Shield. An important component of the collaboration was obtaining ethics approval from the University and Aboriginal community research ethics boards, both of which granted written approval. In addition, the entire research project was then reviewed and supported within WUIR by the Waasa Naabin Youth Services Centre, the Health Services Committee, and through a Band Council Motion. University and community leaders signed a research agreement to ensure responsibilities and expectations were clear, and a community research steering committee (CRSC) was established to both review and guide the research process within the community.

There were three phases to the research. Table 1 provides an outline of these phases and research questions. In Phase 1 we used principles of community-based participatory action research (CBPAR) to refine the OALE program. In Phase 2 and 3 we used a concurrent transformative mixed-method study design (Creswell, 2009) to implement and evaluate the program. Preliminary results will be reported in this paper, and several subsequent papers will present additional detail on the findings.

POPULATION AND SAMPLE

The target population for the intervention was 12 to 18 year old adolescents from one FN reserve (WUIR). The age bracket was identified by WUIR community leaders and was a group at-risk of poor mental health. Given the heterogeneity of FN populations and language groups across Canada, sampling from within one relatively homogeneous community was deemed important for study validity. WUIR was selected because the research team had an established program of research within the community (Schinke, et al., 2009), and there was some pre-existing infrastructure to support youth wilderness programming. Moreover, both WUIR and LU were easily accessible (170 km by road).

WUIR is a progressive reserve with established infrastructure and self-governance in the areas of health, education, policing, and land management. There was a population of 7,272 status Indian members registered in 2009 with a total of 891 youth aged 12-18 (Indian and Northern Affairs Canada, 2009). However, only 442 youth (status Indians) lived on the reserve at one time (Indian and Northern Affairs Canada, 2009), and approximately 1-2% of WUIR is comprised of non-status Indians (Statistics Canada, 2007). Hence, the available population was estimated at approximately 450 status and non-status youth aged 12-18.

The sample was recruited through a community-led promotional campaign utilizing advertising, referral, recruitment and self-selection. Adolescents were primarily recruited through the Waasa Naabin Youth Services Centre, and through several summer youth training and employment initiatives. Thus, the participants were a sample of convenience.

The program was offered free of charge to reduce financial barriers to participation. Exclusion criteria included pre-existing physical and mental health conditions. Physical health was screened through a participant enrolment form and the Physical Activity and Readiness Questionnaire (PAR-Q) (available from Canadian Society for Exercise Physiology, 2002). Mental health was assessed via the Health and Well-Being Questionnaire (see Phase 2 for a description) administered the day before each intervention began. In any cases where these screenings indicated reason for concern, local health care providers were requested to do a more detailed assessment to determine whether it was safe for that participant to proceed with the OALE program, or to intervene clinically to protect the health of the participant.

Table 1 Study design phases and research questions

	Phase 1	Phase 2	Phase 3
Approach	Qualitative	Quantitative	Qualitative
Design	CBPAR	Concurrent Transformative Mixed Method	
Research Question	What is a culturally relevant OALE?	Does the OALE intervention promote resilience and well-being for WUIR adolescents?	How does the OALE promote resilience and well-being?
Follow-up Question	N/A	Are any observed changes in resilience and well-being sustained over 12 months?	To what extent do participants attribute changes in their resilience and well-being scores to the OALE or other intervening factors?

Note. CBPAR = Community-Based Participatory Action Research; OALE = Outdoor Adventure leadership Experience; WUIR = Wikwemikong Unceded Indian Reserve.

Phase 1 Methods: Refining the OALE using CBPAR

The purpose of this phase was to refine a culturally relevant OALE program (intervention) with WUIR through a series of community planning meetings and focus groups. A community-based participatory action research (CBPAR) design was used as this approach was well established in the literature (Caldwell, et al., 2005; Maiter, Simich, Jacobson, & Wise, 2008; Minore, Boone, Katt, Kinch, & Birch, 2004). The principles of CBPAR are rooted in a family of collaborative community-based participatory research (CBPR) approaches gaining currency in health related research (for an overview see Israel, Eng, Schulz, & Parker, 2005; Minkler & Wallerstein, 2008). Over the course of ten months starting in the fall of 2008, the OALE program was developed from our earlier work (Schinke, et al., 2009), and then refined as a prototype intervention program for youth in the community (see Ritchie, et al., 2010).

The collaborative process involved a series of 17 community meetings, presentations, and training sessions; three CRSC meetings; and two targeted focus groups with Elders, seniors and mental health workers (Ritchie, et al., 2010). Prior to implementation, WUIR leaders and assistant leaders were trained to facilitate the OALE program (intervention).

Beyond Phase 1, the following two phases of the research design were considered transformative since the methodology was rooted in a participatory/advocacy worldview (Creswell, 2009), a lens that also reflects the principles of CBPAR and CBPR.

Phase 2 Methods: Outcome Evaluation of OALE Intervention

The purpose of the second phase was to determine empirically whether Aboriginal youths' resilience and well-being improved as a result of the OALE intervention. This was assessed using a Health and Well-Being Questionnaire (HWBQ) that was a combination of 9 previously developed scales and had 78 individual items. The 9 scales were selected based on their relevance to resilience and well-being, their face validity in an Aboriginal context based on the assessment of the CRSC, and the scales' measurement properties. The combined form of the HWBQ was pilot tested before implementation.

We administered the HWBQ to the participants over two summer seasons during the pre-trip preparation day immediately before each OALE program (intervention), and then approximately one month post-intervention. This paper provides a description of the characteristics of the sample and information on self-rated general health and mental health. Further details on the HWBQ questionnaire and results from the resilience and well-being scales will be reported in separate publications.

Phase 3 Methods: Process Evaluation of OALE Intervention

The purpose of this phase was to determine the mechanism through which the OALE relates to and impacts resilience and well-being. Phase 3 was implemented concurrently with Phase 2 (first season only), and adhered to principles of ethnography (Creswell, 2007; Hammersley & Atkinson, 1995; McQuiston, et al., 2005) and critical ethnography (Madison, 2005; Thomas, 1993). We recorded observations using multiple techniques: participant interviews, focus groups, talking circles, journaling, video and photography. Preliminary results from the participant interviews are presented here. More detail will follow in a separate publication.

A total of 14 youth were selected to be interviewed using a stratified purposeful sampling strategy (Creswell, 2007). All interviews occurred in the field during the latter half of each OALE intervention in the first season. These interviews were conducted by the principle investigator (who was not Aboriginal), and were recorded with a digital audio recorder. Interview probes were designed sequentially to focus initially on eliciting reflections on both positive and negative aspects of the OALE experience and then led to more specific probes pertaining to health and aspects of the experience that may have related to changes in resilience and well-being for the youth. Prior to analysis, all audio recordings were transcribed verbatim. Preliminary analysis of the data followed principles of analytic induction (Patton, 2002) categorizing meaning units (Tesch, 1990) according to the five characteristics of resilience originally espoused by Wagnild and Young (1990; 1993). A more detailed inductive analysis of the interviews and all aspects of Phase 3 will be presented in a subsequent publication.

RESULTS

Phase 1 Results: Description of OALE Orogram (Intervention)

The collaborative program development resulted in an evidence-based curriculum for a short-term 10-day OALE intervention. There were three specific goals that guided all aspects of the program for leaders and participants to: (1) prepare youth as leaders; (2) promote culture and community; (3) protect youth through resilience and well-being. The OALE program was implemented experientially in the traditional territory of WUIR during a 100+km canoe excursion homeward toward the Wikwemikong community. The excursion included many natural challenges such as portages, rapids, and waves that were managed in a progressive manner as participant skill acquisition and comfort level improved. Daily themes reflected leadership training modules, and experiential activities reinforced the themes and program goals. Culture was promoted through traditional practices such as prayer, offering tobacco, talking circles, and a smudging ceremony. An Elder shared a teaching at a pre-arranged meeting place of community significance in order to further promote culture and enhance a sense of identity for the youth. Daily debriefs (or talking circles) were held each evening, and a half day solo experience provided personal reflection time.

Leaders were trained to intentionally facilitate the experience such that daily programming decisions would reflect and reinforce the three program goals. Each excursion was planned so that the trip ended in the Wikwemikong community (the journey home). The arrival included a community welcome feast and a graduation ceremony to celebrate success and recognize individual and group (community) accomplishments. Table 2 depicts a breakdown of excursion and intervention groups over two years. All excursions and groups followed the same travel route. All Phase 2 results were compiled from the entire sample over two years (n = 73). Phase 3 results were based on data collected from multiple sources during the first three excursions in the first year (n = 43).

Table 2. Number of participants by sex for each excursion group

	Male Youth	Female Youth	Total Youth	Adult Leaders
Excursion 1				
Group A	6	4	10	5
Group B	7	1	8	6
Excursion 2				
Group A	3	4	7	3
Group B	3	4	7	3
Excursion 3				
Group A	3	3	6	4
Group B	5	0	5	3
Excursion 4				
Group A	3	5	8	5
Group B	5	2	7	4
Excursion 5				
Group A	4	1	5	4
Group B	5	1	6	5
Excursion 6				
Group A	4	0	4	4
Total	48	25	73*	47*

Note: There were six separate excursions over two years with two groups travelling concurrently during each excursion, with the exception of Excursion 6 with only one travel group (A).

*n=73 Total youth only includes unique individuals and does not include several participants that repeated more than one excursion.

*n=47 Adult leaders includes multiple counts since some participated in more than one excursion. There were 26 different adult leaders involved throughout the study.

Phase 2 Results: Outcome Evaluation – Beginning with Characteristics of the Sample

The final sample included 73 participants or 16% of the on reserve population aged 12 -18 years old. Beyond the 73 participants, there were eight youth who completed the program more than once. Only one youth was excluded from participating for physical health reasons identified through a review of the PAR-Q form completed prior to the trip.

There were 25 females (34%) in total. Nine of the eleven excursion groups included male and female participants, and two groups contained all male participants. Table 2 portrays the number of participants by sex in each excursion group. Although 73 youth participated in the OALE intervention and agreed to participate in the study, only 71 completed the program since two youth were evacuated for minor physical health concerns. The mean age on the day of departure was 14.6 years, and there was no difference in mean age by sex. One youth was under the minimum age of twelve on the day of departure.

The OALE excursion groups were supported by a team that included a program coordinator, certified outdoor leaders (guides), assistant leaders employed on a temporary basis (two to twelve months), and permanent youth workers. The non-Aboriginal principle investigator participated in three excursions, and the principle community collaborator participated in the first excursion. There were 26 different adult leaders who participated in at least one of the excursions, and each travel group included at least three adult leaders (see Table 2). Thus the participant to leader ratio was less than 2:1.

The characteristics of the participants in the sample were collected as part of the HWBQ and results were compared to norms where available. The HWBQ was completed by 64 youth prior to departure. There were 58 youth who self-identified as Aboriginal and North American Indian, one who was Métis, two who did not know, and three who did not respond. Only one youth self-identified as a member from a reserve population outside WUIR. In our sample, 41% were from lone-parent families, which is more than twice the average Canadian rate, and substantially higher than the mean rate for FN reserves. Based on the 2006 Census (Statistics Canada, 2008), 17% of Canadian children Table 2. Number of participants by sex for each excursion group 15 514 years and under live in lone parent families, compared to 33% in FN on reserve populations across the country. In response to the question ‘Compared to your classmates, how well do you do at school?’, 31% of the youth responded above or much above average, 63% responded average, and 6% responded below average. In a large scale study of 2,250 American Indian youth (mean age = 16 years) from ten different tribal high schools (reserves) in western United States, Mitchell and O’Nell (1998) used the same education question and published a mean score of 3.25 (SD = 0.74), which is very similar to the mean score of 3.36 (SD = 0.76) in our sample (n = 64).

Slightly more than half the youth from our sample rated their general health (56.3%) and mental health (58.7%) as very good or excellent. Table 3 compares these self-rated perceptions of health from our sample of WUIR youth to the Canadian population and to the North East Local Health Integration Network of Ontario, a large health service region in Ontario that includes the WUIR population (Statistics Canada, 2009). These results indicated that youth from our sample had a substantially lower perception of their general health and mental health compared to a similar population in Canada and compared to other youth from the local geographic region surrounding the reserve.

Table 3. Self-reported health and mental health compared to Canadian and regional populations

	WUIR Sample (Ages 12-18 yrs)	Canadian Population (Ages 12-19 yrs)*	Ontario NE LHIN Population (Ages 12-19 yrs)*
		General Health Rating	
Very Good to Excellent	56.3%	68.7%	64.9%
Good	35.9%	26.4%	28.3%
Fair to Poor	6.3%	4.9%	6.8%
		Mental Health Rating	
Very Good to Excellent	58.7%	78.7%	70.8%
Good	31.8%	18.0%	F*
Fair to Poor	7.9%	3.3%	F*

Note: WUIR = Wikwemikong Unceded Indian Reservation; NE LHIN = Northeast Local Health Integration Network.

*Comparison data (Canada and Ontario NE LHIN) is based on 2008 data from the Canadian Community Health Survey. Statistics Canada (2009). *Table 105-0501 – health indicator profile, annual estimates, by age group and sex. Canada provinces, territories, health region (2007 boundaries) and peer groups, occasional, CANSIM (database).*

*Data was suppressed by Statistics Canada.

Phase 3 Results: Process Evaluation – Did it Work and Why?

Our preliminary qualitative analysis of 14 field interviews indicated that 13 of the 14 youth respondents reported improvements in their resilience and well-being. The age range of respondents was 12–16 years, and 11 were male (78%). The interviews ranged in length from 10-27 minutes. Many of these youth attributed participation in the pro- gram as contributing to specific areas of personal growth (such as confidence, leadership, and community-mindedness). Further analysis yielded 216 meaning units (MUs) categorized into the five characteristics of resilience originally identified by Wagnild and Young (1990): 1) self-reliance generated 35 MUs; 2) meaning generated 103 MUs; 3) equanimity generated 30 MUs; 4) perseverance generated 42 MUs; and 5) existential aloneness generated 4 MUs. According to Wagnild and Young (1990; 1993), self-reliance is a belief in oneself such that personal strengths, capabilities and successes can be leveraged for future successes. One youth reflected on his experience:

> I was thinking that it [the OALE program] changes our point of view and how things go. You cannot rely on others. You have to help yourself and then you can help others. (male, day 5)

Meaning is another characteristic of resilience, and can be defined as having a sense of purpose in life, and that this purpose can be a reason for living. One youth commented:

> Basically I found the importance of life. I am proud of who I am and where I come from. I love it out here, although it's tough. Tomorrow I am going home but I have got a lot of friends and family that need to hear about the trip. I also want to get on the internet and look up Wikwemikong and learn everything about it. (female, day 8)

Equanimity is a concept that is more difficult to grasp. Wagnild and Young (1993) described it is a balanced view of life that allows one to accept the good with the bad, or accept both positive and negative outcomes. It is characteristic of an ability to moderate the extremes of adversity, and it is often accompanied with a keen sense of humor. A youth described developing sense of equanimity:

> ...that's when the bugs were bothering me and I was thinking holy [######], I just feel like sitting down relaxing, and it's kind of hard to sleep because I'm used to sleep[ing] with a fan, and I think it was two days ago from now, that's when I started to sleep good and then last night was good. I was actually having a good nap. So, I'm just starting to enjoy it. (male, day 5)
>
> Perseverance is akin to persistence and determination and refers to the act of continuing despite difficulties, challenges, obstacles, and setbacks. Many of the youth described a developing sense of perseverance in comments such as: 'I feel really determined to finish this trip. (female, day 6)

During a debrief session after the last OALE intervention in 2009, 13 leaders and two youth participants (15 total) unanimously agreed that the OALE program was effective at promoting resilience and well-being for the participants. Some of the adult leaders suggested that the program also had a positive impact on their own resilience and well-being, and that this impact should be considered in future modifications of the program.

Discussion

The study was both challenging and rewarding, as it merged the resources of an Aboriginal community and academia using a CBPAR-type approach. The nature of the approach included community-university collaboration from the early stages of project inception, through research design, program development, data collection, analysis, evaluation, and dissemination stages. The dissemination stage in particular included both co-presenting and co-authoring. Matier et al. (2008) described similar stages of collaboration in their study, characterizing CBPAR as an ethic of reciprocity that reflects an 'ongoing process of exchange with the aim of establishing and maintaining equality between parties' (p. 321). In the spirit of reciprocity, this study evolved from our earlier research (Blodgett, et al., 2010; Schinke, et al., 2009) addressing youth participation and leadership in sport with a focus on mental health promotion.

The anticipated vulnerability of the Aboriginal adolescent population in WUIR was confirmed from our data by the high rate of lone parent families and low self-rated health scores at baseline. The OALE program was designed to address this vulnerability as a short-term intervention focused on promoting resilience and well-being. Preliminary findings provide early insight into OALE program efficacy in terms of resilience.

The interview data confirmed four of the five resilience characteristics (Wagnild & Young, 1990; 1993), but did not provide adequate support for existential aloneness. This may not be surprising given certain qualities of the experience and population. OALE-type interventions have been described as the development of a social microcosm (Williams, 2000) where a group must work together to accomplish necessary tasks each day; this group work may limit the sense of being alone. Additionally, Aboriginal communities have been described as collectivist societies in contrast to the individualistic society characterized by much of mainstream Canada (Government of Canada, 2006, Chap. 12). Hence, a framework of resilience that includes the characteristic of existential aloneness may not reflect some of the unique characteristics of the OALE intervention and the realities of a collectivist culture.

The initial analysis of interview data leads to cautious optimism with respect to the efficacy of the OALE program. However, the characteristics of resilience used for analysis only reflect a positive personality construct and a framework of resilience developed originally from qualitative studies with resilient older women (Wagnild & Young, 1990). Other frameworks reflect broader, more comprehensive perspectives of adolescent resilience that extend beyond the individual. Adolescent resilience is a complex phenomenon that has been described as both a process and outcome (Olsson, Bond, Burns, Vella-Brodrick, & Sawyer, 2003), and as including a multitude of individual, family, community, and socio-economic factors that intersect in the face of risk or adversity (Ahern, 2006; Olsson, et al., 2003; Wright & Masten, 2006).

Fergus and Zimmerman (2005) presented a framework for understanding adolescent resilience and recommended that interventions should focus on life skills and developing resources rather than focusing on risk amelioration. Further, they summarized several models of resilience including the challenge model which may further help explain the positive outcomes associated with the OALE (Fergus & Zimmerman, 2005). The challenge model reflects a belief that small to moderate levels of risk can help adolescents learn how to overcome the risk as long as the exposure is not so high that overcoming it is perceived as impossible. According to Fergus and Zimmerman (2005), the key point is that the level of risk is at an optimum level (not too low or high) so that the youth can practice skills and access resources. Risks that are too high can be debilitating and lead to feelings of hopelessness and distress. Although Fergus and Zimmerman were not describing the challenge model from an outdoor adventure perspective, the concepts appear to be transferable. The perceived risks and natural challenges inherent in the OALE program may have stimulated or promoted a resilience response in the youth participants.

There are several limitations to this study. First, the preliminary qualitative analysis in Phase 3 used an existing non-Aboriginal resilience framework that focused on a positive personality construct that did not address more comprehensive frameworks beyond the individual. Nevertheless, Wagnild and Young's framework was used as the paradigm for analytic deduction in this study since it was also used to develop the Resilience Scale (RS), one of the most prevalent outcome measures of resilience in use in the literature (Wagnild, 2009). It has been used for a variety of populations and age groups including youth (Wagnild, 2009); it is recommended for use with adolescent populations (Ahern, Kiehl, Sole, & Byers, 2006); and it was also used in three outdoor adventure studies (Ewert & Yoshino, 2008; Neill & Dias, 2001; Shellman, 2009). Furthermore, the RS is part of the HWBQ used in Phase 2 of our study.

Second, since the study involved only one community, findings cannot be generalized to other Aboriginal communities. However, targeting one community was purposeful. Tailored interventions focused on one homogenous population were recommended, based on recent results from studying resilience across international cultures (Ungar, et al., 2007), and then within a group of Canadian adolescents including Aboriginal youth (Ungar, et al., 2008).

Third, the qualitative data collection and analysis was completed by an investigative team that included non-Aboriginal researchers interacting with Aboriginal collaborators and study participants. This may have led to a cultural bias (due to differences of perspective) during analysis, although ethnologists have argued that differences of perspective can also be viewed as a methodological strength (Hammersley & Atkinson, 1995; Wolcott, 2008). Nevertheless, to mitigate the risk of cultural bias, the qualitative approach used methodologies such as CBPAR, researcher reflexivity, guidance from the CRSC, and ongoing collaboration with community leaders.

Conclusion

Currently nearly 50% of the Aboriginal population in Canada is under 25 years old (Statistics Canada, 2008). Aboriginal children and youth are one of the fastest growing sectors of Canadian society, and because it is recognized that children and youth are our future, the indicators of mental health challenges in this population are cause for concern (Canadian UNICEF Committee, 2009; FNIAH, 2003; Government of Canada, 2006). Preliminary findings from the OALE resilience study confirmed some of these concerns. The number of youth from lone parent families in our WUIR sample (n = 73) was nearly three times higher than the Canadian population. Compared to the Canadian population in a similar age bracket (12-19 years), 12.5% fewer youth from our WUIR sample (12-18 years) reported their general health as very good or excellent, and 20% fewer youth reported their mental health as very good to excellent. From a 'determinants of health' perspective, these results are not surprising since the First Nations population in Canada has lower levels education, employment, and income compared to the Canadian population (Health Canada, 2005).

To address the mental health need in WUIR, the OALE was developed collaboratively between community leaders and researchers from Laurentian University. Preliminary findings from 14 participant interviews confirmed four of the five characteristics of resilience originally identified by Wagnild and Young (1990; 1993). These preliminary results suggest that the OALE program seemed to provide most of the components necessary to promote resilience. Over two years, nearly one in six youth (12-18 years) on reserve in WUIR participated in the OALE.

Together, these early findings indicated that the program uptake is excellent, and provide encouraging data to support a potentially effective intervention to address the mental health challenge for adolescents in WUIR. The OALE training manual (Ritchie, Wabano, Lawrence, & Young, 2010) described the program in more detail. Subsequent publications will present results from Phase 2 and 3 in more depth.

Future research should explore whether the OALE program and outcomes would be generalizable to other Aboriginal populations, or whether there are significant process or outcome differences in unique programs developed in other Aboriginal communities in Canada, and in different indigenous populations from other countries.

ACKNOWLEDGEMENTS

The collaborative research team would like to thank the WUIR youth and leaders for their participation, motivation, and support of the research associated with their outdoor adventure leadership experience. We would also like to recognize other members of the Community Research Steering Committee in WUIR (Amy Assinewai, Eric Corbiere, Diane Jacko, Daniel Manitowabi, Amanda Richards, Cody Wassengeso-George, and Pierce Wemigwans). Finally, we would like to acknowledge the gracious financial support for this research from the Indigenous Health Research Development Program (www.ihrdp.ca) and the Canada Research Chairs Program.

REFERENCES

Adelson, N. (2005). The embodiment of inequity: Health disparities in Aboriginal Canada. *Canadian Journal of Public Health, 96*, S45-61.

Ahern, N. R. (2006). Adolescent resilience: An evolutionary concept analysis. *Journal of Pediatric Nursing, 21*(3), 175-185.

Ahern, N. R., Kiehl, E. M., Sole, M. L., & Byers, J. (2006). A review of instruments measuring resilience. *Issues in Comprehensive Pediatric Nursing, 29*(2), 103-125.

Berger, R., & McLeod, J. (2006). Incorporating nature into therapy: A framework for practice. *Journal of Systemic Therapies, 25*(2), 80-94.

Beringer, A., & Martin, P. (2003). On adventure therapy and the natural worlds: Respecting nature's healing. *Journal of Adventure Education & Outdoor Learning, 3*(1), 29-39.

Blodgett, A., Schinke, R., Fisher, L., Yungblut, H., Recollet-Saikonnen, D., Peltier, D., Ritchie, S. & Pickard, P. (2010). Praxis and community-level sport programming strategies in a Canadian Aboriginal reserve. *The International Journal of Sport and Exercise Psychology, 8*(3) 262-283.

Brennan, M. A. (2008). Conceptualizing resiliency: An interactional perspective for community and youth development. *Child Care in Practice. Special Issue: Building resilience in children, 14*(1), 55-64.

Caldwell, J. Y., Davis, J. D., Du Bois, B., Echo-Hawk, H., Erickson, J. S., Goins, T. (2005). Culturally competent research with American Indians and Alaskan natives: Findings and recommendations of the first symposium of the work group on American Indian research and program evaluation methodology. *American Indian & Alaska Native Mental Health Research: The Journal of the National Center, 12*(1), 1-21.

Canadian Institute of Child Health. (2000). *The health of Canada's children: A CICH profile* (3rd edition). Ottawa, ON: Author.

Canadian Society for Exercise Physiology. (2002). *Physical activity readiness questionnaire (PAR-Q)*. Retrieved from www.csep.ca/english/view.asp?x=698.

Canadian UNICEF Committee. (2009). *Canadian supplement to the state of the world's children. Aboriginal children's health: Leaving no child behind.* Retrieved from: http://www.nccah-ccnsa.ca/myfiles/SOWC%20Canada%202009%20 Post%20 release%20 Summary%20June%202009%20_4_. pdf.

Clark, J. P., Marmol, L. M., Cooley, R., & Gathercoal, K. (2004). The effects of wilderness therapy on the clinical concerns (on Axes I, II, and IV) of troubled adolescents. *Journal of Experiential Education, 27*(2), 213-232.

Creswell, J. W. (2007). *Qualitative inquiry & research design: Choosing among five approaches* (2nd ed.). Thousand Oaks, CA: Sage Publications.

Creswell, J. W. (2009). *Research design: Qualitative, quantitative, and mixed method approaches* (3rd ed.). Los Angeles, CA: Sage Publications.

Dumont-Smith, C. (2005). *The health status of Canada's First Nations, Métis and Inuit peoples* (A background paper to accompany 'Health care renewal in Canada: Accelerating change'). Toronto, ON: Health Council of Canada.

Ewert, A., & Yoshino, A. (2008). A preliminary exploration of the influence of short term adventure-based expeditions on levels of resilience. *Journal of Experiential Education, 30*(3), 262-266.

Fergus, S., & Zimmerman, M. A. (2005). Adolescent resilience: A framework for understanding healthy development in the face of risk. *Annual Review of Public Health, 26*(1), 399-419.

First Nations Inuit and Aboriginal Health. (2003). *Acting on what we know: Preventing youth suicide in First Nations (the report of the advisory group on suicide prevention).* Retrieved from Health Canada: http://www.hc-sc.gc.ca/fniah-spnia/ pubs/promotion/_suicide/prev_youth-jeunes/index-eng.php.

Foster, A., & Linney, G. (2007). *Reconnecting children through outdoor education: A research summary.* Toronto, ON: The Council of Outdoor Educators of Ontario.

Government of Canada. (2006). *The human face of mental health and mental illness in Canada* (Cat. No. HP5-19/2006E). Retrieved from Public Health Agency of Canada: http://www.phac-aspc.gc.ca/ publicat/human-humain06/pdf/human_face_e. pdf.

Hammersley, M., & Atkinson, P. (1995). *Ethnography: Principles in practice* (2nd ed.). London, UK: Routledge.

Hart, M. A. (1998). Seeking mino-pimatasiwin (the good life): An Aboriginal approach to social work practice. *Native Social Work Journal, 2*(1), 91-112.

Hattie, J., Marsh, H. W., Neill, J. T., & Richards, G. E. (1997). Adventure education and Outward Bound: Out-of-class experiences that make a lasting difference. *Review of Educational Research, 67*(1), 43-87.

Health Canada. (2005). *A statistical proflle on the health of First Nations in Canada for the year 2000* (Cat. H35-4/30-2000). Ottawa, ON: Her Majesty the Queen in Right of Canada.

Hill, D. L. (2006). Sense of belonging as connectedness, American Indian worldview, and mental health. *Psychiatric Nursing, 20*(5), 210-216.

Hunter, E., & Harvey, D. (2002). Indigenous suicide in Australia, New Zealand, Canada and the United States. *Emergency Medicine, 14*(1), 14-23.

Hunter, L. M., Logan, J., Goulet, J.-G., & Barton, S. (2006). Aboriginal healing: Regaining balance and culture. *Journal of Transcultural Nursing, 17*(1), 13-22.

Indian and Northern Affairs Canada. (2004). *Words first: An evolving terminology relating to Aboriginal peoples in Canada (Catalogue No.R2- 236/2002E-IN).* Retrieved from Government of Canada: http://www.collectionscanada.gc.ca/webarchives/20071114213423/http://www.ainc-inac. gc.ca/pr/pub/wf/index_e.html.

Indian and Northern Affairs Canada. (2009). *Registered Indian population by sex and residence 2009: Wikwemikong.* Ottawa, ON: Author. Israel, B. A., Eng, E., Schulz, A. J., & Parker, E. (Eds.). (2005). *Methods in community based participatory research for health.* San Fransisco, CA: Jossey-Bass.

Kirmayer, L. J., Simpson, C., & Cargo, M. (2003). Healing traditions: Culture, community and mental health promotion with Canadian Aboriginal peoples. *Australasian Psychiatry, 11(*Supplement), S15-S23.

Madison, D. S. (2005). *Critical ethnography: Method, ethics, and performance.* Thousand Oaks, CA: Sage Publications.

Maiter, S., Simich, L., Jacobson, N., & Wise, J. (2008). Reciprocity: An ethic for community-based participatory action research. *Action Research, 6*(3), 305- 325.

Martin, A. (2002). Dramaturgy as a method for experiential program design. *Journal of Experiential Education, 25*(1), 196-206.

McQuiston, C., Parrado, E. A., Olmos-Muñiz, J. C., & Bustillo Martinez, A. M. (2005). Community-based participatory research and ethnography. In B. A. Israel, E. Eng, A. J. Schulz & E. Parker (Eds.), *Methods in community-based participatory research for health.* San Fransisco, CA: Jossey-Bass.

Minkler, M., & Wallerstein, N. (Eds.). (2008). *Community-based participatory research for health: From process to outcomes* (2nd ed.). San Francisco, CA: Jossey-Bass.

Minore, B., Boone, M., Katt, M., Kinch, P., & Birch, S. (2004). Addressing the realities of health care in northern Aboriginal communities through participatory action research. *Journal of Interprofessional Care, 18*(4), 360-368.

Mitchell, C. M., & O'Nell, T. D. (1998). Problem and conventional behaviors among American Indian adolescents: Structure and validity. *Journal of Research on Adolescence, 8*(1), 97-122.

Neill, J. T., & Dias, K. L. (2001). Adventure education and resilience: The double-edged sword. *Journal of Adventure Education and Outdoor Learning, 1*(2), 35-42.

Neill, J. T., & Richards, G. E. (1998). Does outdoor education really work? A summary of recent meta-analysis. *Australian Journal of Outdoor Education, 3*(1), 1-9.

Olsson, C. A., Bond, L., Burns, J. M., Vella-Brodrick, D. A., & Sawyer, S. M. (2003). Adolescent resilience: A concept analysis. *Journal of Adolescence, 26*(1), 1-11.

Patton, M. Q. (2002). *Qualitative research and evaluation methods* (3rd ed.). Thousand Oaks, CA: Sage Publications.

Pryor, A., Carpenter, C., & Townsend, M. (2005). Outdoor education and bush adventure therapy: A socio-ecological approach to health and wellbeing. *Australian Journal of Outdoor Education, 9*(1), 177-190.

Quay, J. (2003). Experience and participation: Relating theories and learning. *Journal of Experiential Education, 26*(2), 105-112.

Ritchie, S. D., Wabano, M. J., Lawrence, E., & Young, N. L. (2010). *Wikwemikong outdoor adventure leadership experience: Program manual.* Wikwemikong, ON: Prepared for Waasa Naabin Youth Services Centre (Training Manual).

Ritchie, S. D., Wabano, M. J., Young, N., Schinke, R., Peltier, D., Battochio, R., et al. (2010). Developing a culturally relevant outdoor leadership training program for Aboriginal youth (2009 SEER abstract). *Journal of Experiential Education, 32*(3), 300-304.

Royal Commission on Aboriginal Peoples in Canada. (1996). *Report of the Royal Commission on Aboriginal Peoples*. Retrieved from Indian and Northern Affairs Canada: http://www.ainc-inac.gc.ca/ap/ rrc-eng.asp.

Russell, K. C. (2003). An assessment of outcomes in outdoor behavioral healthcare treatment. *Child and Youth Care Forum, 32*(6), 355-381.

Schinke, R., Peltier, D., Hanrahan, S., Eys, M., Recollet-Saikonnen, D., Yungblut, H., Ritchie, S., Pickard, P. & Michel, G. (2009). The progressive integration of a Canadian indigenous culture within a sport psychology bicultural research team. *International Journal of Sport and Exercise Psychology, 7*(3) 309-322.

Shellman, A. (2009). *Empowerment and resilience: A multi-method approach to understanding processes and outcomes of adventure education program experiences.* Unpublished Doctoral Dissertation, Indiana University, Indiana. Proquest Dissertations and Theses database. (UMI 3354905).

Statistics Canada. (2007). *Wikwemikong Unceded, Ontario (code3551043) (table). 2006 community proflles. 2006 Census.* Retrieved from Statistics Canada: http://www12.statcan.ca/census-recensement/2006/dp-pd/prof/92-591/index.cfm?Lang=E.

Statistics Canada. (2008). *Aboriginal peoples in Canada in 2006: Inuit, Métis and First Nations, 2006 Census: Findings* (Catalogue no. 97-558-XIE). Retrieved from Statistics Canada: http://www12.statcan.ca/english/census06/analysis/aboriginal/index.cfm.

Statistics Canada. (2009). *Table 105-0501: Health indicator proflle, annual estimates, by age group and sex, Canada, provinces, territories, health regions (2007 boundaries) and peer groups, occasional, CANSIM (database).* Retrieved from Statistics Canada: http://cansim2.statcan.gc.ca/cgi-win/cnsmcgi.exe?Lang=E&CNSM-Fi=CII/CII_1-eng.htm.

Tesch, R. (1990) *Qualitative research analysis types and software tools.* New York, NY: Falmer.

Thomas, J. (1993). *Doing critical ethnography.* London, UK: Sage Publications.

Ungar, M., Brown, M., Liebenberg, L., Cheung, M., & Levine, K. (2008). Distinguishing differences in pathways to resilience among Canadian youth. *Canadian Journal of Community Mental Health (Revue canadienne de santé mentale communautaire), 37*(1), 1-13

Ungar, M., Brown, M., Liebenberg, L., Othman, R., Kwong, W. M., Armstrong, M., & Gilgun, J. (2007). Unique pathways to resilience across cultures. *Adolescence, 42*(166) 287-310.

Ungar, M., Dumond, C., & McDonald, W. (2005). Risk, resilience and outdoor programmes for at risk children. *Journal of Social Work, 5*(3), 319-338.

Wagnild, G. M. (2009). *The Resilience Scale user's guide for the US English version of the Resilience Scale and the 14-item Resilience Scale.* Worden, MT: The Resilience Center.

Wagnild, G. M., & Young, H. M. (1990). Resilience among older women. *Image: Journal of Nursing Scholarship, 22*(4), 252-255.

Wagnild, G. M., & Young, H. M. (1993). Development and psychometric evaluation of the Resilience Scale. *Journal of Nursing Measurement, 1*(2), 165-178.

Williams, B. (2000). The treatment of adolescent populations: An institutional vs a wilderness setting. *Journal of Child and Adolescent Group Therapy, 10*(1), 47-56.

Wilson, K. (2003). Therapeutic landscapes and First Nations peoples: An exploration of culture. *Health and Place, 9*(2), 83-93.

Wolcott, H. F. (2008). *Ethnography: A way of seeing* (2nd ed.). Lanham, MD: Altamira Press.

Wright, M. O. D., & Masten, A. S. (2006). Resilience processes in development. In S. Goldstein & R. B. Brooks (Eds.), *Handbook of resilience in children* (pp. 416). New York, NY: Springer.

REFLECTING

Life can only be understood backwards; but it must be lived forwards.

–Soren Kierkegaard

CHAPTER 10

Preliminary Findings* from a Meta-analysis of Adventure Therapy Program Effects

Daniel J. Bowen and James T. Neill

*These preliminary findings of this meta-analysis were originally presented at 6IATC. The final findings have been published in *The Open Psychology Journal.*

INTRODUCTION

Adventure therapy is increasingly being understood as a credible treatment approach for a range of clientele, including youth, adults and families (Gass, Gillis, & Russell, 2012; Pryor, 2009). Adventure therapy programs take many forms and operate in a range of settings around the world (Bandoroff & Newes, 2004; Mitten & Itin, 2009; Pryor, Carpenter, Norton, & Kirchner, 2012). In some cases adventure therapy is used as the primary method of treatment, whilst other times it is utilised as an adjunct to mainstream therapeutic interventions (Newes, 2000). Treatment outcomes that are commonly sought in adventure therapy include the development of personal responsibility, intrapsychic outcomes (e.g., self-awareness, self-efficacy, self-confidence), psychological resilience, cooperation and relationship building, and social skills (Gass et al., 2012).

Adventure therapy has been referred to by a variety of terms, including wilderness therapy (Russell, Hendee, & Phillips-Miller, 2000), wilderness adventure therapy (Crisp, 2006), wilderness experience programs (Friese, Hendee, & Kinziger, 1998), bush adventure therapy (Pryor, Carpenter, & Townsend, 2005), adventure-based counselling (Fletcher & Hinkle, 2002), outdoor adventure intervention (Pryor, 2009), therapeutic camping (Brown, 2005), and outdoor behavioural healthcare (Russell, 2002).

A consistent and accepted definition of adventure therapy is lacking. In exploring a variety of definitions and identifying common components, Gass et al. (2012) proposed that adventure therapy is "the prescriptive use of adventure experiences provided by mental health professionals, often conducted in natural settings that kinaesthetically engage clients on cognitive, affective, and behavioural levels" (p. 1). Alternatively, Neill (2004) defined adventure therapy for psycho-therapeutic purposes.

Adventure therapy programs are designed and developed around therapeutic goals for specific populations (e.g., substance abusers, psychiatric inpatients, disabled children, physical, emotional and sexual abuse victims, sexual perpetrators, at-risk teens, adjudicated youth, couples and families (Cason & Gillis, 1994). The three most common adventure therapy formats are challenge/ropes courses with games, trust activities and initiative experiences, wilderness expeditions, and residential camps (Gillis & Gass, 2003). Although adventure therapy predominantly takes place in the outdoors, programs can also effectively operate indoors (Richards, Carpenter, & Harper, 2011).

Key elements that characterise adventure therapy include a) the positive influence of nature, b) the use of eustress (positive response to stress), c) the active and direct use of client participation and responsibility, d) meaningful involvement in adventure experiences, e) the focus on positive change (present and future functional behaviour), and g) the strong ethic of care and support (Gass et al., 2012). Features that differentiate adventure therapy from other treatment modalities include: a) the emphasis on the effect of the experience; b) the deliberate tempering of perceived risk in order to utilise elevated levels of arousal and eustress; and c) holistic effects on client learning (Crisp, O'Donnell, Kingston, Poot, & Thomas, 2000). In addition, it should be noted that adventure therapy is generally delivered as a group-based intervention and that psychosocial and group processes are often integral to the experience and treatment methodology.

Organisations conducting adventure therapy programs are increasingly expected to provide accountability information and evidence of program effectiveness to boards, treatment facilities, funding bodies, policy makers and consumers. Further, in order to facilitate the development of effective adventure therapy programs to more precisely accommodate client needs, program documentation, evaluation of outcomes, and analysis of factors that contribute to outcomes are needed.

To date, a number of meta-analyses have been published in the areas of education (e.g., Hattie, 1992), psychological training (Lipsey & Wilson, 1993), psychotherapy (Casey & Berman, 1985; Smith, Glass, & Miller, 1980), and outdoor education (Gillis & Speelman, 2008; Hans, 2000; Hattie, Marsh, Neill, & Richards, 1997; Wilson & Lipsey, 2000). However, the outdoor education meta-analyses have predominantly focused on the broader field of adventure programming, with none solely focused on therapeutic programs. Gillis (1992, p.

7) recommended that "someone needs to conduct a meta-analysis of therapeutic aspects of adventure-challenge-outdoor-wilderness" programs. Although several adventure therapy meta-analyses have been conducted, they are unpublished and have notable limitations; one remains incomplete (Staunton, 2003), another was unable to obtain a large number of potential studies due to cost (Baker, 2011), and a third focused specifically on Outdoor Behavioral Healthcare programs for adolescents (George, 2011) (See Table 1 for a summary of previous related meta-analyses). Thus, a comprehensive adventure therapy meta-analysis is needed.

Table 1. Effects Sizes from Outdoor Education, Camping, Adventure and Wilderness Therapy Meta-analyses[a]

Author/Year	Focus	Client Group	No. of Studies	No. of Effects	No. of Participants	ES Baseline (Base-Pre)	ES Program (Pre-Post)	ES Follow-Up (Post-FU)
Baker (2011)	Adventure Therapy	All	18	67	982		.42	
Bedard (2004; 2003)	Wilderness Therapy	Juvenile Delinquents	23	37	2,042		.45	
Bunting & Donley (2002)	Challenge (Ropes) Course	All	15				.55	
Cason (1993; 1994)	Adventure Education	Adolescents	43	147	11,238		.31	
George (2011)	Outdoor Behavioural Healthcare	All	25	233	4,172		.45	
Gillis & Speelman (2008)	Challenge (Ropes) Course	All	44	390	2,796		.43	
Hans (2000)	Adventure Programming (Locus of Control)	All	24	30	1,632		.38	
Hattie et al. (1997)	Outdoor Education	All	96	1,728	12,057	-.05[b]	.34[c]	.17[d]
Marsh (1999)	Camping (Self-Concept & Self-Esteem)	Children/ Adolescents	22	37	1,139		.25	
Staunton (2003)	Adventure Therapy	All	17	95	~1,000		.42	
Wilson & Lipsey (2000)	Wilderness Therapy	Juvenile Delinquents	22	60	~3,000		.18	

Note. *a: Adapted from Neill (2002, 2003, 2009); b Based on 316 effect sizes; c: Based on 1,062 effect sizes; d: Based on 347 effect sizes.*

The current study, therefore, set out to locate empirically-based outcome studies about adventure therapy programs, determine short and longer-term effects of adventure therapy programs compared to alternative and no treatment, and to explore the relationships between sample, program, and participant moderator variables and participant outcomes. It is expected that findings will encourage adventure therapists to examine the impact of their programs and to use findings as a guide for program development.

METHOD

Selection Criteria

Four selection criteria, adapted from (George, 2011; Wilson & Lipsey, 2000), were used to determine the relevance of studies for this adventure therapy meta-analysis:

- The program primarily uses wilderness, adventure or outdoor recreation activities specifically for psychological and/or behavioural therapeutic purposes
- The study reports at least preened post-psychological and/or behavioural outcomes
- The study provides sufficient statistical information to allow calculation of standardised mean effect sizes (e.g., means, standard deviations, and number of participants)
- The study is reported in 1960 or later, and in English.

Search and Coding

A systematic search for relevant adventure therapy studies was conducted between February 2012 and June 2012 of the following sources:

1. Electronic data bases (e.g., PsychInfo, Google Scholar, ERIC, ProQuest Dissertations & Theses A&I) using the search term (adventure OR outdoor OR wilderness OR nature OR eco* OR bush OR experien* OR recreation OR challenge OR rope* OR expedition OR school OR camp) AND (therap* OR psychotherap* OR treatment OR intervention OR counsel* OR healthcare OR program OR education OR course) Related journals (e.g., Journal of Adventure Education and Outdoor Learning, Therapeutic Recreation Journal) Related internet sites (e.g., http://wilderdom.com; http://leegillis.com/AT)
2. Related meta-analyses (e.g, Baker, 2011; Cason & Gillis; George, 2011; Wilson & Lipsey, 2000)
3. Listserv and emails to experts in the field
4. Scanned bibliographies and reference lists

Identified and obtained studies which met the selection criteria were coded using a Coding Manual based on Lipsey and Wilson (2000) and George (2011) (see http://www.danielbowen.com.au/meta-analysis), taking care to avoid duplicate samples.

Data Analysis

This study used meta-analysis to investigate measured impacts of participation in adventure therapy programs. Meta-analysis is "a set of statistical methods for combining quantitative results from multiple studies to produce an overall summary of empirical knowledge on a given topic" (Littell, Corcoran, & Pillai, 2008, p. 1-2). An effect size, a value which reflects the magnitude of the treatment effect, is calculated for each study and the results from each study are then combined to compute a summary effect size (Ellis, 2010). The effect size statistic used in this analysis is Hedges' g (Hedges, 1981) which is the difference between the means of two groups divided (or standardised) by the population standardised deviation [(M1-M2)/SD_{pooled}]. The pooled sample standard deviation was calculated as SD_{pooled} = square root of [(n1 1) * s12 + (n2 1) * s22] / (n1 + n2 2)]. As the population standard deviation is often not available, sample standard deviations were used instead. Hedges' g was used as the effect size statistic because it adjusts for studies with small sample sizes. Cohen's (1988) commonly referred to standards for interpreting effect sizes is 0.20 (small), 0.50 (medium), and 0.80 (large).

This meta-analysis was performed following the methods described by Borenstein, Hedges, Higgins, and Rothstein (2009). This involved:

a) A random-effects model was used. While fixed-effects models assume that there is one true effect size and that all differences in observed effects are due to sampling error, the random-effects model assumes that study outcomes vary across studies, not only because of random sampling effects, but also because there are real differences between the studies (Borenstein, Hedges, Higgins, & Rothstein, 2010).
b) Where available, mean effect sizes were calculated within each sample by treatment group (Adventure Therapy Treatment, Alternative treatment, No Treatment), outcome and outcome category (Academic, Behaviour, Clinical, Family, Morality/Spirituality, Physical, Self-Concept, and Social), and time comparison (Base-Pre; Pre-Post; Post-Follow-Up).

c) A 0.5 correlation between the measurements across time was assumed (since it was rarely reported); and
d) Additional comparisons were conducted to explore the existence of potential sample (publication year, type of publication, sample size, methodological quality), program (funding type, use of adventure, program delivery, group structure, placement type, program type, program model, daily duration and program length) and participant (mean age, sample source, race, gender, population, issue) moderators.

The Methodological Quality Rating Scale (MQRS) was used to rate the overall quality of each study. The MQRS contains 12 items for rating a study, including study design, quality control, follow-up length, and attrition (Littell et al., 2008). Ratings closer to 0 indicate poor methodological quality, while ratings closer to 16 indicate stronger or better quality (Miller & Wilbourne, 2002).

There were three treatment groups: Adventure Therapy Treatment included participants who completed an adventure therapy program, Alternative Treatment included participants in alternative, non-adventure therapy programs, and No Treatment included participants from control groups who did not participate in any form of therapy. There were three time comparisons: Base-Pre (Prior to program (Base) compared with beginning of program (Pre)) which indicates changes leading up to the start of the program; Pre-Post (Beginning of the program (Pre) compared with the end of the program (Post)) which indicates the short-term effect of the program; Post-Follow-Up (End of the program (Post) compared with a subsequent time (Follow-Up)) which indicates the longer term effect of the program.

A software program, Comprehensive Meta-Analysis (CMA) Version 2 (Borenstein, Hedges, Higgins, and Rothstein, (2005), was used to conduct the analysis. CMA provides information regarding the statistical significance of the mean effect size (z score, p value and confidence intervals), variance, standard error, and heterogeneity for each effect. These statistics are briefly described.

The z score, converted from the mean effect size, indicates the magnitude of an effect in terms of standard deviation units (Ellis, 2010). Whether a z score is significant or not depends on whether it exceeds the critical *z* value. If the z score exceeds the critical value (±1.96), it can be concluded that the result is statistically significant at the $p < .05$ level (Card, 2012).

The *p* value indicates the probability of obtaining the finding by chance, and is a measure of how much evidence there is against the null hypothesis (Leandro, 2005). The null hypothesis (H_0) signifies the hypothesis of no change or no effect.

The smaller the p value, the more evidence there is against H_0. However, the p value does not indicate the strength or magnitude of the effect (Littell et al., 2008).

Confidence intervals represent the range of values likely to include the true effect, and thus express the level of certainty associated with the mean effect size estimate (Littell et al., 2008). A wide confidence interval implies poor precision, while a narrow confidence interval implies good precision. Intervals that are very wide indicate that little is known about the effect and that further information is needed. If the interval excludes the null value of zero, then the mean effect size is considered to be statistically significant (Ellis, 2010).

Variance is a measure of dispersion, indicating the extent to which values are spread around a mean or population parameter (Littell et al., 2008).

Standard error is an estimate of the precision of the mean effect size (Card, 2012). A smaller standard error is indicative of a more precise estimate of the mean effect size and narrower confidence interval. Conversely, a larger standard error is indicative of an imprecise estimate of the mean effect size and larger confidence interval (Ellis, 2010).

Heterogeneity refers to the extent of variation in a distribution of effect sizes, which includes both true variance and random error (Borenstein et al., 2009). Heterogeneity includes differences between studies in regards to outcomes (statistical heterogeneity), populations (clinical heterogeneity), and methods (methodological differences) (Littell et al., 2008). By assessing the heterogeneity of the distribution of effect sizes, the question is being asked: Do the individual effect size estimates reflect a common population effect size? (Ellis, 2010).

CMA provides two tests of heterogeneity, the Q statistic and I^2. The Q statistic signifies the amount of heterogeneity in effect sizes amongst studies used to calculate a mean effect size, and thus assesses the null hypothesis of homogeneity versus the alternate hypothesis of heterogeneity (Borenstein et al., 2009). The Q statistic is significant when the associated p value is less than the critical alpha value (.05 in the current study), in which case the null hypothesis of homogeneity can be rejected in favour of the alternate hypothesis of heterogeneity (i.e., the variability across effect sizes is greater than expected from sampling error alone) (Lipsey & Wilson, 2000). The Q statistic is sensitive to the number of studies included in the analysis, is not sensitive to the metric of the effect size index, should be interpreted cautiously if there is inadequate statistical power, and does not provide the magnitude of heterogeneity if it exists (Card, 2012). I^2 is the percentage of variability among effect sizes that exists between studies relative to the total variability among effect sizes (i.e., the ratio of true heterogeneity to total variation in observed effects) (Card, 2012). It indicates how heterogeneous the effect sizes are (the degree of inconsistency across studies) and is not dependent on the scale used in the meta-analysis (Littell et al., 2008). I^2 is expressed as a ratio with a range of 0% to 100%, with low (or zero) values suggesting little or no heterogeneity and larger values representing high heterogeneity (Borenstein et al., 2009). $I^2 \approx 25\%$ is a small amount of heterogeneity, $I^2 \approx 50\%$ is a medium amount of heterogeneity, and $I^2 \approx 75\%$ is a large amount of heterogeneity (Huedo-Medina, Sánchez-Meca, Marín-Martínez, & Botella, (2006). In summary, both Q and I^2 will be low (or zero) if the total dispersion is low relative to the error within studies, and higher if the total dispersion is high, relative to the error within studies (Borenstein et al., 2009).

Results

Results of this meta-analysis are based on 2,356 effect sizes from 175 unique samples located within 166 studies published between 1967 and 2012[1]. The calculated effect sizes pertain to three treatment groups: Adventure Therapy Treatment (1,809; 76.8%), Alternative Treatment (304; 12.9%), and No Treatment (243; 10.3%), and where available are broken down into three time comparisons across four time points (Base, Pre, Post, Follow-Up): Base-Pre (55; 2.3%), Pre-Post (1,831; 77.7%), and Post-Follow-Up (470; 20.0%).

There were 14,554 unique participants (M = 83.2; SD = 137.0 per study), of whom 67% were male and 33% female. The participants ranged in age between 9 and 64 years (M = 17.2; SD = 7.5), and the programs lasted between 1 and 534 days, with a mean of 42.1 days (SD = 66.8), and a median of 22.0 days. The mean length of time between Base and Pre was 20.8 days (SD = 15.3), while the mean length of time between Post and Follow-up was 184.2 days (SD = 287.6). A summary of the sample, program and participant characteristics are presented in Tables 2, 3, and 4, respectively. Caution should be used when interpreting some of the results due to high heterogeneity.

---

[1] At the time of 6IATC, the authors were still in the process of acquiring relevant studies. A final analysis was published in the *The Open Psychology Journal*

Table 2. Adventure Therapy Sample Characteristics

Characteristic	Sample *N* (%)		Participant *N* (%)	
Publication Year				
1960-1969	3	(1.7)	139	(1.0)
1970-1979	12	(6.9)	754	(5.2)
1980-1989	28	(16.0)	1,648	(11.3)
1990-1999	44	(25.1)	2,574	(17.7)
2000-2009	70	(40.0)	7,380	(50.7)
2010-2012	18	(10.3)	2,059	(14.1)
Publication Type				
Published (Article, Book, Report)	83	(47.4)	8,495	(58.4)
Non-published (Thesis or Dissertation)	92	(52.6)	6,059	(41.6)
Study Sample Size				
≤ 50	88	(50.3)	2,142	(14.7)
51-100	52	(29.7)	3,709	(25.5)
101-150	13	(7.4)	1,614	(11.1)
151 +	22	(12.6)	7,089	(48.7)
Methodological Quality Rating Scale (MQRS)				
Study Design				
Single Group (Pre/Post)	95	(54.3)	9,533	(65.5)
Quasi-experimental (W/Control)	65	(37.1)	4,373	(30.0)
Randomisation with Control Group	15	(8.6)	648	(4.5)
Considered Replicable	166	(94.9)	12,515	(86.0)
Baseline Data Reported	175	(100.0)	14,554	(100.0)
Quality Control	169	(96.6)	14,104	(96.9)
Follow-Up Length				
< 6 Months	149	(85.1)	11,483	(78.9)
6-11 Months	11	(6.3)	876	(6.0)
≥12 Months	15	(8.6)	2,195	(15.1)
Follow-Up Rate				
< 70% Completion	156	(89.1)	12,995	(89.3)
70-84% Completion	4	(2.3)	501	(3.4)
>85% Completion	15	(8.6)	1,058	(7.3)
Collaterals Interviewed	15	(8.6)	844	(5.8)
Objective Verification of Self-Report Data	28	(16.0)	1,713	(11.8)
Dropouts Discussed	163	(93.1)	13,667	(93.9)
Independent (Blind)	0	(100.0)	0	(0.0)
Appropriate Analysis	175	(100.0)	14,554	(100.0)
Multisite with Separate Research Teams	0	(100.0)	0	(0.0)
Average MQRS Score = 7.06 (*SD* = 1.82)				

Note**.** *Sample N = 175; Participant N = 14,554.*

Table 3. Adventure Therapy Program Characteristics

Characteristic	Sample *N* (%)		Participant *N* (%)	
Funding Type				
Private	133	(76.0)	12,399	(85.2)
Public	42	(24.0)	2,155	(14.8)
Use of Adventure				
Primary	116	(66.3)	10,228	(70.3)
Adjunctive	59	(33.7)	4,326	(29.7)
Program Delivery				
Continuous	113	(64.6)	10,502	(72.2)
Intermittent	62	(35.4)	4,052	(27.8)
Group Structure				
Closed group	158	(90.3)	11,629	(79.9)
Open group	17	(9.7)	2,925	(20.1)
Placement Type				
Private	146	(83.4)	12,816	(88.1)
Adjudicated	29	(16.6)	1,738	(11.9)
Expedition Program Type				
Contained Expedition	43	(24.6)	2,794	(19.2)
Continuous-Flow Expedition	3	(1.7)	246	(1.7)
Base-camp Expedition	7	(4.0)	295	(2.0)
Residential Expedition	12	(6.9)	849	(5.8)
Mixed (Combination of these Types)	32	(18.3)	5,010	(34.4)
Unspecified/ None of the Above	78	(44.6)	5,360	(36.8)
Program Model				
Base Camp	8	(4.6)	518	(3.6)
Expedition	47	(26.9)	3,161	(21.7)
Residential	7	(4.0)	600	(4.1)
Outpatient	1	(0.6)	33	(0.2)
School	0	(0.0)	0	(0.0)
Integrated Expedition	0	(0.0)	0	(0.0)
Multiple	35	(20.0)	5,003	(34.4)
Ropes Course/Challenge Course/ Adventure Based	77	(44.0)	5,239	(36.0)
Daily Duration				
Residential	103	(58.9)	9,871	(67.8)
Outpatient	28	(16.0)	1,972	(13.5)
Mixed	44	(25.1)	2,711	(18.6)
Program Length				
1-2 Days	16	(9.1)	789	(5.4)
3-7 Days	24	(13.7)	1,528	(10.5)
8-14 Days	20	(11.4)	1,379	(9.5)
15-21 Days	24	(13.7)	1,618	(11.1)
22-45 Days	41	(23.4)	3,072	(21.1)
46-80 Days	27	(15.4)	2,035	(14.0)
81-150 Days	11	(6.3)	893	(6.1)
151+ Days	8	(4.6)	878	(6.0)
Unspecified	4	(2.3)	2,362	(16.2)

***Note**. Sample N = 175; Participant N = 14,554.*

A summary of the overall effect sizes by each treatment group and time comparison is presented in Table 5. A break-down of effect sizes by each outcome category for each treatment group and time comparison are presented in Tables 6 to 12.[2]

Table 4. Adventure Therapy Participant Characteristics

Characteristic	Sample *N* (%)		Participant *N* (%)	
Age				
≤9 Years Old	4	(2.3)	178	(1.2)
10-14 Years Old (Early Adolescents)	56	(32.0)	5.127	(35.2)
15-17 Years Old (Late Adolescents)	65	(37.1)	5,693	(39.1)
18+ Years Old (Adults)	27	(15.4)	1,978	(13.6)
Mixed (e.g., Families)	7	(4.0)	680	(4.7)
Unspecified	16	(9.1)	989	(6.2)
Sample Source				
Asia	7	(4.0)	316	(2.2)
Australia	24	(13.7)	1,103	(7.6)
Canada	6	(3.4)	475	(3.3)
Europe	2	(1.1)	150	(1.0)
New Zealand	3	(1.7)	228	(1.6)
USA	133	(76)	12,282	(84.4)
Predominant Race				
> 60% Caucasian	69	(39.4)	6,452	(44.3)
> 60% Minority	22	(12.6)	1,428	(9.8)
Mixed, No Race > 60%	14	(8.0)	1,104	(7.6)
Unspecified	70	(40.0)	5,570	(38.3)
Predominant Gender				
< 50% Male	31	(17.7)	2,378	(16.3)
> 50% Male	119	(68.0)	10,232	(70.3)
Unspecified	25	(14.3)	1,944	(13.4)
Identified Population				
At-Risk	104	(59.4)	10,139	(69.7)
Clinical	42	(24.0)	2,677	(18.4)
Adjudicated	29	(16.6)	1,738	(11.9)
Identified Focus				
Abuse Victims (Physical, Emotional or Sexual)	4	(2.3)	216	(1.5)
Adjudicated Youth	29	(16.6)	1,738	(11.9)
Behaviour Disordered	16	(9.1)	1,108	(7.6)

[2] Only summary information for outcome categories is provided. A total of 66 distinct outcomes were included in the 8 outcome categories: Academic (*N* = 4); Behavioural (*N* = 8); Clinical (*N* = 30); Family (*N* = 2); Morality/Spirituality (*N* = 1); Physical (*N* = 2); Self-Concept (*N* = 11); Social Development (*N* = 8). For the manuscript submitted for publication, the authors intend to provide summary information for all outcomes included in each outcome category.

Characteristic	Sample N (%)		Participant N (%)	
Disabilities	5	(2.9)	255	(1.8)
Educationally Disengaged	18	(10.3)	1,302	(8.9)
Emotionally Disturbed	6	(3.4)	290	(2.0)
Families	6	(3.4)	708	(4.9)
Mental Health	24	(13.7)	1084	(7.4)
Mixed	32	(18.3)	4,297	(29.5)
Physical (e.g., Brain Injury, Weight-Loss, Etc.)	12	(6.9)	1,656	(11.4)
Substance Abuse	10	(5.7)	1,126	(7.7)
Welfare	13	(7.4)	774	(5.3)

Note. *Sample N = 175; Participant N = 14,554.*

Table 5. Overall Effect Sizes for Treatment Group by Time comparison

	Adventure Therapy Treatment			Alternative Treatment			No Treatment		
Time	*g*	*V*	*N*	*g*	*V*	*N*	*g*	*V*	*N*
Base-Pre	.09	.00	55						
Pre-Post	.47	.00	1424	.13	.00	213	.03	.00	194
Post-FU	.05	.00	330	-.03	.00	91	-.08	.00	49

Note. *g = Hedges' g; V = Variance; N = Number of effect sizes.*

Table 6. Base-Pre Adventure Therapy Treatment Effect Sizes and Summary Information Relating to Outcome Category Variables

Outcome Category	No of Samples	No. of ES	Hedges' *g* (Variance)	Standard Error	95% CI	*z* value (*p* value)	*Q* value (*p* value)	*I*2
Academic	3	8	.26 (.01)	.12	.02-.49	2.12 (.034)	.43 (.808)	.00
Behaviour	2	5	-.10 (.02)	.13	-.36-.15	-.78 (.436)	.00 (.961)	.00
Clinical	6	8	.20 (.01)	.12	-.03-.43	1.68 (.093)	4.13 (.531)	.00
Family Development	1	1	.20 (.02)	.15	-.09-.50	1.35 (.179)		
Morality/Spirituality								
Physical	1	1	.03 (.06)	.24	-.45-.51	.13 (.896)		
Self-Concept	8	19	.05 (.01)	.07	-.09-.18	.70 (.483)	1.38 (.986)	.00
Social Development	5	13	.10 (.01)	.07	-.04-.25	1.40 (.162)	.49 (.974)	.00
Overall	9	55	.09 (.00)	.07	-.04-.22	1.36 (.174)	1.48 .993	.00

Note: *ES = Effect Size; CI = Confidence Interval.*

Table 7. Pre-Post Adventure Therapy Treatment Effect Sizes and Summary Information Relating to Outcome Category Variables

Outcome Category	No of Samples	No. of ES	Hedges' *g* (Variance)	Standard Error	95% CI	*z* value (*p* value)	*Q* value (*p* value)	*I*2
Academic	54	106	.43 (.00)	.05	.33-.52	8.80 (.000)	201.72 (.000)	73.73
Behaviour	68	180	.42 (.00)	.06	.31-.53	7.46 (.000)	497.24 (.000)	86.53
Clinical	116	486	.50 (.00)	.05	.41-.59	10.70 (.000)	1097.09 (.000)	89.52
Family Development	28	92	.37 (.00)	.08	.22-.53	4.74 (.000)	169.52 (.000)	84.07
Morality/Spirituality	4	6	.18 (.05)	.23	-.27-.63	.78 (.437)	8.24 (.041)	63.60
Physical	10	16	.38 (.02)	.12	.14-.63	3.08 (.002)	39.30 (.000)	77.10
Self-Concept	113	310	.41 (.00)	.04	.34-.48	11.71 (.000)	437.34 (.000)	74.39
Social Development	88	228	.42 (.00)	.04	.34-.51	9.78 (.000)	436.83 (.000)	80.08
Overall	174	1424	.47 (.00)	.03	.40-.53	13.77 (.000)	1124.35 (.000)	84.61

Note: *ES = Effect Size; CI = Confidence Interval.*

Table 8. Pre-Post Alternative Treatment Effect Sizes and Summary Information Relating to Outcome Category Variables

Outcome Category	No of Samples	No. of ES	Hedges' *g* (Variance)	Standard Error	95% CI	*z* value (*p* value)	*Q* value (*p* value)	*I*2
Academic	11	13	.14 (.00)	.06	.02-.26	2.22 (.026)	12.56 (.249)	20.39
Behaviour	16	23	.13 (.00)	.06	.00-.25	1.97 (.049)	28.28 (.020)	46.96
Clinical	24	79	.14 (.00)	.07	.01-.27	2.18 (.029)	50.13 (.001)	54.12
Family Development	3	6	-.19 (.03)	.19	-.56-.17	-1.05 (.295)	5.51 (.064)	63.67
Morality/Spirituality								
Physical	3	3	.03 (.02)	.13	-.22-.29	.26 (.795)	2.52 (.283)	20.70
Self-Concept	25	52	.16 (.00)	.06	.04-.27	2.60 (.009)	49.51 (.002)	51.52
Social Development	17	35	.15 (.01)	.08	-.00-.29	1.95 (.051)	36.28 (.003)	55.90
Overall	36	213	.13 (.00)	.04	.06-.20	3.54 (.00)	40.72 (..27)	11.58

Note: *ES = Effect Size; CI = Confidence Interval.*

Table 9. Pre-Post No Treatment Effect Sizes and Summary Information Relating to Outcome Category Variables

Outcome Category	No of Samples	No. of ES	Hedges' *g* (Variance)	Standard Error	95% CI	*z* value (*p* value)	*Q* value (*p* value)	I2
Academic	15	28	-.01 (.00)	.05	-.11- .00	-29 (.772)	8.44 (.865)	.00
Behaviour	11	25	-.05 (.00)	.07	-.19- .09	-.71 (.481)	16.36 (.090)	38.89
Clinical	15	30	.05 (.00)	.05	-.05- .14	.95 (.344)	13.49 (.488)	.00
Family Development	8	17	.06 (.00)	.06	-.06- .19	1.00 (.316)	1.22 (.990)	.00
Morality/Spirituality	2	3	.03 (.31)	.60	-1.06- 1.13	.06 (.956)	8.42 (.004)	88.13
Physical								
Self-Concept	24	49	.01 (.00)	.04	-.09- .09	.23 (.818)	20.25 (.627)	.00
Social Development	18	41	-.02 (.00)	.04	-.10- .07	-.38 (.707)	9.10 (.937)	.00
Overall	33	194	.03 (.00)	.04	-.04- .09	.77 (.44)	20.48 (.942)	.00

Note: *ES = Effect Size; CI = Confidence Interval.*

Table 10. Post-Follow-Up Adventure Therapy Treatment Effect Sizes and Summary Information Relating to Outcome Category Variables

Outcome Category	No of Samples	No. of ES	Hedges' *g* (Variance)	Standard Error	95% CI	*z* value (*p* value)	*Q* value (*p* value)	I2
Academic	15	21	.04 (.00)	.06	-.08- .15	.65 (.517)	21.30 (.094)	34.26
Behaviour	18	40	.23 (.00)	.05	.13- .33	4.64 (.000)	22.31 (.173)	23.81
Clinical	29	88	.02 (.00)	.05	-.09- .12	.31 (.754)	61.25 (.000)	54.29
Family Development	10	16	-.05 (.01)	.07	-.18- .09	-.65 (.519)	14.52 (.105)	38.03
Morality/Spirituality	1	1	.63 (.14)	.37	-.10- 1.35	1.70 (.089)		
Physical	2	2	.19 (.13)	.36	-.52- .90	.52 (.600)	6.82 (.009)	85.35
Self-Concept	36	94	-.01 (.00)	.05	-.11- .08	-.28 (.778)	86.99 (.000)	59.76
Social Development	23	68	-.02 (.00)	.05	-.14- .07	-.52 (.604)	31.79 (.081)	30.80
Overall	49	330	.05 (.00)	.03	-.06- .12	1.51 (.130)	79.53 (.003)	39.65

Note: *ES = Effect Size; CI = Confidence Interval.*

Table 11. Post-Follow-Up Alternative Treatment Effect Sizes and Summary Information Relating to Outcome Category Variables

Outcome Category	No of Samples	No. of ES	Hedges' *g* (Variance)	Standard Error	95% CI	*z* value (*p* value)	*Q* value (*p* value)	I2
Academic	4	4	.00 (.01)	.10	-.20-.21	.02 (.983)	4.08 (.253)	26.54
Behaviour	6	11	.17 (.01)	.10	-.01-.36	1.81 (.070)	8.12 (.150)	38.43
Clinical	9	33	-.11 (.01)	.11	-.32-.10	-1.01 (.312)	16.55 (.035)	51.67
Family Development	2	3	-.06 (.01)	.11	-.28-.16	-.53 (.599)	.30 (.584)	.00
Morality/Spirituality								
Physical	2	2	-.20 (.09)	.29	-.78-.37	-.69 (.492)	4.71 (.030)	78.78
Self-Concept	11	26	-.04 (.01)	.08	-.20-.11	-.56 (.579)	15.42 (.118)	35.14
Social Development	5	12	.00 (.02)	.12	-.24-.24	.00 (1.000)	8.45 (.076)	52.69
Overall	15	91	-.03 (.00)	.05	-.13-.07	-.62 (.537)	10.47 (.727)	.00

***Note:** ES = Effect Size; CI = Confidence Interval.*

Table 12. Post-Follow-Up No Treatment Effect Sizes and Summary Information Relating to Outcome Category Variables

Outcome Category	No of Samples	No. of ES	Hedges' *g* (Variance)	Standard Error	95% CI	*z* value (*p* value)	*Q* value (*p* value)	I2
Academic	2	4	-.14 (.02)	.13	-.41-.12	-1.06 (.290)	.00 (.962)	.00
Behaviour	2	8	-.07 (.02)	.13	-.32-.18	-.57 (.571)	.04 (.838)	.00
Clinical	4	11	-.27 (.05)	.23	-.72-.19	-1.16 (.247)	10.20 (.017)	70.58
Family Development	1	2	.14 (.02)	.14	-.14-.42	.97 (.331)		
Morality/Spirituality								
Physical								
Self-Concept	6	9	-.01 (.01)	.09	-.18-.16	-.10 (.918)	2.02 (.846)	.00
Social Development	3	15	-.04 (.01)	.12	-.26-.19	-.32 (.753)	.30 (.860)	.00
Overall	6	49	-.08 (.01)	.09	-.26-.10	-.89 (.375)	5.33 (.377)	6.23

***Note:** ES = Effect Size; CI = Confidence Interval.*

In addition to the overall effect size and average effect sizes based on outcome category constructs, the role of sample, program, and participant-related moderator variables were analysed for the Adventure Therapy Treatment group between Pre and Post for 174 samples (see Tables 13, 14 and 15 respectively).

In most instances, findings indicated no clear or notable moderator effects. This would suggest that, on the whole, sample, program and participant variables do not greatly moderate the effectiveness of adventure therapy programs.

Discussion

This study aimed to analyse the empirically measured effectiveness of adventure therapy and to examine variation in outcomes across different types of samples, programs and participants. Findings pertain to three treatment groups (Treatment, Alternative Treatment, No Treatment) and, where available, three time comparisons were reported (Base-Pre, Pre-Post, and Post-Follow-Up). Caution should be used when interpreting some of the results due to high heterogeneity.

Outcomes

The Base-Pre time comparison provided an indication of the effect leading up to the start of the program, whereby cognitions and emotions such as anticipation, excitement and/or fear may influence self-perceptions at the start of the program. Base-Pre data was only available for the Adventure Therapy Treatment group, with a small positive overall effect of .09. The greatest effect was on academic outcomes (.26), followed by clinical (.20), family development (.20), social development (.10), self-concept (.05), physical (.03), and behaviour (-.10) outcomes. Although relatively small, the positive overall effect suggests that the lead up to the start of an adventure therapy program is for most participants a positive experience that results in a slight improvement for most outcomes. This finding is in contrast to Hattie et al. (1997) who found a small negative effect (-.05) between Base and Pre for outdoor education.

The Pre-Post time-comparison indicated the short-term effect of the program, with data available for all three treatment groups. Pre-Post outcomes are reasonably consistent across all eight major outcome categories for the Adventure Therapy Treatment group, with the greatest effect on clinical outcomes (.50), followed by academic (.43), social development (.42), behaviour (.42), self-concept (.41), physical (.38), family development (.37), and morality/spirituality (.18) outcomes. These findings, as well as the overall effect of .47, are largely consistent with previous unpublished adventure therapy meta-analyses (mid .4;

Baker, 2011; George, 2011; Staunton, 2003), and compare favourably with outdoor education (mid .3; Cason & Gillis, 1994; Hans, 2000; Hattie et al., 1997). However, findings, for the most part, are not as strong as for one-on-one psychotherapy (see Lipsey & Wilson, 1993). The Alternative Treatment Pre-Post effects for outcome categories ranged from -.19 (family development) to .16 (self-concept), with a relatively small positive overall effect of .13. The No Treatment group Pre-Post effects for outcome categories ranged from -.05 (behaviour) to .06 (family development), with a very small positive overall effect of .03. Thus, the findings for the Adventure Therapy Treatment group compared favourably against the negligible effects of the Alternative and No Treatment groups (< .1), highlighting that on the whole there are beneficial outcomes associated with participating in adventure therapy programs.

The Post-Follow-Up time comparison provided an indication of the longer-term effect of the program, with data obtained for the three treatment groups. The greatest Post-Follow-Up effect of the Adventure Therapy Treatment was on morality/spirituality outcomes (.63), followed by behaviour (.23), physical (.19), academic (.04), clinical (.02), social development (-.02), self-concept (-.01), and family development (-.05) outcomes. Although relatively small (.05), the positive overall effect suggests that, on average, the impact of adventure therapy programs appear to be maintained in the long-term. This finding is lower than Hattie's et al. (1997) previous finding (.17) for outdoor education. In contrast, the Alternative Treatment Post-Follow-Up effects for outcome categories ranged from -.20 (physical) to .17 (behaviour), with a very small negative overall effect of -.03. Similarly, although slightly lower, the No Treatment Post-Follow-Up effects for outcome categories ranged from -.27 (clinical) to .14 (family development), with a very small negative overall effect of -.08. This suggests that for those who participated in alternative treatment, the effects were only partially retained, and on average participants seemed to experience a slight decline in the gained benefits over the long-term. Similarly, for those who did not participate in any treatment, although there was minimal positive change between pre and post, on average participants seemed to experience a slight decline in overall wellbeing and functioning over the long-term. These findings therefore favourably suggest that, on average, adventure therapy is an effective treatment resulting in outcomes, which appear to be maintained over the long-term.

Moderators

The breakdown of overall Pre-Post effect sizes for the Adventure Therapy Treatment by sample, program and participant variables indicated that, in most instances, there are no clear or notable trends. In general, higher effects were found for samples, which were published or had a lower MQRS rating, for participants who were older or female, and for programs whose use of adventure was adjunctive, or had an open group structure or private placement. However, the results indicate that, on the whole, sample, program and participant variables do not greatly moderate the effectiveness of adventure therapy programs. Thus, findings from the moderator analysis provide further support for the overall moderate effectiveness of adventure therapy. Additionally, these results support the use of findings from this study for benchmarking program effectiveness. Neill (2003) suggested that meta-analytic benchmarks be used to provide a systematic means to categorise and evaluate outcomes. Valuable diagnostic information about a program's relative efficacy can be obtained by comparing a particular program's effect sizes with relevant meta-analytic findings. For example, findings from this meta-analysis (based on overall effect size and confidence intervals) suggest that adventure therapy programs which attain an overall effect between 0.4 and 0.6 are within the expected range, with values below this having a weaker effect than expected, and values above this having a stronger effect than expected.

Limitations and Recommendations for Future Research

This meta-analytic study demonstrated that adventure therapy programs are, on the whole, an effective intervention. However, important limitations must be considered when interpreting the results. Limitations pertain to availability of studies, heterogeneity, generalisability, type of data provided by empirical studies (including the provision of sufficient statistical information to calculate effect sizes), and the methodological quality of studies, (including the use of psychometrically validated assessment tools). Each of these are briefly discussed below.

These results are preliminary as the authors are still in the process of obtaining additional existing accessible empirical studies.

A substantial proportion of the findings were heterogeneous, indicating a medium to high degree of variance in the effectiveness of adventure therapy programs, as well as a sizable amount of discrepancy between studies claiming to measure the same outcome.

Only a small percentage of adventure therapy programs undergo empirical program evaluation (Neill (2003) indicates less than 1%). In addition, only studies reported in English were included. However, adventure therapy is increasingly being applied in non-English cultures (Pryor et al., 2012). Thus findings from this meta-analysis may not accurately represent actual adventure therapy program outcomes.

A substantial percentage of studies included in the meta-analysis did not use matched samples when reporting outcomes (i.e., there was a discrepancy between pre N and post N). Very few of these studies also provided matched sample results. For the current study, the smaller N was used in order to be conservative. Although participant attrition is a reality of program evaluation, in order to gain an accurate program evaluation, it is recommended that future empirical studies provide matched sample results. When matched samples are reported, it is important that drop-outs are enumerated, otherwise the results run the risk of selectively reporting on completers only.

Although over 230 studies have been used in previous related meta-analyses (see http://www.danielbowen.com.au/meta-analysis), and over 1,000 related studies were obtained for the current study, many did not provide enough data to calculate effect sizes. In addition, a substantial proportion of studies did not provide adequate demographic information to allow moderator analyses. It is imperative that future empirical studies provide necessary statistics to allow calculation of effect sizes to help reduce sample bias and increase generalisability of findings. Researchers should also, where appropriate, provide sample, program and participant demographics listed in Tables 2, 3, and 4, respectively. Future adventure therapy research should, where possible, capture data about a larger range of outcomes and at multiple time points.

One noteworthy methodological issue is that there are two different kinds of standardised mean effect sizes commonly used in meta-analytic studies. A standardised mean effect size can be calculated as the difference between scores at two different times for a treatment group. Alternatively, a standardised mean difference effect size can be calculated as the difference between post-treatment means for a treatment group and a comparison group. Both methods involve subtracting means and then dividing by the standard deviation, but the pre-post standardised mean effect size indicates the degree of change over time in a single group, while the standardised mean difference effect size provides an indication of the differences between two separate groups. It is not appropriate to combine these two types of effect sizes into one aggregate mean effect size (Lipsey & Wilson, 2000). Although a number of previous meta-analyses in this area of research have combined these two types of effect sizes, this study only used the standardised mean change effect size. This meant that studies which only reported post-test results for the treatment and control groups were not included (N = 47; see http://www.danielbowen.com.au/meta-analysis). Because of this approach, findings may not be representative of all outcomes (e.g., many recidivism studies were not included in the current study).

The average MQRS score was moderate (7.06), with only nine studies achieving a high rating (12-16). High quality research is needed to strengthen the reliability, validity, and usability of these findings. It is recommended that those conducting future research on adventure therapy programs consult such resources as the MQRS when designing research studies. Gass et al. (2012; Appendix D) have also provided a rubric for evidence-based research on adventure programs, which could be similarly used.

Whilst the majority of studies utilised psychometrically validated assessment tools and reported the tools' psychometric properties, several studies used less well-developed assessment tools. It is possible that these less developed tools inflated or reduced the overall effect size depending on the capacity of the tool to assess the specified construct. It is recommended that psychometrically validated assessment tools are used in research on adventure therapy, and that the psychometric properties of tools are reported. It is also recommended that future research develop purpose-built, multidimensional assessment tools using the best available psychometric techniques.

Conclusion

These results provide the most substantial and robust meta-analysis of adventure therapy program outcomes to date and confirm that overall adventure therapy is moderately effective in facilitating positive short-term change in behavioural, emotional, and interpersonal measures which, for available studies, on average appears to be maintained in the long-term. Heterogeneity of outcomes indicates considerable variability, although little of variance appears to be explained by the measured moderators.

References

Baker, D. (2011). *The effects of adventure and wilderness therapy: A meta-analytic review.* (Masters of Psychology), James Cook University, Townsville, Australia.

Bandoroff, S., & Newes, S. L. (Eds.). (2004). *Coming of age: The evolving field of adventure therapy.* Boulder, CO: Association for Experiential Education.

Bedard, R. M. (2004). *Wilderness therapy programs for juvenile delinquents: A meta-analysis.* (Doctor of Philosophy), Colorado State University, Fort Collins, CO.

Bedard, R. M., Rosen, L., & Vacha-Haase, T. (2003). Wilderness therapy programs for juvenile delinquents: A meta-analysis. *Journal of Therapeutic Wilderness Camping, 3*(1), 7-13.

Borenstein, H., Hedges, L. V., Higgins, J. P. T., & Rothstein, H. (2005). *Comprehensive meta-analysis (Version 2).* Englewood, NJ: Biostat.

Borenstein, M., Hedges, L. V., Higgins, J. P. T., & Rothstein, H. R. (2009). *Introduction to meta-analysis.* Chichester, UK: John Wiley & Sons.

Borenstein, M., Hedges, L. V., Higgins, J. P. T., & Rothstein, H. R. (2010). A basic introduction to fixed-effect and random-effects models for meta-analysis. *Research Synthesis Methods, 1*(2), 97-111. doi: 10.1002/jrsm.12

Brown, K. (2005). Therapeutic camping programs. In R. G. Steele & M. C. Roberts (Eds.), *Handbook of mental health services for children, adolescents, and families* (pp. 305-315). New York: Kluwer Academic/Plenum.

Bunting, C. J., & Donley, J. P. (2002). *Ten years of challenge course research: A review of affective outcome studies.* Poster presented at the 6th Coalition for the Education in the Outdoors Research Symposium. Bradford Woods, IN.

Card, N. A. (2012). *Applied meta-analysis for social science research.* New York: The Guilford Press.

Casey, R. J., & Berman, J. S. (1985). The outcome of psychotherapy with children. *Psychological Bulletin, 98*(2), 388-400.

Cason, D. R. (1993). *A meta-analysis of adventure programming with adolescents.* (Master of Science), Georgia College & State University, Milledgeville, GA.

Cason, D. R., & Gillis, H. L. (1994). A meta-analysis of outdoor adventure programming with adolescents. *Journal of Experiential Education, 17*(1), 40-47.

Cohen, J. (1988). *Statistical power analysis for behavioral sciences* (2nd ed.). Hillsdale, NY: Lawrence Erlbaum Associates.

Crisp, S. J. R. (2006). Taking a risk for adolescents: Wilderness adventure therapy. *InPsych: Bulletin of the Australian Psychological Society, 28*(4), 22-23.

Crisp, S. J. R., O'Donnell, M. J., Kingston, L., Poot, A., & Thomas, N. E. (2000). Innovative multi-modal day-patient treatment for severely disordered at risk adolescents. In N. N. Singh, J. P. Leung & A. N. Singh (Eds.), *International Perspectives on Child and Adolescent Mental Health* (Vol. 1, pp. 331-345). Kidlington, United Kingdom: Elsevier.

Ellis, P. D. (2010). *The essential guide to effect sizes: Statistical power, meta-analysis, and the interpretation of research results*. Cambridge, UK: Cambridge University Press.

Fletcher, T. B., & Hinkle, J. S. (2002). Adventure based counseling: An innovation in counseling. *Journal of Counseling & Development, 80*(3), 277-284.

Friese, G. T., Hendee, J. C., & Kinziger, M. (1998). The wilderness experience program industry in the United States: Characteristics and dynamics. *Journal of Experiential Education, 21*(1), 40-45.

Gass, M. A., Gillis, H. L., & Russell, K. C. (2012). *Adventure therapy: Theory, research, and practice*. New York: Routledge.

George, J. T. (2011). *Efficacy of Outdoor Behaviour Healthcare (OBH) for adolescent populations: A meta-analysis.* (Doctor of Psychology), University of Indianapolis, Indianapolis, IN.

Gillis, H. L. (1992). *Therapeutic uses of adventure-challenge-outdoor-wilderness: Theory and research*. Paper presented at the Coalition for Education in the Outdoors Symposium, Martinsville, IN.

Gillis, H. L., & Gass, M. A. (2003). Adventure therapy with groups. In J. L. DeLucia-Waack, D. A. Gerrity, C. R. Kalodner & M. Riva (Eds.), *Handbook of group counseling and psychotherapy*. Thousand Oaks, CA: Sage.

Gillis, L. H., & Speelman, E. (2008). Are challenge (ropes) courses an effective tool? A meta-analysis. *Journal of Experiential Education, 31*(2), 111-135.

Hans, T. A. (2000). A meta-analysis of the effects of adventure programming on locus of control. *Journal of Contemporary Psychotherapy, 30*(1), 33-60.

Hattie, J. A. (1992). *Self-concept*. Hillsdale, NJ: Lawrence Erlbaum.

Hattie, J. M., Marsh, H. W., Neill, J. T., & Richards, G. E. (1997). Adventure education and Outward Bound: Out-of-class experiences that make a lasting difference. *Review of Educational Research, 67*(1), 43-87. doi: 10.3102/00346543067001043

Hedges, L. (1981). Distribution theory for Glass's estimator of effect size and related estimators. *Journal of Educational Statistics, 6*, 107–128.

Huedo-Medina, T. B., Sánchez-Meca, J., Marín-Martínez, F., & Botella, J. (2006). Assessing heterogeneity in meta-analysis: Q statistic or I^2 index? *Psychological Methods, 11*(2), 193-206. doi: 10.1037/1082-989x.11.2.193

Leandro, G. (2005). *Meta-analysis in medical research: The handbook for the understanding and practice of meta-analysis*. Malden, MA: Blackwell.

Lipsey, M. W., & Wilson, D. B. (1993). The efficacy of psychological, educational, and behavioral treatment: Confirmation from meta-analysis. *American psychologist, 48*(12), 1181-1201.

Lipsey, M. W., & Wilson, D. B. (2000). *Practical meta-analysis*. Thousand Oaks, CA: Sage.

Littell, J. H., Corcoran, J., & Pillai, V. K. (2008). *Systematic reviews and meta-analysis*. New York: Oxford University Press.

Marsh, P. E. (1999). *What does camp do for kids? A meta-analysis of the influence of organized camping experience on the self constructs of youth.* (Master of Science), Indiana University, Bloomington, IN.

Miller, W. R., & Wilbourne, P. L. (2002). Mesa Grande: A methodological analysis of clinical trials of treatments for alcohol use disorders. *Addiction, 97*(3), 265-277. doi: 10.1046/j.1360-0443.2002.00019.x

Mitten, D., & Itin, C. M. (Eds.). (2009). *Connecting with the essence: Proceedings of the Fourth International Adventure Therapy Conference*. Boulder, CO: Association for Experiential Education.

Neill, J. T. (2002). *Meta-analytic research on the outcomes of outdoor education.* Paper presented at the Coalition for Education in the Outdoors Research Symposium, Bradford Woods, IN.

Neill, J. T. (2003). Reviewing and benchmarking adventure therapy outcomes: Applications of meta-analysis. *Journal of Experiential Education, 25*(3), 316-321.

Neill, J. T. (2004). Adventure therapy definitions [Web log post]. Retrieved from http://wilderdom.com/adventuretherapy/adventuretherapydefinitions.html

Neill, J. T. (2009). Outdoor education meta-analyses. Retrieved from http://wilderdom.com/research/ResearchReviewsMetaanalysis.html

Newes, S. L. (2000). Adventure-based therapy: Theory, characteristics, ethics, and research. Retrieved from http://wilderdom.com/SandyNewes.htm

Pryor, A. (2009). *Wild adventures in wellbeing: Foundations, features and wellbeing impacts of Australian outdoor adventure interventions (OAI).* (Doctor of Philosophy), Deakin University, Burwood, Australia.

Pryor, A., Carpenter, C., Norton, C. L., & Kirchner, J. (Eds.). (2012). *Emerging insights: Proceedings of the Fifth International Adventure Therapy Conference 2009*. Prague, Czech Republic: European Science and Art.

Pryor, A., Carpenter, C., & Townsend, M. (2005). Outdoor education and bush adventure therapy: A socio-ecological approach to health and wellbeing. *Australian Journal of Outdoor Education, 9*(1), 3-13.

Richards, K, Carpenter, C, & Harper, N. (2011). Looking at the landscape of adventure therapy: Making links to theory and practice. *Journal of Adventure Education & Outdoor Learning, 11*(2), 83-90. doi: 10.1080/14729679.2011.632877

Russell, K. C. (2002). *Longitudinal assessment of treatment outcomes in outdoor behavioral healthcare*. Moscow, ID: University of Idaho.

Russell, K. C., Hendee, J. C., & Phillips-Miller, D. (2000). Wilderness therapy as an intervention and treatment for adolescents with behavioral problems. *Wilderness Science in a Time of Change, 15*(3), 136-141.

Smith, M. L., Glass, G. V., & Miller, T. I. (1980). *The benefits of psychotherapy*. Baltimore, MD: Johns Hopkins University Press.

Staunton, N. (2003). A meta-analysis of adventure therapy program outcomes. Retrieved from http://wilderdom.com/adventuretherapy/Staunton2003ATMeta-analysis_files/frame.htm

Wilson, S. J., & Lipsey, M. W. (2000). Wilderness challenge programs for delinquent youth: A meta-analysis of outcome evaluations. *Evaluation and Program Planning, 23*(1), 1-12.

CHAPTER 11

Integrating Theory with Practice: Applications in Adventure Therapy

Alison Voight and Alan Ewert

INTRODUCTION

Understanding how theories can be applied to practice in the adventure therapy setting provides practitioners with an important foundation from which to establish a sound justification for practice methods, and a means for measuring client improvement. Without a theoretical connection, practice methodologies in the adventure therapy setting can be subject to an agency's philosophy, different adventure settings, or be randomly applied based on staff experience or staff turnover. Understanding the theoretical aspects that underlie human behavior can be an important component of service delivery in the adventure therapy setting. When a theory-based foundation is missing, it might be compared to floating directionless on the ocean. Perhaps Da Vinci said it best in his statement, "He who loves practice without theory is like the sailor who boards a ship without a rudder or compass, and never knows where he may cast" (United Earth, n.d.). Simply providing activities, or establishing a list of outcome measures for clients is not always sufficient. Theory-based practice can help explain dysfunctional behavior and emotions in the identification, assessment and treatment of client dysfunction. These explanations can then provide the basis from which applied methodologies are established. Without this vital underpinning of theoretical knowledge and application, the experiential activities applied in adventure therapy may risk becoming merely diversional exercises.

DEFINING THEORY

Theories are useful in that they help us describe or explain some phenomenon in a systematic or logical way (Kraus & Allen, 1995). Generally speaking, a theory is a proposed explanation whose status is still conjectural and subject to experimentation, in contrast to well-established propositions that are regarded as reporting matters of actual fact (Riddick & Russell, 2008). "A theory can be a particular conception or view of something to be done or of the method of doing it, or regarded as a set of principles on which the practice of an activity is based, such as 'a theory of education,' or 'music theory'" (Merriam-Webster, n.d.). As such, a theoretical foundation can also be applied to the practice of Adventure Therapy. In particular, theories that are based on a social-psychological context can play a critical role in understanding the identification, assessment, development and maintenance of dysfunction, as well as the prevention and treatment of dysfunction in Adventure Therapy.

Theory-based Practice in Adventure Therapy

Theories have played an important role in helping to create an overall philosophical framework from which to conceptually guide adventure therapy practice. For instance Walsh and Gollins' Outward Bound Process Model (1976) has often been used as the structural basis for adventure therapy programs. Their model incorporates a multi-level process in which clients or participants engage, with instructors' guidance, throughout the process. Leaders place their participants in unique physical and social environments, while assigning specific problem-solving tasks to the group, requiring a scaffolding of skill building, often through situations of dissonance and challenge, until a mastery of skills is achieved, relevant to each client, ultimately resulting in increased self-efficacy and self-awareness (Walsh & Gollins). While some critics question the puissance of the model (Gass, Gillis, & Russell, 2012; Sibthorp, 2003), it continues to serve as a strong theoretical framework for program development in outdoor adventure and adventure therapy.

Theory-based practice, using such theories as self-efficacy, motivation, and self-determination, can also help establish and identify specific areas of therapeutic engagement for clients. For example, reviewing previous theoretical research regarding motivation or improving levels of self-efficacy in a client can play an integral role in how a therapeutic intervention is approached or initiated. Gass, Gillis, and Russell (2012) provide some illuminating thoughts on motivation and the role theory plays in adventure therapy practice:

How to motivate people to change has perplexed the psychological community for centuries. And form the basis for several major research initiatives, including that of Deci and Ryan, and others in their development of self-determination theory. Self-determination theory is a macro theory of human motivation that is useful in helping explain how to shift motivation during a therapeutic process from an external source of motivation to an internal one (p. 74).

Gass et al., elaborate on the role of theoretical research in adventure therapy by indicating that, "research and anecdotal evidence suggest the Adventure Therapy experiences foster the development of inherent motivation in individuals to want to change despite low motivations at the onset of treatment (p. 74)."

Kottman, Ashby and DeGraaf, (2001) further defend the use of theory-based practice in adventure activities as an important predictor of human performance, using the basis of Bandura's (1986) social learning theory or self-efficacy. They proffer that adventure activities can expose clients to opportunities for self-efficacy exploration, and through the processes of reflection, generalization, and application, instructors or counsellors can assist clients in making changes in their lives based on increased self-efficacy (Kottman, et al. p. 18). As indicated, understanding and implementing a theoretical-based intervention can be tremendously helpful in better interpreting the behavior of clients, but also in developing realistic client expectations and outcomes of adventure therapy practice.

Theories can be particularly useful in describing a situation or behavior, predicting its occurrence, and understanding how to change or modify that outcome through a selection of a planned intervention (Voight & Ewert, 2007). Theories may also provide an important measuring stick from which to, not only develop interventions, but also from which to judge the effectiveness of outcomes or goals established for clients in Adventure Therapy.

While numerous theories exist that are relevant to the adventure therapy experience, it is beyond the scope of one article to cover them all. However, the basic tenets of two specific theories deemed particularly relevant in the practice of adventure therapy—stress and coping theory, and attribution theory—will be discussed, as well as their direct application in the practice of processing activities, and in providing feedback in adventure learning situations.

Theory of Stress and Coping

Most people are familiar with the term "stress" and its implications in their lives. The concept of stress usually implies something negative or sinister, and should be dealt with or removed from one's life. The dictionary defines stress as, "a physical, chemical, or emotional factor that causes bodily or mental tension and may be a factor in disease causation" (Merriam Webster, n.d.). As an element of stress is introduced into a person's life, whether categorized as immediate or long-term stress, the second half of the "equation" is how one *copes* with that stress. The theory of stress and coping has evolved to try and explain this process.

Lazarus and Folkman (1984), describe "stress" as something that transpires between the person and environmental stimuli, where stress results when demands exceed resources, and coping represents an individual's response to stress. According to Lazarus and Folkman, when a person encounters stress, he or she engages in a four-step process. These steps include the following:

1. Appraisal of stressor
2. Appraisal of resources
3. Carrying out coping strategy
4. Evaluation of coping efforts (Lazarus & Folkman, 1984)

When a person "appraises" or encounters a stressor (e.g., challenge or struggle whether mental or physical), he/she must determine if this stressor can be managed and dealt with. Is the stressor to be met within his or her ability to control or to cope with? Each person appraises a stressor based on many aspects, or the "resources" a person has with which to cope, or face the stressor. Often past successes or failures of managing a stressor play a pivotal role in how that stressor, if encounter again, will be met. Participants, who may fail to meet the challenges of a stressor in their life, find alternative methods to cope, and these methods might be considered negative or destructive (i.e., drugs, alcohol, excess eating, etc.). While coping with a stressor, the person may default to an established coping mechanism, such as taking drugs, or drinking, running away (literally or metaphorically) from an uncomfortable or perceived threatening situation, or becoming aggressive, confrontational, or unstable. More positive reactions to coping with stressors, however, could include "applying" oneself, maintaining discipline, trying harder, talking with people who are supportive, and self-reflection or self-evaluation towards the purpose of self-improvement.

Hood and Carruthers (2002) posit that stress and coping for an individual involves an "assessment of the situation by the person facing it and includes an evaluation of both the demands of the situation and the resources the person brings to bear on that situation" (p. 139). They further indicate that a person's assessment of a stressor sets up a stress-coping mechanism where the individual determines the type of coping mechanism warranted. The coping may warrant different responses, which are dependent on several factors, including a person's perceived emotional responses to the stress-coping situation. Some coping strategies may involve either an emotion-focused or problem-focused approach, where coping styles may include avoidant, or confrontational style (Shank & Coyle, 2002). Being able to use both styles can be beneficial when an individual makes a cognitive appraisal of the stressor interpreting the stressor as unimportant or significant (Shank & Coyle, 2000).

APPLICATION OF STRESS AND COPING THEORY IN ADVENTURE THERAPY

When adventure therapy activities are carefully developed and processed (i.e., debriefed) participants may benefit from a re-appraisal of their coping mechanisms. Most Adventure Therapy programs employ elements of risk that can create a sense of dissonance within the individual. When risk is introduced to create stress, or "eustress" - considered positive stress - (Ellis, 1973), participants are challenged to create new coping methods to deal with the stress. Clients may no longer rely on past coping styles, which may have been detrimental to their health, negative, or inappropriate. When interventions are carefully applied, clients can learn new coping mechanisms in stressful situations (i.e., challenge activities, rock climbing difficult terrain, long distance hiking, etc.) that may be approached in a more positive manner. Clients may also become aware that they possess the confidence and self-efficacy to manage new and stressful situations in constructive, rather than destructive ways. For instance, circumstances for clients in Adventure Therapy might include dealing with cold or wet weather, being hungry, feeling out of their comfort zone, afraid, and feeling extremely tired. Individuals engaging in adventure experiences can: (a) Develop heightened awareness of capabilities and limits, (b) learns new coping skills from participant groups, (c) become aware of emotions and behavior, and (d) identify changes in levels of confidence and self-esteem (Thomas, 2004).

Hood and Carruthers (2002) stated that, "the assessment of the resources a person has for coping is of particular importance for therapeutic recreation interventions" (p. 139). While creating stressful situations for participants through Adventure Therapy can have a constructive impact, it must be managed thoughtfully for clients, taking care not to overstress clients, or create adventure therapy activities that create distress. Experienced and effective professionals delivering Adventure Therapy activities, which employ the use of stress and eustress, can be powerful change agents for clients in the development and/or restructuring of positive coping skills.

ATTRIBUTION THEORY

Attribution theory, first proposed by Heider (1958), attempts to explain how individuals interpret events that transpire in their lives. The theory became a major area of research in social-psychology in the 1970s and 80s, discerning how people attach meaning to their behavior and its outcomes, or why they do what they do (Weiner, 1974, 1986). Attribution theory attempts to explain attributions that people ascribe to the outcomes of their behavior, both good as well as bad outcomes. In other words, how do people explain the success or failure of their actions relative to a given endeavor? The theory expounds that people can make either *internal* or *external* attributions, where internal attributions relate to something that could be caused by the person, and external attributions are attributed to something situational, or external to the person's control. Attribution theory also attempts to qualify attributions as stable or unstable, and global or specific (Peterson & Seligman 1984).

APPLICATION OF ATTRIBUTION THEORY IN ADVENTURE THERAPY

The significance of attribution theory, or how people attribute outcomes of their behavior, is regarding the ability to change negative or pessimistic attributes a person may possess, to something that is recognized to be within the person's control (whether a positive or negative outcome results). For example, many clients that are engaged in Adventure Therapy, particularly youth-at-risk, may feel they have little control in their lives, or any effort produced on their behalf will yield similarly negative results, as it always has. Statements such as, "Everything I do turns out bad" represent internal, stable, global attributions. Internal attributions that are indicative of low self-esteem or low self-efficacy can be challenged when a youth confronts his or her fears in a risk-based activity, and is able to overcome the obstacles. A client can change attributions to more internal, unstable, and specific attributions, such as, "That was a really hard rock climbing route. I wasn't too good this time, but I did better than the last time I tried." Experiencing success through carefully facilitated and processed Adventure Therapy activities can begin to counteract persistent (stable) attributes that may change by situations (specific) when fears or challenges are confronted. Risk is shared with group members, and trying or effort, despite the outcomes, represents the real success. Adventure Therapy programs, where interventions are designed for specific outcomes, can play an essential role in "un-learning" attributions of participants that prevent a sense of accomplish and achievement, and help ameliorate pervasive, or global self-perceptions that are negative and persistent. Adventure therapy provides an excellent platform for development and growth of its participants through activities that scaffold skill-building and are sequentially introduced, provide concrete challenges and decision-making, and where feedback of effort can be immediate. Allowing clients to "reattribute" or make different attributes, despite their past history, through Adventure Therapy activities, can help them to develop more realistic expectations, while attempting to eliminate stable, or persistent attributes that have promulgated negative outcomes in their lives.

Conclusion

Although integrating theory behind every aspect of practice may not always be feasible or necessary, it can serve as a foundational building block, from which to strengthen, re-evaluate and facilitate our interaction with clients. As evidence-based outcomes are often becoming necessary to maintain funding for programs, having a specific theoretical model, from which a program is developed, and from which changes in clients can be measured, provides a powerful tool for Adventure Therapy programmers. Being able to base our practice on sound, social diagnostic theory, such as the two theories discussed in this paper, moves us away from programming as usual, to specifically identifying, classifying, and assessing the behavior and needs of our clients.

Theories are an important means of attempting to understand and predict certain behaviors in our clients. Whether it is the identification of coping patterns of participants to specific stressors, or the personal attributions of clients that have negatively impacted their lives, using a theoretical component in our practice can provide a "benchmark" parameter for diagnosing behavior, as well as implementing specific and relevant interventions. In addition, theoretically-based programming easily lends itself to much needed research in the Adventure Therapy field; research that can be greatly advantageous in enhancing its professional status, and most importantly, measuring both short-term and long-term results of our programs. Ultimately, it is not just about demonstrating positive changes in participants, but documenting how they have changed, and how these changes will impact their future. This is the essence and the efficacy of Adventure Therapy.

REFERENCES

Ellis, M. (1973). *Why people play.* Englewoods Cliff: NJ.

Gass, M., Gillis, L., & Russell, K. (2012). *Adventure Therapy: Theory, Research, and Practice,* New York: Routledge.

Heider, F. (1958). *The psychology of interpersonal relations.* Upper Saddle River, NJ: Prentice-Hall.

Hood, C. D., & Carruthers, C. P. (2002). Coping skills theory as an underlying framework for therapeutic recreation services. *Therapeutic Recreation Journal, 36*(2), 137-153.

Kottman, T., Ashby, J. S., & DeGraaf, D. (2001). *Adventures in guidance: How to integrate fun into your guidance program.* Alexandria, VA: American Counseling Association.

Kraus, R., & Allen, L.R. (1995). *Research and evaluation in recreation, parks, and leisure studies* (2nd ed.). Boston: Allyn & Bacon.

Lazarus, R.S., & Folkman, S. (1984). *Stress, appraisal, and coping*. New York: Springer.

Peterson, *C., &* Seligman, M.E.P. (*1984).* Causal explanations as a risk factor for depression:

Theory and evidence. *Psychological Review, 91*, 347–74.

Riddick, C.C. & Russell, R.V. (2008). *Research in Recreation, Parks, Sport, and Tourism* (2nd ed.). Champaign, IL: Sagamore.

Sibthorp, J. (2003). An empirical look at Walsh and Golins' adventure education process model:

Relationships between antecedent factors, perceptions of characteristics of adventure education experience, and changes in self-efficacy. *Journal of leisure Research, 35*(1), 80-106.

Shank, J. & Coyle, C. (2002). *Therapeutic Recreation in Health Promotion and Rehabilitation.* State College, PA: Venture.

Thomas, M. (2004). The potential unlimited programme: An outdoor experiential education and group work approach that facilitates adjustment to brain injury. *Brain Injury, 18*(12), 1271-1286.

United Earth (n.d.). Retrieved from http://www.unitedearth.com.au/davinci.html

Voight, A., & Ewert, A. (2007). Theory-based Processing in Therapeutic Wilderness Camping:

Facilitation Techniques in Achieving Outcomes. *Journal of Therapeutic Wilderness Camping,6*(1), 13-18.

Walsh, V., & Gollins, G. (1976). *The exploration of the Outward Bound process*. Denver: Colorado Outward Bound School.

Weiner, B. (1974). *Achievement motivation and attribution theory*. Morristown, NJ: General Learning Press.

Weiner, B. (1986). *An attributional theory of motivation and emotion*. New York: Springer-Verlag.

CHAPTER 12

Rethinking Notions of 'Therapeutic Landscapes': A Case Study Exploring Perceptions of a 'Wild Place' Experience (WPE)

Elizabeth Freeman and Jacqui Akhurst

ABSTRACT

This paper examines the nature of therapeutic landscapes and draws from perspectives of participants during a 'Wild Place' Experience (WPE). Two WPEs will be utilised as the basis of the data to be explored. The WPE consisted of a five day journey and involved university students *walking through* and *sitting with* the environment. The paper is ecopsychological as it seeks to explore the relationship between humans and their environments, and is concerned with the therapeutic nature of this relationship. Participant narratives are used to discuss notions of therapeutic landscapes as 'healing places', in relation to natural environments (e.g. wild places), and builds on suggestions made by Baer and Gesler (2004) that therapeutic landscapes are "ambivalent [and] nuanced spaces". This, and the meaning-making journey of people during and after WPEs, is discussed in relation to the influence of cultural artefacts – both physical and metaphorical. To do so, this paper draws from discourses created and collected during interviews, group discussions and journals during and after a WPE. A 'wild place' can be described as an area, or landscape, where natural features are predominant and that is relatively remote from human settlements. In the UK, the size of the country and the imprint of historic activity over the centuries means that locating and being able to have a so-called wilderness experience is different from what might be possible in the USA, Canada, Australia or Africa. This work relates to our exploration of the features of a 'Wild Place' Experience (WPE) in the north of England.

INTRODUCTION

In the past two decades, increasing attention has been paid to the potential restorative aspects of nature, and Baer and Gesler (2004) assert that natural landscapes have, for a long time been viewed as therapeutic landscapes, as 'healing places'. Gesler (1992) had earlier noted that whilst the idea that such places may contribute to human health and well-being is not new, the therapeutic landscape concept is a recent social science construct conceived as a way for academics to frame both real and imagined connections between place and human health. The concept of therapeutic landscapes is similar to humanism and the philosophy of holistic health as it resists and criticises positivist hegemony and positivism "for many of the same reasons that it criticizes the biomedical model itself" (Gesler 1992, p. 744). One of the features of some of the ecopsychology literature is that some of the studies may take a relatively romantic view of 'wild places', without considering the potential difficulties inherent in experiences (Akhurst, 2010). This highlights the need to interrogate the nuanced and complex nature of the ways that people make meaning from their experiences.

Baer and Gesler (2004) discuss he usage of the term 'therapeutic landscapes', and note the following potential shortcomings: that (i) use of the term may raise false expectations; (ii) research often fails to recognise that perceptions about therapeutic landscapes differ over space, time and across individuals; and (iii) no landscape is perfectly 'healthy', thus research findings need to be balanced by a critical view that also mentions unhealthy aspects of wild places.

In this paper, we hope to illustrate the ambivalences and nuanced nature of therapeutic landscapes (TLs), which potentially have many shades of meaning. Drawing from data we show that a landscape's therapeutic quality is changeable over time, person, space and experience; and that a number of factors, qualities, elements and processes are involved in creating and maintaining "ambivalent and nuanced spaces" (Baer & Gesler, 2004, p 411). We will argue that notions of cultural artefacts, both physical and symbolic, help conceptualise and understand participant 'meaning-making' in a natural environment, and illuminate the human-environment interrelationship. Cultural artefacts are used by participants to make sense of their surroundings and their relationship to it. Finally, we highlight some of the positive and negative consequences of these on a person's experience of wild places.

Cultural Artifacts and the Environment

Within this paper the persons' world, their own individual set of beliefs and assumptions and perceptions are foregrounded. Cultural artefacts have been elucidated by Cole (1996) and may be things, a person, a group, and symbolic in the form of ideas and processes. In every environment there are objects that constantly surround us. We interact with pre-existing objects in environments and also bring new objects into environments. We perceive and react to objects, consciously and subconsciously, and use them to suit our purposes in many ways depending on our current and possible future needs. Our reactions can be manifested in an action, a change in mood or emotive response, which can impact on experience of environment and place. In relation to the research to be described, objects were used as reference points and as tools (e.g. equipment).

Cultural artefacts can exist as external, simulated, and internal entities. Within this research both external and internal artefacts are of interest. External objects exist in the landscape, like fences, paths and buildings, and are symbolic in that they are cultural reference points that are used to make meaning of place and experience. Internal artefacts are concepts and ideas that often originate in cultural interactions, and form internalised images. Some physical objects serve as positive reference points and others as negative ones, but all are mediated by cultural repertoires.

In a natural environment a person who comes across a building or walks on an established path may interact with objects in varied and different ways. Interactions with objects-in-the-environment are different for different people and can lead to positive and negative responses and meaning. For example, a person coming across a building or walking on a an established path in a wild place, may have a positive reaction to these objects giving the building and path a practical meaning related to refuge or safe route of passage, or may have a negative reaction, related to the objects' symbolic meaning as a representation of human influence on environment.

This example however illustrates a polarised notion. It may be more useful that the shades of meaning between the two descriptive 'poles' are acknowledged. Baer and Gesler (2004) for example talk of shades of meaning. Lighter (positive) shades are often referred to in the literature; grey shades of meaning however, typically, are not (Gesler 2003; Gesler & Kearns, 2002). Often, it is in these greyer shades of meaning where interesting and surprising things may be found.

Within this paper we will refer to grey shades of meaning and experience, the nuanced and ambivalent. We hope to show that by seeking and acknowledging these greyer shades of meaning, a richer understanding of people's relationship with wild places (bounded within a wild place experience programme context) and the notions of therapeutic landscapes can be explored. In addition, we illustrate that the ideas of 'cultural artefacts' are a useful means to categorise the richness of some of the themes that emerged from the data.

Studies of Two Wild Place Experiences

This paper will draw from data collected on two different (and comparative) wild place experiences (WPEs) studied in England. Following ethical clearance from the appropriate university committee, a grounded theory approach informed the design of the studies. Study 1 was a five-day trip in the Cheviot Hills, in Northumbria (4 participants); and study 2 comprised two successive weekend trips to Upper Nidderdale, in Yorkshire (5 participants). The participants in both studies were volunteers, recruited from a cohort of students on Counselling degree programmes at a university, and there were two participants who took take part in both. The WPEs were designed and facilitated by the first author, with supervision of the research by the second. Each WPE comprised an exploration and journey phase, wild camping, and a solo phase (of 34 – 38 hours).

Research Questions

1. How do people 'make-meaning' of their surroundings?
2. What was the human-landscape interrelationship in wild places (study locations)?
3. What factors and objects were involved in the interrelationship & meaning making, and how do these impact the experiences?
4. How do the findings of this study contribute to the notion of therapeutic landscapes?

Data were collected from multiple sources over the course of both studies, resulting in over 390,000 words, transcribed from source material. The participants were each interviewed before and after their experience, they kept diaries (from which they selected material for inclusion), and focus group discussions were held. The data were coded in nVivo, and analysed following the approach of Thematic Analysis (TA) (Braun & Clarke, 2006). The extracts included below are not interspersed with much interpretation from the writers, to emphasise the participants' words.

Findings

Therapeutic Landscapes (Positive Shades)

The following excerpts from a variety of the data sources illustrate the positive effects experienced by a cross-section of participants:

> It was fantastic it was just that freeing that freedom I felt and that peace of mind just everything. (Alex*; follow-up interview, study 1*)
>
> It feels like a really positive experience it felt like that before and it still does. (Sarah*; post-experience interview, study 2*)
>
> I thought it was just really good for personal reflection you know that kind of thing (…) working with other people that you don't know and you know it's really personal growth. (Nina*; post-experience interview, study 2*)
>
> It is really really freeing really freeing you know and you get a real awareness of you. (Joe*; follow-up interview, study 2*)
>
> It was totally different and I've actually forgotten that I'm an ex-addict which is a real, I've never ever expected… I hadn't forgot my past but it was like somebody else you know. *(Alex; group discussion, study 1*)
>
> I think what I'll keep which is really lovely is that realisation that I have the potential to stand still because I honestly don't do that ever. I can't even remember a time that I've not had anxiety in my life so, just a really nice realisation that like 'awww' it is possible for me because I just assumed it wasn't. … It's nice that there's an outlet that I do feel calm. It's really good 'cos I think it's something to try and incorporate into my life that would be really healthy and that would be really positive. (Sarah; *post-experience interview*)

Common features of the above accounts include the experience as described as different from everyday experiences, with some reporting a deepened sense of self-awareness, a greater sense of freedom and enhanced feelings of calmness.

Therapeutic Landscapes (Negative Shades):

The following more extensive accounts from two participants' journals illustrate the challenges they recorded in initial phases of the WPE.

> Sat on my own in my own head my thoughts started to wander. Oh my god I'm miles away from home – panic was setting in – but I had to think to myself what was I trying to run away from I would feel like this if I was home. Still out of my comfort zone I think that is part of the problem. I feel like no-one understands but I don't open my mouth how will they now. I don't want to look stupid + scared. Just talked a little with someone in the group and feel a little better. … We have fitted the bags, how do I know if it's fitting ok, and I'm a little worried that I'm not going to be able to carry it. Its deffo the calm before the story or at least that's I'm thinking anyway. I'm so anxious/ worried but excited, apprehensive about the next 4 days. Today has seemed one minute like a year and the other minute like we've only just arrived. It feels like it's not real, like I'm not actually here, this is all a dream. (Alex; *journal, study 1*)

> When we started going over rough terrain, I hated it. I kept losing my balance, tripping and falling over. I felt out of control and had to put 100% trust in Lizzie to guide me through until we reached the camp area. … I didn't have a problem putting my trust in Lizzie. The problem was that I didn't feel in control. At times I couldn't see my feet, which added to my frustration. … (Lesley; *journal, study 2*)

Both participants above report uncomfortable feeling states, shaded with anxiety in the first case, and frustration in the second. They illustrate the challenges of the new experiences, in which participants are taken out of their comfort zones, provoking emotive responses.

Therapeutic Landscapes (Positive and Negative Shades):

The following excerpts show the shifting of thoughts reported in some of the accounts.

> …have found my thought wandering on to 'unfinished' around concerns about relationship problems. All this space and no distractions allows

> them to come through... However now I have found this place I feel at more at ease with my thoughts. (Joe; *journal, during 24 hour solo*)
>
> It's funny really the wilderness space persuades thought to come through and for them to feel … At around 10am, I started to feel a bit bored as there was nothing to do. …
>
> The sound of the animals became distant as the sound of the wind became louder at around 11am, I ventured out and sat on the rock near my tent and took some photos this helped to empty my mind of boredom and just enjoy the peace of the outdoors. (Lesley; *journal, study 2*)
>
> Just walked into town and it felt really full – the atmosphere people everywhere – really annoying – and money – I don't need money in the wild place, but here everything stems from money… I also wanted to use the toilet in the supermarket and was pretty pissed off when it was closed – I had to wait till I got home, but the weekend I could go to the toilet whenever I wanted. (Alex; *Journal, study 2*)

In each of the above, shifts from more negative feeling states to more positive ones are illustrated. In addition to the variations in these, many of the accounts included references to 'markers' in the environment that prompted responses, as follows.

Physical Objects.

In study 1, parts of which took place in a designated natural park, two of the participants reported features that they felt compromised the sense of being in a wild place, as follows:

> I think it was just that middle bit where we were kinda along that wooden pathway and stuff like that kinda felt, didn't feel, it still felt like a wilderness [louder voice] don't get me wrong but there was other folk around and stuff like that [tone goes down like sulky] and em so, so it felt like we dipped in and out of it that's what it felt like. (Joe; *Post-experience interview, study 1)*
>
> It felt like it was the first couple of days and then we did that walk and I saw *those* guys eating *cheese* sandwiches with their shorts on. It kind of blew the whole thing up and I thought you know that's really spoilt my

kinda like *fantasy* image of where we were. Then I realised that we were just here, just a few miles from home. ... So that's what spoilt that, other *people* you see *people*. (Alex; *Post-experience interview, study 1)*

More accounts of the sense of human intrusion into the environment, through references to objects, came from the second study, where the wild place was less remote from human settlement.

I felt quite remote when it was the solo period because I couldn't even see the other tents I mean I felt we were in quite a remote place in the first camp but because I kind of knew that a house was just down that hill then it wasn't. But when we were actually climbing and when we camped at the other one I did feel that it was quite remote. (Sam; *Postexperience interview).*

The weather is overcast – cloudy but pastel blue sky scattered here and there – a plane flies over head and I sense that I am only a few miles from home. Whereas last time I knew and could feel I was miles away. This place doesn't seem deserted the land looks different, a fence to the left of me which reminds me that there are farms and farmers close by. ...I feel like I'm in a picture – a painting, the scenery is beautiful. A plane flies overhead, which reminds me I'm still on planet earth. But my thoughts of worries of bills, of life at home seems to have gone – the peace is great. ... "I've walked just up the hill to get a slightly different feel to this experience. Wow the view is fantastic and even though I can see someone and I saw a truck going up the path I'm not disappointed at all. ...The view is fantastic, the open fields with fencing to boarder them – the few sheep I can see are all on the other side of the fence – as if fenced out of this beautiful place. (Alex; *Journal, Study 2).*

I've just been for a walk along the stream, the wind is so cool and refreshing. You especially feel it after being in a stuffy tent. I was really enjoying my walk until I saw an old wire fence curled round the rocks. At first I didn't notice it as it had moss and grass growing on it, it definitely spoils it and must be damaging to the environment and the sheep and rabbits around, even that sheep that is still staring me out. (Nina; *Journal, Study 2).*

> I'm fifty, fifty… I was quite amazed at how remote it was and it wasn't because I see houses that didn't particularly bother me a lot. In some way that kinda helped put it into context to where I was and I think probably and kind of the first campsite as well felt remote even though you know I think there was a house at the bottom of the valley, but there wasn't a connection there kinda mentally. It felt we were in a remote place and that felt *good.* (Joe; *Post-experience interview, study 2).*

Symbolism

The accounts that follow illustrate the ways in which participants drew from their own repertoires of cultural material, as they reported their thoughts about their experiences.

> I know last night I felt quite vulnerable and small insignificant to this huge place. I was quite fearful, but that was my thoughts thinking of horror films I have seen. I have to bring myself back to reality sometimes as the fear seems to get so intense. And in this place when it's cold and dark I hear noise I don't know and the tent slightly blowing I can imagine that there's someone outside or an animal – not sure what animal, but obviously at that time of night_I think it's gonna harm me. …I'm really trying again to connect with this place, this space and allow myself the full benefit of this time alone. My head tends to wander from fantasy to reality. (Alex; *journal, study 1).*

> I found the most amazing mushrooms, the red ones with white spots on, it was like something from a fairytale. It really does remind me of stories or films I'd watched as a child, when I'm out here, and how it links to some of my previous artwork when I explored nature, and the magical aura it has. My sketches were of fairies and mystical creatures that were a part of the environment, such as mother nature herself in different forms, the green man and goblin type things, faces in trees and caves. I'd create characters of my friends, "Peteree the forest keeper," who used to live in Sherwood forest, a friend from college... the forest today opened my imagination and has made me want to pick that back up. (Kit; *journal, study one).*

> That was like the one bit that's put me off the solo experience was like spending the night by myself like in the wilderness sort of thing …. sort of once I got back and then I'd be too scared to come out my tent and

sort of stuff like that (.) erm (.) which I was a bit frightened erm …I know how we were saying before like all the muggers and stuff sort of live (.) are all where other people are (.) erm but I've got the sort of imagination that'll still like you see a horror movie and you think like oh yeah in the wilderness like this crazy man's going to come along …I didn't have a good night that was like the first Friday night I just kept waking up and then I woke up and I needed the loo but I was like no::: I'm going to go outside cos it's pitch black you know (.) what if someone gets me. (Nina; *post-programme interview, study 2.)*

E: What else did you see that can you remember?

S: I have a 3D view as well you get to see like surround you.

E: Yeah.

S: So yeah (.) that was quite fun [laughs] and then also that means it's more scary in the dark coz I can see stuff and over there ,there's a big rock behind you and honest to God if we sit by my tent and I'll try and show you where it is because it looks like a commando like, like a sniper like a man's torso (.) no it's over it's up the hill a bit and like a bit further away which is why I couldn't tell whether it was or not and it just looks like a man like lying there (Sarah; *individual interview, study 2)*.

SUMMARY OF FINDINGS

1. Therapeutic landscapes are shown to be 'ambivalent and nuanced spaces' in the findings reported above.
2. Therapeutic landscapes have many shades of meaning and experience; they can be perceived as healthy and unhealthy at the same time.
3. Being aware of how perceptions of wild places can be de-stabilised or stabilised by cultural objects is important for both the setting up and facilitation of WPEs.
4. There is an interaction and interplay between cultural artifacts (both physical and symbolic) and the nature of therapeutic landscapes. Shades of meaning arise in the different ways individuals perceive and experience them.

Discussion

The above excerpts illustrate both the 'shades' of reported emotional responses during and after WPEs, as well as examples of physical and symbolic artefacts utilised by participants to describe aspects of their meaning-making. One of the emergent themes is the way that the 'markers' of boundaries during the WPE – paths, fences, buildings, other people, and streams – were features of participant accounts. Often participants would use boundary markers to relate to positive, mixed and negative emotions. Physical objects seemed to be an intermediary between participants and the environment, at times connecting them with the environment. Boundary markers were used in discussions about the characteristics of the environment (e.g. whether the environment/location was as remote or wild as they were expecting) and their pre-constructed expectations of what the location would be like and the experience itself (e.g. walking on or off path, getting away from signs of human settlement and achieving remoteness). The outcomes of these thoughts in journal writing or within interviews, or during group discussions appeared to influence being satisfied (expectations met) and not satisfied (expectations not being met).

The meanings associated with physical objects lead to ideas about the identity of the object as created by culture, and illustrate the influence of such *cultural repertoires*. Cole (2005) refers to culture as "socially inherited past human accomplishments that serve as the resources for the current life of a social group" (p.196) and notes the role of symbols for the transmission of cultural behaviour and the embodiment of these in artefacts. Within cultural repertoires, different codes are used, including semiotic codes and collective schemas (Holley, 2011). Cultural experiences are characterised by inconsistencies that are enabling and flexible in their application but that may constrain and limit behaviour. Semiotic codes reflect collective schemas of meaning that are embedded within particular communities. Importantly semiotic codes are components that reflect the experiences that individuals bring with them into any situation or environment, and reflect the choices made by individuals.

The data suggest that those participants who reported more instances of ambivalence seemed to derive this from deciphering the cultural codes in their experiences of the environment. Three particular 'cultures' seemed to influence participants: the *general culture* influencing material that they drew from, the *research or academic culture*, because they were studying counselling and used skills from the reflective processes that this enhances; and then the *group culture* that developed from the dynamics of being in the group together on the WPE.

Each of these cultures contributed to meaning making and behaviour, and had elements that also overlapped with one another.

Concluding Comments

In this paper, we have illustrated some of the points made by Baer and Gesler (2004), which they deduced from a very different context and study. We have raised for discussion issues related to ambivalence, nuances and various shades of therapeutic landscapes, that we believe need to be explored and acknowledged within research. It is clear that the landscapes of our meaning-making, like natural environments, are complex multi-faceted entities. Thus defining, researching, and assessing the efficacy of natural environments is a difficult enterprise. We hope to have illustrated a deeper and critically conscious understanding and conceptualisation of 'wild places' and people's interactions with it – physically and mentally (by embracing an embodied holistic approach). We welcome thoughts and opinions related to this material, drawing from personal experiences and reflections in wild places.

Baer and Gesler (2004) note that "These environments may be therapeutic for some, but not for others; their therapeutic potential may change over time...We need to be open to assessments of the efficacy of therapeutic landscapes by diverse participants in the healing process." (p 410). Through offering extended notions of therapeutic landscapes and human-environment interrelationship theory, we want to emphasise the importance of respecting, acknowledging and attempting to understand the changing relationships that people have with the natural environment. This interrelationship can be deepened through acknowledging both consistency *and* ambiguity, as a 'community of practice' (Wenger, 1999) develops, and is facilitated as people engage together on exploring and experiencing wild places.

References

Akhurst, J. E. (2010). Exploring the nexus between wilderness and therapeutic experiences. *Implicit Religion*, *13*, 3, 295-306.

Baer, L. D. & Gesler, W. M. (2004) .Reconsidering the concept of therapeutic landscapes in J. D. Salinger's 'The Catcher in the Rye. *Area*, *36,* 4, 404-413.

Braun, V. and Clarke, V. (2006) Using thematic analysis in psychology. *Qualitative Research in Psychology*, *3*, 2, 77-101.

Cole, M. (1996). *Cultural psychology*. Cambridge, MA: Harvard University Press.

Cole, M. (2005). Cross-cultural and historical perspectives on the developmental consequences of education. *Human Development, 48,* 195–216.

Gesler, W. M. (2003) *Healing places,* Rowman & Littlefield, Lanham MD

Gesler, W. M. & Kearns R. A. (2002) *Culture/place/health,* Routledge: London

Gesler, W. (1992) 'Therapeutic Landscapes: Medical issues in light of the new cultural geography' Social Science & Medicine 34(7), 735-746

Holley, K. A. (2011). A cultural repertoire of practices in doctoral education. *International Journal of Doctoral Studies*, 6, 79-94.

Wegner, E. (1999). *Communities of practice: learning, meaning, and identity.* Cambridge: Cambridge University Press.

CHAPTER 13

The Role of the Natural Environment for Eudemonic Well-being and Identity During Adventure Experiences

Joe Hinds

ABSTRACT

Two quantitative studies are presented that assessed the extent to which being exposed to the natural environment during adventure experiences could positively affect, as a dual-process model, both psychological wellbeing and environmental identity. Working with the John Muir Trust and their programme of adventure activities in Scotland (e.g. sea kayaking, camping, woodland craft skills, conservation tasks & canoeing), two studies investigated the effects of adventure on participant's eudemonic wellbeing (*self-actualisation* & *personal-expressiveness*), hedonic wellbeing (*satisfaction with life* & *happiness*) and *environmental identity*. Results from Study 1 ($N = 47$) indicated that participants reported significantly greater eudemonic, but not hedonic, wellbeing and stronger *environmental identity* after their adventure experiences. The second study ($N = 44$) compared an Adventure group ($n = 21$), to a Control group ($n = 23$) – matched by mean age and gender in a partial replication of the first study. The findings indicated that the Adventure group reported greater post-experience *self-actualisation* and stronger *environmental identity* than did the control group; but not for the other research variables. The convergences and divergences between both studies and the strengths and limitations of each are considered. Moreover, how outdoor adventure experiences may operate reciprocally, positively affecting participants and the environment (e.g. Totton, 2011), are discussed.

INTRODUCTION: WELL-BEING AND THE NATURAL ENVIRONMENT

There is growing interest in how experiences of the natural environment can impact positive affect (e.g., Kals, Schumaker, & Montada, 1999). The relationship between people's experience of the natural environment (direct and immersed) and their emotional wellbeing is beginning to be better understood (Hinds, 2011a; Sohr, 2001). For instance, Jacob and Brinkerhoff (1999) found that participants exposed to natural environments tended to report experiencing feelings of union with nature, joy, a sense of wonder and peace of mind. Similarly, Eigner (2001) suggests that the well-being associated with immersion in the natural environment may be a qualitatively different, "higher quality" well-being than a more hedonic well-being. Participants active in various voluntary environmental protective behaviours such as the maintenance of local natural environments have reported that the natural environment produced "an amazing feeling of happiness", an "inner sort of calm", and feelings of being "really satisfied", more relaxed and more like themselves (Eigner, 2001, pp. 191-192). These emotional responses mirror those reported during eudemonic experiences including feelings of inner peace, a deep appreciation of life, and feelings of connection (Huta & Ryan, 2010). Moreover, eudemonic wellbeing tends to emphasise personal growth (Ryff & Singer, 2008), self-realisation (Ryan & Deci, 2001) and has been described as the achievement of potential in the individual and the recognition of "the type of life worth living" (Waterman, 1990, p. 55). These eudemonic feeling states are very similar to those states that would be expected in peak experiences as described by Maslow (1964) and therefore has considerable theoretical overlap with eudemonia (Ryff & Singer, 2008). Additionally, some research has suggested that wilderness users may be more self-actualised than non-users (Young & Crandall, 1984) and that natural environments can induce self-transformative experiences similar to those described by self-actualising experiences (Talbot & Kaplan, 1986; Williams & Harvey, 2001).

These reported feelings stand in contrast to the more mainstream measurement of subjective well-being (SWB), which has tended to assess general negative and positive affect and life satisfaction; generically labelled hedonic wellbeing (e.g., Kahneman, Diener, & Schwarz, 1999). There have been criticisms that the SWB measure is an insufficient indicator of the more meaningful and intrinsic aspects of people's well-being: "reports about happiness and satisfaction with one's life are not necessarily valid read-outs of an internal state of personal well-being" (Schwarz & Strack, 1991, p. 28). There is some evidence to suggest that people's assessment of their overall life satisfaction may be positively related to the degree to which they feel a sense of connection with nature (Mayer & Frantz, 2004). Some research has disputed the eudemonic-hedonic distinction and questioned the need to divide well-being into two "constructs that are artificially separated from one another" (Kashdan, Biswas-Diener, & King, 2008, p. 228). However, it has been suggested that the inclusion of both eudemonic and hedonic perspectives within the well-being literature is necessary for a broad and meaningful interpretation of psychological well-being (Boniwell & Henry, 2007).

Adventure Therapy

Implicit in the term 'adventure' is risk and its associated emotions (positive & negative) which help mark out adventure and wilderness therapies from other forms of experiential therapies (Berger, 2008). The activities that are engaged in by participants during adventure programmes are 'real', such as building and using rafts or climbing (Davis-Berman & Berman, 2000). Moreover, these activities often require an element of group assistance or encouragement for success and provide an environment for peer-group interaction, which may contribute positively to a range of psychological benefits (Hattie, Marsh, Neill, & Richards, 1997).

Research suggests that adventure programmes orientated to encouraging human contact with nature can have a variety of psychological benefits such as a greater internal locus of control and higher self-esteem (Hans, 2000), and greater self-efficacy (Hattie et al, 1997). By incorporating specific therapeutic elements within these types of natural environmental encounters there are opportunities to expand on the array of benefits to the human condition (Glass & Jackson, 2008; Totton, 2011). In particular, wilderness therapies have been targeted to foster positive growth in many authentic, emotional and meaningful ways (Annerstedt & Währborg, 2011; Williams, 2000). Cohen (1993), suggests that by relinquishing our hold on our contemporary 'closeted ways' and by re-bonding to the natural environment we can begin to both reduce the frequency and intensity of our collective psychological problems. Nature, in these circumstances maybe conceived as 'intimate other'; the 'third' entity within an outdoor dyadic therapeutic encounter, one in which clients can explore an embodied, multi-sensory, sensuous experience that awakens them to their here-and-now experiencing (Adams, 2010). Others have stressed the importance of exposure to the natural environment to build a sense of self that is orientated around a transpersonal relatedness (Jordan, 2009). Adventure has the potential to foster growth in aspects of the self (e.g., self-confidence) and compassion for other people and the environment in which the adventure takes place (Mortlock, 1984). Healing individual trauma in the wild may liberate people's attention so that they can "reconnect with their innate love and care for the other-than-human" (Totton, 2011, p. 213).

Environmental Identity

There is increasing recognition of the importance of the inclusion of nature within representations of self for pro-environmental attitudes, otherwise termed environmental identity how people see themselves in the context of nature and the natural world (Clayton & Opotow, 2003). Strong correlations have been found between various measures of identity and self-reported environmental behaviours, such as energy efficiency and recycling (Mannetti, Pierro & Livi, 2004). Arguably, the role of experience of the natural environment plays an invaluable part in the construction of environmental identities (Hinds, 2011b), in pro-environmental attitudes and behaviours (Teisl & O'Brien, 2003), and in some cases both wellbeing and identity (Hinds & Sparks, 2009). In line with the eudemonic wellbeing effects (reported above), other research has found that profound experiences (aligned to both eudemonia and Maslow's [1964] concept of peak experiences) with wildlife has the potential to positively transform environmental attitudes (DeMares & Krycka, 1998; Smith, Ham, & Weiler, 2011). Conversely however, overly structured wilderness experiences, such as those with an emphasis on adventure-based activities such as rock climbing may result in *reduced* awareness of the environment in which these activities are conducted (e.g. Haluza-DeLay, 1999).

Dual Process

There is a small but influential corpus of research, which describes a reciprocal relationship between users of natural places and the natural environment in terms of the development of pro-environmental orientations (e.g. Hinds, 2011a). For instance, some evidence suggests that people willing to lead a simple, more sustainable way of life, such as driving less, having smaller houses, and engaging in recycling, tended to be happier and have higher life satisfaction than those in a control group matched on gender, age, and geographic location, who were more not leading simpler lives (Brown & Kasser, 2005). Similarly, people who see greater potential for psychological restoration in natural environments, such as stress reduction, also tend to report increases in ecological behaviour, as with recycling or reduced driving (Hartig, Kaiser,& Bowler, 2001; Hartig, Kaiser & Strumse, 2007).

The Present Research

The present research, based upon the issues outlined above, sought to examine the impact of adventure encounters (specifically the role of the natural environment) on people's well-being. In particular, the inclusion of both eudemonic and hedonic measures were critical for a broader assessment of the influence of the natural environment on well-being. The present research was also designed to gain a better understanding of how exposure to the natural environment may impact upon people's environmental identification.

The present sample, derived from the John Muir Trust's outdoor programme, was chosen because of the Trust's access to areas of wilderness and to qualified outdoor personnel capable of leading small groups within those environments. The range of activities was diverse: sea kayaking, camping, woodland craft skills, conservation tasks and river canoeing. The common denominators for all activities were both the closeness to, and dependency on, the natural environment, and the introduction of conservation-related activities such as restoration of pathways, conducting wildlife surveys, and litter clearances.

After consideration of the evidence reviewed above, it was hypothesised that experience of the natural environment would elicit: (i) greater self-actualisation, (ii) greater personal-expressiveness, (iii) stronger environmental identity, (iv) greater happiness, (v) and greater satisfaction with life.

STUDY 1: METHOD

Participants

Participants (*N* = 47; female = 27; male = 20) represented a convenience sample and were all paying volunteers on a variety of John Muir Trust (JMT) summer programme activities lasting between 3-9 days. Their mean age was 31 years (range 16-62).

Materials and Procedure

Participants were presented with two questionnaires. The first questionnaire was completed approximately one week prior to their JMT experience and the second approximately three weeks after their experience. The second questionnaire was largely a replication of the first but with some additional items. Responses were recorded along fully anchored, 7-point Likert-like scales, unless otherwise indicated. Response scale end-points are indicated in parentheses. Reverse coding of variables was carried out where appropriate. The questionnaires requested information on age and gender before assessing the variables described below and a number of additional measures (which are not reported here).

Well-being

Well-being was measured in four different ways:

1. *Happiness* was measured with the single item, "In general, how happy or unhappy do you usually feel?" (Fordyce, 1988). Responses were recorded on an 11-point scale (*extremely unhappy* [1] to *extremely happy* [11]).
2. *Satisfaction with life* (Diener, Emmons, Larson, & Griffin, 1985) was measured with 5-items: "In most ways my life is close to my ideal", "The conditions of my life are excellent", "I am satisfied with my life", "So far I have achieved the important things I want in life" and "If I could live my life again, I would change almost nothing" (*strongly disagree* [1] to *strongly agree* [7]). The mean of these items was used to form a composite measure of *Satisfaction with life* (Time 1, α = .86; Time 2, α = .90).
3. *Self-actualisation* (adapted from Sheldon et al., 2001) was measured with 3 items: "Being in the natural environment gives me a sense of being who I really am", "Being in the natural environment gives me a sense of a deeper purpose in life" and "Being in the natural environment gives me a deeper understanding of myself and my place in the universe" (*strongly disagree* [1] to *strongly agree* [7]). The mean of these items was used to form a composite measure of *Self-actualisation* (Time 1, α = .90; Time 2, α = .85).
4. *Personal-expressiveness* (adapted from Waterman, 1990) was measured with 5 items: "Being in the natural environment gives me my greatest feeling of really being alive", "Being in the natural environment gives me a feeling that this is what I was meant to do", "Being in the natural environment gives me my greatest pleasure", "I feel more complete or fulfilled when engaged with the natural environment than I do when engaged in most other activities" and "I feel a special fit or meshing when engaged in the natural environment" (*strongly disagree* [1] to

strongly agree [7]). The mean of these items was used to form a composite measure of *Personal-expressiveness* (Time 1, α = .83; Time 2, α = .89).

Environmental Identity

Environmental identity (adapted from Stets & Biga, 2003) was measured with 10 items: 'To what extent do you think of yourself as [x] the natural environment?' and assessed, '*detached from*' '*connected to*', '*respectful of*', '*concerned about*', '*disinterested in*', '*passionate about*', '*independent from*', '*superior to*', '*in competition with*', and '*protective of*' (5-point scale: *not at all* [1] to *extremely* [5]). The mean of these items was used to form a composite measure of *environmental identity* (Time 1, α = .77; Time 2, α = .84).

Results

A series of paired-samples t-tests were conducted to determine any significant changes in the dependent variables between Time 1 and Time 2. Inter-correlations, means and standard deviations for these variables are presented for both time points (see Table 1). Participants reported an increase in self-actualisation, $t(46) = -2.22$, $p = .032$, and greater personal-expressiveness, $t(46) = -2.14$, $p = .038$. They also reported a significantly stronger identification with the natural environment, $t(46) = 4.94$, $p < .001$. There were no changes in Happiness, $t(46) = -.06$, $p = .96$ or Satisfaction with life, $t(46) = -.35$, $p = .73$.

Table 1. Study 1 inter-correlations, means and standard deviations for the research variables (*N* = 47): Time 1 appears above the diagonal and Time 2 below.

	1	2	3	4	5	*M*	SD
1. General Happiness	_	.43**	.09	.14	.34*	8.04	2.32
2. Satisfaction With Life	.45**	_	.07	.02	.25	4.86	1.31
3. Self-Actualisation	-.09	-.01	_	.70***	.37**	5.48	1.25
4. Personal-Expressiveness	-.09	.03	.71***	_	.53***	5.40	1.07
5. Environmental Identity	.07	.25	.30*	.46**	_	3.89	0.47
M	8.06	4.89	5.77	5.62	4.07		
SD	2.43	1.38	1.08	1.15	0.54		

* $p < .05$; ** $p < .01$; *** $p < .001$

Discussion

Despite past research indicating satisfaction with life and happiness being sensitive to life events, there were no significant time differences for these variables. However, in line with the remaining hypotheses, results indicated that participants reported developing a stronger sense of environmental identity, improved self-actualisation, and a heightened sense of personal-expressiveness following a 3-9 day exposure to the natural environment. Although encouraging, these findings might be the result of change over time (for a variety of reasons) rather than as a direct effect of the natural-environment experiences *per se*. Thus, in order to draw firmer research conclusions, the second study incorporated a control group.

STUDY 2: METHOD

Study 2 followed a similar format to that of the Study 1 but with the inclusion of the aforementioned control group. It was again hypothesised that, in comparison to a control group, experience of the natural environment would elicit: (i) greater self-actualisation, (ii) greater personal-expressiveness, and (iii) stronger environmental identity. Given the non-significant results of Study 1, no a priori hypotheses were generated for the remaining variables.

Participants

Participants (N = 44) consisted of two groups matched by mean age and gender ratio. The first, an *experiential* group (n = 21; female = 16; male = 5), were paying volunteers on a variety of JMT summer programme activities. Their mean age was 26 years (range 15-60). The second, *control* group (n = 23; female = 18; male = 5), were undergraduate social science students at Sussex University, UK. Their mean age was 26 years (range 20 43). Sussex University is situated within the South Downs National Park in east Sussex and is recognised as an area of outstanding beauty.

Materials and Procedure

The *experiential* group was presented with two on-line questionnaires. The first questionnaire was completed approximately two weeks prior to the natural environment experience and the second approximately three weeks after the experience. The *control* group were presented with paper versions of the same questionnaires in the same time frame. The questionnaires followed a similar format as Study 1. All variables were constructed as in Study 1 with the exception of the following: *Satisfaction with life* which was measured with the single item: "I am satisfied with my life" (strongly disagree to strongly agree) and *Environmental identity* which was measured with 8 items: 'To what extent do you think of yourself as [x] the natural environment?' and included, '*respectful* of', '*concerned* about', '*disinterested* in', '*passionate* about', '*independent* from', '*superior* to', and '*protective* of' (*not at all* [1] to *extremely* [5]). The mean of these items was used to form a composite measure of *environmental identity* (Time 1, α = .80; Time 2, α = .87). Inter-item reliabilities for the remaining measures, retained in their original form, were: *personal-expressiveness* (Time 1, α = .92; Time 2, α = .95) and *self-actualisation* (Time 1, α = .93; Time 2, α = .92).

Results

Group Differences

Inter-correlations between the variables for the control group and the experiential group at both time points are presented, as are means and standard deviations (see Table's 2 & 3 respectively). A series of ANCOVAs were performed to assess group (experiential vs. control) differences on the variables at Time 2, controlling for Time 1 scores. Levene's test of equality of error variances was non-significant in all instances.

There was a significant main effect of Group on *Self-Actualisation* $F(1,41) = 4.71$, $p = .036$, with the experiential group reporting being more self-actualised ($M = 5.83$; SD = 0.95) than did the control group ($M = 5.30$; SD = 1.21). However, there were no effects for *Personal-Expressiveness*, $F(1,41) = 4.71$, $p = .34$, *Happiness*, $F(1,40) = 0.10$, $p = .75$, or *Satisfaction With Life*, $F(1,41) = 0.54$, $p = .47$. There was a significant main effect of group for *Environmental Identity* $F(1,41) = 5.18$, $p = .028$, with the experiential group reporting stronger environmental identities ($M = 3.94$; SD = 0.58) than the control group ($M = 3.63$; SD = 0.57).

Table 2. Study 2 control group ($N = 23$) inter-correlations for the research variables. Time 1 correlations appear above the diagonal and Time 2 below.

	1	2	3	4	5	*M*	SD
1. General Happiness	_	.58**	-.22	-.01	.20	7.78	2.21
2. Satisfaction With Life	.80***	_	-.23	-.01	.31	5.00	1.35
3. Self-Actualisation	-.09	.01	_	.81***	.53**	5.23	1.35
4. Personal-Expressiveness	-.10	.01	.75***	_	.55**	4.64	1.44
5. Environmental Identity	.03	.10	.36	.67**	_	3.59	0.51
M	8.26	5.35	5.07	4.57	3.48		
SD	1.66	1.37	1.21	1.49	0.57		

** $p < .01$; *** $p < .001$

Table 3. Study 2 experiential group (N = 21) inter-correlations for the research variables: Time 1 correlations appear above the diagonal and Time 2 below.

	1	2	3	4	5	*M*	SD
1. General Happiness	_	.75***	.08	.01	.41	8.57	1.47
2. Satisfaction With Life	.16	_	.22	.03	.26	6.00	1.00
3. Self-Actualisation	.04	-.02	_	.54*	.47*	5.92	0.83
4. Personal-Expressiveness	-.06	-.05	.89***	_	.48*	5.72	0.81
5. Environmental Identity	.05	.32	.70***	.77***	_	3.98	0.48
M	8.35	6.14	6.08	5.70	4.10		
SD	2.28	0.85	0.95	1.14	0.58		

* $p < .05$; *** $p < .001$

General Discussion

The results from these two studies provide cumulative support for some of the hypotheses. First, Study 1 showed that participants involved in an Adventure experience reported significant and positive changes in self-actualisation. In comparison to a control group, the experiential group in Study 2 also reported greater Time 2 self-actualisation. The present self-actualisation findings, whilst not unique (see Young & Crandall, 1984), certainly present a relatively novel addition to the understanding as to the effects the natural environment may have on well-being. As self-actualisation in relation to the natural environment has tended to be researched within a qualitative paradigm, the present study complements this existing work (Eigner, 2001; Williams & Harvey, 2001).

Second, the present research also provides important empirical support for theoretical standpoints regarding the importance of the direct experience of the natural environment in forming environmental identities (Hinds, 2011b). Adjunct research has suggested that an environmental identity may have a role to play in predicting pro-environmental behaviours (Clayton & Opotow, 2003). Although research has shown that direct experience of the natural environment can be influential in determining (self-reported) pro-environmental behaviours (Teisl & O'Brien, 2003), it remains to be seen if experience of the natural environment under similar conditions to those of the present research can lead to actual quantifiable pro-environmental behaviour changes mediated by environmental identity.

Although differences over time were detected for personal-expressiveness in Study 1, no differences were apparent between the experiential and control groups for personal-expressiveness in Study 2. This finding was surprising given the strong correlations between these variables found here and elsewhere (e.g.,

Waterman, 1990). Further research, incorporating both experimental and regression methods may help to determine any distinction between these measures and decide how each of them contributes to environment-related eudemonic well-being.

Moreover, there were no apparent effects of the natural environment on happiness or satisfaction with life (SWL). These results stand in contrast with the limited research on SWL and the natural environment (Mayer & Frantz, 2004). The non-significant effects on happiness and satisfaction with life may be accounted for by their particular trait or global nature. In other words, those aspects of well-being may tend to capture trait-like aspects of human functioning that tend to be resistant to change. This stands in contrast to self-actualisation, which was conceived of as a goal that people are motivated to move towards (Maslow, 1964). It is therefore possible that the natural environment, under specific conditions, can readily engender eudemonic well-being but not necessarily hedonic well-being (cf. Kashdan et al, 2008). Moreover, from a theoretical perspective, eudemonia and hedonism were found to be empirically distinct here; there were no significant relationships between eudemonia (self-actualisation & personal-expressiveness) and hedonia (SWL and happiness). However, the scientific understanding and conceptualisation of eudemonia is still in its infancy and awaits further and more detailed investigation before definitive conclusions can be arrived at (Boniwell & Henry, 2007).

Due to the broad nature of the study encapsulating various activities, it is impossible to determine in the present study the individual effects of specific activities (e.g., canoeing or camping) on the results. Moreover, the small sample sizes representing each separate activity would make analysis problematic. As well as problems of drawing any general conclusions from a study with a small sample, the inherent bias in the experiential group composition should also be flagged. Participants in both studies were self-selecting individuals; they not only chose to be involved with the natural environment but also had a choice of activity. There is therefore the potential for these participants to be predisposed to have natural-environment preferences that allow them to develop, for example, an environmental identity more readily than a randomly-selected sample. Although the results were encouraging with regards to the benefits to (eudemonic) wellbeing, it remains to be seen if similar results can be obtained by utilising a non-clinical sample with an explicit therapeutic element. In addition, there are difficulties in recognising and securing an appropriate control group. Further research may wish to utilise control groups involved in alternative programmes of activities in order to further explore the effects discovered here.

Collectively the results from both studies would seem to indicate that extended experiential encounters with the natural environment within an adventure programme incorporating an environmental aspect (cf. Haluza-DeLay, 1999) can engender greater eudemonic well-being and a greater sense of identification with the environment, thus supporting research indicating a similar dual process (e.g.,Hartig et al, 2007; Hinds 2011a). With careful considerations for the environment and with a sensitive and skilful approach to the introduction of people to the natural environment, the present findings may provide a fertile ground for reciprocal interventions addressing not only people's well-being but also environmental identities (e.g. Totton, 2011). At the very least the present research maybe considered a further impetus towards a broadening of the understanding of positive well-being, and the relative measurement instrumentation required, within adventure experiences.

REFERENCES

Adams, W. W. (2010). Basho's therapy for Narcissus: Nature as intimate other and transpersonal self. *Journal of Humanistic Psychology, 50*, 38-64.

Annerstedt, M. & Wahrborg, P. (2011). Nature assisted therapy: Systematic review of controlled and observational studies. *Scandinavian Journal of Public Health, 39*, 371-388.

Berger, R. (2008). Building a home in nature: An innovative framework for practice. *Journal of Humanistic Psychology, 48*, 264-279.

Boniwell, I., & Henry, J. (2007). Developing conceptions of well-being: Advancing subjective, hedonic and eudaimonic theories. *Social Psychological Review, 9*, 3-18.

Brown, K. W., & Kasser, T. (2005). Are psychological and ecological well-being compatible? The role of values, mindfulness, and lifestyle. *Social Indicators Research, 74*, 349-368.

Clayton, S. (2003). Environmental identity: A conceptual and operational definition. In S.

Clayton & S. Opotow (Eds.), *Identity and the natural environment: The psychological significance of nature* (pp. 45-65). Cambridge, MA: MIT Press.

Clayton, S., & Opotow, S. (2003). Introduction: Identity and the natural environment. In S.

Clayton & S. Opotow (Eds.), *Identity and the natural environment: The psychological significance of nature* (pp. 1-24). Cambridge, MA: MIT Press.

Cohen, M. J. (1993). Counselling with nature: Catalyzing sensory moments that let earth nurture. *Counselling Psychology Quarterly, 6,* 39-52.

Davis-Berman, J., & Berman, D. S. (1989). The wilderness therapy program: An empirical study of its effects with adolescents in an outpatient setting. *Journal of Contemporary Psychotherapy, 19*, 271-281.

DeMares R, Krycka K. 1998. Wild animal triggered peak experiences: transpersonal aspects. *The Journal of Transpersonal Psychology, 30*,161–177.

Diener, E., Emmons, R. A., Larson, R. J., & Griffin, S. (1985). The satisfaction with life scale. *Journal of Personality Assessment, 49*, 71-75.

Eigner, S. (2001). The relationship between "protecting the environment" as a dominant life goal and subjective well-being. In P. Schmuck & K. M. Sheldon (Eds.) *Life goals and well-being: Towards a positive psychology of human striving* (pp. 182-201).

Hogrefe and Huber: Göttingen Fordyce, M. W. (1988). A review of research on the happiness measures: A sixty second index of happiness and mental health. *Social Indicators Research, 20*, 355-381.

Glass, J. S. & Jackson, J. (2008). Connecting theory to programming: Using existentialism and adventure based counselling with adolescents. *International Journal of Existential Psychology and Psychotherapy, 2*, 1-11.

Haluza-Delay, R. (1999). The culture that constrains: Experience of "nature" as part of a wilderness adventure program. *The Journal of Experiential Education, 22*,129-137.

Hans, T. A. (2000). A meta-analysis of the effects of adventure programming on locus of control. *Journal of Contemporary Psychotherapy, 30*, 33-60.

Hartig, T., Kaiser, F. G., & Bowler, P. A. (2001).Psychological restoration in nature as a positive motivation for ecological behaviour. *Environment and Behavior, 33*, 590-607.

Hartig, T., Kaiser, F. G., and Strumse, E. (2007). Psychological restoration in nature as a source of motivation for ecological behavior. *Environmental Conservation, 34*, 291-299.

Hattie, J., Marsh, H. W., Neill, J. T., & Richards, G. E. (1997). Adventure education and outward bound: Out-of-class experiences that make a lasting difference. *Review of Educational Research, 67,* 43-87.

Hinds, J., & Sparks, P. (2008). Engaging with the natural environment: The role of affective connection and identity. *Journal of Environmental Psychology, 28*, 109-120.

Hinds, J. (2011a). Exploring the psychological rewards of a wilderness experience: An interpretive phenomenological analysis. *The Humanistic Psychologist, 39*, 189-205.

Hinds, J. (2011b). Woodland adventure for marginalized adolescents: Environmental attitudes, identity and competence. *Applied Environmental Education and Communication, 10,* 228-237.

Huta, V. M. & Ryan, R. M. (2010). Pursuing pleasure versus virtue: The differential and overlapping well-being benefits of hedonic and eudaimonic motives. *Journal of Happiness Studies, 11*, 735–762.

Jacob, J. C., & Brinkerhoff, M. B. (1999). Mindfulness and subjective well-being in the sustainability movement: A further elaboration of multiple discrepancies theory. *Social Indicators Research, 46*, 341-368.

Jordan, M. (2009). Back to Nature. *Therapy Today, 20*, 28–30.

Kals, E., Schumaker, D., & Montada, L. (1999). Emotional affinity toward nature as a motivational basis to protect nature. *Environment and Behavior, 31*, 178-202.

Kashdan, T. B., Biswas-Diener, R., & King, L. A. (2008). Reconsidering happiness: The costs of distinguishing between hedonics and eudemonia. *The Journal of Positive Psychology, 3*, 219-233.

Mannetti, L., Pierro, A., & Livi, S. (2004). Recycling: Planned and self-expressive behaviour. *Journal of Environmental Psychology, 24*, 227-236.

Maslow, A. H. (1964). *Religions, values, and peak-experiences*. New York: Penguin.

Mayer, F. S., & Frantz, C. M. (2004). The connectedness to nature scale: A measure of individuals' feeling in community with nature. *Journal of Environmental Psychology,24*, 503-515.

Mortlock, C. (1984). *The Adventure Alternative.* Milnthorpe, Cumbria: Cicerone Press.

Ryan, R. M., & Deci, E. L. (2001). On happiness and human potentials: A review of research on hedonic and eudaimonic well-being. *Annual Review of Psychology, 52*, 141-166.

Ryff, C., & Singer, B. H. (2008). Know thyself and become what you are: A eudaimonic approach to psychological well-being. *Journal of Happiness Studies, 9*, 13-39.

Schwarz, N., & Strack, F. (1991). Evaluating one's life: A judgmental model of subjective well-being. In F. Strack, M. Argyle, & N. Schwarz (Eds.), *Subjective well-being: An interdisciplinary perspective* (pp.27-47). Oxford: Pergamon Press.

Sheldon, K. N., Elliot, A. J., Kim, Y., & Kasser, T. (2001). What is satisfying about satisfying events? Testing 10 candidate psychological needs. *Journal of Personality and Social Psychology, 80*, 325-339.

Smith, L. D. G., Ham, S. H., & Weiler, B. V. (2011). The Impacts of Profound Wildlife Experiences. *Anthrozoös, 24*, 51–64.

So Shr, S. (2001). Eco-activism and well-being: Between flow and burnout. In P. Schmuck & K. M. Sheldon (Eds.) *Life goals and well-being: Towards a positive psychology of human striving* (pp. 182-201). Hogrefe and Huber: Göttingen.

Stets, J. E., & Biga, C. F. (2003). Bringing identity theory into environmental sociology. *Sociological Theory, 21*, 398-423.

Talbot, J. F., & Kaplan, S. (1986). Perspectives on wilderness: Re-examining the value of extended wilderness experiences. *Journal of Environmental Psychology, 6*, 177-188.

Teisl, M. F., & O'Brien, K. (2003). Who cares and who acts? Outdoor recreationists exhibit different levels of environmental concern and behavior. *Environment and Behavior, 35*, 506-522.

Totton, N. (2011). *Wild therapy: Undomesticating inner and outer worlds*. PCCS Books: Ross-on-Wye.

Waterman, A. S. (1990). Personal expressiveness: Philosophical and psychological foundations. *Journal of Mind and Behaviour, 11*, 47-74.

Williams, K., & Harvey, D. (2001). Transcendent experience in forest environments. *Journal of Environmental Psychology, 21*, 249-260.

Young, R. A., & Crandall, R. (1984). Wilderness use and self-actualisation. *Journal of Leisure Research, 16*, 149-160.

CHAPTER 14

Adventure Therapy in Spain: Lights and Shadows

Alexander Rose

ABSTRACT

Analyzing determinant factors prior to starting to design a therapeutic intervention program based on adventure is necessary, especially, if there are no such programs traditionally. This paper dissects factors related to adventure and wilderness therapy in Spain, such as major approaches in psychology and psychotherapy and also experiential education, specific facilities, access to the land, social security and private insurance coverages, laws related to our field, etc.

INTRODUCTION

The most important aim of this paper is to analyze the factors related to Adventure therapy (AT) in order to introduce this therapy approach in Spain. Thereby we will proceed to introduce briefly general facts about the country to illustrate a complete framework of the country.

To start defining the context, Spain is a South European country divided politically in 17 autonomous communities. Despite the existence of general laws of the state, each region has considerable autonomy of decision on issues of health, education or land management. The Spanish highest law, the Constitution, guarantees a public social security system for all citizens, though a remarkable offer of private therapeutic programs also exists.

At present, world's socioeconomic crisis and the politicians' decisions are threatening the Spanish welfare system, specially increasing (youth) unemployment and suppressing labour and civil rights.

Gass, Gillis & Russell (2012) start their new book with the following definition of Adventure Therapy: "(AT) is the prescriptive use of adventure experiences provided by mental health professionals, often conducted in natural settings that kinaesthetically engage clients on cognitive, affective and behavioural levels". This definition helps us to establish the three cornerstones for the present communication: adventure experiences, prescriptive use provided by mental health professionals and natural settings.

Adventure Therapy Related Factors

Experiential and Adventure Education in Spain

In this section, we need to distinguish between formal and non-formal education. Traditionally, non-formal educative intervention in Spain is mostly designed using French patterns. Due to the dictatorial regime in Spain (1939-1975) few educational innovative approaches merged during that time (Trilla, 1997). Commonly researchers and intellectuals migrated to France and were trained in *Animación sociocultural*, bringing back and adopting further on this model in Spain (Senent, 1998). As opposed to the Experiential model, this approach places more emphasis on community education, improving the level of social welfare and with goals more focused on creating group dynamics through cultural and art activities (Trilla, 1997). The most similar intervention model to Experiential education, is the subtype of Free time pedagogies (*pedagogía del tiempo libre*), with stress on developing individual capabilities through group activities in natural settings (Martínez Rico, 2003).

The model of *animación sociocultural* has been perpetuated in training in outdoor schools, vocational trainings and in most of the interventions addressed to non-formal education. Therefore, the mid and northern European experiential education's approach was unusual until the nineties, where outdoor training and experiential team building was introduced in sports and business environments (Anglada, 2007). In the last ten years users of active tourism have increased, and, slightly, educational institutions are coming closer to this current although only from a recreational point of view (Anglada, 2007).

Other institutions related to this business, like the Spanish Mountaineering Federation (*Federación Española de Deportes de Montaña y Escalada*) only offer activities with emphasis on developing sport skills. On the other hand, the Professional association for rope courses (*Asociación Española de Parques de Aventura*), founded in 2007, has among its goals to start training professionals in 2013.

Related to this, each country of the European Union (EU), coordinated by Cedefop (European Centre for the Development of Vocational Training), is going through an evaluating process in order to establish all competencies in vocational training, including (adventure) sports. Both federations as private sport training centres are included in the sport education in special regime category.

On the other hand, formal education is also reproducing the French model. Subjects and contents related to experiential education are predominantly taught at Social education, Social work and Teacher training faculties.

Mental Health and Psychological Therapy

Article 41 of the Spanish Constitution states that the public authorities shall maintain a public social security system for all citizens [...] and that the support and additional benefits shall be free. The service portfolio of national health system includes mental health interventions but, nowadays, demand exceeds the system's capacity.

In Spain, mental health interventions are developed interdisciplinarily by many different professionals: physicians, psychologists, social workers, physiotherapists, occupational therapists... Nevertheless, psychiatrists and clinical psychologists are the only professionals with competencies for clinical mental health therapy.

In order to prescribe psychological therapy, social security physicians refer patients directly to the mental health specialists, usually psychiatrists, to proceed with the evaluation and search for the most appropriate treatment, resource or facility. This is the normal procedure with both adolescents and adults. When justice comes into play, both juveniles and adults are taken to rehabilitation centres after a court ruling.

Nowadays, Psychology is undergoing a thorough process of change, both formative and professional. On one hand, in order to become a licensed clinical psychologist (General Health Psychologist) one has to complete four years at University (240 ECTS[1]), and study an Official Master's degree in Clinical and Health Psychology (90 ECTS[2]), including no less than 750 hours of practical training. To become a Specialist in Health Psychology, with competencies for severe mental health treatment, in addition, one needs to pass a competitive exam and to accomplish a two year long internship.

On the other hand, this change will affect the labour market, where there will soon be three levels of specialization in clinical and health Psychology. Although

---

[1] ECTS: European Credit Transfer System. 1 ECTS equals 25 hours of dedication. 240 ECTS equals 6.000 training hours.

[2] 90 ECTS equal 2.250 hours.

its role is determined by different laws (Ordination of health professions act 44/2003, approved November 21st, Social economy act 5/2011, published March 29th and Public Health Act, which in its seventh additional provision regulates health psychology, Law 33/2011 of October 4th), specific competencies are not explained clearly enough.

Also, in order to work as a Psychologist in Spain you need to become a member of your autonomous community's professional association (*Colegio Oficial de Psicólogos*). In year 2011, there were 54.594 affiliates all over the country.

Last research about professional's profile was done by Fernández, Berdullas, Santolaya and Muñiz (2000), with 27.787 affiliates, and reflected the following panorama: Clinical and Health Psychology division was integrated by 68.36% of the members, 15.29% were affiliated to the Educational & School Psychology division, 8.05% to Work and Organizational Psychology division, 4.40% belonged to the Social Psychology division, 1.63% to the Traffic Psychology division, 1.15% to Legal Psychology, 0.35% to Sport Psychology and 0.25% to Military Psychology.

The same research also referred the most common currents followed by psychologists in Spain (Fernández et al., 2002):

Fig. 1. Adapted from Fernández et al. (2000)

Psychological Current	Percentage
Cognitive Behavioural	49.08
Behaviour modification	14.12
Eclecticism	12.80
Psychoanalysis approaches	9.48
Systemic approach	5.45
Humanistic approach	4.16
Orthodox Psychoanalysis	3.88
Transactional analysis	0.57
Phenomenological - Existential models	0.20
Gestalt therapy	0.20
Others	0.07

Finally, about research and divulgation of AT in Spain (*terapia a través de la aventura – terapia de aventura*), few references appear in Spanish (Kraft, 1990; Fonseca Agosto, 2010), and only a dozen papers presented in international and national conferences in Spain. In the same way, there is no specific training in AT in Spain. Nevertheless, many web pages mention both terms, mostly from south and central America due to the recent celebration of AEE conferences in Mexico and Colombia, in 2001 and 2012 respectively.

Access to the Land

Spain, geographically, is a very rich country: surrounded by the sea, with many mountain ranges and highest elevation is above 3.400 meters (11.100 feet), deserts, rivers and lakes... According to the data of the Spanish Forestry Strategy (2010), mountains or forest lands occupy about 26 million hectares, 51.4% of total area. Nonetheless, it is very infrequent to find wild or uninhabited areas. Conditioning also the introduction of Wilderness therapy programs, campfires and free camping are prohibited in most of the autonomous regions, allowing only bivouacs above a certain altitude in National Parks.

Conclusions

After analyzing the conditioning factors in order to introduce AT in Spain, the first conclusion is that there is still a steep and long, while exciting, way to go.

Primarily, efforts should be made towards accessing specific AT and experiential education knowledge. Publications are crucial to making our field in Spain known. To publish books, articles and to submit experiences and research at conferences can lead to this. To conduct research in collaboration with universities is also necessary to become an evidence-based programme, in order to be considered a facility in agreement with the National Health Services.

Using networking can help to create international programs under EU funding, and also train professionals in our field using experiences from other EU countries. This last question is relevant because the program has to be designed and managed by qualified psychologists, preferably with specific AT training.

Subsequent to the prior facts, it is complicated to implement a pure model of AT programme based on the classification of Gass (1993b): Wilderness therapy, Adventure based-therapy or Long term residential camping. Access and availability of wilderness and limited specific facilities determine location and length, being easier to develop short time programs, combined with residential camping or adventure based-therapy.

References

Anglada, P. (2007). Estudio sobre constatación del cumplimiento de objetivos de un programa de formación para el desarrollo de la capacidad de trabajo en equipo en adultos a través del modelo "adventure based counseling" (asesoramiento basado en la aventura). Doctoral Thesis. UNED. Madrid.

Anglada, P. (2008). Orígenes de los programas de aventura en la naturaleza con fines educativos. Córdoba: IV Congreso Internacional y XXV Nacional de Eduación Física. Comunicación.

Fernández Hermida, J.R., Berdullas Temes, M., Santolaya Ochando, F. & Muñiz, J. (2000). Unpublished.

Fonseca Agosto, M. (2010): Educación aventurera y sus efectos en el desarrollo afectivo de los estudiantes de Educación Física. Universidad Metropolitana: Bayamón, Puerto Rico.

Gass, M. Gillis, H.L. & Russell, K.C. (2012). Adventure Therapy: Theory, Research, and Practice. New York: Routledge.

Gass, M. A. (1993). Adventure in therapy: Therapeutic applications of adventure programming. Boulder, CO: Association for Experiential Education.

Gass, M. (1993b). Foundations of adventure therapy. In M. Gass, Adventure Therapy: Therapeutic applications of adventure programming. Dubuque, Iowa: Kendall / Hunt publishing company.

Jiménez Martín, P. & Gómez Encinas, V. (2006). Turismo activo y outdoor training. Kronos nº 9, pp. 45-53,

Karft, R. J. (1990). Terapia de aventura, una nueva forma de intervención. Orientación Educacional núm. 6. Santiago de Chile, Chile, pp. 29-33.

Ochando, F.S., Temes, M.B., Hermida, J.R.F. (2002). La década 1989-1998 en la psicología española: análisis del desarrollo de la psicología profesional en España. Papeles del psicólogo n1 82, pp. 65-82.

Martínez Rico, G. (2003). Orientación y cartografía desde la intervención socioeducativa. Cuadernos de Animación Sociocultural nº 2.Valencia: Ed. Edetania ediciones.

Rose, A. & Sánchez, V. (2006). La evolución del uso de las actividades en el medio natural como instrumento educativo y/o terapéutico. Una perspectiva a partir de la educación social: desde Kurt Hahn a la actualidad. Actas IV Congreso Internacional: El aula naturaleza en la EF escolar. Escuela Universitaria de Educación, Universidad de Valladolid, Palencia.

Santolaya Ochando, F., Berdullas Temes, M, y Fernández Hermida, J.R. (2002). La década1989- 1998 en la psicología española: análisis del desarrollo de la psicología profesional en España. Papeles del psicólogo, junio, nº 82.

Senent, J.M. (Coord.) (1998). Animación y Pedagogía del Tiempo Libre. Valencia: Edetania Ediciones.

Trilla, J. (coord.) (1997). Animación sociocultural. Barcelona: Ariel.

CHAPTER 15

New Directions: Adventure Therapy with Special Populations
Part I: Adaptive Adventure Therapy

Carinna Kenigsberg and Megan Millar

INTRODUCTION

Adaptive adventure therapy meets the physical, emotional and psychological needs of clients with disabilities. In doing so, adaptive adventure therapy utilizes a strengths-based approach that focuses on capacity and ability, rather than simply focusing on limitations. Power to Be Adventure Therapy Society (Power to Be) is an adaptive adventure therapy program that inspires youth and families in need of support to discover their limitless abilities through nature-based programs. Since 1998, Power To Be has been working with their community to support people that are typically underserviced. Power To Be does this under two program streams; the Adaptive Recreation Program and the Wilderness School. In the fall of 2012, Power To Be had the opportunity to attend the International Adventure Therapy conference and both participate as well as contribute to the rich learning community created.

Power To Be's 'Adaptive Recreation Program' is a positive response to the community need for inclusive, nature-based recreation activities and therapeutic opportunities for people living with a barrier or disability. The goal of this paper is to share the Adaptive Recreation program practices and highlight the subsequent impact on participants and their families. In particular, this paper explores how the combination of nature, adventure, long-term client investment, inter-program peer mentoring, adaptive equipment and a family systems approach achieve outcomes in the following nine areas:

(a) Environmental awareness and stewardship
(b) Interpersonal skills
(c) Access to outdoor recreation
(d) Community engagement

(e) Life skills and personal development
(f) Community contribution
(g) Physical health and well-being
(h) Leadership and mentorship
(i) Family connectedness

Within the Adaptive Recreation Program, Power To Be services a wide range of people to explore and discover their unique abilities. From children and youth with autism, families living with an acquired brain injury, families at risk emotionally, people who are deaf or hard of hearing, people living with type 1 diabetes, oncology patients, to youth and adults living with developmental, cognitive or physical disabilities. Power To Be's trained Therapeutic Adventurists provide access to a world that was previously closed, through focusing on abilities and tapping into participants' ingenuity and tenacious spirits.

Adaptive Recreation

According to Miller and Katz (2002), inclusion involves a number of social processes such as: i) feeling respected, ii) being valued for who you are; and iii) feeling a level of supportive energy and commitment from others so that you can do your best work. At Power To Be, it is believed that Inclusion leads to a sense of belonging and that is what guides Power To Be's philosophy of support. Further, reaching personal competent skills and abilities are essential for the development of a healthy identity and personal well-being (Groff & Kleiber, 2001) and Power To Be's fosters this self-development through adventure activities like; kayaking, hiking, rock-climbing, canoeing and camping. It is key that researchers and practitioners who work with individuals with diverse needs or barriers need to collaborate, and share ideas to have a better understanding of what type of programs, adaptations and experiences can contribute to optimal development.

Program Goals

Power To Be is guided by the unique goals, dreams and abilities of the participants they aim to serve. One of the main goals of therapeutic recreation is to empower participants to overcome perceptions of low self-efficacy, and to re-focus participants' attention away from limitations and towards their capabilities (House & Paisley, 2008). Thus, the workshop promoted this idea of an ability-centered perspective (Blinde & McClungs, 1997) by creating an inspiring atmosphere to stretch people's realms of therapeutic outlets through engaging in interactive and visual exercises and discussions. The workshop also discussed adventure therapy practices that employ adaptation and innovation to eliminate barriers and foster nature-based experiences for the populations mentioned above.

Trainings and Workshops

Through trainings for professionals, Power to Be staff simulate a sense of what our clients live with every day, while creating an opportunity for professionals in the adventure therapy community, to expand their vision of accessibility and adventure. Power To Be's offers examples, tools, perspectives and solutions in the hopes that workshop participants could leave inspired to bridge the gaps back in their own community by increasing access to therapeutic, nature-based recreation opportunities.

Power to Be Sensitivity Trainings

Trainings begin in a circle, to model and create an equal space for everyone from the beginning. Power To Be sessions begin and end in a circle, to start as one inclusive group and return that way. Following introductions, we use an activity called the “YES game.” With an emphasis on the power of the word YES the group is guided to focus on what can be accomplished and experienced if you begin with the mind-set of "I can" vs. “I can't”. This experiential activity is followed with a Power Point presentation to illustrate the program's demographics, activities, and impact while educating around our programming and funding structures. The third layer involves walking through a few of Power To Be's outcomes. Engaging in experiential activities assists the group to think beyond the typical scope that they are accustomed to and bring fresh perspectives and solutions to reduce barriers in their communities. As facilitators at Power To Be, we find personally, that the biggest impact is in hearing stories of change from our participants who have lived a life saturated by "No” and “You Can't". It is hoped that our workshops will inspire other outdoor professionals to realize how they can be catalysts of change in the area of accessible outdoor recreation. The following quote is from a program participant and highlights this message:

A Power To Be Testimonial:

> I love teaching others what Power To Be has taught me. I love watching Power To Be work with others and watching others grow like how I have and still have. Power To Be teaches me to never give up, to be who

I am. A little saying I have now is 'Dream what you wanna dream, go where you wanna go, love who you need to love, Know what you wanna know, think what you're gonna think, say what you're gonna Say who you wanna be, forever and always'. I thank Power To Be everyday of my life.

POWER TO BE PARTICIPANT PROGRAM OUTCOMES

As mentioned above, in order to fullfill the mission of Power To Be, programs aim to meet the the following nine outcomes, or a portion of them:

(a) Environmental awareness and stewardship
(b) Interpersonal skills
(c) Access to outdoor recreation
(d) Community engagement
(e) Life skills and personal development
(f) Community contribution
(g) Physical health and well-being
(h) Leadership and mentorship
(i) Family connectedness

Outcome 1. Environmental Education and Stewardship

Participants increase their knowledge, understanding, care and connection with nature.

Activities: Environmental education and stewardship initiatives; wilderness expeditions; solo and quiet time in nature; interactions with animals; gardening; and outdoor activities such as beach cleanups, invasive species identification and removal, and planting native species

Goal: To explore the activities of environmental stewardship the group discussed two limitations or barriers they would envision when supporting people with complex neurological and cognitive barriers. As well as to brainstorm options, adaptations and language modifications that can be used to increase access to these activities in the locations that the professionals reside in.

Outcome 2. Interpersonal Skills

Participants strengthen their social networks and increase interpersonal skills including communication, trust building, conflict resolution, teamwork, and maintaining positive relationships.

Activities: Pro-social group process through intentional activities, discussions and debriefs; psycho-education; immediate feedback; role modeling; mentorship opportunities within Power To Be as well as within our community.

Goal: To share the voices of Power To Be' participants and how they developed their interpersonal skills while reflecting on a time when our interpersonal skills have been challenged and shaped by an experience.

A Power To Be Testimonial:

> There's so much about Power To Be Adventure Therapy that I could write a book about. When I first met Power To Be I was a nervous kid, but now that I've gotten to know Power To Be I've become a strong guy and become the person I've always wished to be. There's so much I thought I would never have been able to do, I never thought of myself as a kayaker, a rock climber, a canoer, a snowboarder or any of those adventurous things. I was always told that there's so much I couldn't do, but with Power To Be I've learned that people told me wrong, with Power To Be they told me that I can do these things if I set my mind to it. Even though I have autism 24/7 they respect autism and also teach that I can set my mind to anything.

FERNS & FIDDLEHEADS PARTICIPANT IN THE AUTISM PROGRAM

Outcome 3. Access to Outdoor Recreation

Participants experience increased ability to access natural environments and outdoor recreation opportunities.

Activities: utilizing adaptive equipment and communication modifications; day, weekend and expedition trips; education and connection to local resources, opportunities and natural environments.

Goal: Power To Be looks at our clients comfort physically and emotionally, their mobility, and their stability within every activity, location and equipment. There is a presumption that creating access to therapeutic and nature based opportunities is only associated to physical limitations; however many of the tools help people who have invisible barriers as well. To explore this concept small groups reviewed the photos of adaptive equipment, such as a TrailRider and Pontoons, as well as communication tools and modifications that can be used when a program is geared around the individuals abilities. The group discussed the many options of simple and complex adaptive tools that could be used as a support towards individuals with anxiety, trauma, illness, cognitive and physical limitations. By matching different adaptive photos with a scenario the group was able to see how interchangeable the support systems can be used to offer a wide scope of clients the opportunity to access nature-based activities and locations.

Examples of a few common adaptive tools are illustrated below; the TrailRider is typically used for all terrain adventures, the aqua chair is used for water based activities, the pontoons are used to enhance the safety and mobility of a kayak and the ear defenders are commonly used for people who find certain sounds over stimulating.

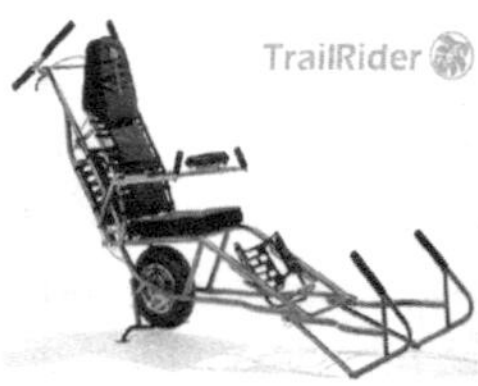

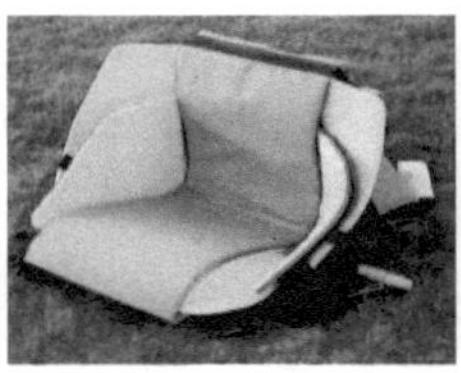
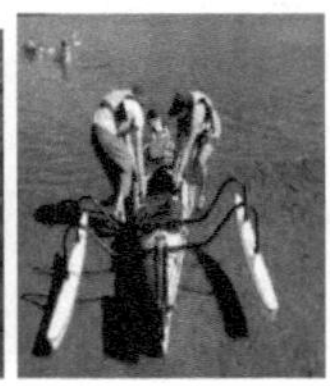
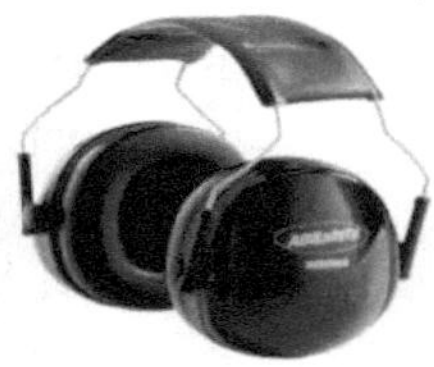

A Power To Be Testimonial:

> Power To Be has so much to offer to me and to others. People who meet Power To Be should feel as honoured as I do, because of Power To Be I'm able to trust and feel confident in myself, I've learned to try new things and to accept life the way it is.

PARTICIPANT IN OUR ADAPTIVE RECREATION PROGRAM

Outcome 6. Community Contribution

Participants cultivate the importance of giving back and working with their community.

Activities: Service learning projects; community events; inter-mentorship opportunities.

Goal: A circle of connectivity in an experiential fashion by discussing the different elements of a program design that incorporates community aspects such as site locations, support staff, stakeholders, family members, and partners locally and around the globe. The group created a literal web with string and labels of all the components necessary for an inclusive community. Through tugging on different areas of the string the goal was for the group to feel how valuable each roles plays and the type of impact that happens when one element is missing or being stretched.

Power To Be has built up an amazing community. It is Power To Be's strong emphasis on community collaboration that has allowed Power To Be to be diverse with the nature and adventure based opportunities we offer. This success was highlighted in the workshop by describing how Power To Be's private donors and foundations support 92% of the annual costs; therefore, allowing Power To Be to have the freedom to design safe, impactful, and community based programming per a needs basis versus being stricken by the grants restrictions and limitations. It takes a group of passionate people to paddle a voyageur canoe, but it takes a community to make lasting change around the world.

Outcome 9. Family Connectedness

Participants experience an increase in their understanding and connection with their family.

Activities: Family camping trips; family days; parent nights; graduations.

Goal: To identify all the components that require therapeutic support when engaging a family based program. Most families have the luxury of acting on the desire to go camping together. However if you are a family with a child with an illness, or a parent with an acquired brain injury, what are the extra considerations to think about? With every extra consideration that was suggested a rock was added into an empty backpack to signify the extra weight their families wear. How heavy is the backpack going to be, and can that family carry it? Power To Be envisions a world where outdoor recreation is accessible to all, and by taking a family living with barriers needs into consideration and finding solutions and creative modifications, there is more freedom for the family to just be together in natures pristine settings.

Conclusion

Power to Be helps participants examine the words *adaptation* and *barriers* more closely, so that participants develop the perception of YES, and have creative ideas and inspiration regarding how to approach new populations with an accessibility mind-set. This frame of mind is key when forming relationships and building identity. Power To Be has long-term programs, it is not a onetime event, but a process of ongoing self-discovery, connecting with others, dealing with adversities and frustrations, and achieving goals (Dorris, 2012). To highlight the steps to foster change Power To Be uses principles to promote successful therapeutic opportunities, identify the comfort, mobility and stability of the client and adapting as necessary to suit the individual needs, as well as language techniques to offer calm guidance and emotional support.

Power To Be creates and evaluates all programs based on our mission to inspire youth and families in need of support to discover their limitless abilities through nature-based programs. Power To Be's mission is guided by our nine outcomes. We outline these outcomes through visual and hands on techniques, with the end result illuminating that adaptations are everywhere. People wear glasses, learn through hands on techniques, modify rules to games, use slang and other idiosyncratic language and use specialized devices such as pontoons or TrailRiders. When one focuses on abilities, it allows one's gifts and strengths to become the focus thus inviting the field of adventure therapy to make a profound impact on those who currently are not able to access the healing power of outdoor adventure (Blinde & McClung, 1997).

A Power To Be Testimonial:

> Power To Be provides opportunities and experiences that are enabling and inclusive, allowing me to forget about my disabilities and focus on my strengths; not only as a participant, but also a father and a husband. All of the activities have been wonderful. Prior to my accident I was quite active in the outdoor setting. Power to be has provided the opportunity to be outdoors again! Kayaking, Rock Climbing and Camping are my favorites! The outdoors provides an experience that no hospital or other institution can provide Freedom, Adventure, Strength and Happiness. I can't thank this group, and the staff and volunteers enough; their hard work, drive and dedication are honourable and representative of the Power To Be brand – true ambassadors.
>
> - Acquired Brain Injury Family Program Participant

Power To Be envisions a community where the power of nature is accessible to all, and it is hoped that Power To Be's vision will be passed on globally through other like-minded Adventure Therapy professionals.

REFERENCES

Blinde, E., & McClung, L. (1997). Enhancing the physical and social self through recreational activity: Accounts of individuals with physical disabilities. *Adapted Physical Activity Quarterly, 14*, 327-344.

Dorris, R. (2012). *The power to adapt: A case study of special needs youth who have participated in an adaptive recreation program*. University of Victoria: Unpublished Master's thesis.

Groff, D. G., & Kleiber, D. A. (2001). Exploring the identity formation of youth involved in an adapted sports program. *Therapeutic Recreation Journal, 35*, 318-332.

House, M., & Paisley, K. (2008). An empowerment theory approach to adventure programming for adults with disabilities. *Therapeutic Recreation Journal, 42*, 89-102.

King, G., Law, M., King, S., Rosenbaum, P., Kertoy, M.K., & Young, N.L, (2003). A conceptual model of the factors affecting the recreation and leisure participation of children with disabilities. *Physical and Occupational Therapy in Pediatrics, 23*, 63–90.

Miller and Katz (2003). The Inclusion Breakthrough: Unleashing the Real Power of Diversity

Rimmer, J. A., & Rowland, J. L. (2008). Physical activity for youth with disabilities: A critical need in an underserved population, *Developmental Neurorehabilitation, 11*, 141-148.

CHAPTER 16

New Directions: Adventure Therapy with Special Populations
Part II: Adventure Therapy through Sailing for People with Chemical Dependency

Richard Lannowe Hall and Sue Parker Hall

INTRODUCTION

Sailing can be understood as a metaphor for life. The process of acclimatizing to ever changing landscapes, sea states and weather conditions is likened to the need to adjust to the ongoing emotional and practical challenges of life. Quantitative and qualitative research data show evidence how participants experience and benefit from the Sailaday OK experience and how they integrate learning into life ashore. The Charity Sailaday OK offers marine Adventure therapy to participants who are recovering from chemical addictions, abuse and trauma and are in the potentially difficult transition from intensive residential drug and alcohol treatment centres to living in the community. Our program sails from Falmouth, Cornwall, UK for 4 to 5 days and nights at a time and in groups of four.

THEORETICAL UNDERPINNING

Addiction is conceptualised as a coping mechanism for trauma, usually archaic, dating back to early life (Parker Hall, 2008). We understand that trauma arrests the development of, or undermines the functioning of, an individual's Adult ego state (Berne, 1957); when traumatised, we can only respond to today's events in a way that is unhelpfully influenced by our past.

Addiction serves to keep raw, unprocessed emotional experience out of awareness because of an inability to process it, to feel it through, to come to terms with what has happened. Unfortunately, people who are traumatised are not only unable to process the experience which afflicted them in the first place but frequently have been unable to process many subsequent life events, resulting in a multiple pile up of emotional experience which has never been expressed (Parker Hall, 2008).

We know from neuroscience that, in order to process trauma, both left and right brain need to be engaged at the same time (Schore, 1994). EMDR (Shapiro, 1989, 2012) uses bilateral stimulation (eye movement or taps) because you cannot *not* process whatever material you are focussing on when both right brain and left brain are being stimulated at the same time. Bi-lateral stimulation can happen in other ways; for example through experiencing an empathic relationship which encourages the processing of emotion through using left brain language to express right brain experience; this is at the heart of psychotherapy.

It also occurs when sailing; steering and using a compass often involves behaving counter-intuitively and performing any task aboard you have to think and feel at the same time. Sitting on the bows viewing the seascape the eye is constantly in motion, scanning.

It follows then that combining an empathic psychotherapeutic relationship with sailing creates an optimum environment for stimulating an individual's latent organismic capacity to regulate and process their here-and-now emotional experience, but also any archaic experience which may surface during the exercise.

This capacity is a primary function of the integrating Adult ego state (Tudor, 2002) and, once developed, a person can then deal with the backlog of unprocessed archaic emotional material that was lodged in their Child ego state. As a result, their Adult ego state is strengthened and expanded; the energy which was used to repress the organism's trauma is now available to them in the here-and-now, they are more present to their experience, are able to reflect on their present situation and to think usefully and feel at the same time; they are better able to do the necessary emotional processing in any given situation, to weigh up their circumstances accurately, to realistically assess risk and make good decisions about what is required in order to proceed safely and effectively. This capacity greatly improves people's view of themselves so it increases their confidence and self-esteem, they are more likely feel 'I'm OK' and 'You're OK' (Berne, 1962, 1976), and enhances our ability to negotiate, collaborate and work as a team.

Those suffering from addiction are likely to have early developmental deficits. The Sailaday OK activity consciously addresses the first three developmental stages:

1. Being- expanding self-awareness to all the sensations and feelings and being in the world
2. Doing- participating in the experience
3. Thinking- processing and using metaphors to make sense of the experience (Clarke & Dawson,1998; Erickson, 1950).

Kahlil Gibran likes metaphors. He articulates, powerfully and persuasively, the 'integrating Adult ego state' (2002) in action, the right brain and left brain operating in unison; he speaks to us of Reason and Passion in his poem 'The Prophet' (1923):

> Your reason and passion is the rudder and the sails of your seafaring soul.
>
> If either your sails or your rudder be broken, you can but toss and drift, or else be held at a standstill in mid-seas. reason, ruling alone, is a force confining; and passion, unattended, is a flame that burns to its own destruction.

The metaphor is a useful way of condensing and communicating complex ideas; in psychotherapy it is used to engage the Adult ego state in a reflecting process and in order to think and make meaning of experiences (right brain and left brain functioning together).

Sailing is understood here as a metaphor that is steeped in useful wisdom that is easily transferrable to recovery from addiction and to life in general. Staying afloat and managing ever changing weather, sea and emotional states, often beyond an individual's control, requires the same high degree of Adult present awareness, ability to reflect and make meaning and to manage emotional experience as does adjusting to the ongoing practical and emotional challenges of recovery and life.

All the exercises / interventions are designed to expand and strengthen the integrating Adult which we understand to be arrested when a person is traumatised and/or using alcohol & drugs.

A skipper / facilitator models an integrating Adult by being authentic, boundaried and by maintaining safety. In Rogerian terms they strive to create the optimum environment in which an organism can grow and thrive (Rogers, 1980); they engender the conditions in which both left-brain and right brain activity is bilaterally stimulated. The skipper / facilitator informs about and directs the exercise but also encourages participants to notice and reflect on their thoughts and feelings, both the more debilitating archaic feelings that are not congruent to the immediate task such as powerlessness, uselessness and stupidity as well as appropriate feelings for example, a degree of anxiety, fear and excitement. There is also encouragement to take pleasure in the 'wow' factor, the thrill of the experience.

The purpose of the exercise is to have a new experience; Relational Analysts believe this is the foundation for internal change.

> It is likely that we cannot understand a thing until we have experienced it inwardly. (Carl Jung)

A tick list is as necessary for a sailing journey as it is equally relevant to existential or practical journeys.

- Have I considered where I am (my start point) and identified my goal.
- Is this goal achievable?
- A chart for me is like a manual, a narrative, written by those who have been here before me. This narrative is like any manual or therapeutic relationship, mentor, sponsor that can help; advise us to have a successful voyage.
- We prepare our course one step at a time move one step (waypoint) at a time. All 12 step fellowship programmes (AA. NA etc.) will encourage you to follow this way to manage your new life and recovery
- Have I considered my condition, am I fit (physically, emotionally and mentally), do I Have the means, resources and tools.
- Am I prepared to ask for help and cooperation? (Be part of)?
- Do I have the flexibility required; do I accept that when the conditions change, I need to make some changes; or if my condition changes, I need to respond?
- How will I know when I have achieved my goal?

Researching Sailaday OK Process and Outcomes

We collect quantitative and qualitative data to measure effectiveness and to develop the project. The quantitative data is generated by feedback forms. However, because Sailaday OK is a process and a phenomenological experience, we also want to understand the unique meaning that each individual makes of it so we also collect qualitative data through asking some open questions which invites their reflection. Figures 1, 2 and 3 demonstrate some of the data we've collected on our program, showing that clients' confidence about staying drug/alcohol free improves as a result of the sailing program, and they also connect deeply with the idea of sailing as a metaphor for life.

Figures 1-3. Sailaday Outcomes

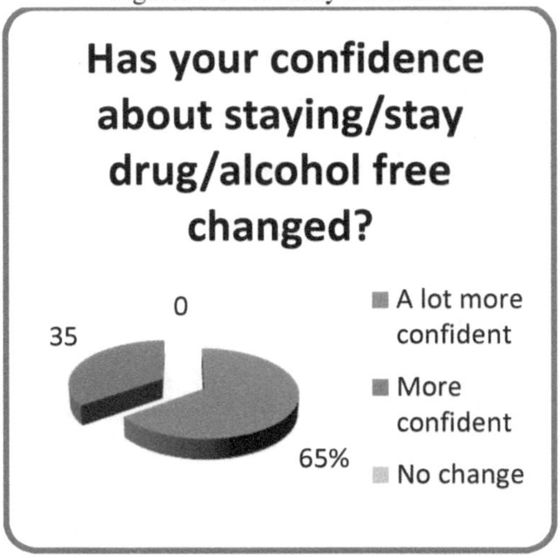
Has your confidence about staying/stay drug/alcohol free changed?
0
35
65%
A lot more confident
More confident
No change

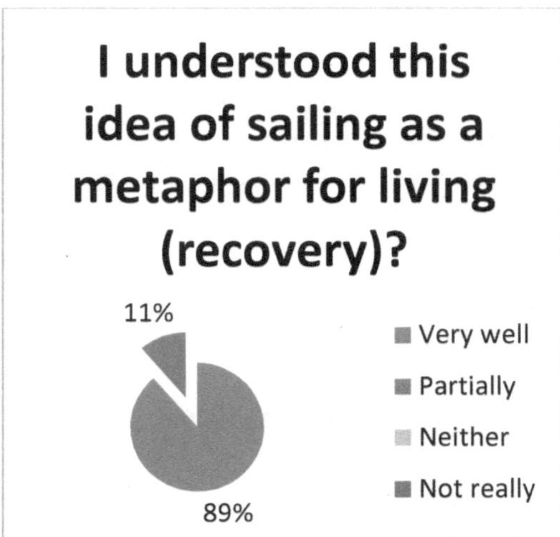

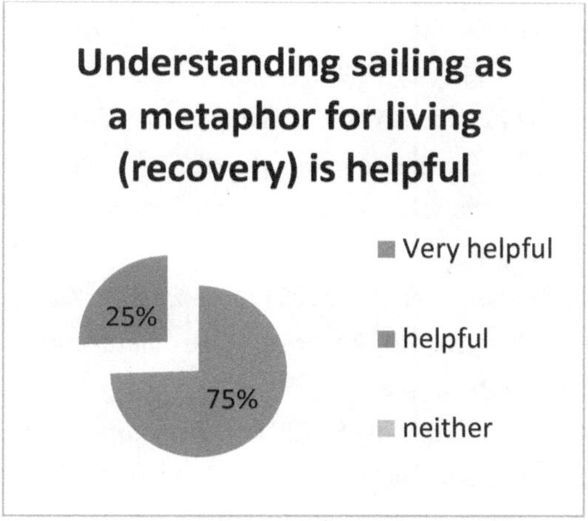

Conclusion

Jeremy Holmes presents a metaphor describing both the process and outcomes of psychotherapy:

> On weighing the anchor, every sailor must take with him the best possible technical and cultural equipment for coping with the perils of the sea, but the expert sailor knows that he must adapt his techniques to the sea and the weather and that every voyage will to some extent be unpredictable and at any rate different from its predecessors. It is precisely this awareness, no less than the skills acquired that distinguishes his approach from the rigid illusions nurtured by the beginner (Bolognini, 1997).

Although Bolognini is talking about psychotherapy, we hope we have demonstrated that this metaphor can equally be applied to sailing and recovery from addiction.

References

Berne E, (1957). Ego states in psychotherapy, *American Journal of Psychotherapy*, 11(2), 293-309.

Berne, E. (1976). Classification of positions, *Transactional Analysis Bulletin Selected Articles from Volumes 1 through 9,* 3. San Francisco, TA Press (Original work published 1962).

Bologniini, S. (1997). Empathy And 'Empathism', *Inernational Journal of Psycho-Analysis*, 78, 279-293.

Gibran, K. (1923). *The Prophet*, Alfred A Knopf, New York.

Holmes, J. (1998). *The British Journal of Medical Psychology*, The changing aims of psychoanalytical psychotherapy, an integrative perspective, 70, 231/248.

Lannowe Hall, R., & Parker Hall, S. (2011). *Addiction Today*, 'Even when it's dark, I don't have to be lost: Two therapeutic interventions for wilderness therapy at sea.

Lannowe Hall, R., & Parker Hall, S. (2011). *International Stress Management Magazine,* Sailaday OK: Analysis of the role of a marine wilderness therapeutic activity in stress management.

Lannowe Hall, R., & Parker Hall, S. (2008). *Addiction Today*, Analysis of a marine wilderness therapeutic activity .

Parker Hall, S. (2008). *Anger, Rage and Relationship: An Empathic Approach to Anger Management*, London: Routledge.

Rogers, C. R. (1980), *A Way of Being*, Mariner Books

Schore, A. (1994). *Affect Regulation and the Origin of Self*, New Jersey, Laurence Erlbaum Associates

Shapiro, F. (1989). Efficacy of the eye movement desensitisation procedure in the treatment of traumatic memories, *Journal of Traumatic Stress,* 2, 199-223. 2012, Getting Past Your Past: Take Control of Your Life with Self-Help Techniques from EMDR Therapy, New York: Rodale.

Tudor, K. (2002). Neopsyche In Hargaden & Sills (Eds.), *Ego States (Key Concepts in Transactional Analysis).* Location: Worth Publishers.

CHAPTER 17

A Practical Model for Adventure Therapy

Stephan Natynczuk

INTRODUCTION

The intrinsic therapeutic qualities of adventure activities are described in a wide range of literature (e.g. Mortlock, 1984; Miles & Priest, 1999; Schoel & Maizell, 2002; Gass, Gillis & Russell, 2012), and are routinely used in the UK to help with personal and social skills development among disaffected and vulnerable young people (Ogilvie, 2013). It can be argued that, because adventure activities have their own intrinsic therapeutic qualities, they do not necessarily have to be consciously managed to have a positive effect. There are commonly accepted benefits in terms of increased sense of wellbeing from just being outdoors, increased fitness, companionship and common objectives. Just being outdoors seems to help boys learn more effectively. Gustafsson, Szczepanski, Nelson, & Gustafsson (2012) found that didactic teaching outdoors using natural materials (during afternoon lessons over 15 days spread over 6 months) led to moderate improvements in boys' mental health as measured by parents' responses to a strengths and difficulties questionnaire. My own work in education since 1988 has been primarily based outdoors and, since 1995, has been mostly focused on re-engaging vulnerable young people with education through outdoor adventure activities. In the early days I was most influenced by existential approaches, humanistic approaches, active and experiential learning models and biological theories about survival and adaptation. I weaved useful theories and practice into my work and began using a solution-focused approach as soon as I learned that what I had been working towards already existed as solution focused brief therapy.

Adventure Therapy (AT) is a term that is not always easy to define. An adventure can be viewed as any undertaking with an uncertain outcome and therapy as a process by which some healing comes about. Their combination to form adventure therapy has been defined by Gillis and Ringer (1999) as "the deliberate, strategic combination of adventure activities with therapeutic change processes with the goal of making lasting changes in the lives of participants". Neill (2004) elaborated the definition of AT to "the use of adventure-based activities and/or adventure-based theory to provide people with emotional and/or behavioural problems with experiences which lead to positive change in their lives".

Adventure therapy has been critiqued as experience rich and theory poor (Glass & Jackson, 2008). There is no doubt that understanding the mechanisms and influences on the effectiveness of AT would facilitate the testing of therapeutic models. In this paper I propose a therapeutic model, with an existing, and evidenced theoretical basis that would appear relatively simple for outdoor instructors to use during adventure activities and wilderness journeys. I will draw on personal experiences of successful therapeutic outcomes both with vulnerable adolescents exhibiting emotional, behavioural and social difficulties during adventure activities (Natynczuk, 2012).

Applying Theory to Practice

There is much literature on solution focused brief therapy (SFBT); however, this article will only deal briefly with the background to this approach. SFBT is a model that is radical in its approach (McKergow, 2009) as it focuses on strengths and problem-solving capacity, not simply pathology. Although SFBT continues to evolve, it is increasingly becoming more robust through evidenced and theory backed practice (see, for example, Simm, Andrew, Brogan, & Slinger, 2010; Shennan & Iveson, 2011; Macdonald, 2011) and seems particularly useful for children and young people (Hackett & Shannon 2007; Simm, Andrew, Brogan, & Slinger, 2010).

This approach began when Steve de Shazer developed the work of Erikson and in turn hugely influenced the development of SFBT (de Shazer, Berg, Lipchick et al., 1986; de Shazer, 1994; O'Hanlon, 1987). Ratner (2006) reviews de Shazer's innovations and the development of SFBT. Solution focused Brief Therapy is so called because the average number of sessions to bring about change is small (Gingerich & Eisengart, 2000), the approach taking as few sessions to bring about change as is needed, and not one session more, indeed Ockham's Razor is a guiding philosophy in this work (Iveson, George & Ratner, 2012, p.8) who wrote "What can be achieved by fewer means should not be achieved by many. This requires the constant examination of assumptions and a preparedness to abandon even the most sacred of cows if a desired outcome can be achieved without them…[and] this has led us to some remarkable discoveries about the process of change." Such a short intervention could arguably be very helpful when considering merging a therapeutic approach with an adventure or wilderness experience at the point of practice.

In solution focused brief therapy the worker and client co-construct a preferred future in which whatever brought the client to therapy is no longer present or, at the very least, they are able to cope. At times, the preferred future can be made a reality through careful design of the programme (for example, from personal SFBT work, where the problem was travel anxiety and a programme based on cave explorations, requiring much travel throughout the UK, moved to a preferred future when travel was not an impediment to doing something the client wanted to do and enjoyed very much as a new activity). The worker asks future focused questions and listens with a constructive ear while the client works to visualise their preferred future from their own and others' perspectives in small detail, as well as identifying instances when their preferred future already exists and identifying what skills and strengths they already use to cope and could use to move forward (Ratner, George & Iveson, 2012).

It is the use of simple to ask, future focused, questions and conversations that enable instructors to work with the client to enhance the intrinsic therapeutic qualities of adventure activities. Therapeutic conversations can be had at appropriate and natural times as the activity or expedition unfolds, and without a need to break the flow of events with a distinct stand-alone therapy sessions that can make the whole adventure therapy process somewhat disconnected and clunky.

SF therapeutic conversations follow the process laid out by George, Iveson and Ratner (1999) and Ratner, George & Iveson (2012). Typical techniques are scaling, third-person perspectives and questions that prompt thinking about a preferred future (Briefer, 2009; O'Connell, 2005). Detail is encouraged through questions such as "What difference would that make to you?" and "What might you notice instead…?" Emotions and feelings are generally left out of solution focused sessions, unless they are helpful to the client (Miller & de Shazer, 2000). While SFBT has been criticised for ignoring emotions (Schwartz & Johnson, 2000; Piercy, Lipchik & Kiser, 2000), I would suggest that not inviting emotions into a conversation, for example "How does that make you feel?" can help make the experience safer for instructors who may not be trained counsellors and may not have any useful way of dealing with emotional burdens additional to those that arise through dysfunctional thoughts and behaviours that routinely occur and at a time when the instructor has wider responsibilities to others in the group. I would also suggest that returning from an expedition when clients have unburdened themselves of emotion and transferred them to an instructor can lead to stresses that can contribute to burnout among staff especially when no clinical supervision is at hand (personal observations). Indeed the worker deliberately acts as not needing to know the background to the client's problem and, unless the client can say how it would be helpful to them if the worker listened to it, the worker keeps the conversation future focussed and thus keeps the problem out of the conversation, instead concentrating on a future where the 'problem' no longer exists. In this way the worker helps the client take responsibility for their own role in finding their own solutions.

The techniques of solution focused therapy seem surprisingly simple yet they can be very challenging for the client. The questions firmly put the ability to change in the hands of the client who must be trusted to know what is best for them. Anything less is considered solution forced and can result from misunderstanding good practice or having an agenda that is not necessarily in the client's best interests (Nylund & Corsiglia, 1994)—that is, the best interests of the client are superseded by those of others (Iveson, George & Ratner, 2012). Solution forced agendas are quite common, one example of being "This boy is a nuisance in school and we want you to sort it out". Initial questions establish what the client wants to achieve for themselves and what their best hopes for this conversation are. Questions about what difference something would make, or what might be noticed instead, keep a client future focused and keep the client in a position of doing the work for themselves. These questions also keep the worker away from giving advice. If asked for advice the worker could ask in turn, "What difference would having that advice make to you?" and thus, respectfully hand the power for change to the client, increasing the client's autonomy and responsibility for change (Iveson, George & Ratner, 2012).

Scales, where zero is the worst things could get and ten the best, help a client explore where they are now, what strengths and resources they have that they can use, or build on, to bring about change, and what they would notice when things are better. The worker always asks for signs of things being better, and avoids to-do lists and talk of steps, in order to keep the conversation future focused and client centred. Asking 'the tomorrow question' helps quickly take the client to a time when the problem they struggle with is absent, and can be useful to avoid getting stuck. The client is asked to imagine that they wake up tomorrow and their problem has gone. What would the very first sign be that it had gone? What would they notice? Asking "What else?" respectfully, a number of times, takes a client to the smallest of details of this change. These small details are examples of the preferred future that are more easily realisable and are more likely to help the desire change come about (Ratner, George & Iveson, 2012).

A User-friendly Model for Outdoor Adventure Instructors

To aid outdoor instructors' understanding of SF therapy there are a few good metaphors that present themselves using aspects of good practice in delivering adventure activities. For example, low visibility navigation, duty of care, and leave no trace. Co-construction of a preferred future is similar, in many ways, to night navigation or low visibility navigation. On a mountain at night, or in bad visibility, we should have a good idea of where we are, certainly of where we have been, and should be able to point to our position on a map. We also know where we want to get to and we can plan a route to get there – so many paces, so many minutes on a given compass bearing. Next we need to visualise from the map what it will look like when we arrive so that we can be sure we have arrived at the right place – slope aspect, interpretation of contours, proximity to certain landscape features etc. Not being able to do this can be potentially lethal, for example, putting us over a cliff or on to an avalanche prone slope or might just mean we descend the wrong side of the mountain causing great inconvenience. The concept of an adventurous journey as a metaphor for change is also obvious (Allin & Humberstone, 2010).

Creating a Climate of Competence

On first meeting a new client the ensuing conversation is problem free and explores existing competencies and strengths. These illustrate that there are times when things go well and help build a climate of competence. We have these problem free conversations whilst walking in the countryside, usually to a high place with a good view, subtly suggesting a process of new perspectives. We are also evaluating a client's fitness and general outdoors capability as part of a risk assessment. Ratner, George and Iveson (2012, pp.49-51) write of problem free talk as something developed from ordinary conversational skills, a simple process with three purposes:

1) To meet the person rather than the problem within the first few minutes.
2) To allow the therapist to 'choose' the client with whom they are going to work.
3) To begin a process of 'resource-gathering', which will equip the therapist with the necessary means to solve whatever problems have brought them together.

Low Visibility Navigation

This metaphor resonates with working towards a client's preferred future we know what it looks like because we explore in our conversation the signs of arriving there, both from the client's perspective and from the perspective of others. With full knowledge of the signs of arriving at his or her preferred future the client identifies a time when therapy is no longer needed. Just as the outdoor instructor draws on strengths built on experience, our client draws on strengths identified has those that have helped him/her cope with and survive difficult and challenging times. Alternatively, a client has survived thus far so they must have been doing something right. Questions such as, "Things seem pretty bad for you at the moment. How have you coped?" acknowledge the client's difficulties and focus instead on strengths and resources that can be built on to get the client to their preferred future.

Leave No Trace

Talking about the signs of having made changes towards a preferred future and not the steps that might be needed to be made (giving advice) keeps the therapist neutral and minimises any impact on the client's decision making. The SF model is underpinned by the principle of letting the client do the work, with their own interest upper most. This is regarded as good practice (Macdonald, 2011; Ratner, George and Iveson, 2012). Therapy is not something that is done to a client; rather it is a process or a journey (both real & metaphorically) undertaken by the client. The principle of minimal impact on the environment is familiar to many outdoor adventure and wilderness instructors and the idea of leave no trace is a well-known and generally respected aspect of outdoor and wilderness leadership.

Talking about signs, and asking questions such as "What would you notice when…", rather than discussing steps or things that could be done to bring about a change, helps keep the worker distant from the client's problem by prompting the client to actually do the work and keeping the worker away from offering advice. According to the SF model advice leaves a trace of the worker's intervention that can backfire, being solution forced (Nylund & Corsiglia, 1994) and can damage the therapeutic alliance between the worker and the client as well as challenge some of the ethical issues specific to SFBT (Macdonald, 2011).

Duty of Care

Duty of care in the UK is a responsibility that instructors and coaches have to uphold to ensure that their clients come to no harm during adventure activities and coaching sessions and is particularly explicit in training courses offered by UK national governing bodies for outdoor adventure activities such as caving, paddle sports and mountaineering. Duty of care includes all aspects of safe practice including compiling risk assessments, providing appropriate safety equipment and clothing, supervision of activities and child protection procedures. Working with vulnerable children and adults demands an enhanced duty of care that will be familiar to instructors following UK national governing body (NGB) awards.

Protecting ourselves and making sure it is safe to approach a casualty, then making sure we do no harm, are among the first rules of immediate and temporary care, as First Aid is now known. In the UK a valid and current First Aid certificate is mandatory for holders of NGB awards. Incorporating a therapeutic duty of care (or maintaining therapeutic core conditions) should not then be a difficult transition for outdoor activity instructors. Maintaining the client's confidentiality (unless there is good reason to believe the client will harm themselves or someone else), respecting the client's narrative and trusting them as the expert on their story, and doing no harm through poor therapeutic practice, which includes being solution forced instead of being solution focused, should be easily understood by NGB award holders. A SF approach would give credibility first and foremost to the client's own perspective and interpretation of goals, barriers and solutions and would work towards giving the client control and ownership of any preferred future, focusing on strengths rather than deficits. This positive and affirmative approach parallels much work that an outdoor practitioner would seek to achieve with any client in the outdoor activity setting and again, should not be a difficult transition.

Being Useful

Outdoor instructors are also familiar with the idea of being useful as a component of customer care. Taking time to help a stuck participant, being reassuring, having a tool to hand to make simple repairs, encouraging participation, effort and endurance, making sure everyone enjoys a suitably challenging, educational, fun and safe experience, and being mindful of changing weather and other physical conditions such as ice under foot and water levels. Being able to ask questions useful to a client as they work towards a preferred future should not be an alien concept to outdoor instructors used to coaching as part of their leadership toolbox.

WIDER PARALLELS

Evolutionary theory tells us that organisms survive by continually doing what they are good at in a given environment (Clutton-Brock & Harvey, 1984). Any animal that starts to concentrate on what it is not good at is likely to not last very long being killed by a rival, starving or eaten. I see this premise underpinning the SF model where the worker asks questions to identify the client's strengths, personal qualities and ways of coping. These abilities are what have helped the client survive in difficult times and challenging circumstances. Drawing on this interpretation the qualities and strengths that have enabled survival thus far, can be used to bring about change towards the client's preferred future.

A technique that helps us examine those survival strengths is scaling whereby zero might be the worst something could be and ten the best. Somewhere in between is "good enough". The scale might be confidence, competence, or a measure of distance travelled towards a preferred future and therefore a time when therapy is no longer needed. A client is asked where they are now on the scale and asked to give a personally significant number between zero and ten. The follow up question is key to the worker as it explores what motivated the client to give that particular number. Strengths are identified in some detail before the client is asked what they would notice about themselves when they move up the scale and perhaps what others would notice about them too. This brings the conversation back once more to a future focus and to a time when the problem that brought them to therapy is less of a problem or subject to improved coping skills. This is a significant step towards a time when the problem no longer exists.

It is often part of an instructor's role to coach skills and improve technique for example, ice-axe arrests, J-strokes, rigging ropes, and so on. Increasingly, UK instructor training incorporates coaching methods. Solution focused techniques can easily be used for coaching hard skills required to, for example, safely navigate a rapid. "What would you notice when you make that turn, just behind that boulder?" This is a question demanding visualisation of a technique, the components of which are, in broad terms, body, boat, blade—coaching emphases that would be familiar to any canoe or kayak coach. The language is important. Asking questions that demand an answer with reference to future performance helps the instructor frame things so that the client's best interest are kept in mind: "At the end of today what will tell you it's been a good day?" "How will you know this expedition has been useful?" "What will you notice about yourself when…?" "What would your social worker notice that told her this had been a useful experience for you?"

Debriefing with clients and also between staff once the clients have left can easily focus on the things that went well, looking for positives in term of successes and improvements things that we were pleased to notice. If things did not go so well we can ask what stopped them getting worse and in that way paying attention to strengths, skills, experience and judgement that helped prevent events becoming worse and reminds instructors of their own competence in keeping everyone safe.

Conclusion

SFBT is noted for the simplicity of its questions and is often used for coaching as well as therapy. Its language is based on everyday conversation and its techniques translate well in to coaching improvement in outdoor skills. The SF approach, while taking years to hone, can easily be initially taught in a short course and it is not a difficult transition for outdoor instructors to undertake. Indeed, my professional work with My Big Adventure CIC is an example of a social enterprise that works with school age young people who, for various reasons, do not attend school or are at risk of exclusion from school and are often at risk of social exclusion. Practitioners here are routinely trained in SFBT and incorporate the model in their day-to-day work. Because SF conversational skills translate easily to coaching they can be seamlessly used in therapeutic conversations in the course of adventure activities or wilderness expeditions without stopping or pausing the adventure experience for therapy.

[An earlier version of this paper was presented at the Sixth International Adventure Therapy Conference]..

References

Allin, L., & Humberstone, B. (2010). Introducing 'Journey(s)' in adventure and outdoor learning research. *Journal of Adventure Education and outdoor Learning, 10 (2),* 71-75.

BRIEFER (2009). *A solution focused practice manual*. London: BRIEF.

Clutton-Brock, T.H. & Harvey, P.H. (1984). Comparative approaches to investigating adaptation. In J.R. Krebs and N.B. Davies (Eds). *Behavioral Ecology: An Evolutionary Approach.* Oxford: Blackwell Scientific Publications.

de Shazer, S., Berg, I.K., Lipchick, E., Nunnally, E., Molnar, A., Gingerich, W. and Weiner-Davis, M. (1986). Brief therapy: Focused solution development. *Family Process,* 25, pp 207-221.

de Shazer, S. (1994). *Words were originally magic.* New York, W.W. Norton & Co., Inc.

George, E., Iveson, C., and Ratner, H. (1999). *Problem to solution.* London: BT Press.

Gingerich, W. and Eisengart, S. (2000). Solution focused brief therapy: A review of the outcome research. *Family Process*, 39 (4), 477 – 498.

Gass, M.A, Gillis, H.L. and Russell, K.C., (2012). *Adventure Therapy*. New York: Routledge.

Gillis, H.L. and Ringer, T.M. (1999). Therapeutic adventure programs adventure programming. In S. Priest & J. Miles (Eds), *Adventure Education.* State College, PA: Venture Publications.

Glass, J.S. and Jackson, J. (2008). Connecting theory to programming: Using existentialism and adventure based counselling with adolescents. *International Journal of Existential Psychology and Psychotherapy, 2*(1), 1-11.

Hackett, P. and Shennan, G. (2007). Solution focused work with children and young people. *Handbook of Solution Focused Brief Therapy: Clinical Applications*. Philadelphia, PA, Hawthorne Press.

Iveson, C., George, E., Ratner, H. (2012). *Brief Coaching: A Solution Focused Approach.* London and New York, Routledge.

Gustafsson. P.E., Szczepanski. A., Nelson, N., and Gustafsson, P.E. (2012). Effects of an outdoor education intervention on the mental health of school children. *Journal of Adventure Education and Outdoor Learning, 12 (1)*, 63-80.

Macdonald, A. (2011). *Solution-focused Therapy: Theory, Research and Practice*. London, Sage.

McKergow, M. (2009). In between – Neither inside nor outside: The radical simplicity of Solution Focused Brief Therapy. *Journal of Systematic Therapies, 2(28)*, 34-49.

Miles, J.C., and Priest, S. (1999). *Adventure Programming*. State College, PA: Venture Publishing Inc.

Mortlock, C. (1984). *The Adventure Alternative*. Milnthorpe, Cumbria, UK: Cicerone Press.

Natynczuk, S., (2012). Solution focused practice outdoors or "If it works well let's have some morefl" *Horizons, Institute for Outdoor Learning Magazine,* Issue 58, Summer, 56-58.

Neill, J.T., (2004). Adventure therapy definitions [Weblog post]. Retrieved 7/15/12http://wilderdom.com/adventuretherapy/adventuretherapydefinitions.html

Nylund, D., & Corsiglia, V. (1994). Becoming solution-focused forced in brief therapy: Remembering something important we already knew. *Journal of Systemic Therapies, 13 (1),* 5-12.

O'Connell, B. (2005). *Solution-focused Therapy*. London, Sage Publications.

O'Hanlon, W. H. (1987). Groundwork: Introduction to Erikson's work. *Taproots: Underlying Principles of Milton Erikson's Therapy and Hypnosis*. New York: W.W. Norton.

Ogilvie, K. (2013). *Roots and Wings: A History of Outdoor Education and Outdoor Learning in the UK*. Cumbria: Institute for Outdoor Learning.

Ratner. H., George, E. and Iveson, C. (2012). *Solution Focused Brief Therapy: 100 Key Points and Techniques*. London and New York: Routledge.

Percy, F.P., Lipchik, E., and Iser, D., (2000). Miller and de Shazer's article on "Emotions in Solution-Focused Therapy". *Family Process*, *1*(39), 25-28.

Ratner, H. (2006). The therapist doesn't have the magic, the client has the magic! The legacy of Steve de Shazer. *Context*, 84, 39-41.

Schoel, J., and Maizell, R.S. (2002). *Exploring Islands of Healing: New Perspectives on Adventure Based Counselling*. Beverly MA, USA: Project Adventure Inc.

Schwenk, E. and Natynczuk, S. (2015). Supervision and adventure therapy: Fighting burnout and providing emotional First Aid for practitioners. In A. Pryor, C. Carpenter, C.L. Norton (Eds.), *Explorations of Adventure Therapy around the Globe*. Champaign, IL: Common Ground Publishing.

Simm, R., Andrew. R., Brogan, S., and Slinger, R. (2010). Auditing the effectiveness of solution-focused brief therapy in a child and family psychology service. *Clinical Psychology Forum, 210*, 11-15.

ADAPTING

> *Continuity gives us roots; change gives us branches, letting us stretch and grow and reach new heights.*
>
> -Pauline R. Kezer

CHAPTER 18

Motivational Interviewing and Adventure Therapy: Enhancing Approaches to Resolving Client Ambivalence

Bonnie Dyck

ABSTRACT

Therapists professing to be eclectic develop their practice from more than one theoretical framework and use techniques from various theories that may or may not have similar tenets (Corey, 2001). This technical eclecticism may reflect an attempt to more deeply engage the client and become more client-centered. Theoretical integration explores commonalities between theories, and synthesizes them with the goal of creating an approach that will be richer than either of the theories alone (Corey, 2001). This paper draws on this integrative approach by examining the basic principles of motivational interviewing (MI) and adventure therapy (AT) and the connection between the two. A case study demonstrates how MI and AT enhance each other in assisting clients to resolve their ambivalence towards change. The author's overall intention is to encourage adventure therapists to reflect upon their own practice to gain increased awareness about the connection between their use of adventure therapy activities and their other theoretical frameworks, in particular MI.

INTRODUCTION

Early on in my career as a therapist, I reflected on what client groups I was drawn to working with, and what approaches and techniques I wished to incorporate in my practice. As my career developed, I became more specialized in the application of particular theories and approaches that I believed to be effective in assisting clients progress towards desired change. Several realizations occurred during this process, one of which is that the tenets of certain theories and approaches seem to be closely linked with those of others. As my practice evolved, I also began to see instances where techniques from outside of the methodology of one theory may actually enhance the practical application of that theory.

This is supported by Wallbridge (1995) who discussed how therapist adaptability may be beneficial when therapeutic problems develop, and states that his predominant theory has become 'the core around which he has collected a toolbox of other ideas and techniques' (p.112). I began to realize that integrating theories and approaches may help to enhance my work with clients. Norcross (2005) described theoretical integration as a situation where two or more therapies are integrated in the hope that the result will be better than the constituent therapies alone. I remained cautious however in altering theories, as maintaining the core or spirit of the theory seemed to yield great significance. This is especially true of motivational interviewing, a clearly outlined approach to resolving client ambivalence.

In a study presented by Boardman, Catley, Grobe, Little, and Ahluwalia (2006), results indicated that engagement and alliance with the therapist was predicted by the therapists' adherence to the spirit of MI. Though motivational interviewing on its own can have positive results, when used in partnership with other clinical approaches it may be found to be even more effective.

Based on my experiences as an adventure therapist, along with documentation in the literature, this paper proposes that AT practice can enhance the MI approach in helping clients to resolve ambivalence towards change. Furthermore, AT practitioners may likely enhance their AT practice by becoming more conscious of the presence of MI principles in their facilitation and processing of AT activities. This paper examines the basic premises of MI as a clinical approach, explores the connection between AT and MI, and uses a case example to illustrate the presence of MI principles in AT facilitation.

MOTIVATIONAL INTERVIEWING

It is not uncommon for therapists to be faced with clients who present as ambivalent towards change, vacillating between wanting to modify their lives and resisting any shifts in their behavior (Shebib, 2000). Shebib (1997) suggested several essential elements in high client motivation including: a willingness to engage in counseling; a commitment to doing the work involved in creating change; and the ability to sustain efforts when faced with challenges. In times when clients are presenting with lower levels of motivation, they can have a tendency to be more challenging to engage in the treatment process and can also have more difficulty maintaining change. Assisting these clients to resolve this ambivalence and increase motivation for change is an important step in the therapeutic process.

Motivational interviewing, as defined by Miller and Rollnick (2002) is a 'client-centered directive method for enhancing intrinsic motivation to change by exploring and resolving ambivalence (p.25). Goldstein (2001) talks about core tactics of motivational interviewing involving 'generous use of open-ended questions; reflective listening to affirm client effort; and, especially, therapist attempts to elicit, support, and encourage self-motivational statements by the clients' (p.27). The aspect of eliciting change talk is fundamental in the motivational interviewing approach.

Miller and Rollnick (2002) identify expressing empathy, developing discrepancy, rolling with resistance, and supporting self-efficacy as the four basic principles of MI. Miller and Rollnick suggest expressing empathy involves normalizing client ambivalence, reflective listening, and demonstrating acacceptance. It entails bringing awareness to where the client is currently at in terms of their change process, rather than trying to move them forward. Developing discrepancy involves the client identifying a difference between their present behavior and their goals. This principle has more to do with using discrepancy to help the client explore possible reasons for change. The third principle, rolling with resistance, relates to the therapist's response to client resistance. Miller and Rollnick suggest that resistance should not be directly opposed and should rather be viewed as an invitation for the therapist to respond differently. Relevant to this principle, is the idea of accessing the client as the primary resource for finding solutions. Resistance may be experienced when the therapist takes on the role of problem-solver or is perceived as having an agenda for the client's change process. The final principle Miller and Rollnick introduce, supporting self-efficacy, suggests that the client's and therapist's belief in the client's ability to change is instrumental. They also suggest here, that it is the client who is ultimately responsible for identifying what they wish to change and how they plan to do so. The principles of MI emphasize that the change process belongs to the client, not the therapist.

In describing what something is, it is also helpful to explore what it is not. Miller and Rollnick (2009) provided a list of what MI is not. MI is not: derived from the trans-theoretical model of change; a method used to coerce an unwilling client; a technique or theory; simply the use of exercises of decisional balance; what practitioners inherently do; or a 'cure all'. MI is also not adventure therapy; however the principles of MI can often be found in the facilitation of AT activities. It is necessary to understand the true nature of MI (both what it is and is not) if one is to suggest that use of adventure therapy practice can enhance a use of MI.

The efficacy of MI for increasing motivation for change has been supported by a number of studies. Arkowitz, Westra, Miller, & Rollnick (2008) make reference to over 100 randomized clinical trials examining the efficacy of MI, and from the literature conclude that there is strong evidence that MI can be effective in triggering change. The usefulness of MI in motivating ambivalent clients has led to exploration about further applications. Arkowitz et al. (2008) suggest that MI has the potential for enhancing the effectiveness of other therapies. This paper proposes that not only does the presence of MI principles in AT facilitation enhance AT practice, but also that AT has the potential to enhance the effectiveness of MI.

Adventure Therapy

There has been a long standing debate regarding the definition of AT that continues to this day. For the purpose of this paper a definition put forth by the Adventure Therapy International Committee will be used, which states: 'AT involves the combination of physically and psychologically demanding activities, usually (but not always) conducted in a group setting. Adventure therapy is usually based on the principles of experiential education, but draws on traditions from counseling, psychology, social work, and education' (5IATC, 2009). Since there continue to be differing views regarding the definition of AT, it is very difficult to define what it is not. Discussions during the 5IATC suggested AT should continue to be defined very broadly, so as not to be exclusive as the community of AT practitioners continues to grapple with its identity.

Ringer (2003) outlined five definitional points of AT. Four of these have particular relevance to this paper. The first highlights AT as an experiential approach to group or family counseling. This relates to Ringer's second point, that AT involves the utilization of an activity base such as cooperative games, problem solving initiatives, ropes courses, outdoor pursuits, or wilderness expeditions. Activity becomes the experience through which clients actualize their change process. For this to occur, clients need to be given an opportunity to make meaning of the experience through verbal and/or non-verbal processing of the adventure experience, which is the fourth point Ringer presents. The final definitional point that has relevance here entails the use of isomorphic metaphor to support the transfer of client learning into change in client behavior. Ringer suggests that this involves matching the structure of the activity with the resolution of the problem. Gass (1993) suggests that isomorphic connections embedded in the facilitation of the adventure activity itself, rather than in the debriefing of the activity, is what makes metaphoric transfer possible and influences client change.

Connection between Motivational Interviewing and Adventure Therapy

Facilitation of AT activities lends itself to incorporating principles of MI. It is the interplay between the use of isomorphic metaphor in AT facilitation and the adherence to MI principles that I believe can have a profound effect on assisting clients in resolving ambivalence towards change. Knott (2004) outlined a protocol whereby MI components are embedded within the facilitation of AT activities through the use of specific questions and the stance of the facilitator.

Knott suggested that asking about potential risks symbolized in an activity can help the client to identify personal risk or problem behaviors in their life. In doing so, the facilitator begins to engage the use of isomorphic metaphor and involves the client in exploring ambivalence towards change. Knott also suggested that clients should reflect these risk behaviors back to the group. This provides the opportunity for the client to hear their own words, which is important in the process of working through ambivalence. It also allows the group to empathize with the client and normalize what has been expressed. When benefits and costs of the risk or problem behavior are asked about, Knott suggested that the client is able to weigh the pros and cons of changing the behavior and begin developing discrepancies between this behavior and their personal goals. To engage isomorphic metaphor here, the facilitator creates a parallel process between what is happening in the activity and the client's process of exploring their problem behavior. Knott (2004) highlighted that it is 'crucial that the facilitator be open to recognizing the potential benefits of the problem behavior to affirm the youth and the difficulty surrounding changing risk behavior' (p.240). In doing so, the facilitator is engaging the MI principle of rolling with resistance. This principle is reinforced in the activity when the facilitator ensures that they do not have a personal agenda for the client in the activity, and does not help the client find success in the activity through problem-solving for them.

Other techniques that Knott suggested are helpful to include in the facilitation of AT activities include reflecting the client's ambivalence regarding their behavior, and conveying to the client that they are capable of change. These reflect the MI principles of rolling with resistance and supporting self-efficacy. Knott suggested that when clients engage with and observe others during participation in AT activities, they have the opportunity to build new skills and experience what they are capable of. This in turn builds client self-efficacy. Isomorphic metaphor can be used to make a clear link between the skills the client used in the activity and the relevance of these skills to resolving the client's problem areas.

Case Example: Working with an Ambivalent Family in a Youth Residential Drug and Alcohol Program

The Client

A 16 year old girl, Sara (not real name), has been admitted into a three-month youth residential treatment program. The family is asked to attend the first day of the program and participate in a group introduction to family counseling. Sara has a history of depression, Attention Deficit Hyperactivity Disorder (ADHD), and substance use. She began using alcohol and marijuana at the age of 14, and her use has escalated to daily use. All family members express that there is a great deal of conflict in the home as a result of Sara's substance use. Sara presents as having low motivation for treatment and the motivation that is present is external. She states that her parents feel she has a problem and that she is only here because she was told she would not be allowed to live at home if she did not complete this program. Her parents state that Sara is the one who needs to change, but that they are willing to participate in the program if it will help her.

Initial Assessment of Client Motivation

Because this is a family-centered program, the family is seen as the client. All family members present with low motivation for working on individual change, while having a higher motivation for change to occur with other family members. Sara presents with the treatment goal of completing this program to rebuild some trust with her parents so she is allowed to remain in the family home. Parents' treatment goals at intake are based on change they would like to see with their daughter Sara. They would like to see her stop using substances, follow through on expectations, and be a happier member of the family.

Introduction of Stepping Stones Activity

The stepping stones activity is introduced to the family. Family members are each given a foam block. Their task is to get from one side of a room to the other, as a group, with only the blocks being able to touch the floor. If anyone steps off the blocks, it is classified as a slip up. At this point the family is given a choice to either end the activity or take one big step back, whatever they determine that to be, and carry on from that point. The activity ends when the family has either chosen to end the activity or have successfully crossed the room using the blocks (adapted from Rohnke & Butler, 1995). The goals of the activity are to assist the family to more clearly understand their treatment goals, to explore steps they have already started to take in the direction of their goals, and to begin to address and resolve any ambivalence they may have towards individual and family change. The nature of the activity provides opportunities to explore concepts of trust, participation, and follow-through, which have been expressed as important topics of focus for this family.

Discussion

The application of this activity with this family demonstrates how MI and AT can be integrated to enhance the clients' treatment goals. The activity begins when family members are asked to think about personal strengths that have helped them through tough times in their lives and to write these on the foam blocks. In doing so, the therapist is relaying to clients a belief that they have already developed strengths that are applicable and transferable to their current situation. This taps into the ability aspect of change, and is reflective of the MI principle of supporting self-efficacy.

The family is then asked to stand behind a line marked on the floor. Another line is marked on the floor about 10 feet ahead. The therapist states 'be as specific as possible and tell me what it is you see on the floor in front of the line'. Family members are then asked to stay where they are and explain what they see in front of the line 10 feet away. The next question asked is 'what is different between what you see here and what you can see 10 feet away?'. In asking this question, the therapist introduces another principle of MI, which is assisting clients to develop discrepancy between where they are and where they are heading. The family is then asked to describe the nature of their current situation, the line they are currently standing behind. Following these descriptions, the family is asked 'if this line is Family Welcome Day, and the line down there is the last day of the program, what would you like to be different in your life or the life of your family three months from now? These questions involve the introduction of isomorphic metaphor to help the clients link the activity to their actual change process, highlighting the discrepancy between where they are as a family today and where they would like to be. Luckner & Nadler (1992) stated, 'when you use metaphorical communication, participants are compelled to think and listen in symbols and soon learn to make bridges from the experience to their life' (p.142). Now that this isomorphic metaphor has been introduced, it is maintained through the activity (e.g. 'the task is to work together to get from where you are today to three months from now, using your strengths and the strengths of other family members' – a statement that includes MI principles of developing discrepancy and supporting self-efficacy). Reflecting back to the clients their identified goals reinforces that they are in treatment to address what they would like to, and keeps these goals forefront in their minds.

As the therapist continues to frame the activity for the family, additional MI principles emerge. The therapist informs the family of when a 'stop' will be called in the activity: ('If there is a slip up during the activity, I will call 'stop'. At that point you will have a decision to make. You can either end the activity, end treatment, or take one big step back, whatever you interpret one big step to be, and carry on from that point forward. I will not be a part of that decision and whatever decision you make will be respected.'

This framing introduces the MI principle of expressing empathy. If a slip up does occur in the activity, it allows the therapist the opportunity to normalize slip ups and empathize with the client if they feel ambivalent about continuing (e.g. 'how many of us have slipped up when working towards something that is important to us? What are common feelings that come up when we do slip up? Has anyone ever felt like giving up when they have had a slip up?'. The therapist can then reflect back what they are hearing from the clients as they answer these questions and make the decision whether or not to carry on.

Again, isomorphic metaphor is used to link the clients' experience in the activity to times they believe they may feel like giving up in treatment. The therapist remains neutral in the clients' decision, expressing empathy, and supporting the client's choice. The MI principle of rolling with resistance presents itself if a slip up occurs and the family chooses to end the activity. The therapist does not argue for reasons to continue the activity or resist the decision that has been made. Instead the therapist may give the family the option of coming back to the activity at a later date (starting from where they left off), or ask, 'are your three month goals still of importance to you, and if so is there anything I can do differently to better support you in reaching these goals/completing the activity?'. This engages the MI principle that resistance is a signal for the therapist to respond differently.

The MI principle of supporting self-efficacy is present in the next part of framing the activity. The family is informed that the activity will also be stopped if the therapist has a question, or sees something interesting. Stopping the activity early on provides an opportunity to highlight progress (e.g. 'I stopped the activity because you have three people who have taken steps forward and entered treatment. What that tells me is that things are working for you. Can you tell me what is working for you so far?'). Doing so gives client's an opportunity to identify skills that they are currently using that are resulting in recognized progress. Recognition of skills and progress can have an impact on the clients' belief in the possibility of change. It can also assist in developing discrepancy between the family's current behavior of finding success together, and previous beliefs that they were not able to make progress as a family. In stopping the process early on, the family is able to experience a sense of success, regardless of whether or not they complete the activity and/or complete the treatment program as a family at this time.

Gass (1993) suggests that isomorphic connections embedded in the facilitation of the adventure activity itself, rather than in the debriefing, is what makes metaphoric transfer possible and influences client change. However, this author believes that reflecting on the nature of the role of therapist in the debriefing of the activity can highlight client's personal agency in creating their success. In this scenario, after the activity, the therapist may ask, 'what role, did I play in the activity?. What did and didn't I do?' As clients identify that the therapist did not tell them how to do the activity, it brings to light the MI principle of rolling with resistance. It leads clients to identify that they were the primary resource in finding their solutions and carrying out the process of using their strengths to progress towards change. The use of isomorphic metaphor throughout helps clients link how they can, and maybe already are, starting to find solutions for their goals.

Outcomes for Case Study Family

Sara engaged in the Stepping Stones activity. Her defensive affect seemed to dissipate as she was provided with choices and as she recognized that the therapist had no agenda as to what she wanted to see from Sara in the activity or in the program. This seemed to allow Sara to begin to explore her ambivalence towards treatment. During the debrief of the activity, Sara stated that to be successful, her family had needed to 'trust each other and communicate'. At the end of the day Sara expressed that she felt better about her decision to come to treatment. Sara's parents began the activity by focusing on the changes they would like to see Sara make. As the activity progressed and they experienced that Sara could not reach the other side of the room without them, they began to take active steps to support both her progress and their own. During the debrief of the activity, when asked what the relationship between the activity and family counseling was they responded, 'we must work together and all do our part for change to occur'.

Conclusion

Research shows that motivational interviewing enhances intrinsic motivation to change by exploring and resolving ambivalence. However, this paper shows how adventure therapy activities can also help clients to explore their process of change. As clients are given experiential opportunities to act out new patterns of behavior, they create real time discrepancy, which in turn supports their self-efficacy. When MI principles are embedded in the facilitation of AT activities and coupled with the use of isomorphic metaphor, what emerges is an enhanced integrative approach for resolving client ambivalence towards change. Clients are able to link their 'here and now' experiences in the activity with their process of addressing their 'real life' dilemmas.

The discussions above are just a beginning for reflections on how AT and MI may be integrated in helping clients to resolve ambivalence towards change. It is hoped that ideas presented in this paper will encourage other therapists to reflect upon their use of adventure therapy and the connection it has with other theoretical frameworks that inform their practice, especially motivational interviewing.

References

Adventure Therapy International Committee. (2009). Retrieved on 2/1/10 from: http://www.bacp.co.uk/5iatc/definitions.php.

Arkowitz, H., & Miller, W.R. (2008). *Learning, applying, and extending motivational interviewing: Motivational interviewing in the treatment of psychological problems.* New York: The Guilford Press.

Boardman, T., Catley, D., Grove, J. E., Little, T. D., & Ahluwalia, J. S. (2006). Using motivational interviewing with smokers: Do therapist behaviours relate to engagement and therapeutic alliance? *Journal of Substance Abuse Treatment, 31*, 329-339.

Cory, G. (2001). *Theory and practice of counselling and psychotherapy* (6th ed.). USA: Brooks/Cole.

Gass, M.A. (1993). Enhancing metaphor development in adventure therapy programs. *Adventure therapy: Therapeutic applications of adventure programming.* Iowa: Kendall/Hunt Publishing Company.

Goldstein, A. (2001). *Reducing resistance: Methods for enhancing openness to change.* Champaign, IL:Research Press.

Knott, J. (2004). *Self-efficacy and motivation to change among chronic youth offenders: An exploratory examination of the efficacy of an experiential learning, motivation enhancement intervention.* Unpublished Doctoral Dissertation in Counselling Psychology: University of Oregon.

Miller, W.R. & Rollnick, S. (2002). *Motivational interviewing: Preparing people for change* (2nd ed.). New York: The Guilford Press.

Miller, W.R. & Rollnick, S. (2009). Ten things that motivational interviewing is not. *Behavioural and Cognitive Psychotherapy, 37*, 129-140.

Norcross, J.C. (2005). A primer on psychotherapy integration. *Handbook of Psychotherapy Integration* (2nd ed.). New York: Oxford.

Ringer, M. (2003). Adventure therapy: A description. *Therapy within adventure: Proceedings of the second international adventure therapy conference.* Augsburg: Ziel.

Rohnke, K. & Butler, S. (1995). *Quicksilver: Adventure games, initiative problems, trust activities, and a guide to effective leadership.* Iowa: Kendall/Hunt Publishing Company.

Shebib, B. (2000). *Choices: Practical interviewing and counselling skills.* Canada: Prentice Hall/Allyn and Bacon.

Shebib, B. (1997). *Counselling Skills.* Victoria: Province of British Columbia, Ministry of Education, Skills and Training.

Wallbridge, H. (1995). Difficult issues for new therapists. *Basics of clinical practice: A guidebook for trainees in the helping professions.* Prospect Heights, IL: Waveland Press, Inc.

CHAPTER 19

Building Bridges: Using Adventure to Enhance the Therapeutic Relationship Cross-culturally

Christine Lynn Norton

ABSTRACT

This paper examines the importance of the therapeutic relationship, and the need for cultural competence in adventure therapy. Cultural differences between the counselor and the client can sometimes result in possible misinterpretation and conflict, which can lead to clients prematurely dropping out of treatment. This paper builds on current research in adventure education and therapy on 'cultural competence' and multicultural factors, and clarifies the role that adventure can play in 'cultural bridging' and enhancing the therapeutic relationship. A new framework, the ABC model, is presented for developing the therapeutic relationship cross-culturally in adventure therapy.

INTRODUCTION

It is well-known in counseling literature that the therapeutic relationship between counselor and client is one of the most important factors in the change process (Lambert & Barley, 2001). Regardless of the counselor's theoretical orientation, the quality of the relationship that a counselor builds with a client can be predictive of the outcomes of treatment (McCabe, 2004). However, one of the biggest barriers to the establishment of an effective therapeutic relationship is a lack of cultural competence on the part of the counselor. Cultural competence can be defined as the ability to work effectively across cultures (Olsen, Bhattacharya, & Scharf, 2006). Often, when cultural differences exist between a counselor and client, it can result in misinterpretation and conflict. This may, in turn, lead clients to prematurely terminate counseling or to drop out of counseling at a high rate (Sue, Fujino, Takeuchi, Hu, & Zane, 1991).

It has been shown that conflict between individuals from different cultural groups is often a result of differences in their concept of worldview, and more specifically in the different dimensions of their worldviews (Brown & Landrum-Brown, 1995; Myers, 1991; Nichols, 1976; Nobles, 1972). For this reason, counselors must learn to be effective with clients from different cultural backgrounds. To do so, they must be aware of and understand not only the client's perspective of the world but also their own worldview (Sue, 1981). By comparing worldviews, the counselor is then able to examine possible misinterpretations that can arise in a therapeutic situation in which the counselor and client are from different cultural backgrounds.

This is especially important in an adventure therapy context if the cultural backgrounds of the adventure therapist and the client are different. When this occurs, not only can these differences cause the client to feel disconnected from the therapist, but the unfamiliarity of the environment used in many adventure therapy contexts can also create an unproductive level of disequilibrium. Fabrizio and Neill (2005) wrote that in many ways, entering an outdoor program is like entering another country and requires a lot of adaptation on the part of the client, making the therapeutic relationship even more essential.

The purpose of this paper is to build upon current research in adventure education and therapy on cultural competence and multicultural factors (Brookes, 2003; Crisp, 1996; Cummings, 2004; Mitten, 1994; Warren, 1999; 2002; 2005; Wright, 1997) and to clarify the role that adventure can play in enhancing the therapeutic relationship through cultural bridging. A new framework, the ABC model, is presented as a tool for developing the therapeutic relationship cross-culturally in adventure therapy.

Defining Key Terms

In order to understand the impact of adventure on the therapeutic relationship, we must first understand and define several key terms. This section will examine what is meant by the terms therapeutic relationship, cultural competence and adventure.

The therapeutic relationship can be defined as a supporting and trusting relationship that is built between a counselor and the client. It is an alliance that should be based on unconditional positive regard (Rogers, 1957). Unconditional positive regard does not mean that the relationship will be easy or conflict free, but rather that the therapist will not impinge the client's motives, and will focus on the client's strengths. In this sense, the therapeutic relationship does not automatically exist; rather, it must be cultivated over time in order to establish a relationship that involves a high level of support and authenticity. Once a therapeutic relationship is established, it can provide a corrective emotional experience for the client. The therapeutic relationship in adventure therapy is especially unique and powerful because it is built on closeness and shared experiences which fosters a high level of therapist-client communication and often 'minimizes a sense of counter-therapeutic hierarchy' (Kimball & Bacon, 1993, p. 33).

Cultural competence is the ability to work effectively across cultural differences and divides. Cultural divides should be viewed in the broadest context, since our work with clients most often includes a multitude of differences ranging from obvious differences such as nationality, race, ethnicity, and gender, to more subtle yet no less important differences such as socioeconomic status, levels of education, literacy, as well as sub-cultural differences, like youth culture, street cultures, or cultures of addiction for example. More specifically, in a counseling setting, cultural competence involves the ability to engage the client, assess the client in terms of multicultural factors, and develop a treatment plan that includes culturally sensitive and relevant intervention and evaluation strategies. According to Kleinman (2004), counselors must avoid stereotyping clients, and evaluate the culturally relevant aspects of the stresses and support in the life of clients. Attention should also be paid to the ways in which culture can impact the therapeutic relationship (Kleinman, 2004).

When defining adventure, we often think of physically challenging activities such as climbing a mountain or paddling a rapid river. However, this paper seeks to define adventure by its most common elements (rather than in terms of specific activities). Wright's (2004) definition of adventure as a shared experience that includes challenges and peak experiences does just that. 'Peak experience' is a term created by Maslow (1970) that embodies the concept that there are certain experiences we have in life that bring us a sense of joy, wonder, and even awe. Adventure also involves mutual engagement in acts of meaning, like community service, activism and social justice. Finally, adventure is a form of co-created play. It is a process of incorporating positive risk-taking and physical, mental and emotional challenges in a developmentally appropriate manner.

Cultural Competence and Multicultural Factors in Adventure Therapy: A Brief Review of the Literature

In order to understand multicultural factors in adventure therapy, we first need to look at the area of cultural research in outdoor and adventure education. Purdie and Neill (1999) wrote about cross-cultural difficulties that students on outdoor programs can face when program activities go against the client's cultural world view. They later advocated for greater understanding of the impact of cultural identity on outdoor education experiences (Purdie, Neill & Richards, 2002).

Despite these few studies, there have been criticisms that both outdoor education and adventure therapy have done little to address the need for adventure-based educators and counselors to competently and effectively treat diverse populations (Warren, 1999). Likewise, Mitten (1994) and Warren (2000) encourage practitioners to adapt intervention strategies and methods of treatment to meet the unique needs of diverse populations, as well as increase knowledge and experience in order to engage effectively with these clients. This combination of enhancing cultural competence in outdoor education and adventure therapy through increased knowledge, awareness and skills was validated by Cummings (2004).

In response to these concerns and the need for more guidance in these areas, the Therapeutic Adventure Professional Group (TAPG), an interdisciplinary sub-group of professionals who utilize adventure for therapeutic purposes in the United States, developed a set of ethical guidelines that addressed the issue of cultural competence. They consulted with the American Psychological Association (APA) and the Association of Marriage and Family Therapists (AAMFT), and other professionals in the field of therapeutic adventure, along with consulting literature in this area (TAPG, 2002). While not all of these are unique to adventure therapy, TAPG highlighted the following considerations on their 'Best Practices' website:

- Awareness of particular factors regarding culture/ethnicity that may be related to a particular setting/environment (e.g. African Americans from Washington, D.C. going to a wilderness area near a white supremacist community in West Virginia).
- Given the ease with which practitioners and organizations in all professions assume cultural biases unknowingly, it is essential to continually ask 'what do culturally competent/appropriate/responsive practitioners and/or organizations look like?
- It is important that awareness be maintained of the potential cultural parity of practitioners in comparison to clients.
- It is important that practitioners adjust adventure activities and realize that different cultural groups have very different perceptions of the same activities/environments. Central to this is that practitioners continually examine their own biases and those that might be embedded in an AT

activity, particularly assumptions about client reactions to particular activities and how those may/may not be associated with positive/culturally relevant therapeutic outcomes.

- Practitioners should continually challenge themselves to understand how cultural beliefs about adventure or environment shape experiences, for both themselves and clients. Although there are many, areas to explore might include how cultural values and beliefs are shaped, identification of relevant cultural barriers, skills that enhance open communication, culturally appropriate assumptions regarding levels of self-disclosure, effective techniques for particular client populations (e.g. working with interpreters), role of cultural upbringing and how that relates to communication style/conflict resolution, etc.
- Practitioners should continue to educate themselves about culturally relevant outcomes, in order to avoid making what may be misassumptions about treatment success or non-success (TAPG, 2002)

While this information has been helpful in building awareness and knowledge of ethical and cultural issues in adventure therapy, very little has been written to help practitioners know how to engage in culturally competent practice. This paper aims to add to the guidelines set forth by TAPG and other professional organizations, to provide practitioners of adventure therapy with a multicultural practice model that utilizes adventure as a bridge to develop and enhance the therapeutic relationship. This paper builds on Wright's (1997) model in which he used 'shared adventure' as a means of increasing multicultural competence with outdoor professionals. Wright created a multicultural adventure program based on the goal of increasing awareness of one's own personal identity and creating positive regard for others through interpersonal encounter and community formation. In Wright's model, key program components included: a diverse group of participants; challenge or risk; shared cooperative tasks; supportive context; dialogue; and reflection. Wright found that these components led to program outcomes of self-discovery, self-disclosure, identity formation, and community formation, which in turn led to intercultural dialogue and increased tolerance and understanding.

Creating a multicultural practice model is especially important in outdoor education and adventure therapy because the foundations of these educational and therapeutic approaches are generally based on a white, male model of Western cultural interaction (Brookes, 2003; Warren, 2005). Therefore in order to develop cultural competence in adventure therapy, the practitioner may need to 'de-centre' from his/her own cultural world view and begin to see the adventure experience from the perspective of the client.

Creating a Foundation for Adventure

Adventure involves physical risk, emotional risk, and interpersonal risk. Perceptions of whether an adventure activity is high-risk or low-risk is personally and culturally determined. If adventure is to be used effectively, one has to assess what level of risk the client applies to the activity; the activity can only be applied in a context of trust. In order for adventure to be a cultural bridge that enhances the therapeutic relationship, there are three things that must be present: safety, choice and empathy. These things create a foundation for being able to use adventure as a therapist and the client, especially when cultural differences are present.

Safety

In an adventure therapy context, physical and emotional safety is paramount. It is essential to consider and preserve the health and well-being of participants, both clients and staff. Likewise, safety related to the gear, facilities and logistics must always be taken into consideration. Risk management is a critical component to mitigate actual risk, so that clients can deal with their perceived risk for therapeutic purposes. Of course, emotional safety in adventure therapy is also critical. Much has been discussed about how to create emotional safety in adventure therapy, including specific techniques used by instructors, instructor skills and abilities, the physical environment, and group compositions (Vincent, 1995).

The field of adventure therapy has responded to the need for physical and emotional safety by tightening up procedures related to assessment and screening, as well as emergency medical and clinical first responder skills to maintain client safety once participating in the program. Staff training in many adventure therapy programs involves training in crisis intervention and de-escalation skills; however, little mention has been made of multicultural factors and issues of power and privilege in facilitating safety during an adventure therapy program. Yet if the atmosphere of an adventure therapy program or group replicates the dominant culture in a way that, at the very least, lacks awareness of the importance of multicultural issues, and at worst is oppressive, then clients will not feel safe and therapeutic outcomes may suffer.

Choice

The issue of client choice in counseling has often been defined as the 'client's right to self-determination' (Floyd Taylor, 2006). In adventure therapy, the concept of 'challenge by has been identified as an important way of respecting client autonomy. It is a way of avoiding coercion and helping clients decide upon their level of participation, while still encouraging them to add something of value to the group. While a full review of the concept of challenge by choice is beyond the scope of this paper, it is important to acknowledge some of the controversy around this concept. Some advocate for what I might call 'complete choice' in adventure therapy settings, which includes the freedom to come and go, to participate or not, to decide on the level of challenge and self-expression. However, some realize that because many adventure therapy clients are young people who we might consider to be involuntary clients, challenge by choice is often limited. Regardless of whether one's stance on challenge by choice involves complete or limited choice, the concept of choice must be present to a certain extent if a client is to fully engage in the therapeutic process.

Empathy

The final component that must be in place in order to use adventure as a bridge to enhance the therapeutic relationship is empathy. Empathy is the ability to feel what someone else is feeling and to be aware of the how one's actions affect another. Ibrahim (1991) identified the need to 'convey empathy in a culturally consistent and meaningful manner' (p. 18) when working with culturally diverse groups. In a preliminary study by Sue, Yau, and Mao (1995), it was found that counselors' credibility with a client was increased if they demonstrated and communicated an understanding of the client's worldview and acknowledged the cultural differences between them. This can lead to what is known as cultural empathy. David and Erickson (1990) provided a framework for cultural empathy, defining it as the counselor possessing competencies or attitudes that begin to bridge the cultural gap between counselor and client. Therefore, when using adventure to enhance the therapeutic relationship, cultural empathy not just empathy is required as a way of relating interpersonally as well as understanding and communicating across cultures (Chung & Bemak, 2002). Fortunately, ethnic similarity is not necessary to achieve cultural empathy (Chung & Bemak, 2002); however, a multicultural practice model assists the worker to convey this type of empathy and enhance the therapeutic relationship cross-culturally.

ABC: An Adventure-based Framework for Developing the Therapeutic Relationship Cross-culturally

This paper presents the ABC model as an adventure-based framework for developing the therapeutic relationship cross-culturally. Similar to Wright's (1997) multicultural model of adventure education, the ABC model combines the intentional use of shared adventures as a means of bridging the cultural divides between the adventure therapist and the client. It is an experiential model in which adventure activities can lead to cultural bridging and an enhanced connection in the therapeutic relationship.

Adventure

Adventure has been defined in this paper as a shared experience (Wright, 1997). The idea of shared adventure experiences mirrors Alvarez's (2002) model of adventure-based practice. According to Alvarez (2002), adventure-based practice is a form of practice with the following common elements: it explores the unknown; is action oriented; explores challenges and difficulty for the purpose of change; offers an active stance for the practitioner; and offers the opportunity for genuine community participation (as cited in Aylward, 2005). When adventure is used intentionally for these purposes, it becomes a shared experience between the adventure therapist and the client that offers multiple opportunities for personal growth. In the ABC model, adventure-based activities should be used to fit the client's cultural background and treatment goals.

Bridging

Cultural bridging involves creating a shared understanding that involves 'constructively engaging with difference, as well as similarity' (Mason & Sawyerr, 2002, p. xxi). Once the adventure therapist and the client have engaged in a shared adventure experience, they have the possibility of understanding one another better. This bridging process occurs when:

- The counselor expresses a genuine interest in learning more about the client's culture;
- The counselor demonstrates an awareness and sensitivity about some aspects of the client's culture but not necessarily in all areas;
- The counselor shows a genuine appreciation for cultural differences between the client and counselor, and an openness to finding common ground as well;

- Culturally appropriate help-seeking behaviors and treatment outcome expectations will be incorporated into the counseling process as needed (ChiYing Chung & Bemak, 2002).

In other words, cultural bridging allows the client to collaborate with the therapist to infuse the treatment process with culturally relevant information that can help adapt the treatment process to meet the client's needs, rather than pushing the therapist's cultural agenda.

Connection

As a result of engaging in shared adventure experiences and utilizing strategies for cultural bridging, it is hoped that the end result is a greater connection between the adventure therapist and the client. This connection can be seen through a greater awareness of interdependence, and increased levels of trust and respect. It does not mean that the adventure therapist and the client will become friends or even like one another, but rather realize that their well-being is connected to one another. This deeper level of connection is a result of increased empathy as well.

Overview of the ABC Model: A Case Study

The ABC model is built upon a foundation of physical and emotional safety, choice, and cultural empathy. Once this foundation is established, adventure can be utilized in the form of shared challenges and peak experiences, mutual engagement in acts of meaning, and co-created play. This shared adventure experience may lead to cultural bridging and create greater connection and common ground between the adventure therapist and the client. A cross-cultural case study is presented to better illustrate this model.

Case Study

Several years ago, I served as a consultant for a newly developing therapeutic adventure program in Croatia. As an American, I tried to be highly conscious of my biases and Western approaches to mental health and adventure therapy work. I worked hard to listen to the Croatian staff and gain insight from their cultural nearness to the adolescent clients with whom we worked. For the most part, I was able to form good relationships with the clients, in spite of the cultural and language barriers. I demonstrated unconditional positive regard and empathy and found these basic counselling skills work well at solidifying the therapeutic relationships I was trying to build.

However, there was one client, a 15 year old Croatian girl with a history of trauma who had grown up in residential treatment who acted in a very hostile manner towards me. There were many factors impinging on this girl's ability to trust me or form a positive relationship with me, including attachment issues impacted by her developmental history. But these psychodevelopmental factors were compounded by the cultural differences that existed between us. As an American, I represented cultural archetypes that she found threatening. Often she would say 'America! Svana!' which translates 'America is shit.' I didn't take this personally, as I was aware that there were probably transference issues that were a factor in the situation, given her history of abuse and neglect. I was also aware of and able to own, the negative impact of American foreign policy in various parts of the world.

Every morning, I would wake up and do my best to greet her in her native language, and every morning she would curse at me with bold Croatian swears. Nothing I did made any positive difference in our relationship. The harder I tried to connect interpersonally, the angrier and more distant she became. I sought consultation from the Croatian staff, and one of them had a wonderful idea that led to the creation of the model I have presented in this article.

On the day that we were to go rock climbing, this particular staff member set it up so that I could belay this client. At first, the girl balked at the idea, stating in Croatian something equivalent to there was no way in hell she would let me be responsible for her safety. The instructor explained to her that I was highly trained and that she could have a peer serve as a back-up belayer if that would make her more comfortable. In this way, the instructor was trying to create a sense of safety for the client. Next, she reminded the client that ultimately, it was her choice, and that she could climb with another belayer but that she would have to wait until the other belayers were available. Lastly, the instructor empathized with how uncomfortable the client felt, and then offered to role model climbing while I belayed her so the client could actually see how safe it was.

After seeing the staff person climb with me, the girl reluctantly agreed to allow me to belay her on her climb. As she climbed, we had a translator help me respond to her needs for slack in the rope or to make the rope tighter, among other things. This shared adventure experience ended with her making it to the top of the climb, rappelling down, and having me say 'Bravo!' enthusiastically. Still, she seemed unimpressed and distant.

That night at our group meeting, I asked a staff person to translate for me while I thanked this girl for taking the risk of trusting me, and pushing herself beyond her limits physically and emotionally. I told her about how scared I was the first time I climbed (trying to find some common ground) and how inspired I was by her courage. I also told her that I was not offended by her anger towards Americans and that I knew that American foreign policy often hurt people in other parts of the world. I told her that if she ever wanted to talk to me more about this, I would be open to it. This attempt at cultural bridging yielded nothing more than a nod. Still, that was better than being cursed at.

The next morning, I awoke as always expecting a bad Croatian greeting, only this time, I was merely ignored and not verbally attacked. At breakfast, I went to refill my water bottle with one of the larger jugs, when suddenly this young girl yelled out to me, 'no!' and followed with something in Croatian. Upon speaking with one of the Croatian staff, I discovered that the girl had stopped me from using the non-potable water, and told me I needed to use the good water instead so I didn't get sick. I was astounded; given her hostile behaviour towards me throughout the trip, I assumed that she would actually enjoy watching me drink the wrong water and get sick. This may have clearly been a negative assumption on my part, but after the climbing day and our talk that followed, this incident confirmed for me that something had shifted. It is hard to know what occurred, but it seemed like there was now a modicum of trust between us, enough so that this girl no longer felt threatened by me and may have actually cared about my well-being.

From then on, this client and I were able to co-exist peaceably on the trip. Her hostile behaviour subsided, and we began to interact through small talk and humour, as best we could, given our language barrier. What was noticeable, however, was not just her openness with me, but she became less caustic with the entire group and with her trip leaders as well. It is fair to say that the ABC model not only enhanced the therapeutic relationship, but also the level of emotional safety the client felt on the trip as a whole.

Conclusion

While I realize that this case study presents only one example of using adventure to enhance the therapeutic relationship, the ABC model is one that can be used in multiple settings and should be further applied and tested. The model draws awareness to the need for shared adventure experiences, cultural bridging and greater connection in adventure therapy, and clears the way 'for situationist approaches to outdoor education (and therapy) that bring much needed sensitivity to cultural, regional, historical, and social contexts' (Brookes, 2003, p. 119). Clearly, there is a need for more research and theory building on the impact of shared adventure and cultural bridging. Likewise, there is a need for more research on the importance of the therapeutic relationship in adventure therapy. Despite the need for further research in these areas, one thing is clear; adventure can be a powerful tool for enhancing the therapeutic relationship cross-culturally.

REFERENCES

Aylward, T. (2005). *Outdoor Education; A resource for Social Care Education.* Presented at a Lecture in the Health & Leisure Dept. at the Institute of Technology, Tralee to the Irish Association of Social Care Educators Annual Conference; 'New directions in Social Care Education and Practice' 21st October 2005.

Bemak, F. (1998). Interdisciplinary collaboration for social change: Redefining the counsellor profession. In C. C. Lee & G. R. Walz (Eds.), *Social action: A mandate for counsellors* (pp. 279–292). Alexandria, VA: American Counselling Association/ERIC Counselling and Student Services Clearinghouse.

Bemak, E, Chung, R. C-Y., & Pedersen, P. (2003). *Counselling refugees: A psychosocial cultural approach to innovative multicultural interventions.* Hartford, CT: Greenwood Publishing.

Berry, J.W. (1997). Individual and group relations in plural societies. In C. S. Granrose & S. Oskamp (Eds.), *Cross-cultural group works* (17–35). Thousand Oaks, CA: Sage.

Brookes, A. (2003). A critique of neo-Hahnian outdoor education theory. Part two: 'The fundamental attribution error' in contemporary outdoor education. *Journal of Adventure Education & Outdoor Learning, 3*(2), 119-132.

Brown, M.T., & Landrum-Brown, J. (1995). Counsellor supervision: Cross-cultural perspectives. In J. G. Ponterotto, J. M. Casas, L. A. Suzuki & C. M. Alexande (Eds.), *Handbook of multicultural Counselling* (pp. 263–286). Thousand Oaks, CA: Sage.

Chi-Ying Chung, R. & Bemak, F. (2002) The relationship of culture and empathy in cross-cultural counselling. *Journal of Counselling & Development, 80*(2), 154-160.

Crisp. S. (1996) *Churchill Fellowship Report: International models of best practice in wilderness and adventure therapy*. Retrieved on 8/24/2009 from:
http://www.churchilltrust.com.au/res/File/Fellow_
Reports/Crisp%20Simon%20196.pdf .

Cummings, D. (2004) *Multicultural competence and levels of effectiveness in adventure based counselling.* Unpublished dissertation: West Virginia University College of Human Resources and Education.

David, A. B., & Erickson, C. A. (1990). Ethnicity and the therapist's use of self. *Family Therapy,* 17, 211–216.

Fabrizio, S., & Neill, J.T. (2005). Cultural adaptation in outdoor programming. *Australian Journal of Outdoor Education, 9*(2), 44-56.

Floyd Taylor, M. (2006). Is self-determination still important? What experienced mental health social workers are saying. *Journal of Social Work Values and Ethics, 3*(1).

Ibrahim, F. A. (1991). Contribution of cultural worldview to generic counselling and development. *Journal of Counselling & Development, 70*, 13–19.

Kimball, R.O., & Bacon, S.B. (1993). The wilderness challenge model. In M. Gass (Ed.), *Adventure therapy: Therapeutic applications of adventure programming* (pp. 11-41). Dubuque, IA: Kendall/Hunt Publishing.

Lambert, M.J., & Barley, D.E. (2001). Research summary on the therapeutic relationship and psychotherapy outcomes. *Psychotherapy: Theory, Research, Practice, Training, 38*(4), 357-361.

Maslow, A. (1970). *Religion, values and peak experiences.* New York: Viking.

Mason, Barry & Sawyerr, Alice. (2002). *Exploring the unsaid: Creativity, risks and dilemmas in working cross-culturally*. London: H. Karnac (Books) Ltd.

McCabe, R. (2004). The therapeutic relationship in the treatment of severe mental illness: A review of methods and findings. *International Journal of Social Psychiatry, 50*(2), pp. 115-128.

Mitten, D. (1994). Ethical considerations in adventure therapy. *Women and Therapy, 15*(3), pp. 55–84.

Myers, L. J. (1991). Expanding the psychology of knowledge optimally: The importance of worldview revisited. In R. L. Jones (Ed.), *Black psychology,* 3rd ed. (pp. 15-28). Berkeley, CA: Cobb & Henry.

Neill, J. (2008). *Challenge by choice.* Retrieved on 8/24/2009 from: http://wilderdom.com/ABC/ChallengeByChoice.html.

Nichols, E. (1976, October). *The philosophical aspects of cultural differences.* Paper presented at the conference of the World Psychiatric Association. Ibadan, Nigeria.

Nobles, W. (1972). African philosophy: Foundation for Black psychology. In R. L. Jones (Ed.), *Black psychology* (1st ed.) (pp. 18–32). New York: Harper & Row.

Olsen, L., Bhattacharya, J., Scharf, A. (2006). *Cultural competency: What it is and why it matters?* California Tomorrow: Lucile Packard Foundation for Children's Health.

Pedersen, P. (1991). Multiculturalism as a generic approach to counselling. *Journal of Counselling & Development, 70*, 6–12.

Project Adventure. (2004). *Challenge by choice.* Retrieved on 3/3/10 from: http://www.pa.org/about/ glossary.phpff.

Purdie, N., & Neill, J.T. (1999). Japanese students down-under: Is Australian outdoor education relevant to other cultures? *Australian Journal of Outdoor Education, 4*(1), pp. 48-57.

Purdie, N., Neill, J.T., & Richards, G.E. (2002). Australian identity and the effects of an outdoor program. *Australian Journal of Psychology, 54*(1).

Ridley, C. R., & Lingle, D.W. (1996). Cultural empathy in multicultural counselling: A multidimensional process model. In P. B. Pedersen, J. G. Draguns, W. J. Lonner, & J. E. Trimble (Eds.), *Counselling across cultures,* 4th ed. (pp. 21-46). Thousand Oaks, CA: Sage.

Robinson, T. L., & Ginter, G. L. (Eds.). (1999). Racism: Healing its effects [Specia issue]. *Journal of Counselling & Development, 77*(1).

Rogers, C. R. (1957). The necessary and sufficient conditions for therapeutic personality change. *Journal of Consulting Psychology*, 21, 95–103.

Stewart, E. C. (1981). Cultural sensitivities in counselling. In P. B. Pedersen, J.G. Draguns, W. J. Lonner, & J. E. Trimble (Eds.), *Counselling across cultures* (pp. 61–68). Honolulu: University Press of Hawaii.

Sue, D. W. (1981). *Counselling the culturally different*. New York: Wiley.

Sue, D., & Sundberg, N. D. (1996). Research and research hypotheses about effectiveness in intercultural counselling. In P. B. Pedersen, J. G. Draguns, W. J. Lonner, & J. E. Trimble (Eds.), *Counselling across cultures*, 4th ed. (pp. 323-352). Thousand Oaks, CA: Sage.

Sue, D., Yau, T. Y., & Mao, J. (1995). *Microskills in multicultural counselling.* Unpublished manuscript.

Sue, D. W., Bingham, R. P., Porche-Burke, L., & Vasquez, M. (1999). The diversification of psychology: A multicultural revolution. *American Psychologist, 54*, 1061–1069.

Sue, D. W., & Sue, D. (1990). *Counselling the culturally different: Theory and practice* (2nd ed.). New York: Wiley.

Sue, S., Fujino, D., Takeuchi, D., Hu, L-T., & Zane, N. (1991). Community mental health services for ethnic minority groups: A test of the cultural responsive hypothesis. *Journal of Consulting and Clinical Psychology, 59*, 533–540.

Therapeutic Adventure Professional Group. (2002). *Ethical Guidelines*. Retrieved on 3/2/2010 from: http://tapg.aee.org/tapg/ethicalguidelines.

Vincent, S. (1995). Emotional safety in adventure therapy programs: Can it be defined? *Journal of Experiential Education, 18*(2), 76-81.

Warren, K. (1999). *Unpacking the knapsack of outdoor experiential education: Race, gender, and class sensitive outdoor leadership.* Unpublished doctoral dissertation, Graduate School of The Union Institute, Cincinnati, Ohio.

Warren, K. (2002). Preparing the next generation: Social justice in outdoor leadership, education and training. *Journal of Experiential Education, 25*(1), 231-239.

Warren, K. (2005). A path worth taking: The development of social justice in outdoor experiential education. *Equity & Excellence in Education, 38*(1), 89-99.

Wright, A. (1997). Multicultural education through shared adventure. *Journal of Outdoor Education, 27*, 4-15.

CHAPTER 20

Finding the Extraordinary in the Ordinary: Reflections on Working in the Outdoors with Adults with Severe Mental Health Problems

David Stacey

ABSTRACT

This paper explores themes that have developed as part of my experiences as an outdoor practitioner working with adults with severe and enduring mental health problems. They have particularly developed as part of looking at the field of adventure therapy and trying to understand where, if anywhere, my work may fit within this field. While this paper is based largely on personal reflections, it also includes perspectives shared by conference attendees within the related workshop delivered by the author at the 5IATC, using references from related literature as a means of shaping this process. Points that unfold are not presented as 'rigorously argued and verified conclusions'; rather, they should be considered as way-markers to help clarify how my own and others' areas of work may fit within the adventure therapy field.

INTRODUCTION

> 'There are many ways to skin a cat: therapeutic outcomes are not solely obtained by engaging in therapy. Sometimes it is healthy not to focus on the problem, but rather be distracted by focusing on participation in challenging, yet enjoyable activities designed to ensure success experiences. When designing programmes we must be able to make this distinction' (Van de Graaf, 2003).

For over fifteen years I have worked with adults with severe and enduring mental health problems within the Community of St Antony and St Elias, based in Devon,

England. The organisation offers residential support and rehabilitation for clients who often have complex placement needs. Our work centres on creating ordinary, domestic, non-institutional living environments in relatively small homes, with high levels of staff support. Although not a medical organisation, we work closely with medical services and aim to complement the on-going medical support (psychiatric and otherwise) required by a client. The core of this work centres on living in a domestic environment and involving clients in the social dynamics and activities that form part of this.

In addition, the organisation runs an extensive activity programme, open to both clients and staff. A large part of this entails outdoor activities, including walking, canoeing, caving, overnight trips and surfing, amongst other activities.

Typically, groups are relatively small, between four to eight persons, including staff support for residents. Initially the purpose of running these activities was to provide physical activity, fun and creative life experiences. However, as the activities have developed, we would argue that they also provide additional benefits such as social interaction, learning new skills and abilities, and developing flexible ways of coping. Although working with a specialised client group, a key feature of the activities is that they are not focused on problems or illness, but on supporting and enabling those taking part to have positive experiences and a sense of achievement. On a basic level, it is a varied programme of activities that we tailor to the needs/ability levels of those living in the Community, and could be considered primarily 'recreational'. However anecdotal feedback, particularly from past clients who have moved on, suggests that for some, it has had a more significant impact, as illustrated by the following two examples.

The Extraordinary in the Ordinary: Therapeutic Case Studies of Clients' Participation in Outdoor Activities

1.

A young woman with a background of mental health and substance misuse problems was referred to the Community at short notice due to the breakdown of her previous placement. During the initial weeks of the placement she expressed an interest in trying canoeing, and a short trip was arranged on the river estuary nearby. It was a small group, including one other resident who enjoyed canoeing plus a couple of staff members who the person related well to, led by myself as the instructor. It was a warm, sunny summer's day and part way through the paddle she asked if she could jump in for a swim. Although not a typical request and not an ideal area due to the tide, we were able to find a spot to do this where she could then just swim from the canoe to the riverside, where we would join her for a lunch break.

She jumped in and enjoyed swimming and drifting in the river, with much whooping and swearing, eventually making it to the river beach for drying off and food. After a relaxed lunch we headed back. Over the coming months this resident carried on with canoeing, tried many other activities, and became a regular participant in the activity programme. However, after a couple of years, and after she had moved on to more independent living, she explained in her own inimitable style, the impact of that day as follows:

> The first time canoeing I had a 'spiritual' high rather than 'drug induced' high – peaceful, clarity, fun, companionship'. The activities had been a big factor in her being able to settle into the placement and look ahead to the future. '[They] helped me to change... took away the focus from my problems and I began to build a picture of what I wanted in life and I could plan for the future.

2.

A week-long camping and canoeing trip to a river on the borders of England and Wales was run, involving six residents, three staff and myself. All had been involved in half-day or day-long canoeing trips throughout the year before the trip. Due to heavy rain, the river was at a higher level than usual, making what would have been a relaxed journey on a placid river something a little more challenging. It was still a realistic activity, but getting on the river had to be assessed on a day-by day basis. The trip proved to be one of those where the combination of conditions, the individual's approaches, and group support, all combined to make it both memorable and successful. Everyone, in some way, had overcome a particular challenge or fear on the journey. One young person, prior to going on the trip, had a history of persistent and frequent self harm. On returning, this stopped for a period of over four months.

Emerging Questions and Themes

> 'As I understand it, one emphasis is on the adventure and the therapeutic gain is implicit, the other is on the therapy and therapeutic gain is explicit. The outcome may be the same' (Aldridge, 2009).

Although as an organisation we are confident about the positive values of the activities we provide, we are keen to develop our understanding of why this may be. In fact, it is essential that we do. As one workshop participant challenged me afterwards, 'You need to understand better what you do so as to explain it to those purchasing the service'.

So, this paper looks at taking some steps in this process, primarily by focusing on two questions that have developed in exploring my own working experience and the field of adventure therapy:

- Firstly, while not being adventure therapy, this area has the potential for therapeutic outcomes. Paradoxically, part of its effectiveness is precisely because it is not perceived or presented as being 'therapy'. Why is this so?
- Secondly, are some outdoor practitioners working in certain ways with certain client groups where the 'ordinary' engagement and involvement with outdoor/adventurous activities is 'extraordinary' for those taking part?

These two themes were incorporated into the workshop I delivered at the 5IATC. They formed the basis of a lively group discussion, shaped as follows:

'Therapy is in the outcome, not just in the intent'

The area in which I work is not adventure therapy, but does that mean it is not therapeutic in some way? What if this is never made explicit but remains an implicit quality of the work? In addition, are there occasions/situations in which the use of 'therapy' language may actually be a block or counterproductive?

'What can outdoor practitioners bring to this area and why is it of value?'

An initial response to this question may be very obvious – the ability to take groups into wilderness or outdoors environments. But are there parallels to how outdoor practitioners work with individuals/groups and the core qualities/characteristics that form part of a therapeutic relationship (albeit in a different context and with different aims)?

An exploration of these themes follows; first, an overview of some adventure therapy terminology is provided.

ADVENTURE THERAPY VERSUS 'RECREATIONAL' OUTDOOR ACTIVITIES – IS THERE ANY COMMON GROUND?

Initially, I felt quite daunted at the prospect of looking at the field of adventure therapy because of my own preconceptions that the practice originates solely from a therapeutic starting point. My working background and experiences of being an outdoor practitioner did not fit with this perspective. In addition, the organisation I work for has often described itself as a 'lay' organisation with aims of creating an 'ordinary' domestic living environment. The activities provided are to complement the support given to clients already under medical care, and therefore are not described in therapeutic or medical language. The boundaries between professional tasks and responsibilities are clearly recognised and delineated.

However, the fact that we are approaching from the 'adventure' direction does not necessarily exclude the potential for therapeutic outcomes to occur. In Figure 1, Itin (2003) gives a helpful triangular model, with adventure and therapy each occupying a base corner, and adventure therapy at the apex.

Figure 1. Itin's adventure therapy model

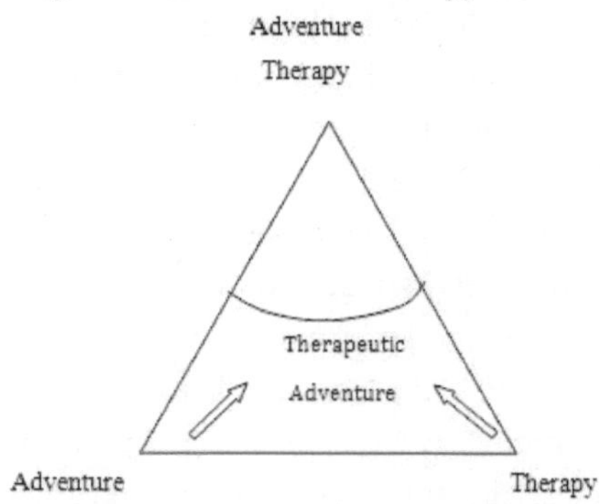

Within this model, adventure therapy is understood as a purposeful change process directed at meta level change through the use of adventure activities (Itin, 2003). From this perspective, it is a process that involves both the therapy and the adventure. (Meta level change relates to unconscious or other processes not easily addressed, hence requiring specific skills of therapy to address). On the other hand, therapeutic work is directed at the level of increasing healthy behaviour and decreasing unhealthy behaviour something can be therapeutic if it helps a person move in the direction of healthy change (Itin, 2003). In Itin's model, the therapeutic use of adventure can be approached from the adventure corner or the therapy corner, and occupies the 'lower' levels. However, at some point a threshold is passed where the two combine to form a specific area of adventure therapy.

A second potentially helpful approach to clarifying this area is shown by Crisp (1999) shown in Table 1. Crisp uses an adventure based practice continuum as a means of looking at the depth of therapeutic input within a programme.

Although this approach uses the terms 'recreation' and 'enrichment' to describe the shallower end of potentially therapeutic work, it shares with Itin's model the recognition that therapy is aimed at changing the underlying cause of a problem. Both of these models help to explain the breadth of the therapeutic use of adventure, and offer a context in which to situate our work. They will be referred to in more detail later in this paper.

Exploring the Themes

The exploration of these themes draws on points made within the workshop discussion, from my own experience, and insights from adventure therapy literature.

Within the workshop there was limited discussion on what outdoor practitioners could bring to this area. However, the discussion did generate some forthright comments: 'Almost nothing' was one summary (this was made in relation to the outdoor activity instructor who is centre-based and who runs short, activity focused sessions). An additional point was made that it is with increased experience and reflection on the use/purpose of activities that an appreciation of the wider potential of the activities develops. While it may be reasonable to see the validity of the initial point about outdoor activity instructors working with a specific activity focus, when the context is broadened to the larger field of outdoor/experiential learning it becomes more interesting. In considering the foundations of adventure therapy, Gass (1993) makes the point that 'while the area of adventure therapy has developed as a discrete addition to the mental health field, many of the origins, principles and philosophies of adventure therapy are founded in the field of experiential education' (Gass, 1993, p.3). From this starting point, key elements within experiential learning include:

1. The learner is a participant rather than a spectator in learning;
2. The learning activities require personal motivation in the form of energy, involvement and responsibility;
3. The learning activity is real and meaningful in terms of natural consequences for the learner;
4. Reflection is a critical element of the learning process; and

5. Learning must have present, as well as future relevance for the learner and the society in which he/she is a member.

These are translated over to the adventure therapy context as follows:

1. The client becomes a participant rather than a spectator in therapy;
2. Therapeutic activities require client motivation in the form of energy, involvement and responsibility;
3. Therapeutic activities are real and meaningful in terms of natural consequences for the client;
4. Reflection is a critical element of the therapeutic process; and
5. Functional change must have present as well as future relevance for clients and their society (Gass, 1993, p3-

The following key point is also highlighted:

> [experiential learning] is also predicated on the belief that change occurs when people are placed outside of positions of comfort (e.g. homeostasis, acquiescence) and into states of dissonance. In these states, participants are challenged by the adaptations necessary to reach equilibrium. Reaching these self-directed states necessitates change with its resultant growth and learning (Gass, 1993, p4). The cross reference to adventure therapy is clear to see.

Relating these points to the question 'What can outdoor practitioners bring to this area?' at a very basic level, activity instructors bring very little, as their training, skills and working environment are primarily 'activity focused'. However, broader training programmes (e.g. graduate or postgraduate level) or other work contexts may bring in wider aspects, including experiential education. If I look back to my own formal training, a postgraduate teacher-training course in outdoor education, it was a practical, broad-ranging course that included experiences of Outward Bound and a range of outdoor work placements (not just school environments). Although I do not recall much directly about the philosophy/ theory of experiential learning, I suspect I was 'soaking it up' without necessarily knowing it. This process then continued into early work experiences. So, without being aware of it, I was building foundations in outdoor/experiential education that are partly shared or translatable into adventure therapy.

Table 1. Crisp's adventure therapy model

Recreation	***Enrichment***	***Therapy***
The extension of an individual's normal functioning to greater levels of achievement based on a spontaneous learning process.	The provision of a positive and potentially beneficial experience which can enhance the client's position relative to their disorder or dysfunction, but does not directly address the underlying cause of a client's problem	The treatment of an underlying dysfunction, which seeks a specific change following a diagnostic analysis of a long standing problem or behavioural pattern

Within the range of professional experiences carried by workshop participants, it was interesting to hear how the therapeutic element of the work was presented to programme participants. In some cases a clear theoretical framework/therapeutic model was presented, and the fact that participants were taking part in an adventure therapy programme was made explicit throughout. However, several workshop participants who worked within the mental health field noted that in their work, although there was an acknowledgement of the therapeutic value and purpose of the activities, the activities or programmes were not presented as being 'therapy'. This was predominantly because potential participants would have found this off-putting and meant they would not have taken part. However, this was not considered to be a problem. In one case, explaining the purposes and potential benefits to others (including professionals) was done through the language of 'mental health care/wellbeing', as opposed to that of 'therapy'.

In light of these points, it is valuable to consider the earlier frameworks provided by Itin (2003) and Crisp (1999). Both models outline differing degrees of intervention, and the comments above can be related to different parts of both. Some interventions are in the context of specific adventure therapy programmes, following a particular therapeutic approach. Within these, one would expect staff to be trained and skilled in this approach, and to work ethically in a manner that is explicitly therapeutic. These interventions would be at the apex of the triangular model used by Itin (2003). In this area, more than just outdoor practitioner skills are needed. But what of interventions where adventure is being used in a therapeutic way, as opposed to specifically addressing meta-level behaviour or dysfunction? Here, the aims may be broader and more general. It is in this area that a different language may be more suitable to describe the overall purpose of an activity. For example, in the UK the concept of 'recovery' is currently a key element within mental and social care services, outlined as follows:

- Recovery is about building a meaningful and satisfying life as defined by the person themselves, whether or not there are ongoing symptoms or problems.
- Recovery represents a movement away from focusing solely on pathology, illness and symptoms to health, strengths and wellness.
- Recovery is about discovering and often re-discovering a sense of personal identity, separate from illness or disability (Recovery, Devon, 2010).

In use of 'recovery' terminology the presence of ongoing or longer-term problems/illness is acknowledged, but the orientation focuses on wellbeing, strengths, health etc. If designing an activity programme to embody these principals, it would be reasonable to argue that such an intervention would fall into the recreation or enrichment categories of Crisp's continuum not adventure therapy but valuable in other ways, and able to be presented in the context and language of mental health recovery.

The observation by workshop participants who worked in the mental health field, of the negative effects on participants when describing the context of their work as 'therapy' echoes my own experience. Often, therapy is associated with being in hospital or institutional care and when the resident was particularly ill a stage they now feel they have moved on from. Perhaps the stigma associated with use of the term 'therapy' points to a paradoxical element within this area. Namely, that while recognising the potential for engaging outdoor activities to be therapeutic for this client group, it may be that this is partly because these activities are not considered to be or presented as therapy at all. Likewise, the perception of the activity leader not being a therapist or even from a 'healthcare' background, can actually have a positive role in helping reduce the distance between leader and participant. Therapeutic participation in 'ordinary' adventure activities, affirms an unspoken message regarding social inclusion to those taking part. As one outdoor practitioner described their experience to me after the conference, 'they see me as an ordinary person as opposed to a 'white coat'.

Perhaps this highlights the range of factors that need to be considered when designing activity programmes. Regarding attendance at the First South Pacific Wilderness Adventure Therapy Forum in 2002, Pryor, Carpenter and Townsend (2005) made the observation that: 'although a reasonable percentage of practitioners (more than half) had undertaken training in therapeutic techniques or held recognised clinical therapy qualifications, the terms therapy or therapeutic were very rarely used by practitioners to describe their work' (Pryor, et al., 2005, p.7). Programmes could be framed in a range from educational to therapeutic, with consideration given to factors including, 'the nature and rationale of the intervention, the expertise and approach used by the practitioner, and the needs and vulnerabilities of the participants' (Pryor, et al., 2005, p.7).

Within the workshop discussion, a point was also made that approaching the work from an outdoor instructor/practitioner perspective, could mean a lack of awareness of therapeutic issues, such that potential opportunities for areas to explore may be missed, or warning signs go unheeded. Several conference participants highlighted the value of a therapy/training background in giving a necessary framework for staff awareness of their professional relationship and responsibilities to clients, particularly working in a field that can be personally demanding and where complex interpersonal dynamics may be encountered. These comments are important and point towards that extra level of insight that specific therapeutic training and experience can provide.

However, to respond from my own experience and working context: as well as adventurous activities taking place within the standards and guidelines of the relevant governing bodies for an activity, they are designed with considerable personal knowledge of the individuals who will be involved. This includes awareness of an individual's care plan aims, risk management issues and appropriate staff support. In short, there is a professional framework surrounding the running of activities that while not having a specific therapy basis, probably has considerable shared ground with other safe therapeutic endeavours.

Further Reflections

The workshop discussion generated some valuable contributions. My own thoughts on this subject include experiences related specifically to the organisation I work for, and result from a research study I undertook to identify key elements within its functioning (Stacey, 2003). Within the environment created by the community, several core elements were identified as important, including: building trusting relationships, creating a 'safe space' to work in, honest and open dialogue, respect and non-judgment. These are also recognised as elements identified as important within a therapeutic relationship (Bateman, Brown, & Pedder, 2000). Although this comparison was made in relation to the general work of the community, it could be reasonable to extend these qualities to the delivery of outdoor activities, as this is a part of the community's overall work. Similarly, these are important qualities that have a part to play in working with individuals or groups in the outdoors at large, and an outdoor practitioner would be looking to foster many if not all of these elements within the atmosphere of the group in order to create a supportive, enabling environment in which another person is able to feel safe, secure and able to participate in the activity.

Some of these skills may be functioning tacitly, and may not yet have been made or need to be made, explicit (Claxton, 1998). For example in looking at the process of therapeutic change, Nadler (1993) highlighted several elements important to this, one of which was trust, 'this condition is the result of an appropriate reliance and confident dependence on others, one's self, the leader and the experience. The more trust that exists from these four sources, the easier it is for clients to make focused efforts during tasks or endure the tension of being in disequilibrium'(cited in Gass, 1993, p.65). Nadler also explains ways of enhancing the conditions in an adventure therapy context, such as talking about trust in the group, or using specific exercises or tasks that focus on this area.

However, within my own working context, while recognising trust as a vital element that builds up as relationships develop and experiences are shared, it is very rarely explicitly mentioned. Here again is an area of potential overlap, and one in which insights from the field of therapy could be valuable.

Concluding Thoughts: So What is the Extraordinary in the Ordinary?

At the end of this paper, am I any nearer to reaching an informed explanation of the use of activities within my workplace, why they are of value, and where they may fit within the wider field of an international adventure therapy?

I would say 'yes', and referring to the original two themes, I would summarise these as follows:

First, though not specifically adventure therapy, our use of outdoor activities does have a place within the wider spectrum of adventure therapy in that it is providing recreation and enrichment, and in doing so, recognises the potential for the existence of therapeutic elements. Although there is no intent to 'do' adventure therapy, we are doing the activities with an intention to provide a broad, flexible programme. Offering recreation and enrichment provides the possibility of a therapeutic outcome for some individuals.

Second, as adventure therapy shares some common foundations with experiential learning, outdoor practitioners trained and experienced in this area may be utilising some shared skills and qualities, thus bringing diverse elements that relate to the careful use of activities, engaging participants in them and creating a positive group environment in which they take place.

Within my own working context, a big emphasis is placed on 'ordinariness', whether this be trying to create an ordinary domestic living environment, facilitate the ordinary dynamics of human interactions, or take part in ordinary adventurous activities. However, the insights and ideas encountered from within the field of adventure therapy help to shed some light on why these 'ordinary' outdoor activities can be 'extraordinary' for some.

References

Aldridge, S. (2009) Adventure therapy as an emerging approach: Towards a profession. Abstract booklet. BACP.

Bateman, A., Brown, D., & Pedder, J. (2000). *Introduction to psychotherapy: An outline of psychodynamic principles and practice* (3rd ed). Routledge, London.

Claxton, G. (1998) Investigating human intuition: Knowing without knowing why. *The Psychologist*, 11(5), 217-220.

Crisp, S. (1999). International models of best practice in wilderness and adventure therapy. In Itin, C. (Ed), *Exploring the boundaries of adventure therapy* (pp. 201-212). Proceedings of the 1st International Adventure Therapy Conference. Boulder, CO: Association of Experimental Education.

Gass, M. (1993). *Adventure therapy: Therapeutic applications of adventure programming*. Dubuque, Iowa, USA: Kendall/Hunt Publishing.

Gillis, H. L. (1995). If I conduct outdoor pursuits with clinical populations, am I an adventure therapist? *Journal of Leisurability*, 22(2).

Itin, C. (2003). Adventure therapy vs. therapeutic adventure? In K. Richards & B. Smith (Eds.), *Therapy within Adventure.* Proceedings of the 2nd International Adventure Therapy Conference. Augsburg: Ziel.

Pryor, A., Carpenter, C., & Townsend, M. (2005). Outdoor education and bush adventure therapy: A socio-ecological approach to health and wellbeing. *Australian Journal of Outdoor Education*, 9(1), 3-13,2005.

Recovery Devon. Putting recovery at the heart of all we do. (2010). Retrieved on 12/1/10 from: www.recoverydevon.co.uk.

Stacey, D. L. (2003) Method and mystery: Clarifying the ethos of the community of St. Antony and St. Elias. Unpublished Dissertation: University of Exeter.

Van de Graaf, H. (2003). Thank God you're not therapists! (Paradigm lost). Paper presented at the MHS Conference, Canberra, Australia.

CHAPTER 21

A Review of an Introductory Tertiary Course in Adventure Therapy

Scott Polley

ABSTRACT

In 2007, the University of South Australia conducted its first 'Introduction to Adventure Therapy' course as part of a study stream in Outdoor Education. This paper reports on the process of developing the curriculum for this course, the resultant learning program, and evaluations by students, staff and employment providers. Implications for future introductory adventure therapy courses for tertiary students are discussed.

INTRODUCTION

This paper discusses the implementation of an introductory course in adventure therapy at the University of South Australia. The term 'course' is used throughout this paper, but for many institutions 'subject' would better describe the studies described here. The term 'course' is used by University of South Australia to describe 4.5 units of study, with 8 courses or 36 units making up one year of full-time study. This course is a component of a larger degree program, which consists of 24 courses, 8 per year, in a Bachelor Program. This paper includes a discussion of the process of curriculum design in adventure therapy how the learning program was organised, and a review of the feedback from students, staff and local providers of therapeutic adventure in the community. It is hoped that some of the issues identified will assist others who are designing introductory-oriented adventure therapy curriculum for tertiary programs.

When considering what might be included in in introductory adventure therapy curriculum, Reddrop (1997) noted the following: 'Despite the important role staff play, relatively little research has been done on the qualities or qualifications of effective outdoor leaders' (p.108). No specific guidelines for the development and professional recognition of adventure therapists could be found, much as no singular definition of the field could be found (Gillis, in Itin, 1997). However, three categories of professional education for outdoor leaders were identified for this course and can be summarised as follows:

1. *Therapist with outdoor leadership skills.* This approach involves the education of counselors and psychologists in outdoor leadership. In this way, the therapist is able to conduct outdoor activities as a forum to use established therapeutic modalities to achieve therapeutic outcomes. Institutions that have degree programs in counseling and psychology as well as pathways in outdoor leadership appear to be well placed to produce such graduates. This approach is advocated by Itin (2001) for professionals to describe themselves as adventure therapists.
2. *Outdoor leader with counseling or therapy skills.* This approach would appear to be supported by Priest and Gass (2005) who describe the need for more skills in the use of more sophisticated techniques for outdoor leaders, such as a range of ways of debriefing, to achieve therapeutic outcomes. This approach is criticised by Crisp (in Itin, 1997) who argues that unless a person is a trained and accredited counselor and/or therapist they should not be engaging in therapy.
3. *Outdoor leader with skills to support a counselor and/or therapist.* This approach is supported by Davis-Berman and Berman (1994) who advocated 'bifurcated staff in which there are different criteria for those coordinating the physical components of the program and those coordinating the counseling components' (p.141). The rationale for this includes the ability to manage a psychological crisis in the field and to maximise the opportunity for therapeutic outcomes in the field.

As a result of discussion with local providers of adventure therapy in South Austraila, this course focused on the preparation of professionals for the third model – 'Outdoor Leader with skills to support a counselor and/or therapist'. In retrospect, it might have been better to title the course 'Introduction to Therapeutic Adventure' to more correctly describe the content, however 'adventure therapy' appeared to be the most commonly used title, as evidenced by IATC Proceedings.

THE UNIVERSITY OF SOUTH AUSTRALIA

Historically, the University of South Australia (UniSA) has had a pathway in Outdoor Pursuits originally available only to Health and Physical Education students (since 1970). Since 1997, UniSA has had a pathway in Outdoor Education available to all degree programs, but primarily for Human Movement students. (Human Movement replaced Exercise and Sports Science as well as the Health and Physical Education program in 1997. Those students wanting to become teachers from this time completed postgraduate qualifications in Education).

As an evolution of previous study pathways in outdoor leadership, in 2005 a decision was made at the School of Health Science to offer a minor, sub-major and major in Outdoor Education. This study pathway would also be offered to other degree students, such as those in Recreation, Business, Education, Psychology, Tourism and Hospitality, Aboriginal Studies and others. The primary purpose of the Outdoor Education study pathway was to prepare students for future professional roles in Outdoor Education, Adventure Therapy and Nature-based tourism. The majority of students undertaking this Outdoor Education study pathway were completing a combined Outdoor Education and Physical Education pathway in preparation for a post graduate Bachelor of Education. Other students were completing Bachelor of Youth Studies, Psychology, Education and Business.

During the curriculum investigation phase of the Outdoor Education specialist pathway, a number of representatives from local providers identified the need for more highly educated staff in the adventure therapy field. As a result, a decision was made in 2006 to include an 'Introduction to Adventure Therapy' course as one of the options within the Outdoor Education pathway (see Table 1). Up until this point, adventure therapy had been a topic within another course (Wilderness and Adventure Education) and students could elect to do an essay further researching the topic if they so choose. Students in the Outdoor Education study stream could choose other elective alternatives such as Aboriginal Studies, Alpine Journeys (a 30 day field trip to New Zealand), Environmental Studies or other related courses (see Table 1).

Thirty students took part in the 'Introduction to Adventure Therapy' course; they came from a variety of backgrounds. Eighteen students were studying a Bachelor of Human Movement and were in their final year of three years study; three students were undertaking a Bachelor of Youth Work at another institution and were undertaking this course as cross-institutional study; two students were completing a Bachelor of Education; and five students were on exchange from

Norway, completing a Bachelor of Physical Education in their own country. One student was completing a Bachelor of Psychology. Students were mostly in the final year of study, and all had at least completed foundational studies in outdoor leadership in the course 'Introduction to Outdoor Leadership', with some undertaking further courses in the discipline to form a major study pathway.

Course Objectives

Designing the curriculum using an action research process, a decision was made by the author to keep the focus of this new adventure therapy course grounded in professional practice. That is, theoretical content needed to have a practical application. To this end, the central question that was applied throughout the process of writing the curriculum was: 'How will the knowledge and skills taught contribute to the development of a future professional in an adventure therapy context?' (This is very similar to other competency-based approaches to higher education in other disciplines such as education, counseling and social work).

The University of South Australia bases course provision on a course statement that requires course objectives. The final course objectives that were created reflect the competencies needed as an outdoor leader with skills to support a counselor and/or therapist, as follows:
On completion of this course, students should be able to:

- Plan and conduct an adventure based activity that supports a theoretically grounded therapeutic intervention;
- Evaluate the effectiveness of an adventure-based activity in supporting therapy;
- Recognize and respond to a range of common dysfunctional behaviours that occur with different client groups;
- Demonstrate knowledge of specialist referral services and processes (University of South Australia, 2006).

Selecting Course Readings

As stated previously, time constraints necessitated a restricted review of the literature during the curriculum development phase. Key texts were identified based on availability, on reviewing of IATC Proceedings (1997; 2000), and a selection of journal articles written for the Australian Journal of Outdoor Education. Volumes cited frequently and available in the University of South Australia library were reviewed for recommendations regarding the body of knowledge and the methodology of preparing professionals. Key volumes identified were:

Table1.UoiSA Outdoor Education Pathway
(Each course = 100-157.5 hours, with 8 courses in a full year fuII time study load).

Course title	Brief description of content	Normal study sequence
Introduction to Outdoor Leadership	Basic Skills in Kayaking, 3-day kayaking and 3-day bushwalking field trip focus on safe leadership of expeditions, foundational topics such as leadership, risk management, weather, equipment, legal and environmental interpretation.	1
Wilderness and Adventure Education	Approaches to environment, conservation, relationship of art and literature to approaches to adventure, 4-day field experience focused on meaning of participation in adventurous activities in nature.	2
Aquatic Journeys	Aquatics instruction, Sailing, kayaking, sea kayaking, canoeing, snorkeling	3
Outdoor Leadership Praxis	Practices in professional outdoor leadership, planning and organization of outdoor education.	4
Mountain Journeys	Mountain instruction, Bushwalking, Rock climbing, XC skiing, Steep Terrain, high ropes.	5
Outdoor Leadership Philosophy and Issues	Philosophical approaches to adventure and wilderness, relationship between philosophy and practice, leadership, programming evaluation.	6
Effective 1	Either: Introduction to Adventure Therapy Alpine Journeys Aboriginal Studies Global and Local Environment courses Other negotiated electives	7
Effective 2		8

- Davis-Berman, J. & Berman, D. (1994). Wilderness therapy: Foundations, theory, and research.
- Gass, M, (1993). Therapeutic application of adventure programming.
- Nadler, R. & Luckner, J. (1992). Processing the adventure experience.
- Schoel, J., Prouty, D. & Radcliff, P. (1988). Islands of healing: A guide to adventure based counselling.

The key volumes reviewed described programs, programming issues, methodologies, professional issues and philosophies relating to therapeutic adventure. However, none of these texts provided clear recommendations regarding how to best to prepare professionals to work in an adventure therapy setting. This gap, along with some of the dated material in these texts reflects the need for ongoing research in this area. Gillis and Ringer (in Miles & Priest, 1999) reiterate this idea:

> Once adventure therapists have gained more clarity about what works with which client groups, there will be an urgent need to clarify the nature of skills and knowledge required by practitioners in order to provide quality leadership. (Miles & Priest, 1999, p.34)

Despite the apparent lack of clarity regarding qualifications and skills for professionals in adventure therapy and therapeutic adventure, these volumes provided a useful guide to the theoretical content of the course.

Curriculum Design

The curriculum design process for an introductory course in adventure therapy broadly followed the advice of Davis-Berman and Berman's (1994) approach in the design of a Wilderness Therapy intervention. The steps in this sequence were: 1. Needs analysis; 2. Staff capacity analysis; 3. Client analysis; 4. Assessment; 5. Follow-up; 6. and Program evaluation.

Needs Analysis

It was hoped that graduates would be prepared for employment in therapeutic applications of adventure in local settings. Four key providers were identified, based on the author's prior knowledge of programs in the state of South Australia. Each provider was asked details about their program, and each was asked in informal meetings what should be included in such an introductory course. This information was recorded in a journal, and referred to from time to time during the curriculum design phase. Towards the end of the process each provider was contacted, provided verbal detail of the program and asked whether they might suggest any changes. Each provider supported the general structure, given constraints of time and resources.

Staff Capacity Analysis

As this was an introductory course, it was clear that the main outcome of undertaking study in adventure therapy was to prepare professionals who would provide support to therapeutic interventions, and not 'undo' the work of other health professionals. Davis-Berman and Berman (1994) stated that wilderness therapy professionals ought to have a minimum of wilderness skills so they can focus on the needs of their clients, have the ability to take over the physical aspects of the program in an emergency, and provide first aid with CPR training (p.140). These authors recommended that programs where clients had mental health issues should provide the 'same rigorous standards that would apply in other settings' (p.141). This view suggested the need for the curriculum to include training in ensuring that clients with mental health issues did not have other therapeutic interventions 'undone' by trained therapists.

Using Gillis, et al.'s (1991, cited in Gass, 1993) continuum of levels of therapeutic intervention (see Figure 1), it was clear that the focus of this course was on a use of outdoor experiences to provide an adjunct (or support) for other interventions, using either a recreational, enrichment or adjunctive approach. It was not realistic to attempt to prepare professionals for primary therapy within the one course. However, those students completing this as part of a psychology degree were well placed to consider this as a future option.

Figure 1. Depth of intervention continuum

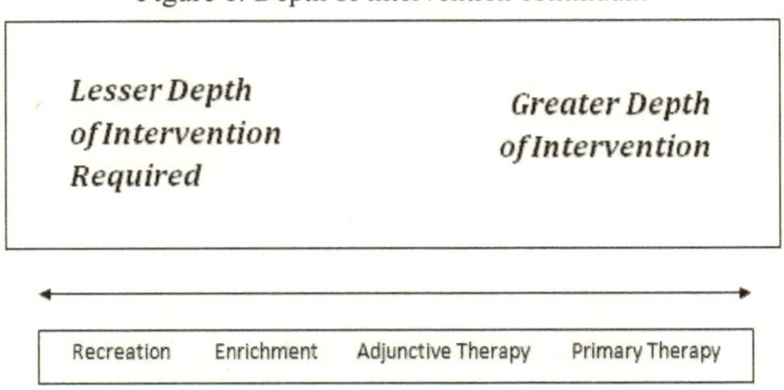

Client Analysis

The client analysis aspect of curriculum design considers the actual clients who receive adventure therapy services, and also considers the students' needs. This analysis involves careful consideration of the theoretical approaches used by local programs, as well as an analysis of the client populations with whom adventure-based interventions are being utilised. Based on the needs of the client populations students would encounter, in the community basic skills training in mental health and direct practice experience in therapeutic settings were also incorporated into the course.

Theoretical Approaches

Early in the curriculum development process, three therapeutic adventure providers were contacted to engage in the curriculum development process, and as possible providers of direct practice experience for students undertaking the course. Questions were asked about providers' use of theoretical frameworks in order to guide curriculum development. Discussion with representatives of these three local providers revealed a conscious use of Gestalt Theory and Cognitive Behavioral Therapy by one (Parker, personal communication, 2006), with other providers not having a clearly stated theoretical approach (The Forensic and Applied Psychology Group, 2001). The programs without clearly stated theoretical approaches were examined, and compared with key literature (Gass, 1993; Davis-Berman and Berman, 1994; Gillis and Ringer, in Miles and Priest, 1999) to determine theoretical approaches of best fit. From the providers' descriptions, they appeared to use a 'behaviorist approach'. According to these authors, behaviorist therapeutic adventure interventions 'use both the natural environment and the human interaction to provide concrete 'natural consequences' and 'logical consequences' for participants 'maladaptive behavior' (p.32).

The original intention to ground the curriculum in theoretical knowledge and practice was challenged by the lack of breadth of theoretical application by local providers. After selective reviewing of the literature, there appeared to be scope to expose students to a broader range of therapeutic approaches than those currently offered locally so that they might contribute to the future development of the field. In addition to Gestalt approaches and Cognitive Behavioural Therapy, a decision was made to introduce students to the use of Narrative approaches, as described by Stolz (1998), and Psychoanalytical approaches as described by Ringer (2002). Secondary sources for the application of these approaches were considered appropriate at this level.

Client Populations

As stated previously, an examination of the populations more likely to use adventure as part of a therapeutic program in South Australia revealed 'youth at risk' as the most prominent client group. Two providers used adventure activities as recreation with intellectually disabled people, and one used adventure activities as recreation with physically disabled people. No programs that focused on mental health could be found in South Australia. Subsequently, the main client population focus of the course was 'youth at risk'.

Despite an apparent lack of programs in South Australia specifically designed to address the needs of mental health patients, discussions with providers noted the high incidence of mental health problems among their clients. Davis-Berman and Berman's (1994) recommendations regarding ensuring mental health clients received the same therapeutic standards as any other setting suggested training in mental health might be a critical component of an introductory course. In order to address this issue, it was decided to include basic first responder skills in relation to mental health issues within the course.

Basic Skills Training in Mental Health

Prior to the curriculum design process for this offering, the author had been responsible for hosting the delivery of a course offered by Crisp, called 'Psychological First Responder' training. This course was offered for the first time in South Australia in 2005. This course uses a model similar to that of a first aid course that attempts to equip participants with foundational knowledge to deal with medical emergencies until more professional assistance can be found. The Psychological First Responder course focused on detection, initial response and referral of common mental health issues. This three-day course was theoretically and practically grounded, and included a systematic approach to managing potential mental health issues by non-professionals (Crisp, 2006a; Crisp 2006b). Crisp conducted the Psychological First Responder as part of the study program. This three-day course has a central theme of 'do no harm' a concept that was adopted as a central theme to the Introduction to Adventure Therapy course.

In discussion with providers of adventure therapy in South Australia, experience, personal qualities and communication skills were highlighted as important criteria for future employees in this field. These qualities appeared to be valued even more highly than outdoor leadership qualifications or therapeutic theoretical knowledge. Providers were anxious that early career staff did not impact negatively on their clients. When developing the curriculum, it became obvious that experiences within the course of study that promoted the development of personal skills and knowledge of personal qualities would be needed to ensure that negative impacts were less likely to occur.

The inclusion of the Psychological First Responder course sought to give basic theory and practical skills in avoiding psychological harm when engaging with clients with mental illness or psychological issues. The course achieved this by using face-to-face role-plays, and focused on basic counseling skills when faced with particular mental health issues. This 'mini' course was delivered early in the students' study program, prior to any field experiences. In addition Facilitation Workshop, based on the work by Schoel, Prouty & Radcliff (1988) was also included. This workshop involved role-plays and used peers as 'pretend clients', to facilitate 'Project Adventure' style activities (such as icebreakers, group initiative tasks, and co-operative games). This workshop focussed on basic facilitation skills, sequencing of initiative activities, and ensuring physical and psychological safety. These skill-based workshops were supported by introductory lectures to students about theoretical approaches, a review of the programs and practices of local service providers (including speakers from these organisations), and seminar discussions.

It was hoped that following the examination of theoretical approaches, completion of the Psychological First Responder, and participation in the Facilitation Workshop, that students would be ready to observe or assist a local adventure therapy program, and 'do no harm'.

Direct Practice Experience in Therapeutic Settings

Students were asked to gain experience in a therapeutic setting (with a minimum of 16 hours and a maximum of 50 hours) to meet the study requirements as set by the University of South Australia. Students gained placements with government organizations, not-for-profit organisations, church based organizations, schools, private companies and others. Some of the students were international students that completed the course whilst in Australia, but completed the practical and subsequent report in their home country (Norway).

Out of these students, 20 were able to obtain placements with either a not-for-profit non-government organisation, or a government-funded organisation. The students were always placed in contexts where they were not given any direct responsibility for clients, and were not included in any supervision ratios. The providers drew their own conclusions regarding the students and the clients in deciding whether it was appropriate for them to take any minor roles within the program. Table 2 shows the types of programs in which students were placed.

Table 2. Student practical experiences for HLTH 1023 Introduction to Adventure Therapy

Practical Experience	N =
Youth at Risk	
a. Family and Youth Services	5
b. Operation Flinders	1
c. Baptist Community Services	5
Tall ships (Norway)	1
Residential Camp	2
School	7
Intellectually disabled	1
Physically disabled	1
Peer directed counseling alternative	7

Five students spent time with one of the state government agencies responsible for case-management of students with difficult experiences of the law, homelessness or behaviours. These experiences were sometimes with one young person each time, and largely recreational in nature. The focus was on engagement and relationship-building, to learn to develop trust. One student participated in a 10-day expedition in the Arid Lands of South Australia. He was given the title of 'assistant mentor', and travelled with a group of students that had been referred by their school counsellors. Five students spent time with a non-government Anglican Church program that ran weekend outdoor experiences, also with the aim of building relationships and developing trust. The students participated in either a weekend camp, or a day of mountain biking, rock climbing or bushwalking. Local church groups or other agencies referred clients, but participation was voluntary. Consequently the activity was cancelled on at least one occasion due to lack of numbers. Students stayed as a group trekking, abseiling, camping and taking part in an Indigenous cultural experience.

Two participants were Norwegian exchange students who undertook their experience whilst in Norway. One student went with a group of youth at risk on a traditional sailing ship journey, whilst the other took part in a walking trip. One student negotiated to undertake a practicum placement with a school that was conducting a senior school retreat that used adventure activities as a forum for developing skills, relationships and educating young adolescents about the impact of a range of possible lifestyle choices. The three-day residential program involved group counselling and discussion of adolescent issues. Another student participated in a residential holiday program provided by a local non-government agency. Many of the children at the camp were in foster care.

An additional seven students attended school-based field trips, and were asked to analyse these expeditions through an adventure therapy lens. Although they did not observe the conscious use of therapeutic approaches, their reports indicated that they could see possibilities to apply therapeutic approaches learned in the tutorials with these clients also. Two students participated in field trips with a local private provider of disability services that conducted recreational and respite activities with clients that had intellectual and/or physical disabilities. These experiences included walks in local national parks and other non-nature based recreation, such as swimming in the local pool. Although the provider did not state they provided adventure therapy, the experience gave these students time with these client groups and allowed them to have more insight into their needs. (A number of students that took part in these experiences subsequently gained part-time or full-time employment with two of the agencies).

Finding placements for students – or finding dates that were compatible with student timetables and work/life was problematic. Seven students were not able to arrange a suitable experience by the deadline. As a result, a 16-hour alternative peer-led counseling program was constructed that required students to role-play different scenarios provided to students, videotape them, then critically analyse each other's performance.

Assessment of the Course

Students were assessed on their learning using three assessment items. The first was a 20-item test included as part of the Psychological First Responder course (15%). This assessed foundational knowledge and safe practices when responding to psychological issues and emergencies as a non-trained therapist. The second assessment item (35%) was the delivery of a tutorial to the class. Topics included therapeutic approaches that might be used in an adventure therapy or therapeutic adventure context such as Cognitive Behavioural Therapy, Narrative Therapy, Family therapy, Psycho-analytical and Gestalt. Other topics were related to specific populations outside of 'youth at risk'. Finally, the third item (50%) asked students to report on their field experience, and to relate their observations to established literature.

Evaluation of the Course

A number of tools were used to review whether the course had achieved course objectives. These tools included student reports of practical experiences submitted as part of their assessment requirements, informal discussions with direct practice experience providers, UniSA formalised student evaluations and staff reflective self-evaluation. This self-evaluation consisted of returning to the course objectives, and asking honest questions about whether what was learned in the course matched this list.

FINDINGS

As mentioned previously, various elements of the course were assessed specifically; however, not all of the results of these assessments are included in this paper. Instead, the overall course evaluation findings are presented, along with findings from a brief verbal review of the course on the final day. Student feedback is presented from students' written reports of their direct practice experience in mental health settings. Likewise, feedback was gained from providers to gain their perspective about the direct practice experience. Finally, brief findings are presented from the review of the peer-led counselling workshops in which only seven of the students participated. These findings are included because they have important implications for better preparing students for professional practice in the future.

Online Course Evaluation

Thirteen out of thirty students completed a 10-item on-line Course Evaluation Instrument (CEI) that could be completed remotely. The response rate is a result of the evaluation being voluntary, with no consequences if students chose not to undertake this component. Students received an email in the week following the final compulsory attendance day, and were given a month to respond. Using a Likert Scale, scores are attributed to each response and the mean value is calculated as part of the computer software where: Strongly agree = +100; Agree = +50; Neutral = 0; Disagree = -50 and Strongly Disagree = -100. The results are indicated in Table 3. In addition to the Likert Scale responses, students were asked to respond using text to two additional questions relating the strengths and weaknesses of the course. Not all respondents chose to do this, but the responses are provided in Table 4.

The text-based responses appear to give mixed support to the course structure, with compression of the tutorial and seminar program helpful to some students, but less helpful to those that required more time to process the content.

Verbal Review of Course Delivery

In addition to an on-line review, a verbal review of the course delivery was conducted during the final teaching week, with twenty four of the thirty class members present. Key points made during this review indicated that the Psychological First Responder was a strength of the course; the tutorials on different counseling methods needed to be followed up by more practical application; the Facilitation Workshop could have been expanded, but was very valuable; and that a class field trip might have improved their understanding and confidence as potential facilitators in a therapeutic adventure setting. Most students thought that their practical experience was extremely valuable, and that it provided much learning about potential clients and professional expectations (personal journal).

Written Report of Direct Practice Experience

As stated previously, students were asked to prepare a written report of their direct practice experiences in community settings as one of their assessment items. As a component of this, students were asked to write what they learned from the practical experience. Learning described in the reports where students undertook a practicum with youth at risk is synthesized into themes:

- *Insight into difficulties of working with youth at risk.* This included such things as: short attention span; health related issues such as diet, smoking and drugs; behavior standards including language, spitting and put downs; safety issues related to adherence to instructions and threats of physical harm against staff and peers; and the possible impact on the psychological health of staff.
- *Observation of apparent change of behavior during program.* These included relationship building; improvements in behavior; and increased engagement with staff and other participants.
- *Issues associated with programming.* Such experiences, included: absences due to court appearances; being extremely late; or not showing up.

The following excerpt, from one student's report, was typical of many of the responses to their direct experience with clients:

> Taking part in this fairly short, but intense program really gave me a lot of input. Some harder to process than others, but all in all I really learned a lot, especially how to act, and react while being around 'youth at risk'. Working with these kind of participants seemed really difficult in the beginning… For further investigation I would like find out more about the participants' behavior before, during and after the program. (Student, 2007)

Students who worked with different client groups, including school groups, physically and intellectually disabled also reflected on having new insights into the needs of their participants.

Feedback from Providers

Where possible, the provider of practical experiences was contacted, with most providers indicating that they had felt the student experience was valuable, and that the student had made a contribution at their level of learning. One student was able to participate in a 10-day 'Operation Flinders' program with a former graduate as mentor. This student was offered employment as a mentor on future programs. In addition, it was of great benefit for the student to be able to refer to a research-based evaluation of the program for their written report about the direct practice experience (The Forensic and Applied Psychology Research Group, 2001).

Review of Peer Counseling Workshops

The seven students that completed the peer led counseling workshops participated in a separate review of this component of the course. Their comments indicated that this kind of activity might well form part of the curriculum, as the students that participated in this program felt far more prepared to work positively with challenging situations that might be encountered with clients such as 'youth at risk'.

Looking Back: Critical Self-evaluation

When constructing the teaching, learning and assessment structure for this introductory adventure therapy course, the author was influenced by the thinking of educational writer Garth Boomer (Boomer, et al. 1992), who advocated a participatory action-research process in curriculum design and implementation. Boomer's ideas include the notion that curriculum should: be negotiated with students to maximize engagement; enhance opportunities for independent learning; acknowledge limitations of teaching staff, unequal power relations and learning structures; and promote critical thinking. A number of aspects of the course supported Boomer's concepts.

Table 3. CEI results for HLTH 1023 Introduction to Adventure Therapy

Question		SD -100	D -50	N 0	A +50	SA +100	Mean
1.	I have a clear idea of what is expected of me in the course		3	2	7	1	23.08
2.	The ways in which I was taught provided me with opportunities to pursue my own learning			2	6	5	61.54
3.	The courses enabled me to develop and/or strengthen the qualities of a UniSA graduate			1	10	2	53.85
4.	I felt there was a genuine interest in my learning needs and progress			1	4	8	76.92
5.	The course developed my understanding of concepts and principles		1	1	6	5	57.69
6.	The workload for this course was reasonable given my other study commitments		1	1	8	3	50
7.	I have received feedback that was constructive and helpful			4	7	2	42.31
8.	The assessment tasks were related to the qualities of a UniSA graduate			2	9	2	50
9.	The staff teaching this course showed a genuine interest in their teaching				4	9	84.62
10.	Overall I was satisfied with the quality of this course		1	1	7	4	53.85

Table 4. CEI – Text based questions and responses

1. Overall, what are the strengths of this course?	2. Are there any ways this course could be improved?
Great course that allowed a fantastic insight into the field and gave genuine hands on experience	
Having time off at the end of the semester to pursue practical experiences.	*Timetabling - clashes with other courses in Human Movement degree*
Very hands on	*Finding field (sic) work was hard especially as we have no experience in adventure therapy. Working with youths at risk is extremely daunting. Could there be other options?*
There are a lot of practical components which allow further development of skills	*Perhaps set aside certain weekends where a lot of this practical stuff could be done, as opposed to every weekend*
Scott Polley, the guest workshops and the networking opportunities	*More time frames for tutorial options*
Introduces students to different forms of outdoor education and teaches aspects of this medium.	*Try to avoid an overload of information at the start of the course.*

- *Negotiated curriculum to maximize engagement.* Students were able to choose counseling topics and placement locations. An extended period of time would be needed to allow more extensive negotiation of curriculum. It is suggested that the structure allow sufficient time for students to grasp the proposed curriculum and assessment items and then time to discuss possible alternatives. An initial problem was the impending birth of the author's (and course teacher's) child, which necessitated compressing the course into 6 x 4 hours of initial class contact and abandoning a planned class field trip. This compression of the course may have inhibited time for deeper reflection and discussion of ideas. In addition, students had difficulty in researching topics for their presentations on different counseling methods, with some of the presentations lacking depth of knowledge. With more time to research and better guidance, this might have been assisted.
- *Enhance opportunities for independent learning.* Students were asked to conduct independent research on counseling methods for their tutorial assessment task, in addition to research for the practical experience write

up. For those that did not take part in the practical component, a peer workshop was constructed for students to research counseling methods and apply them in role-play scenarios. In general, these methods worked well to promote independent learning, but as stated above, more time and greater guidance in all these aspects would have enhanced the learning outcomes.

- *Acknowledge limitations of teaching state.* Students were advised that the course teacher had been part of a number of youth at risk programs, but that these experiences were conducted without reference to any theoretical framework, and were not therapeutically related. Students were told that they would likely be 'teaching the teacher' at times. A number of provider representatives kindly provided 'guest speaker' roles to discuss their programs, and this assisted greatly with increased depth and relevance of the course for students.
- *Unequal power relations and learning structures*. Boomer suggested that empowering students can increase their learning, and is best achieved by teaching structures that break down the usually unequal power relations between student and teacher. It might have been ideal to address this more in the teaching and learning arrangements, but a choice was made to accept that unequal power relations were going to exist, and likely made worse by the time restrictions on the course delivery.
- *Promote critical thinking.* This was a thematic aspect to the course not highlighted in the objectives listed in the course statement. This was an oversight that might be corrected for future courses. Each theory class time was allocated to critically analyse practice, including the showing of 1970's footage of an Outward Bound program, and a YouTube clip of a practitioner demonstrating 'edge work'. The use of these visual examples promoted some excellent discussion and critical analysis, as well as possible alternative practices. In addition, students were asked to critically reflect on the programs they observed (using literature where possible), and student assignments generally demonstrated some useful analysis and ideas for future practice.

Although the participatory action research approach worked relatively well, there was a miss-match between one of the course objectives and the academic program. The objective: 'Plan and conduct an adventure based activity that supports a theoretically grounded therapeutic intervention' (University of South Australia, 2006) was not achieved. Future courses would need to change objectives or modify the curriculum and assessment tasks to better support this learning. The other three objectives (described earlier) appear to have been met. However, a class-designed field trip that incorporated activities, facilitation and follow up for peers might have been a useful first step and opportunity to evaluate the possibility of achieving this objective. Ideally the author would have been able to allocate more time to the writing of the curriculum, and to research the underpinning body of knowledge more thoroughly. Conversely, the results from student assignments suggested that a number of them struggled with the theoretical aspects as they were presented, so caution is advised before introducing too much complexity.

RECOMMENDATIONS

Based on the findings from the online course evaluations, the verbal reviews of the course, students' written reports of their direct practice experience, feedback from providers, and the reviews of the peer-led counselling workshops, as well as the critical self-evaluation by the author and course designer and instructor, six recommendations are provided for future courses of this nature:

1. *Ensure adequate outdoor skills prior to practicum.* Prior to undertaking this course students had at least undertaken a foundational course, 'Introduction to Outdoor Leadership'. The fact that students had adequate outdoor skills to participate in the practicum suggested that this strategy was effective.
2. *Set achievable objectives.* The positioning of the students as a future provider of therapeutic adventure in conjunction with a trained and qualified counselor and/or therapist appeared to be a realistic objective, although most students were not able to obtain a practical experience within this kind of context.
3. *Depth of knowledge.* Ideally the course lecturer would have substantial theoretical depth of knowledge in addition to experience in the field. Having guest speakers or mini-courses conducted by professionals that have such knowledge depth can assist to ameliorate such deficiencies to some degree.
4. *Grounding in practice.* Grounding the program in practice appeared to give the course cohesion, and a sense of 'real world' application. A lack of theoretical foundations to some programs made it problematic for students to analyse. Conversely it helped to highlight one of the issues

faced by adventure therapy as a professional pursuit, whereby well-researched theoretical frameworks may not always be in use.

5. *Psychological First Responder.* The incorporation of the Psychological First Responder Course was well supported by students and providers, and similar program would be advised if any practicum with clients is involved.
6. *Peer-led counseling workshop.* Participants supported the use of a peer-led workshop to practice and review techniques of counseling using different approaches. Further exploration of this kind of workshop in assisting students to develop professional skills when encountering 'at risk' clients appears warranted.

Conclusion

This course provided an opportunity to develop future outdoor leaders with skills to support a counselor and/or therapist in an adventure therapy setting. Course objectives centered on building competencies related to both outdoor facilitation skills, and also basic adventure therapy skills in order to be able to deal with psychological crises that might arise in the field. Course design followed Davis-Berman and Berman's (1994) approach to the design of a wilderness therapy intervention, and utilised a participatory action research approach to fully engage students and critically evaluate the process in an ongoing manner. Student and provider feedback from course assessments and evaluations provided important information about the course elements that were most useful; however, a weakness of the course evaluation process was the failure to conduct a formal follow-up of the students regarding their understandings and knowledge of adventure therapy. It would be useful to contact graduates and seek input into providing future courses.

Likewise, in designing future courses, it would be important to begin the course design and implementation process with the final evaluation in mind. Due to the paucity of research into the effectiveness of teaching adventure therapy at a tertiary level, it is important to consider and evaluate best practices in order to develop more research in this area. Courses such as this are highly relevant and can offer future professionals with insight and knowledge for practice, and potential foundations for research.

REFERENCES

Boomer, G., Lester, N., Onore, C. & Cook, J. (1992). *Negotiating the curriculum: Education for the 21st Century.* London: Falmer.

Crisp, S. (2007). International models of best practice in wilderness and adventure therapy. In C. Itin (Ed.), *Exploring the boundaries: International perspectives.* Proceedings of the 1st International Adventure Therapy Conference held in Perth, Australia on 1-5 July 1997, (56-74). Boulder, CO: Association of Experimental Education.

Crisp, S. (2006a). *Psychfirst response: Adolescents. Course manual*. Melbourne: Neopsychology.

Crisp, S. (2006b). *Psychfirst response: Adolescents. Training manual.* Melbourne: Neopsychology.

Davis-Berman, J. & Berman, D. (1994). *Wilderness therapy: Foundations, theory, and research.* Dubuque: Kendall/Hunt.

Gass, M. (1993). *Therapeutic applications of adventure programming.* Dubuque: Kendall/Hunt.

Gillis, L. (1997). The journey in Oz: From activity based psychotherapy to adventure therapy in C. Itin (Ed.), *Exploring the boundaries: International perspectives.* Proceedings of the 1st International Adventure Therapy Conference held in Perth, Australia on 1-5 July 1997, (9-20). Boulder, CO: Association of Experimental Education.

Itin, C. (Ed). (1997). *Exploring the boundaries: International perspectives*. Proceedings of the 1st International Adventure Therapy Conference held in Perth, Australia on 1-5 July 1997. Boulder, CO: Association of Experimental Education.

Itin, C. (2001). Adventure therapy – Critical questions. *Journal of Experiential Education, 24*(2), 80-84.

Kemmis, S. & R. McTaggart. (2005). Participatory action research: Communicative action and the public sphere. In N. Denzin & Y. Lincoln, (Eds.), *Handbook of qualitative research,* 3rd ed. (pp. 556–604). Thousand Oaks, CA: Sage.

Miles, J. C. & Priest, S. (1999). *Adventure programming*. State College, PA: Venture.

Nadler, R. & Luckner, J. (1992). *Processing the adventure experience.* Dubuque: Kendall/Hunt.

Priest, S. & Gass, M. (2005). *Effective leadership in adventure programming* (2nd ed.). Champaign: Human Kinetics.

Redrop, S. (1997). *Outdoor programs for young offenders in detention.* Hobart: NCYS.

Ringer, M. (2002). Group action: *The dynamics of groups in educational, corporate and therapeutic settings.* London: Jessica Kinsley.

Schoel, J., Prouty, D. & Radcliff, P. (1988). *Islands of healing: A guide to adventure based counselling.* Hamilton: Project Adventure.

Stolz, P. (1997). Stories of change. In C. Itin (Ed.), *Exploring the boundaries: International perspectives.* Proceedings of the 1st International Adventure Therapy Conference held in Perth, Australia on 1-5 July 1997 (149-152). Boulder, CO: Association of Experimental Education.

The Forensic and Applied Psychology Research Group. (2001). *Evaluation of Operation Flinders wilderness-adventure program for youth at risk.* Adelaide: Forensic and Applied Psychology Research Group University of South Australia.

University of South Australia. (2006) *Course statement: Introduction to Adventure Therapy.* Unpublished record. Available from author on request.

CHAPTER 22

Using Adventure in Professional Counselling Psychology Training in South Africa

Lourens Human and Hendrik Kriek

ABSTRACT

This paper focuses on a use of adventure-based experiential learning in the professional development of postgraduate counselling psychology students at a University in South Africa. Nineteen students were taken on a week-long adventure experience, and asked to reflect on their adventure experience in writing. These written responses were analysed by means of the Duquesne Phenomenological Research Method (DPRM). It was found that students experienced learning during the adventure experience, with specific reference to the themes of awareness, boundaries, uniqueness, trust and cohesion.

INTRODUCTION

The Department of Psychology at the University of Pretoria (UP) South Africa (SA), offers three professional training programmes in psychology: MA (Clinical Psychology), MA (Counselling Psychology) and MA (Research Psychology). After successfully completing any one of these programmes, students can register as psychologists with the Health Professions Council of South Africa (HPCSA). The focus of this paper is on the MA (Counselling Psychology) programme, which runs over a two-year period and is based on three pillars.

The first pillar focuses on psychological theory. Students receive theoretical training in the following subjects: Fundamental psychology, Counselling psychology, Career psychology and Community psychology. The second pillar relates to psychological skills. In the first year of the MA, students undertake practical work at various organizations that are accredited with the HPCSA and that render psychological services to the public. In the second year of the MA, students undertake a one-year full-time internship at an organization that is also accredited with the HPCSA. The third pillar pertains to professional development, which focuses on the 'person' of the student. This pillar is seen as a very important part of the training of students (Corey, 1996; George & Christiani, 1990). It emphasises the trainee psychologist's understanding of his/her role(s), position(s) and service(s) as a psychologist, as well as the importance of knowing yourself. This is consistent with the views of Simons and Andersen (1995) who stated that the most important part of being a psychologist is to 'know thyself'.

As part of their professional development, students receive weekly supervision and go on a week-long adventure experience. The goal of the adventure experience is to address the professional development of the students through an adventure-based experiential learning process, an alternative learning approach to traditional didactic instruction (Coleman, 1979; DeLay, 1996; Kirk, 1987; Priest & Gass, 1997; Schoel, Prouty & Radcliffe, 1988; Snow; 1992). Although adventure-based experiential learning has been employed with mentally retarded youth (Vidolovitis-Moore, 1979), organisational managers (Dainty & Lucas, 1992), war veterans (Hyer, Boyd, Scurfield & Smith, 1992), first year college students (Devlin, 1996) and human movement teaching students (Carlson & McKenna, 2000), and other target groups, there is limited research on the use of adventure-based experiential learning within the field of professional counselling psychology training. Exceptions include Wheeler, Goldie and Hicks (1998) who implemented a quantitative study of 17 graduate counselling students, and Hatch and McCarthy (2003) who conducted a quantitative study of 12 graduate counselling students. Human (2006) implemented a qualitative study (phenomenological study) with 6 postgraduate counselling psychology students, and Human (2008) conducted another qualitative study (narrative approach) with 6 postgraduate counselling psychology students. From these studies in the area of professional counselling psychology training, it was found that adventure-based experiential learning had a positive influence on self-esteem, self-confidence, team co-operation, team building, building trust, setting boundaries and group cohesiveness of the students.

The goal of this paper is to describe the experiences of 19 postgraduate counselling psychology students who participated in a weeklong adventure experience as part of their professional development during a MA (Counselling Psychology) programme.

METHOD

Participants

Two groups of students from the UP in SA participated in this research. The sampling method used in this study was convenient sampling, as participation in the adventure experience was a compulsory part of their professional counselling psychology training (Whitley, 2002). The ethics regarding the participation of the students in a compulsory adventure experience and their participation in the research project will be discussed later on in this paper.

Group 1 (G1) did their MA (Counselling Psychology) degree from 2005 to 2006. Their adventure experience was in May 2005. This group consisted of eight students (N=8). Six were female and two were male. The average age of this group was 30 years.

Group 2 (G2) did their MA (Counselling Psychology) degree from 2006 to 2007. Their adventure experience was held in May 2006. This group consisted of eleven students (N=11). Nine were female and two were male. The average age of this group was 30 years.

As all the students participated in the adventure experience, they were all suitable to participate in the research, because in phenomenological research 'participants are either living the experience or have lived the experience' (Wilson & Washington, 2007, p.64).

Clinical and counselling psychologists acted as facilitators during the adventure experience. The facilitators were male; the clinical psychologist had 30 years' experience in group work, and the counselling psychologist had 10 years' experience in group work and adventure-based experiential learning. Both facilitators are linked to the Department of Psychology at the UP.

Context

The adventure experience for both MA (Counselling Psychology) groups was run by Ecoventures, in the province of KwaZulu/ Natal in SA. Ecoventures is an accredited adventure service provider with the Adventure Recreation Association in SA (Adventure Recreation Association, 2009). An ARA qualified adventure instructor from Ecoventures was responsible for setting up and delivering the adventure activities.

The adventure experience for both groups occurred from Sunday to Friday. On the Sunday, the students and facilitators travelled separately to Ecoventures, 800 km from the UP. The adventure experience ran from Monday to Thursday, and Friday was used to travel the 800 km back to the UP. G1 and G2 both participated in the following programme.

The adventure programme for both groups of students was based on the Briefing-Activity-Debriefing model.

Briefing: The process of briefing implies the act of giving information to the students. Firstly, they were given non-negotiable safety information. Secondly, they were given information that directly related to the upcoming adventure activity (Gillis & Thomsen, 1996; Rohnke, 1989; Schoel et al., 1988).

Table 1. Programme

Time Group 1 (G1) & Group 2 (G2)	Activity Group 1 (G1) & Group 2 (G2)	Comments Group 1 (G1) & Group 2 (G2)	
07:00-07:30	Coffee		
07:30-10:00	Group Debriefing Session	Based on the principles of interactional group work (Yalom, 1995)	
10:00-11:00	Brunch		
11:00-16:00	Adventure Activity	Monday: Tuesday: Wednesday: Thursday:	Archery Obstacle Course Sea Rafting Abseiling
16:00-18:00	Recreation Activity	Free-time for group to use at their own discretion	
18:00-19:00	Supper		
19:00-22:00	Group Debriefing Session	Based on the principles of interactional group work (Yalom, 1995)	

Activity: Adventure activities entail real and/ or perceived physical and/or psychological risk, whereby participants are taken out of their comfort zone into their 'stretch zone', but not into their 'panic zone'. It is within the realm of the 'stretch zone' that personal and interpersonal growth can emerge (Gillis & Thomsen, 1996; Priest & Gass, 1997; Sheldon & Arthur, 2001), which is important for the professional development of the students. For this reason the 'challenge-by-choice' principle was followed, whereby participants can choose to what degree they would like to participate in the adventure activities. The activities employed during the adventure programme are listed in Table 1. The students' experiences of these adventure activities were used for the research project.

Debriefing: Debriefing is the process during which the participants discuss and evaluate what happened during the adventure activities. Schoel et al. (1988) give the following examples of questions to be discussed during the debriefing process: 'What did we do? What does it mean? What are we going to do about it? and What are we going to do next?' (p.32) Rohnke (1989) described debriefing as 'sitting down with a group to talk about what it all means' (p.21). Priest and Gass (1997) explain that 'reflection on experience is a necessary precursor to learning, for without reflection, learning loses much of its potential value' (p.17). In this study, debriefing was done in the format of group sessions, which were guided by the principles and practices of interactional group work (Yalom, 1995).

Design

The research design used in this research project falls within the framework of qualitative research. Qualitative research is sensitive to the context in which people live, and requires the researcher to move out of the laboratory and into the context where phenomena are studied (Creswell, 1998; Kvale, 1996). There are various research designs that align with qualitative research, for example, ethnography, ethnomethodology, phenomenology, symbolic interactionism and grounded theory (De Vos & Fouché, 1998; Fouché, 2002). In this study, phenomenology was used, as the focus was on the adventure experience of the students.

Phenomenological research is divided into two main schools, descriptive and hermeneutical phenomenology. Descriptive phenomenology stems from the work of Husserl, and focuses on the 'essence' of a phenomenon, while hermeneutical phenomenology is informed by the work of Heidegger and Gademer, and focuses on how people 'interpret' a phenomenon (Annells, 1996; Giorgi & Giorgi, 2008; Ryba, 2008). In this study, a descriptive phenomenological approach was followed, as it allowed the researcher to focus on the essence of the phenomenon, being the students' adventure experience.

DATA

Producing

The data used in this research was the written accounts of the students' adventure experience. During the four day adventure experience, they diarized their daily experiences. After the adventure experience they were asked to reflect on the adventure experience as a whole, in writing. A written reflection is seen as a primary material source as it contains the author's own observations and experiences (De Vos, 2002; Giorgi, 1997, 2008; Giorgi & Giorgi, 2008; Strydom & Delport, 2002). The following task was posed to guide their reflections: Write an essay in which you reflect, in as much detail as possible, on the adventure experience.

Analysing

The Duquesne Phenomenological Research Method (DPRM) was used to analyse the material, as it allowed the researcher to study the essence of the adventure experiences of the students (Giorgi, 1985; Giorgi, 1997, 2008; Giorgi & Giorgi, 2008; Van Vuuren, 1989; Von Echartsberg, 1998). This phenomenological analysis method entails the following steps:

- Step 1. Reading the data as a whole.
- Step 2. Identifying meaning units in the data. Step 3. Connecting meaning units with one another and with the whole.
- Step 4. Transforming the descriptions of the concrete experiences into scientific language.
- Step 5. Integrating the results of the project and presenting them to the scientific community.

During the material analysis process the strategy of 'coding-recoding' was employed. The researchers analysed the material at a certain point in time, left it for a certain time, and then analysed the material once again. The two sets of data analysis were then compared with one another (Krefting, 1991).

Quality

The quality of the research was enhanced by applying the criteria of credibility, transferability, dependability and confirmability. Credibility was established by means of participant-checking and peer evaluation. Member-checking was done by allowing the students who participated in the study to view the analysis. Peer-evaluation was done by requesting two independent researchers in the Department of Psychology at the UP in SA to review the analysis. Transferability was obtained by providing a description of the students as participants and the research context. Dependability was gained by giving a description of the material collection and analysis processes. Confirmability was established through researcher reflexivity (Good, Herrera, Good & Cooper, 1985; Krefting, 1991; Lincoln & Guba, 1985).

Ethics

Ethical clearance was received from the Ethics Committee of the Faculty of Humanities at the UP in SA. The main aspects that were addressed in the ethical clearance were: informed consent, participant confidentiality, voluntarily participation (participation in the adventure experience was compulsory, while participation in the adventure activities was voluntarily according to the 'challenge-by choice' principle); and material storage. All the students from G1 and G2 volunteered to participate in the study, which was conducted after the adventure experience.

Results

From the analysis of the students' written accounts, it appears that the adventure experience created an opportunity for the students to learn about themselves. This is apparent from both G1 and G2:

> By this I mean that I want to be more able to explore the things in my life that are perceived as risky or difficult and getting out of my comfort zone more. As we learned this week, adventure is a state of mind and I would like to be open to exploring different experiences in my life with different people in my life. *[G1, S4 (F)]*

> I learned more about myself in that I learned that I don't always have to be right. In the beginning of my diary I wrote more about what physically happened and as the week progressed I looked more into what I was feeling when things happened. *[G2, S13 (F)]*

The learning that took place in G1 and G2 seemed to be in accordance with other studies showing that learning is a fundamental aspect of an adventure experience

(Dwyer, 2006; Eilers, 1997; Hatch & McCarthy, 2005; Holman & McAvoy, 2005; Human, 2006; 2008; Loe'er, 2005; Martin & Leberman, 2005; Nadler, 1995). From the analysis, it seems that students gained deeper knowledge about themselves during the adventure experience in the areas of: awareness, boundaries, uniqueness, trust and cohesion.

Theme 1: Awareness

The adventure experience enhanced the students' awareness of themselves. Experiencing awareness is a fundamental aspect of an adventure experience, as portrayed in previous research (Carlson & McKenna, 2000; Eilers, 1997; Holman & McAvoy, 2005; Human, 2006, 2008; Loe'er, 2005; Martin & Leberman, 2005). The enhanced awareness of the students can be seen in the following extracts from their written accounts:

> This morning the thing that struck me the most in group was the fact that I lost the impetus of being the architect of my life. I am so busy with the dream that I have that I lost the being. *[G1, S3 (F)]*
>
> I remember having the sense that although I am in a group setting, I am working hard on myself and perhaps I am not sharing it with others. For me to keep things to myself, is all too familiar... it is really an old friend of mine. Silencing some of my experiences became a way that I showed I am strong and independent, but only created in the long run, a person who achieved a lot yet cheated myself from taking that leap of expressing how I feel. I have, for too long, depended too much on myself, and I chose in that moment, to learn to let go. *[G2, S10 (F)]*

Learning about awareness is an important aspect of professional development in a graduate/postgraduate counselling training programme, as it enables students to better 'continuously' be aware of who they are in relation to others and their world (Human, 2006; 2008; Johns, 1996; Wheeler, 1996).

Theme 2: Boundaries

Knowing your personal boundaries is an important aspect of professional development that needs to be addressed in a graduate/postgraduate counselling training programme (Human, 2006; 2008; Johns, 1996; Wheeler, 1996). The students experienced that their boundaries were challenged during the adventure experience. In the context of an adventure experience, these boundaries can pertain to physical-, personal or interpersonal boundaries (Goldberg, Klenosky, O'Leary & Templin, 2000; Human 2006). The challenging of boundaries concurs with previous research that indicates that challenging boundaries is a fundamental aspect of an adventure experience (Carlson & McKenna, 2000; Eilers, 1997; Human, 2006; 2008; Martin & Leberman, 2005).

The students' experiences regarding the challenging of boundaries can be seen in the following extracts from their written accounts:

> Okay, in the sense of understanding that sometimes discomfort is very important. The big wave that was going to break on the kayak was symbolic to me as facing my fears. The fact that I was able to face my fear head on meant that I need to challenge myself daily to face whatever fear I have head on. *[G1, S6 (F)]*
>
> I challenged myself to risk more in that moment. I put anxiety in its place and walked up to the adventure, believing... truly believing that I could do this one... the one that counts. As I geared up and I felt anxiety take a hold of me, I posed a sensible question to myself: Why do people abseil anyway? As I leaned back and exhaled, I let go of fear and left everything at the top of the cliff. *[G2, S16 (F)]*

The adventure activities allow students the opportunity to face boundaries they might not have considered before that (of a physical-, personal or interpersonal nature). This experience can be used to help students be aware of the variety of boundaries that could impact on them as psychologists. These include, but are not limited to: interdisciplinary boundaries, boundaries between a client and a psychologist, and other systemic boundaries like personal life and professional life, family life and work life.

Theme 3: Uniqueness

The adventure experience allowed the students to experience their own uniqueness, as well as that of their fellow students. The students' experience of uniqueness is supported by other studies that show that discovering your own and other people's uniqueness is a fundamental aspect of an adventure experience (Eilers, 1997; Goldberg et al., 2000; Human, 2006, 2008; Priest & Gass, 1997).

The discovery of their own and fellow students' uniqueness can be seen in the following extracts from their written accounts:

> I will have to acknowledge that all clients are different and that it will have to be my challenge to motivate them to deal with their difficulties by getting them into contact with themselves. *[G1, S5 (F)]*

> I believe there is room too for experimenting with what can be therapeutic for each individual – from poetry, to writing, to music, to making visual representations of the problem, to using nature and other metaphors. To use my senses in a different way, and use what the client has given – and to go with it, and trust it. *[G2, S17 (F)]*

Learning that each person is different and therefore unique is an important aspect of personal growth and professional development in a graduate/postgraduate counselling training programme (Giorgi & Gallegos, 2005; Johns, 1996; Wheeler, 1996). This will allow students to develop an appreciation for diversity, which is very important in the South African context and in professional roles.

Theme 4: Trust

The students experienced trust during their participation in the adventure experience. Trust is essential to the relationship between a psychologist and a client (Giorgi & Gallegos, 2005; Yalom, 1995). The students' experience of trust is in accordance with previous research that indicates that experiencing trust is a fundamental aspect of an adventure experience (Eilers, 1997; Goldberg et al., 2000; Human, 2006; 2008).

The following extracts from the students' written accounts illustrate their experience of trust during the adventure experience:

> It was amazing in the sense that we all trusted each other so easily and that we trusted in the process as well. In a therapeutic context that would be an essential ingredient for both the client and the therapist and in the past I used to focus more in the trust that the client has to have in the therapist. *[G1, S8 (M)]*

> 'Through letting go of assumptions, and exploring more the stories less travelled; trusting more in the client and what they are giving me in the moment; and risking more as a professional, is something that I take with me and I have begun to be more courageous in putting into practice. *[G2, S12 (F)]*

Trust is an important aspect of professional development that students need to learn about in a graduate/postgraduate counselling training programme (Giorgi & Gallegos, 2005; Human, 2006; 2008; Johns, 1996; Wheeler, 1996). This will enable students to develop the ability to develop and maintain trust with a client as a psychologist, so that this can be transferred to the broader South African society, which needs to grow from distrusting one another to trusting each other.

Theme 5: Cohesion

The adventure experience afforded the students the opportunity to experience cohesion. From previous research, it is evident that cohesion forms an integral part of an adventure experience (Eilers, 1997; Human, 2006; 2008; Loe'er, 2005; Martin & Leberman, 2005; Wheeler, 1996; Wheeler, Goldie & Hicks, 1998). It has also been found that using adventure activities in experiential group work expedites the formation of cohesion in comparison to the formation of cohesion in traditional group work (Hatch & McCarthy, 2003).

The students' experience of cohesion during the adventure experience can be seen in the following extracts from their written accounts:

> The challenges got progressively more difficult, but in the beginning the focus was on the physical ability of the group. The reflection thereafter appeared to be more superficial. One thing this did do was to 'kick-start' some group cohesion because we had to help each other with a common goal in mind. In the group discussions, personal issues began emerging when there seemed to be more trust as a result of cohesion. *[G1, S2 (F)]*

> 'It was amazing to be able to feel the group bonding, and I am 100% certain that this would not have happened if we were to be back in Pretoria. I was amazed at how we managed to stand together as a group, and motivate each other to continue, even if the task at hand seemed impossible. The group served as a safety net when I needed them most, and I realised that it is not necessary to always have a façade of being strong. The physical activities served the purpose of reinforcing group cohesion, and forced us to work together as a group in order to reach our goal. *[G2, S18 (F)]*

Learning about cohesion is an important aspect of professional development of students and needs to be addressed in graduate/postgraduate counselling training programmes (Hatch & McCarthy, 2003; Human, 2008; Wheeler, 1996). For example, cohesion is a fundamental aspect of group psychotherapy (Yalom, 1995). Experience of and reflection on cohesion as part of the adventure experience (Human, 2006) creates opportunities for students to be cognisance of, and become proficient in the use of cohesion as a psychotherapeutic practice. This is important with specific reference to working with diverse groups in the South African context, where the establishment of cohesion is fundamental in allowing people to address issues relating to the history of South Africa.

Discussion

From these results, it appears that the students experienced learning during the adventure experience. This learning pertained to the themes of awareness, boundaries, uniqueness, trust and cohesion. One of the fundamental characteristics of an adventure experience is that the learning that takes place through the adventure experience needs to be transferred to and applied in other contexts (Gillis & Thomsen, 1996; Priest & Gass, 1997). In this study, students were expected to transfer and apply the learning that occurred during the adventure experience to the tertiary education context. In particular (as will be explained), they were required to use the adventure experience as an academic reflection opportunity, as well as a resource during practical work.

Reflection

The training philosophy of the MA (Counselling Psychology) programme at the UP encourages reflection by the students, and therefore goes beyond the mere acquisition of knowledge or meeting the minimum academic standards associated with gaining a degree. Reflections on who they are as individuals (personal reflection) and as psychologists (professional reflection) are encouraged by highlighting the interplay between academic material and experiential learning. On the one hand, this is accomplished by creating the opportunity, through an adventure experience, for students to experience awareness, boundaries, uniqueness, trust and cohesion. On the other hand, the students are expected to study the academic literature on these themes and to reflect on them, based on what they learnt about these themes through the adventure experience. This interplay allows for an understanding that is academically-grounded and experientially-based on these themes.

Resource

This academically-grounded and experientially-based understanding (and reflection) can then be used as a resource during the practical work students undertake with clients. For example, students can use their heightened awareness, challenging of boundaries, appreciation of uniqueness, experience of trust, and creation of cohesion as resources at the various HPCSA accredited organisations where they will undertake their respective internships. For example, heightened awareness of self, other, group dynamics and interaction can be valuable resources during psychological assessment of clients. Furthermore, counselling sessions might be enhanced through the use of trust, and challenge of boundaries as available resource sets, while education can be augmented through application of appreciation of uniqueness or heightened awareness.

Conclusion

From this research it seems that the adventure experience added value to the professional development of the students. One student wrote 'as I left Glenmore I thought to myself how privileged I was to have had this opportunity to explore my strengths and weaknesses so that I can utilize them effectively in my career in helping others' (G1, S2). Another student stated 'this week meant a lot to me personally and professionally and it is something I can use in future' (G2, S14). While this exploratory research attempted to fill the relative void of research on the use of adventure in professional counselling psychology training of students, it opens opportunity for further research within the field. The positive outcomes of the use of adventure activities reported by students could be explored for use in developing other aspects of professional counsellors' development, for example in ethics and personal growth.

Acknowledgement

The authors want to acknowledge Elri Martins, a postgraduate counselling psychology student, for her involvement in this research project.

References

Annells, M. (1996). Hermeneutic phenomenology: Philosophical perspectives and current use in nursing research. *Journal of Advanced Nursing, 23,* 705-713.

Adventure Recreation Association [ARA]. (2009). *Accreditation.* Retrieved on 11/5/09 from http://www. ara.org.za.

Carlson, T. B., & McKenna, P. (2000). A reflective adventure for student teachers. *Journal of Experiential Education, 23*, 17-23.

Coleman, J. S. (1979). Experiential learning and information assimilation: Towards an appropriate mix. J*ournal of Experiential Education, 2*, 6-9.

Corey, G. (1996). *Theory and practice of counselling and psychotherapy* (5th ed.). New York, NY: Brooks/ Cole.

Creswell, J. W. (1998). *Qualitative inquiry and research design: Choosing among five traditions.* Thousand Oaks, CA: Sage.

Dainty, P., & Lucas, D. (1992). Clarifying the confusion: A practical framework for evaluating outdoor development programmes for managers. *Management Education and Development, 23*, 106-122.

DeLay, R. (1996). Forming knowledge: Constructivist learning and experiential education. The *Journal of Experiential Education, 19*, 76-81.

Devlin, A.S. (1996). Survival skills training during freshmen orientation: Its role in college adjustment. *Journal of College Student Development, 37,* 324-333.

De Vos, A. S. (2002). Qualitative data analysis and interpretation. In A. S. de Vos, H. Strydom, C. B. Fouche & C. S. L. Delport. (Eds.), *Research at grass roots, for the social sciences and human service professions* (339-355). Pretoria, South Africa: Van Schaik.

De Vos, A. S., & Fouché, C. B. (1998). General introduction to research design, data collection methods and data analysis. In A. S. de Vos (Ed.), *Research at grass roots: A primer for the caring professions* (76-94). Pretoria, South Africa: Van Schaik.

Dwyer, R. J. (2006). Adventure education? A new way to confront reality! *Development and Learning in Organizations: An International Journal, 20,* 12-15.

Eilers, G. M. (1997). My lessons from adventure therapy. *Journal of Experiential Education, 20*, 61-65.

Fouche, C. B. (2002). Research strategies. In A. S. de Vos, H. Strydom, C. B. Fouche & C. S. L. Delport. (Eds.), *Research at grass roots, for the social sciences and human service professions* (pp. 270-277). Pretoria, South Africa: Van Schaik.

George, R. L., & Christiani, T. S. (1990). *Counselling. Theory and practice* (3rd ed.). Englewood Cliffs, NJ: Prentice-Hall.

Gillis, H. L., & Thomsen, D. (1996). *A research update (1992-1995) of adventure therapy: Challenge activities and ropes courses, wilderness expeditions & residential camping programs*. Indiana University: Coalition for Education in the Outdoors Symposium Proceedings.

Giorgi, A. (Ed.) (1985). *Phenomenology and psychological research.* Pittsburgh, PA: Duquesne University Press.

Giorgi, A. (1997). The theory, practice and evaluation of the phenomenological method as a qualitative research procedure. *Journal of Phenomenological Psychology, 28*, 235-261.

Giorgi, A. (2008). Concerning a serious misunderstanding of the essence of the phenomenological method in psychology. *Journal of Phenomenological Psychology, 39*, 33–58.

Giorgi, A., & Gallegos, N. (2005). Living through some positive experiences of psychotherapy. *Journal of Phenomenological Psychology, 36,* 195-218.

Giorgi, A., & Giorgi, B. (2008). Phenomenological psychology. In C. Willig & W. Stainton-Rogers (Eds.), *The SAGE handbook of qualitative research in psychology* (pp. 165-178). London, England: Sage.

Goldberg, M. A., Klenosky, D. B., O'Leary, J. T., & Templin, T. J. (2000). A means-end investigation into ropes course experiences. *Journal of Leisure Research, 32*, 208-225.

Good, B. J., Herrera, H., Good, M., & Cooper, J. (1985). Reflexivity: Counter transference and clinical ethnography. A case from a psychiatric cultural consultation clinic. In R. Hahn & A. Gaines (Eds.), *Physicians of Western medicine* (pp.193-221). Boston, MA: D. Reidel.

Hatch, K. D., & McCarthy, C. J. (2003). Challenge course participation as a component of experiential groups for counsellors in training. *Journal for Specialists in Group Work, 28*, 199-214.

Hatch, K. D., & McCarthy, C. J. (2005). Exploration of challenge courses' long-term effects on members of college student organizations. *Journal of Experiential Education, 27*, 245-264.

Holman, T., & McAvoy, L. H. (2005). Transferring benefits of participation in an integrated wilderness adventure program to daily life. *Journal of Experiential Education, 27*, 322-325.

Human, L. H. (2006). Adventure-based experiences during professional training in psychology. *South African Journal of Psychology, 36*, 215-231.

Human, L. H. (2008). Unique outcomes in professional psychology training through an adventure experience. *Acta Acedemia, 4*, 151-174.

Hyer, L., Boyd, S., Scurfield, R., & Smith, D. (1996). Effects of Outward Bound experience as an adjunct to inpatient PSTD treatment of war veterans. *Journal of Clinical Psychology, 52*, 263-278.

Johns, H. (1996). *Personal development in counsellor training.* London, England: Cassell.

Kirk, R. (1987). *Learning in action: Activities for personal & group development.* Oxford, England: Basil Blackwell.

Krefting, L. (1991). Rigor in qualitative research: The assessment of trustworthiness. *The American Journal of Occupational Therapy, 45*, 214-222.

Kvale, S. (1996). *Interviews. An introduction to qualitative research interviewing.* Thousand Oaks, CA: Sage.

Lincoln, Y. S., & Guba, E. A. (1985). *Naturalistic inquiry.* Beverly Hills, CA: Sage.

Loe'er, T. A. (2005). Looking deeply in: using photo-elicitation to explore meanings of outdoor education experiences. *Journal of Experiential Education, 27*, 343-346.

Martin, A. J., & Leberman, S. I. (2005). Personal learning or prescribed educational outcomes: A case study of the Outward Bound experience. *Journal of Experiential Education, 28*, 44-59.

Nadler, R. S. (1995). Edgework: Stretching boundaries and generalizing experiences. *Journal of Experiential Education, 18*, 52-55.

Priest, S., & Gass, M. (1997). *Effective leadership in adventure programming.* Champaign, IL: Human Kinetics.

Rohnke, K. (1989). *Cowstails and cobras II. A guide to games, initiatives, ropes courses and adventure curriculum.* Dubuque, IA: Project Adventure & Kendall/Hunt.

Ryba, T. V. (2008). Researching children in sport: Methodological reflections. *Journal of Applied Sport Psychology, 20*, 334-348.

Schoel, J., Prouty, D., & Radcliffe, P. (1988). *Islands of healing. A guide to adventure based counselling.* Hamilton, MA: Project Adventure.

Sheldon, N. M., & Arthur, N. (2001). Adding adventure to therapy. *Guidance & Counselling, 16,* 67-73.

Simons, J. P., & Andersen, M. B. (1995). The development of consulting practice in applied sport psychology: Some personal perspectives. *The Sport Psychologist, 9*, 449-468.

Strydom, H., & Delport, C. S. L. (2002). Information collection: Document study and secondary analysis. In A.S. de Vos, H. Strydom, C.B. Fouche & C.S.L. Delport. (Eds.), *Research at grass roots, for the social sciences and human service professions* (pp. 321-332). Pretoria, South Africa: Van Schaik.

Snow, H. (1992). *The power of team building: Using ropes techniques.* Amsterdam, Netherlands: Pfeiffer.

Van Vuuren, R. J. (1989). An exploration of the role of description in psychology as a descriptive science. *South African Journal of Psychology, 19*, 65-74.

Vidolovitis-Moore, A. (1979). *The effects of an outdoor adventure program on the self-concept of educable mentally retarded/slow learning children.* Unpublished Dissertation. United States of America: Boston University.

Von Echartsberg, R. (1998). Existential-phenomenological research. In R. Valle (Ed.), *Phenomenological inquiry in psychology. Existential and transpersonal dimensions* (21-61). New York, NY: Plenum Press.

Wheeler, S. J. (1996). *Training counsellors: the assessment of competence.* London, England: Cassell.

Wheeler, S., Goldie, J., & Hicks, C. (1998). Counsellor training: An evaluation of the effectiveness of a residential outdoor pursuits activity weekend on the personal development of trainee counsellors. *Counselling Psychology Quarterly, 11*, 391405.

Whitley, B. E. (2002). *Principles of research in behavioral science* (2nd ed.). New York, NY: McGraw-Hill.

Wilson, D. W., & Washington, G. (2007). Retooling phenomenology: Relevant methods for conducting research with African American women. *Journal of Theory Construction & Testing, 11*, 63-66.

Yalom, I. D. (1995). *The theory and practice of group psychotherapy* (4th ed.). New York, NY: Basic Books.

CHAPTER 23

The Power of Storytelling in Adventure Therapy

Tonia Gray and Karen Stuart

ABSTRACT

While universal across human cultures, storytelling has especially entered into educational and therapeutic practice as a technique for self-reflection and growth. The authors propose a pedagogical approach to using story that is developmental and cross-disciplinary. The research upon which this paper is based adopted a phenomenological case study approach in evaluating the benefits of storytelling. Findings show that the pedagogies appeal to our primeval sense of story, to our innate need to 'story' our lives, and potentially provide opportunities for participants of all ages, in all sectors of society to understand themselves and the world around them, and to complete developmental tasks on the basis of this understanding.

INTRODUCTION

> Stories are the closest we can come to experience as we and others tell our experience. A story has a sense of being full, a sense of coming out of a personal and social history… Experience... is the stories people live. People live stories and in the telling of them reaffirm them, modify them, and create new ones. (Clandinin & Connelly, 1994, p.415)

A good story moves us, teaches us, and transforms us (Campbell, 1968; Chisholm, 2000; Kouzes & Posner, 2003; Mitchell, 2005). By providing metaphors to challenge behaviour, Vogler (2007) maintains that stories become almost alive for listeners, who participate in the creation of a dramatic experience. The inherent power of stories is well known within child development and educational research (Bettleheim, 1976). Stories are also used as a tool for adult learning (Parkins, 2001), organisational development (Denning, 2005; Mitchell, 2005) and even as a discrete mode of research (Clandinin & Connelly, 2000). Narrative is particularly useful across all these contexts to access affective dimensions of experience (Thomas & Killick, 2007).

Storytelling is a powerful facilitation technique for outdoor adventure (Gray & Birrell, 2000), but the need to consider the therapeutic implications and rationale for including storytelling in adventure therapy contexts exists. With narratives or stories, the salient message is retained without the 'teller' being perceived as authoritarian, dictatorial or prescriptive. Because the interpretation of storytelling is open and creative, participants can bring their own experiences and modes of understanding to the reflective process.

Playwrites and authors use metaphorical stories to allow children and adults to make sense of unresolved issues or thoughts in a safe, abstract environment (Bettelheim, 1976; Vogler, 2007). Stories have the potential to transform painful, personal and professional stories into a medium that is safe for us to share, discuss and perhaps even resolve. Throughout this paper, storytelling is shown to be an aid to personal growth from pedagogical, therapeutic or developmental perspectives. Narrative reflection allows participants to extract interpretations from their personal experience while transforming that experience into a meaningful story, one that may be recounted repeatedly with new layers of significance, achieving transformative learning (Moon, 1999).

This paper introduces the theoretical rationale for using stories and narratives in some educational, outdoor adventure, therapeutic and inquiry based fields. By describing two practical therapeutic uses of stories, one using the cycle of development, the other using experiential life storying, this paper will argue for a deeper appreciation of how storytelling can augment day-to-day practice in these various fields.

Use of Narratives

Humans have told stories for millennia, and indeed used them to pass on the heritage of their own cultures (Chisholm, 2000). As individuals we experience stories from childhood; for many people, they act as one of our earliest forms of education, encouraging us to develop an ethical sense and to see relationships between our lives and the wisdom of others. Even if we are not told stories at home, we are exposed to them in school, among peers and colleagues, and through popular culture (for instance, on television, computer and radio). We use stories as 'sense making' tools; Boje describes storytelling as 'the preferred sense making currency of human relationships' (cited in Simpson 2008, p. 106). The authors attribute this to our cultural experiences of stories, as they are 'intrinsic parts of being human' (Maguire 1998, p. xiv).

Individuals embrace stories as a mechanism to represent and to make sense of who they are. As stories are read, we relate to different characters and situations, exploring how they represent who we were, who we are, and who we might be. In the course of our development, fairy tales, poems, songs, Aesop's fables and family legends may have informed our way of being in the world. Three noteworthy stories that exemplify this concept in western cultures are *The Boy Who Cried Wolf, Three Little Pigs* and *The Hare and the Tortoise* (see Figure 1). The salient messages embedded within these stories are enduring and profound; although simple, the stories allow us to see analogues in many facets of our lives. For example, these stories remind us: not to tell lies because they undermine our credibility; to build out of strong and long-lasting materials; and to notice that persistence often trumps short-term enthusiasm. The story provides an 'anchor' for lifelong memory and a ready-made rich 'pool' of metaphor.

The stories we choose to read tell us something about who we are. As McAdams (1993) poignantly says: 'If you want to know me, then you must know my story, for my story defines who I am' (p.11). The stories we listen to, create and recount have the potential to initiate attitudinal and behaviour change. This notion was carried to further magnitude by Koch (1998) when she wrote:

> People live stories, and in their telling of them, reaffirm them, modify them, and create new ones. Constructions of experience are always on the move. Stories, when well crafted, are spurs to the imagination, and through our imaginative participation in the created worlds, empathetic forms of understanding are advanced. (p. 1183)

Here we begin to show the developmental aspect to stories. Stories are not fixed; they can be changed. Modifying the events or ending of a story can metaphorically open new ways of thinking and new possibilities to individuals and groups, helping to create personal and professional development. Development and transformation are possible, therefore, in the transition from lived experience to story, and to new versions of the same story.

Bettelheim (1976) first wrote of the developmental scope of enchanted stories for children: 'by dealing with universal human problems, particularly those which preoccupy the child's mind, these stories speak to his budding ego and encourage its development, while at the same time relieving preconscious and unconscious pressures' (p.6). Stories legitimise early childhood emotions and experiences, for example, understanding feelings of hatred towards our own mother as hatred and fear of the evil stepmother. Bettelheim's approach links to early work by Freud on the metaphors that the unconscious mind uses to represent unresolved issues a starting point for psychoanalysis. Transactional analysis (TA) holds that at an early age, we develop a life story or 'script' (Steiner, 1974) that we then endeavour to live out – this can explain some of our repetitive life patterns. Life scripts are used by therapeutic, developmental and organisational TA to expose the unconscious 'script' that is being lived out, to enable greater awareness and autonomy (Berne, 1976).

On the basis of this technique, individuals or organizations might choose to 're-parent' themselves, re-writing a new ending to their own autobiographical stories. This reinterpretation is the power of the method described here. The opportunity to rewrite endings is supported from a TA perspective by Illsley-Clarke and Dawson (1989), and from a narrative inquiry perspective by Clandinin and Connelly (1994). Stories are deeply personal, but 'just as the tiniest sample from your living body can reveal the DNA of your whole biological person, so a brief, well-chosen story can shed light on your entire life history. When you tell a story about an apparently trivial incident, it exposes the entire fabric of your character' (Denning 2007, p. 82).

Figure 1. The boy who cried wolf, Three little pigs and The hare and the tortoise pictures

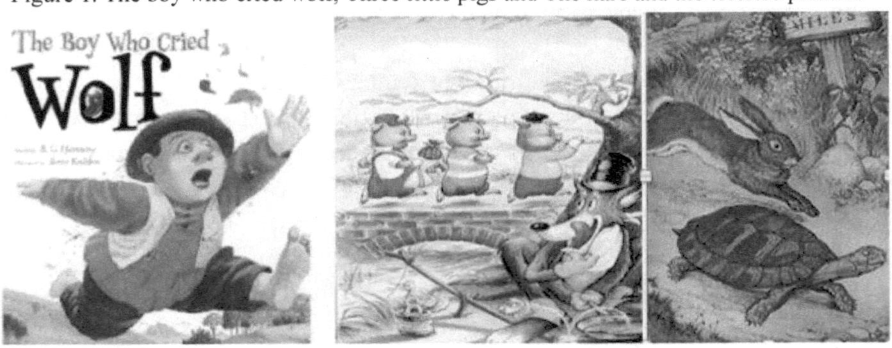

from Gettyimages.com

Working at a metaphorical rather than a literal level is both practical and powerful in adventure therapy (Gass, 1993; Loynes, 1999; Ringer, 2002). The use of metaphorical narratives allows participants to access deeper, more affective and unconscious levels of thinking. Stories work between the personal and professional domains, and additionally place clients in a solution-focussed space, as authors of the story. Finally, stories can potentially protect confidentiality in the discussion process as participants do not have to disclose what the literal situation was, or who was involved.

Narrative therapy is used widely in adventure therapy contexts – whether to 'frontload' an experience with a tale, or whether deconstructing tales of what happened, or listening to stories of others experiences. From this context, as Alice Morgan (2011) stated, 'Narrative therapy is sometimes known as involving 're-authoring' or 're-storying' conversations' (p.12). Adventure contexts offer many opportunities for re-authoring the self, hence its use of narratives. Like other therapeutic approaches, narrative therapy seeks to be a respectful, non-blaming approach which centres people as the experts in their own lives. It views problems as separate from people, and assumes people have many skills, competencies, beliefs, values, commitments and abilities that will assist them to reduce the influence of problems in their lives. The pedagogical tools (experiential workshop and experiential life storying) that we advocate are largely interactive and dialogical in nature, and can be used across the fields of storytelling already discussed.

PEDAGOGICAL APPROACH 1: STORYTELLING WITH THE CYCLE OF DEVELOPMENT

The authors have developed a storytelling approach that is explicitly developmental. This has been achieved by incorporating a model from Transactional Analysis into a storytelling session. Levin's (1982) 'Cycle of Development' has been used as an individual and organisational developmental model. Here we extended its use and applied it to a therapeutic narrative approach appropriate to adventure therapy. The model outlined in Figure 2 uses the cycle of development to promote reflective learning through narrative. The cycle of development (Levin 1982, p.34) is a Transactional Analysis model that accounts for the process of developing from child to adult. The concept is cyclical rather than linear, a reoccurrence stimulated by a new thirteen year chronological cycle, or triggered by a major change in life circumstance.

Figure 2. Levin's cycle of development **(1982)**

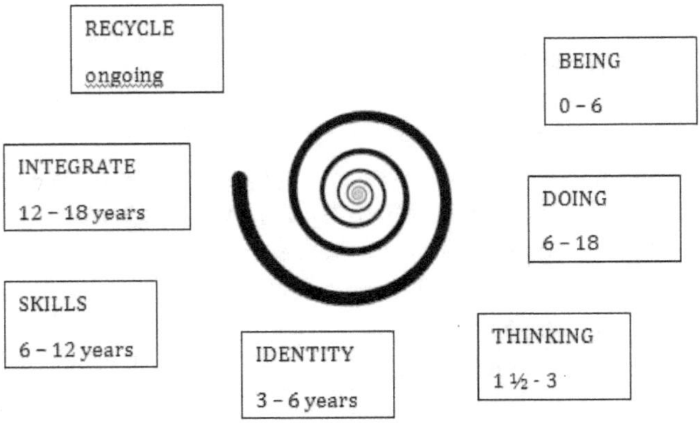

The cycle of development is a model that describes development from ages 0 – 18 years. The model presents repeated cycles of learning, as triggered by significant life events, for instance, a life threatening illness, change of job, divorce and so on. Levin's cycle is a model of life-long learning, or of response to change. The model demonstrates a range of stages that an individual progresses through in order to become a functional autonomous adult. These are age related up to the age of eighteen, but not age related from then on.

In each stage there are key tasks for the individual, for example to experience the world, to experiment with risk-taking behaviour – and key tasks for care-givers, such as providing stimulus and safety. We may not have been able to complete all of the tasks we require in each developmental stage for a range of reasons (post-natal illness, traumatic injury and convalescence for example), or we may have had care givers who were not able to meet our needs in each stage (e.g. post natal depression). In addition, we may have received injunctions against completing a task.

In childhood, comments such as, 'stop asking questions, it just is!' discourage children from thinking. Such injunctions prevent us from completing the developmental tasks in that stage when we progress to the next one. As adults, we can revisit these stages and complete the developmental activity required. One of the authors skipped 'being' as she spent the first four months of her life in an incubator in intensive care. Nowadays, she continually reminds herself that 'it is OK to stand still and just relax and be, I don't need to always be doing.'

In addition, Figure 2 enables the conceptualisation of development that is ongoing and solution focused, allowing adults to locate their personal and professional development on a cyclical spectrum. Additionally, the cycle accounts for how people are in different stages developmentally, in different circumstances. They may, for example, be fully integrated at work, but in a phase of 'being' in their private lives due to a recent divorce. The model allows reflection on the self and others in different contexts, and can offer interventions for both. Levin's cycle is used therapeutically to guide personal, professional and organizational development. It is useful in offering a way for people to anticipate their own and others' reactions to change, and the actions to take in order to move through these stages (Clarke & Dawson, 1998).

The model also offers a clear guide to interventions and roles of care-givers (such as parents, teachers, therapists, or even line managers). The Cycle of Development has been used to plan workplace induction processes as it shows what new employees might be thinking and feeling, the tasks that they need to complete, and significantly, what their managers need to do to enable their development to happen.

The authors have used the approach described in this paper in varying contexts, including:

- An international adventure therapy conference with a range of 12 professionals.
- A multidisciplinary international experiential learning conference with 38 delegates.
- A workshop with 20 multi-disciplinary managers from children's services in the UK.

The next section describes the impact of this pedagogical approach with this range of audiences. The approach that we used was the same in each context and as such the findings are reported together.

USING THE MODEL

After welcoming the participants and engaging in a range of story-related ice breaker activities, delegates were asked to 'en-story' an experience with which they wanted to work. Having encoded the experiences into stories, the authors introduced the Cycle of Development by describing each stage of Levin's model and how the cycle can repeat. Cards were placed on the floor in a spiral. Walking the cycle and describing the different stages helped to bring the spiral metaphor to life. After foreshadowing the model, we allowed the participants to revisit the characters in the stories they had previously encoded. They were invited to reflect on the developmental tasks of the characters and what was needed to allow them to complete those tasks. This reflective process allowed the delegates to reframe the story and the characters within it, and place them in a solution-focused space. After participants had conducted this inventory, we asked them to write a new ending to the stories if they wished to, with the new awareness that participants in the workshop had gained. The rewriting task represented a shift from what 'is' to 'what could be', from 'stuck-ness' and struggle to movement and 'solutions'. The identification of developmental tasks encouraged the participants to be empathetic and caring to their story characters rather than critical.

Critique of the Pedagogical Approach

One valid critique of the method above is that the workshop referred to well-known and established stories in western cultural contexts. The inherent difficulty here is that these particular stories may reinforce some of the grand narratives that exist in society, such as sexual hierarchy, hetero-normativity, and other moral models. The question is whether asking people to refer to cultural stories reinforces notions of masculinity, heroism and 'great man' theory that were often included in those folk tales. Storytelling must also then include a critical dialogue to expose the underlying power dynamics and grand narratives that may be subtly woven into a familiar tale. This critique is not to say that the stories are inaccurate representations of the individual's experiences, but that they may tell us more than appears on the surface. As Willis and Bondi (2009) suggest, the other implication for us as 'story-weavers' is to provide a range of alternative stories to the people with whom we work, so success is not always attached to heroism, and the quiet path is as valid as the epic.

We found that in whatever setting it was delivered, the session transcended personal, professional and cultural differences. In fact it was found to enhance inter-professional learning when used in a UK-based Inter-Professional Education session (with professionals from across the children's workforce). Given our personal belief in the inherent value of narratives, we have reported the findings with excerpts from the delegates' stories. These have mainly been drawn from feedback gained at the 2008 International Consortium of Experiential Learning (ICEL), but not exclusively.

The forty international delegates at the 2008 ICEL did not know each other, had different cultural storytelling norms and all had different conceptions and experiences of learning. Feedback from the session showed that all of the delegates found the experience useful, and that some individuals found the experience especially powerful:

'Our workshop helped me to come to a life decision that I have struggled with for years – I have just rung my husband and told him I am retiring!'

'I use storytelling to 'frontload' or foreshadow an experience/field trip that the class may be going on. Students also love just 'stories' (something which has been lost in our cyberspace world). They learn from oral traditional storytelling being passed down from generation to generation (akin to indigenous learning, which is also (sadly) being phased out). I really enjoyed this workshop and it adds to my enthusiasm to continue to use story.'

'At the conference I was affected by a keynote presentation. I had some unresolved feelings about several things when I walked in to your session. In truth I probably needed to stop have a brew and get my act together – I was feeling pretty empty and unsure about lots of stuff all at once. I entered your session in a daze and was again into another experience. When you asked us to tell a story to a partner that was relevant, it was natural to discuss where I was at after X's session. So I jumped at it, and through the fairytale, without giving away too much to my partner, I told a story which described my complete sense of hopelessness and fear. For me the emotion attached to the things I was reflecting on from the previous session were big and through the storytelling experience I had with you I was able to quickly talk about them safely (manage them without losing). The smart bit in the process was in the next section when we had to come up with the end of the story in the second phase. This helped me stack pack and rack both my experience and emotion, attaching some meaning and guidance on how to proceed. (I had an action plan) In many ways the keynote session opened some big stuff for me that I was afraid I could not cope with but I was able to close it through your session.'

It was solution focused (we could choose the ending to the story) which in turn produced a reversed metaphor). In essence the solution to what I needed to do I took from the ending I had come up with. What was truly great and safe about the whole process was my partner in the discussion was intrigued by the story we shared, and there was no need to disclose which character represented me. My partner was entertained (or pretended they were) and once each story had been shared and the links made in the mind of the storyteller, each person tended to treat each

> *other's story with respect. It was like an unconscious recognition of the depth of the connection between the character and the person within their own story. Making up my own ending to a story for me now is a coping strategy for things that stress me out.'*

The delegates' excerpts clearly convey the potential transformative power of stories across educational, therapeutic and developmental contexts. The authors had hoped that fellow professionals attending would be inspired and stimulated by the session and take the tools away to use themselves. The results surpassed our expectations, leading to significant changes for some individuals. These experiences confirmed the authors' belief in this as a multi-levelled pedagogical method.

Although we have not tested this in an outdoor setting, we believe this is a rich and highly 'portable' developmental narrative technique that may enhance any adventure therapist's toolkit. It offers a pedagogical structure to help ensure development and learning do take place within a narrative session.

Pedagogical Approach 2: Experiential Life Storying

For some adventure therapy practitioners, storytelling is an integral component in their program. At the 2IATC conference in Germany, Gray and Birrell (2000) outlined how this teaching and learning medium can augment behavioural change. Built on the premise that our lives are enstoried, Gray and Birrell (2000) showed how stories can be incorporated as a non-authoritarian strategy to share beliefs, ideals, values and experience. In this earlier presentation, they shared the wide-ranging challenges that were encountered by previous groups and the resultant learning and behaviour change.

Storytelling allows the facilitator to 'frontload' an adventure therapy experience, thereby allowing participants to conceptualise themselves in an adventurous setting prior to the experience. The Bonnum Pic Fairytale (shown in Figure 3) illustrates how a facilitator has used story to communicate the key issues prior to an expedition, in a non-threatening but educative manner.

Figure 3. Front and final page of the Bonnum Pic Fairytale (Gray & Birrell, 2000)

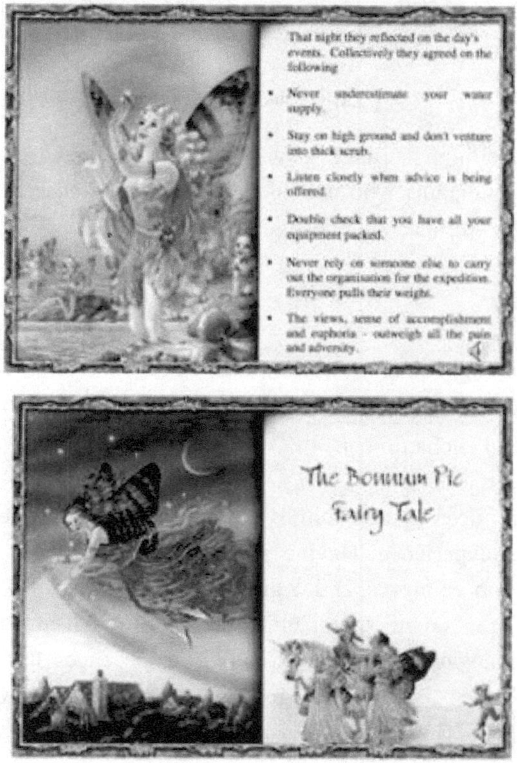
That night they reflected on the day's events. Collectively they agreed on the following
• Never underestimate your water supply.
• Stay on high ground and don't venture into thick scrub.
• Listen closely when advice is being offered.
• Double check that you have all your equipment packed.
• Never rely on someone else to carry out the organisation for the expedition. Everyone pulls their weight.
• The views, sense of accomplishment and euphoria - outweigh all the pain and adversity.
The Bonnum Pic
Fairy Tale

This pedagogical approach has been used in an ongoing tertiary Outdoor Education subject with 25 participants per year since inception in 1999. Previous groups of students on the expedition had encountered hardship and adversity, such as:

1. Running out of water
2. Navigating into overgrown creek gullies and crevices
3. Some group members being unprepared and allowing others in the group to 'carry' the weight of the planning phase on their shoulders.

The use of the Bonnum Pic Fairytale (Gray & Birrell, 2000) allowed the next cohort of student on expedition to learn from these mistakes without being 'lectured' on them. They would then go on to make their own mistakes that they could relay in their own stories, full of the triumph and exhilaration that immediately follows the state of dissonance and disequilibrium contained within that experience, and the sense that learning from experience is without doubt worth the effort.

Emergent Themes

How does storytelling facilitate development and change? In studying the feedback from participants who used both of the approaches, we have identified five ways in which stories create change:

- Validation
- Reframing
- Connects on an unconscious level
- 'New'
- Magic and enchantment

By *validation*, we mean that by telling a story and being listened to, participants have a validating experience. Having a peer listen to and play back a story ('I heard that …') can reinforce and legitimate the storyteller's experience. This validation alone can create therapeutic change and be life altering: 'through transforming our negative, painful or chaotic experiences into stories, we take responsibility for them, and we bring them to bear more constructively on our lives' (Maguire 1998, p.17).

A story can also *reframe* the experience that an individual or group has had. Experience may be reframed by the 'moral' of the story, by the events or characters in the narrative, or through listening and comparing with others' stories. An intimidating life obstacle may seem less significant in the light of others' stories or their perspectives. Once reframed, a change can then occur. Metaphor allows us to conceptualise the familiar in a new way, adding shades of meaning. A well told metaphorical story about teamwork can help a corporate team identify how they function (leading to development): a story with subtle meaning is more palatable than being told you are 'dysfunctional' or given other pointed criticism.

Metaphor may reframe experience, and can offer the safety and distance to allow us to share events that would otherwise remain private. This potential to confront intimacy has been our experience when using stories in multi professional settings; participants often find it easier to talk about the difficulties of the 'Prince trying to get to Snow White' than of the endless hurdles of own professional lives. As Broussine (2008) posits:

> Metaphor provides a description of something by reference to another object that is different to, but analogous to, the 'something' originally described. This is particularly valuable when researching organisational experience, because metaphors can act as a container for emotional and unconscious force at work. *(p.26)*

Because each participant can be applying the common metaphor to slightly different experiences, they need not argue about a particular event, who was to blame or responsible, but can instead focus on the deeper personality, and on social dynamics.

Metaphors have potential for us to make *connections on an unconscious level.* Speaking to us on a number of levels, metaphors can be processed on a conscious and unconscious level. The unconscious connections are often experienced as 'aha' moments, when previously unknown material surfaces from the unconscious into the conscious (for example. the leader who realised he felt as oppressed as 'Cinderella'). This new self-awareness opens up possibilities for change.

By *new* we infer that people often learn, relearn or realize new things through listening to and telling stories. We are often more open to new knowledge in a story format than when it is delivered by a parent or teacher. This is perhaps the most straightforward use. A nurse might tell a story about how an injection went horribly wrong to an apprentice, introducing new knowledge to them about how to and not to inject a patient; a young person might tell a friend what happened last Friday night in town, passing on learning through experience.

Finally, stories can hold an element of magic or enchantment, *and as Denning (2005) articulated 'an appropriately told story had the power to do what rigorous analysis couldn't* – to communicate a strange new idea easily and naturally and quickly get people into enthusiastic action' (p.xii). So by magic and enchantment, we refer to the power of stories to convince and persuade hearers, to 'get them on board' – the territory of political speakers and neuro-linguistic programming (Bandler & Grindler (1979).

Conclusion

The pedagogical approach that we have described, using storytelling and the cycle of development, offers facilitators of adventure therapy a simple developmental model that can be delivered to young people and adults anywhere in the world. The model works on a number of levels, explaining what happened to participants as children and what they are experiencing now. This flexible method offers new awareness and insight into behavioural patterns, and an open-ended method to understand some of the drivers of participants' behaviours today. The model provides opportunities for ongoing development because the technique does not arbitrarily label or categorise; narrative interpretation describes a temporary state, liable to revision and increased reflection. The model tells us to nurture ourselves and allow ourselves to grow and develop, claiming our own locus of control.

Combining narrative reflection with an awareness of the developmental cycles offers much to adventure therapy in many contexts. Explaining current behaviours, conceptualising historic influences on the people with whom we work, anticipating reactions to change (for example going on an adventure), and enabling individuals to take ownership of their own futures and needs are useful for many and varied target groups. For these reasons, we recommend storytelling as a key concept for adventure therapy and we look forward to hearing how other practitioners use storytelling in their practice.

References

Bandler, R. (1979). *Frogs into princes: Neurolinguistic programming*. Moab, Utah: Real People Press.

Bettleheim, B. (1976). *The uses of enchantment: The meaning and importance of Fairy tales.* Knopf, New York.

Broussine, M. (2008). *Creative methods in organizational research.* London: SAGE.

Campbell, J. (1968). *The hero with a thousand faces.* Princeton, NJ: Princeton University Press.

Chisholm, L. (2000). *Charting a hero's journey.* New York, NY: The International Partnership for Service-Learning.

Clandinin, D. & Connelly, F. (2000). *Narrative inquiry.* San Francisco: Jossey Bass.

Denning, S. (2005). *The leaders guide to storytelling.* San Francisco: Jossey Bass.

Gass, M. (Ed.). (1993). *Adventure therapy: Therapeutic applications of adventure programming.* Dubuque, IA: Kendall/Hunt.

Gray T, & Birrell, C. (2000). Fairytales and adventure therapy: I would like to see that! *Proceedings from the Second International Adventure Therapy Conference*, Augsburg, Germany.

Illsley Clarke, J. & Dawson, C. (1998). *Growing up again*, 2nd ed. MN: Hazleden.

Kouzes, J. & Posner, B. (2003). *Encouraging the heart: A leader's guide t rewarding and recognizing others.* San Francisco: Jossey-Bass.

Levin, P. (1982). The cycle of development. *Transactional Analysis Journal, 12*(2), 129-139.

Loynes, C. (1999). Once upon a time. In *The Human Face of Outdoor Education.* Perth, Australia: Australian Outdoor Education Council.

Maguire, J. (1998). *The power of personal storytelling.* New York: Penguin Putnam.

McAdams, D. (1993). *The stories we live by*. London: Guildford Press.

Mitchell, H. (2005). Knowledge sharing: The value of storytelling. *International Journal of Organisational Behaviour, 9*(5), 632-641.

Moon, J. (1999). *The role of reflection in learning and professional development.* Oxon: Routledge Farmer.

Morgan, A. (2000). *What is narrative therapy?* Adelaide: Dulwich Centre Publications.

Ringer, M. (2002). *Group action: The dynamics of groups in therapeutic, educational and corporate settings.* London, Jessica Kingsley.

Steiner, C. (1974). *Scripts people live.* New York: Grove Press.

Stewart, I. & Joines, V. (1987). *TA Today.* Nottingham: Lifespace Publishing.

Thomas, T., & Killick, S. (2007). *Telling tales: Storytelling as emotional literacy.* Blackburn: Educational Printing Services.

Vogler, C. (2007). *The writer's journey: Mythic structure for storytellers and screenwriters.* Michael Wiese Productions

Willis, A. & Bondi, L. (2009). *Troubling adventure therapy: Constructing and consuming Wilderness?* A paper presented at the 5th International Adventure Therapy Conference, 7– 11 September 2009 Edinburgh, London: BACP

CHAPTER 24

The Ecology of Adventure Therapy: An Integral Systems Approach to Therapeutic Change[1]

Duncan Taylor, David Segal and Nevin Harper

ABSTRACT

Currently a fragmentation in ideas exists regarding understanding psychological wellness and preferred routes to healing. This is evident in current adventure therapy (AT) literature, where unique combinations of experiential learning, challenge activities, novel experiences, group work, and other psychological theories are often used to account for positive outcomes and to explain mechanisms for change. Rarely is contact with wilderness environments included as an important variable associated with positive outcomes and change. AT has been rightly criticized for not recognizing the ecological paradigm of therapy conducted in wild nature. By including principles from integral systems theory, we offer AT therapists a map, allowing for these seemingly disparate parts to fit together into a coherent whole. In addition, we propose that wilderness is a crucial co-facilitator in the change process. If seriously considered, these ideas pose a number of important questions for AT theory and practice.

INTRODUCTION

In recent years, integral systems theory has been increasingly used in both the natural and social sciences to improve understanding of how human and biophysical systems undergo change and transformation. A child of complexity and evolutionary systems theory, integral theory offers important insights for fields as traditionally diverse as forest ecology, developmental psychology, and psychotherapy. Further, there are new arguments that suggest immersion in wilderness environments or wild nature during adventure therapy (AT) to be a

[1] Previously published in Ecopsychology, Vol. 2 No. 2 June 2010. Reprinted with permission from Mary Ann Liebert Inc. Publishers (www.liebertpub.com/eco).

crucial factor in facilitating lasting change (Nicholls & Gray, 2007; Trace, 2002) a profoundly integrating force in stabilizing transformation following disequilibrium. AT is being defined broadly as a therapeutic approach utilizing challenge and experiential learning in conjunction with therapist-determined techniques. Moreover, despite our advocating the use of wild nature in AT, we are not limiting our definition to Wilderness AT (WAT). Instead, we wish to reach the broad AT audience and argue for the integration of the natural environment in the AT process.

In light of the nature of open systems (all living systems maintain their integrity as a result of exchanging energy with the environment), the context in which therapy occurs is a crucial variable. Thus, AT that ignores the potential therapeutic benefits of wild nature could be failing to utilize a valuable context. In this article we examine AT in light of integral systems theory. We make the argument that it is a useful model with which to examine the practice of AT – both in terms of how the wilderness adventure experience is a crucial component in facilitating individual change and reorganization, as well as the use of these theories in generating critical questions for further research.

Further, AT theorists have been criticized for their reluctance, or oversight, to connect wild nature to therapeutic change processes; AT theory has primarily developed in the context, dominant discourse, and territorialism of conventional psychological approaches (Beringer, 2004). Thus, limited AT literature exists in which therapeutic values of the 'wilderness experience' in this type of approach are expressed (e.g., Greenway, 1995; Henderson, 1999; Miles, 1987). For the purposes of this article the authors are including contact with wild nature as a key component of AT, whereas current AT definitions often do not the latter postulating greater influence by experiential learning practices and challenge/risk constructs, along with conventional 'clinical' approaches, in therapeutic change. With our inclusion of wild nature in AT, this approach may be considered an ideal expression of ecopsychology in action—a fertile ground for application of ecological thought in psychotherapeutic practice.

We have titled this paper *The Ecology of Adventure Therapy* for the following reasons:

I. The term 'ecology' is from the Greek 'oikos' meaning house or home and 'logos' meaning the study of—hence, the study of our home. This is our extended abode where we all live and upon which our lives and economies ('household management') are utterly dependent (Barber, 1998, p. 442).

II. 'Adventure' – is from the Latin 'adventura' and 'advenire' ('ad' meaning 'to' and 'venire' meaning 'arrive') – hence, 'to arrive.'

III. AT practice often includes the use of wilderness or similar outdoor environments in its definition. 'Wilderness' is from the Old English 'wild-deor' meaning wild animal. It is the abode of the non-domesticated and is out of the control of humans. Wilderness, then, is a place or context that is chaotic, unruly, and disordered, and where people often feel out of control. 'Wild' is also etymologically related to 'will' and 'willful' – hence, uncontrollable, chaotic, and without order (Nash, 1979, p. 1).

IV. 'Therapy' is from the Greek 'herapeia' meaning 'curing' and 'healing.'

The title of this paper relates to the idea that within wilderness places or contexts (our extended home) where we are 'out of control' or which is often 'chaotic', there exists a profound potential for arriving at a new level of wholeness or healing.

THE RISE OF SYSTEMS THINKING

> When we try to pick out anything by itself, we find it hitched to everything else in the universe. (John Muir, My First Summer in the Sierra, 1911/1996)

Ecological perspectives and their application to human systems and therapeutic change emerged largely as a response to the growing influence of scientific reductionism in the social sciences. The work of Bertalanffy (1968) and Laszlo (1996) introduced 'general system theory' to return science and scientists to a holistic, unified way of thinking. By assuming the existence of structural uniformities at all levels of systemic inquiry, the systems theorist is able to recognize similarities and connections between otherwise disparate types of phenomena. The concept of 'system' becomes an invariant facilitating the movement from one field of investigation to another, without losing one frame of reference or having to adopt another. The result is a significant impact on the conceptualization of physical and social sciences ranging from biologists to political theorists, to mental health professionals. Since that time, advancements in systems thinking has brought with it a deep understanding of how systems undergo change and transformation. In recent years, much of this has been synthesized and articulated in integral systems theory.

INTEGRAL SYSTEMS THEORY

Integral systems theory regards the world in which we live as a self-organizing complex, consisting of a myriad number of systems or 'wholes', all of which are interconnected and interlocked. Within this perspective, an individual system—whether an atom, cell, plant, animal, human, community, or nation—is seen to interact with its environment by means of 'feedback' mechanisms. It cannot therefore be properly understood separate from its relationship with the environment of which it is a part (Wilber, 2001).

An integral systems perspective sets out to demonstrate that the world in which we live is not some chaotic heap or aggregate of parts, but is instead an organized and highly elegant structure in which order and structural regularities are always in operation. The traditional systems theorists have typically looked at the implications of systems for the social domain (e.g. Psychology: Bateson, 1972; Political Theory: Taylor, 1999), whereas the integral systems approach also recognizes the importance of the biophysical context, in which human individual and social systems are embedded.

The interconnectedness and co-evolutionary nature of both biophysical and social systems is a cornerstone of integral theory. Common to all natural systems are the following properties (see Laszlo, 1996; Taylor, 1999; Wilber, 1996).

Agency and Communion

All natural systems are relative wholes, 'holons' in systems terminology (Koestler, 1967; Wilber, 2001). Holons are embedded in, and continuously exchange, energy and information with other larger natural systems and environmental contexts. Consequently, a holon has both 'agency' or relative identity, as well as 'communion' insofar as it is also a part of a larger holon or context. An atom, for example, is part of a molecule and a child is part of a family. The two principles that operate to maintain balance between 'agency' and 'communion' are discussed in the following paragraph.

Stabilization and Transcendence

Holons attempt to maintain themselves with respect to their larger environment. All living systems are open with respect to energy and information from their surrounding environment. Despite this continual flow-through of matter energy and information, and indeed because of that capacity, systems can self-regulate to compensate for changing conditions in their environment. Examples of this homeostasis can be found in biological systems, such as the regulative mechanisms in animals which maintain body temperature, blood pressure, sugar and insulin levels, and so on, notwithstanding variations in the surrounding environment.

Open systems tend to return to a level of steady-state following disturbances or perturbations, internally and externally, in their environment. However, at times, when challenges from the environment persist, they can fall apart (dissolution) or evolve (transcendence or self-organization) in response to these perturbations to a new level of complexity with new emergent properties.

The Four-quadrant Model

All humans, and arguably all sentient beings, have both agency and communion. At the level of agency, we all have 'exteriority' or physicality as well as 'interiority'—thoughts, feelings, perceptions, and so on. At the level of communion, we live in larger social and biophysical contexts of interobjectivity. And at the intersubjective level, we inhabit a world of cultural meanings, world views, values, and language. These four areas are referred to as the four-quadrant model (Esbjorn-Hargens & Zimmerman, 2009; Taylor, 2001; Wilber, 2001). Largely attributed to the work of Wilber (2001) the four-quadrant model is a map of reality that encompasses all possible perspectives in which a system exists in the world. Thus, it allows for the most integrated investigation of any holon.

Figure 1. The four quadrant model

	Interior	**Exterior**
	Subjective	**Objective**
Agency (Individual Systems)	Individual phenomenological experiences: E.g. individual thoughts, memories, emotions, perceptions, values etc.	Individual systems that you can observe: E.g. the physical body, behaviours, diet, one's health, etc.
	Intersubjective	**Interobjective**
Communion (Collective Systems)	Collective interior experiences: E.g. meaning-making, social norms, languages, relationships, cultural backgrounds, narratives, etc.	Interacting systems that you can observe: E.g. the biophysical environment, the social environment, technologies and infrastructure.

The Self-system

Sato (2003a) refers to the self as the self-system. This is defined by 'anything I feel a sense of unity with, whether it is a person, object, a place, an abstract concept, or a set of procedures' (p. 86). The self-system's identification range can be from just one's physical body and psychological states to one's larger social group and biophysical world (Taylor, 1991). The Norwegian philosopher and deep ecologist Naess (2008) has defined the 'self' in very similar terms. In turn, we have found it useful to regard the self-system as that which one is emotionally and cognitively attached to and strongly identifies with in each of the four quadrants.

Sato (2003b) underscores this point by arguing that 'the wider the variety of experiences we have, the more our self-system develops...although every response we make is guided by the self-system, every experience including the response and its consequence modifies the self-system as well' (p. 39). In essence, we create a conceptual system that allows us to relate to the world in a way we feel comfortable and are able to protect ourselves.

From this perspective the self-system is a process, or a verb, not an entity or noun (Davies, 2000). It is not separate or isolated, but instead 'a fluid coherence of perspective from which we experience... and the sense of self emerges and changes primarily in relationship' (Mahoney, 2003, p. 7). The self-system is central to counselling and psychotherapy as it is the 'dynamic and usually tacit process that holds together the sundry developmental lines, constructing something of a cohesive whole that recursively serves as each person's psychological universe' (Marquis, 2008, p. 153).

Again, the first tendency of all systems, including the self-system, is for self-preservation—to maintain its relative autonomy and agency in the face of changing environmental circumstances, stress, and perturbations. In terms of the client experience in AT, this could be described as stabilization or 'client resistance'. Although discussions pertaining to client resistance to change is commonplace in therapeutic literature, there is little agreement on the details. Viewing resistance through an integral systems lens offers a promising perspective to understand resistance and breakthrough (or 'transcendence') in the context of AT.

When clients encounter a novel experience they often find themselves resisting the influence of the experience. The self-system is trying to make sense of a novel experience with its current mode of knowing. However, it will only be successful in integrating the experience by reorganizing itself in such a way as to be able to include it (Sato, 2003a). Thus, self-transformation first involves a form of surrender, which usually occurs after all previous resources for resistance have been exhausted in attempts to diminish the new experience. Indeed, transcendence involves disidentifying with that which has previously defined us.

Adventure Therapy in Light of Integral Systems Theory

When individual and group systems are highly unstable, both individual and group encouragement and focused intention can make a difference. Like a ball bearing perched on a mountain top, the smallest perturbation can send it into very different valleys. According to Corey and Corey (2006), group cohesion is not a static state, but instead a 'process of solidarity that members earn through the risks they take with one another' (p. 152). Further, they explain that as a climate of trust is gradually created, members' willingness to take risks will increase the likelihood that others will do the same. In AT the role of the small group is critical. These experiences serve as turning points in establishing increasingly greater degrees of trust and therefore can often springboard other group members level of readiness for challenge and change.

The Chaos State

The psychology of chaos and its relevance for the practice of psychotherapy has been articulated most notably through the work of and Mahoney and Moes (1998). Crisis, from the Greek krisis, means a turning point or time of decision. Thus, a crisis is an opportunity for something new to emerge. Mahoney (2003) explains when working with clients in the chaos state it is critical to communicate empathy and understanding for the importance of disequilibrium for potential breakthroughs versus merely breakdowns. In light of integral theory, adventure therapists and group members are crucially interlocked systems as they serve as a gravitational force attracting those whom are emerging from the chaos point towards transformation as opposed to dissolution. Thus, the chaos state also suggests that AT participants will likely undergo a period of state regression before reorganization occurs. Managing this process warrants further investigation and training as it is crucial that adventure therapists be cognizant of this stage, which may be very 'healthy' and preclude a major breakthrough.

The following narrative is from one of the author's journal following a participant's experience of 'crisis':

> The 15 year old appeared very tense. The others in his group had already balanced their way along the log that provided the only way of crossing the stream. But he was 'different' – having been born with no feet and only one hand, he was the 'crippled kid.' We all waited. Some shouted words of encouragement and others just held their hands in anxious expectation. For the past three days he had seem to have gone out of his

> way to show his unhappiness with the entire trip. In turn, he had been chided for having brought along his I-Pod. Having had it removed only upped his feelings of being thoroughly pissed off. Now he was being asked to cross this. What would be the repercussions if he fell? On –on-slowly-stop, a slight stumble, now a lurch – he had done it! All at once the collective tension broke into cheers and hugs. Later around the campfire our new hero's tale was told over and over. It began to take on an almost Homeric life of its own and began to be owned by everyone there. Indeed it was a pivotal event that allowed others to partake of a new identity and more courage collective 'self'.

Witnessing the instability of the chaos state and the appearance of recovery, on the part of the teenage boy was a catalyst for others to let go in turn. But what about the process of reorganization? In terms of integral theory, nature is not just a backdrop to AT, but is a connected larger 'holon' that embraces the individual and group system. In this way, the reorganization of both the smaller individual and group systems are facilitated by the support of the AT practitioner as well as the larger biophysical systems of nature in which these experiences are given context.

Nature as Partner in AT

'In wildness is the preservation of the world' (Thoreau, Walking, 1862, cited in Nash, 1979).

In recent years, there has been increasing evidence suggesting that the natural world can act as a powerful forum for healing—for all of us—and in particular, in the therapy of individuals with physical and psychological challenges. The rationale for this is underscored by integral systems theory, which views humans and their social and biophysical environments as comprising inextricably connected and interdependent wholes. For example, just as a grizzly bear cannot be separated from its larger context—metaphorically it is 5% claws, teeth, fur, and bone and 95% forest, salmon rivers, ocean beach, and alpine meadow—so too, we are very much emergent properties comprising both biophysical and societal contexts. Upon commencing AT in wild nature, most clients are still in the metaphorically 95% habituated urban context. Placing them in a very different environmental and cultural context becomes a key element in their disequilibrium and eventual reorganization process.

All human systems are open, having the potential to adapt and reorganize with respect to the larger environment. There is now mounting evidence that supports the thesis that natural environments in themselves are contexts for healing and potential therapeutic transformation. The interest in this thesis is becoming more apparent in psychological treatment literature. For example, Berger and McLeod (2006) suggest that nature is more than just a setting but can be an active catalyst and co-facilitator during therapeutic transformation.

These findings are echoed in the Scandinavian literature of 'friluftsliv' or 'free air life' which shows that human internal rhythms and cycles begin to mirror natural cycles after periods spent in wilderness (Gelter, 2000). In turn, studies by Taylor and her colleagues (2001) at the University of Illinois have confirmed that contact with nature supports attention functioning in children, while an array of other studies suggest that contact with nature has beneficial impacts on both adults as well as children with respect to a range of physical and psychological indices (e.g., Frumkin & Louv, 2009).

Currently, most depictions of AT do not consider our connection with nature nor the role it plays in the therapeutic process. In addition to the facilitator-initiated 'reflective debrief' session, the research of both Trace (2002) and Nicholls and Gray (2007) suggest that allowing participants quiet time to engage in 'mindfulness' of their own thoughts and sensations and just experiencing nature without focus may be a vital and underutilized component of processing and integrating change following disequilibrium. There is little doubt that incorporating nature into the client-therapist-environment mix has numerous benefits, although current empirical efforts to understand these relationships seem to result in more questions than answers (Harper, 2009). Consequently, more studies need to take place as to how nature can be most effectively utilized in the AT context.

THE AT PROCESS

In light of our discussion regarding the implications for AT of both integral systems theory and the human-nature connection, we propose a model to map out this process in Figure 2.

1. Accumulation phase

The self-system is already encountering limits in its ability to maintain balance given its individual and collective social realities.

2. Novel experience

The introduction of manageable novelties is the basis for all therapeutic change. These might be novel social and environmental contexts.

3. Disequilibrium (The decision window or edge)

The demands of the situation faced are too much for the current self-system. At this point the self-system's capacity to maintain its configuration in light of the novelties require it to enter into a period of collapse-regression, also known as 'springboard downward.' Facilitators of the AT experience aim to compel the participant into a state of imbalance. The need for support is critical here as the fragile self-system can bifurcate – sometimes referred to as the 'springboard effect'.

4. The Between – falling into a hole (Springboard down)

The self-system, being forced to collapse, is now at a critical juncture. Its reorganization is dependent upon its level of individual resilience as well as the support of the peers, facilitators, and the ability of the participant to access the transformative potential of nature.

5. New Level of complexity phase (reorganization/ transcendence springboard up)

The reconfigured self-system has potentially experienced new ways for dealing with the stresses that helped to lead to its collapse. It has become more complex with a greater degree of differentiation. There is an opportunity for a new level of dynamic homeostasis and the reorganization of existing ideas and information. Conversely, self-stabilization forces may be too strong to allow for change.

Afterwards, the world and self-system may be experienced in a slightly different way. For many clients this will be a transitory 'state' experience that is contingent upon this particular context. Upon arriving home, the negative feedback from habituated patterns of living and previous social relationships, commonly force the client into entrenched patterns. For the reorganization state to be stabilized, it may take a four-quadrant approach over an extended period of time. Lack of this integrated approach has been recognized as an issue in wilderness AT practice (Harper & Russell, 2008). Broader interventions including the family, community and other systems of influence are required.

Figure 2. The adventure therapy process

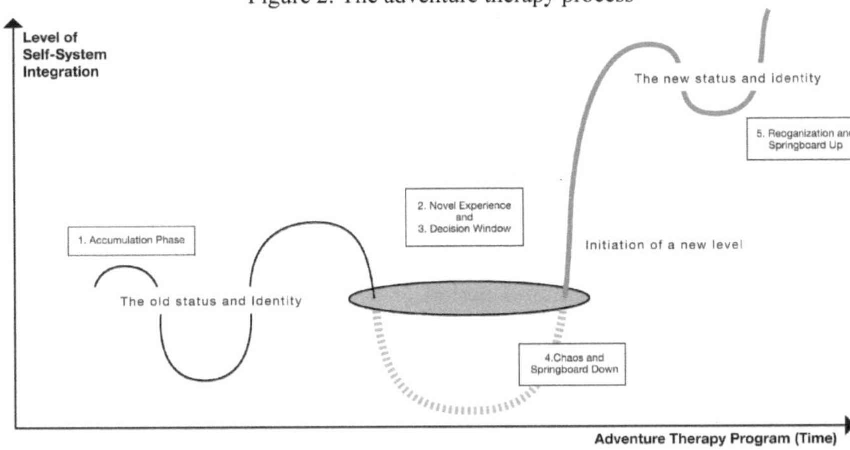

Conclusion

Currently a fragmentation in ideas exists regarding understanding psychological wellness and preferred routes to healing. This is evident in current adventure therapy literature, where unique combinations of experiential learning, challenge activities, novel experiences, group work, and other psychological theories are often used to account for positive outcomes and to explain mechanisms for change. Rarely, is contact with wild nature included as an important variable associated with positive outcomes and change. Recent research in integral systems theory demonstrates the profound impact of the larger social and biophysical contexts, suggesting AT practitioners consider the following questions:

a) How can adventure therapists effectively midwife clients through the chaos state?
b) What role does nature play in self-stabilization?
c) To what extent is the wilderness experience itself a powerful force for reorganization or transcendence?
d) To what extent have the 'quadrants' of the integral approach been investigated in respect to each AT participant?

Further, facilitators cannot consider themselves isolated from this process. Gass (1993) and Norris (2009) have pointed out the importance of the change agents in AT, as they need to possess specific skill sets in the areas of therapeutic change as well as adventure pursuits. Having an appreciation and understanding of the importance of chaos in a person's change process is invaluable. Recognizing the self as an open system requires an understanding that therapists themselves will undergo change as a result of changes in people and contexts around them. In agreement with Mahoney (2003), adventure therapists facilitate change by being open to change themselves. In light of the aforementioned implications, how do we reassess the role of the AT practitioner both as a subject and agent of change?

When we recognize that all systems are open, we are compelled to recognize the importance of nature. How willing are conventional therapists, and even office-based ecopsychologists, to venture beyond the walls of their office and encounter the potential for chaos? As we know, wildness is the realm of the unpredictable and loss of control. It is also the primordial and creative force of the universe that allows for both destruction and rebirth.

References

Bandoroff, S., & Scherer, D.G. (1994). Wilderness family therapy: An innovative treatment approach for problem youth. *Journal of Child and Family Studies, 3(*2), 175-191.

Barber, K. (Ed.) (1998). *The Canadian Oxford Dictionary.* Toronto: Oxford University Press.

Bateson, G. (1972). *Steps towards an ecology of mind.* San Francisco: Chandler Publishing.

Berger, R. & McLeod, J. (2006). Incorporating nature into therapy: A framework for practice. *Journal of Systemic Therapies, 25*(2), 80–94.

Beringer, A. (2004). Toward an ecological paradigm in adventure programming. *Journal of Experiential Education, 27*(1), 51-66.

Bertalanffy, L. V. (1968). *General systems theory: Foundations, development, applications.* New York: George Braziller, Inc.

Corey, M. S. & Corey, G. (2006). *Process and Practice of Groups*. Belmont, CA: Thomson Books.

Crisp, S. (1998). International models of best practices in wilderness and adventure therapy. In C. Itin (Ed.), *Exploring boundaries of adventure therapy,* (pp. 56–74). Boulder, CO: Association for Experiential Education.

Davis, B. (2000). *A body of writing, 1990-1999*. Walnut Creek: Alta Mira Press.

Davis-Berman, J., Berman, D.S., & Capone, L. (1994). Therapeutic wilderness programs: A national survey. *Journal of Experiential Education, 17*(2), 49-53.

Esbjorn-Hargens, S., & Zimmerman, M. (2009). *Integral ecology: Uniting multiple perspectives in a natural world.* Boston: Integral Books.

Frumkin, H. & Louv, R. (2009). The powerful link between conserving land and preserving health. In A. Drengson & D. Taylor (Eds.), *Wild foresting: Practicing nature's wisdom* (pp. 161-164). Gabriola Island, BC: New Society Publishers.

Gass, M. (1993). The foundations of adventure therapy. In M. Gass (Ed.), *Adventure therapy: Therapeutic application of adventure programming* (pp.123-139). Boulder, CO: Association for Experiential Education.

Gelter, H. (2000). Friluftsliv: The Scandinavian philosophy of outdoor life. *Canadian Journal of Environmental Education, 5,* 77-90.

Greenway, R. (1995). The wilderness effect and ecopsychology. In T. Roszak, M. E. Gomes & A. D. Kanner (Eds.), *Ecopsychology: Restoring the earth, healing the mind* (pp. 122-135). Berkeley, CA: Sierra Club.

Harper, N. J. (2009). The relationship of therapeutic alliance to outcome in wilderness treatment. *Journal of Adventure Education and Outdoor Learning, 9*(1), 45-59.

Harper, N. J., & Russell, K. C. (2008). Family involvement and outcome in adolescent wilderness treatment: A mixed-methods evaluation. *International Journal of Child and Family Welfare, 1*, 19-36.

Henderson, B. (1999). The place of deep ecology in adventure education. In J. C. Miles & S. Priest (Eds.), *Adventure programming* (2 ed.) (pp. 439-444). State College, PA: Venture.

Koestler, A. (1967). *Ghost in the machine.* London: Arkana.

Laszlo, E. (1996). *The systems view of the world: A holistic vision for our time.* Cresskill, NJ: Hampton.

Mahoney, M. (2003). *Constructive psychotherapy: A practical guide.* New York: Guilford Press.

Mahoney, M., & Moes, A. J. (1998). Complexity and psychotherapy: Promising dialogues and practical issues. In F. Masterpasqua & P. Perna (Eds.), *The psychological meaning of chaosTranslating theory into practice* (pp. 177-198). New York: American Psychological Association.

Marquis, A. (2008). *The integral intake: A guide to comprehensive idiographic assessment in integral psychotherapy.* New York: Routledge.

Miles, J. C. (1987). Wilderness as healing place. *Journal of Experiential Education,* 10(3), 4-10.

Muir, J. (1996). My first summer in the Sierra. In G. White (Ed.). J*ohn Muir: The wilderness journeys* (p. 91). Edinburgh: Cannongate Classic Books.

Naess, A. (2008). Self-Realization: An ecological approach to being in the world. In A. Drengson and B. Devall (Eds.), *The ecology of wisdom: Writings by Arne Naess* (pp. 81-98). Berkley: Counterpoint.

Nash, R. (1979). *Wilderness and the American Mind.* New Haven: Yale University Press.

Nicholls, V. & Gray, T. (2007). The role of stillness and quiet when developing human/nature relationships. *Australian Journal of Outdoor Education, 11*(1), 32-43.

Norris, J. (2009). *Devoured by a mountain lion: Original nature and the social ecology of adventure therapy.* Keynote lecture at the 5th International Adventure Therapy Conference. September 5th-11th, 2009. Edinburgh, Scotland.

Ray, P. H., & Anderson, S. R. (2000). *Cultural creatives.* New York, NY: Three Rivers Press.

Sato, T. (2003a). *Rhythm, relationships and transcendence: Patterns in the complex web of life.* New York: Writers Club Press.

Sato, T. (2003b). *The ever-transcending spirit: The psychology of human relationships, consciousness, and development.* New York: iUniverse, Inc.

Taylor, A.F., Kuo, F.E., & Sullivan, W.C. (2001). Coping with ADD: The surprising connection to green play settings. *Environment and Behavior, 33*(1), 54-77.

Taylor, A. M. (1999). Time –space-techniques: The evolution of societal systems and worldviews. *World Futures: The Journal of General Evolution,* 54(1), 21-102.

Taylor, A. M. (2001). Ken Wilber's A theory of everything: Some societal and political implications. *World Futures: The Journal of General Evolution, 57,* 213-237.

Taylor, D.M. (1991). Nature as a reflection of self and society. *International Bulletin of Morita Therapy, 4(*1,2), 47-52.

Trace, N. (2002). Adventure therapy as intentional self-recreation in a novel context. *B.C. Counsellor, 25*(1), 91-118.

Wilber, K. (1996). *A Brief History of Everything.* Boston: Shambhala.

Wilber, K. (2001). *Sex, ecology and spirituality: The evolution of spirit.* Boston: Shambhala.

**Ecopsychology has been questioned in the past for its lack of practical guidelines. This appears to be changing with the release of the recent anthology, Ecotherapy: Healing with Nature in Mind (2009), edited by Linda Buzzell and Craig Chalquist. It is noteworthy that Adventure Therapy, which occurs in a wilderness context, is perhaps one of the best articulations of ecotherapy as an application of ecopsychology. Usually referred to as Wilderness Adventure Therapy, there currently exists a large body of research regarding the use of wilderness environments in terms of therapeutic change (e.g., Bandoroff & Scherer, 1994; Crisp, 1998, Davis-Berman et al. 1994. Harper, 2009).*

**Integral systems theory, although largely attribut3ed to the works of Ken Wilber (2001), has also been used in a number of different ways by such scholars as Haridas Chaudhuri and Ervin Laszlo. In this article, we draw on the works of Wilber (2001), Laszlo (1996) and Mahoney (2003) to articulate our own synthesis of ideas in light of Adventure Therapy.*

CHAPTER 25

Naturally Mindful: Using Mindfulness-based Approaches in Adventure Therapy - A Deeper More Sustainable Approach

Stephen Johnson

> *Go climb the mountains and get their glad tidings. Nature's peace will flow into you as sunshine flows into trees. The winds will blow their own freshness into you and the storms their energy. While cares will drop off like autumn leaves.*
>
> \- John Muir, Environmentalist 1838-1914

INTRODUCTION

Mindfulness based (MB) approaches are gaining wider recognition in physical, mental and emotional healthcare provision. Programmes usually range from stand-alone Mindfulness-based stress reduction (MBSR) programmes (Kabatt-Zinn 1990) to combination mindfulness and CBT programmes (Segal et al 2002). These Mindfulness Based CBT approaches are included within the treatment guidelines set by the UK National Institute for Health and Clinical Excellence (NICE 2007) for those patients identified as currently well but with a history of three or more depressive episodes. More recently though mindfulness based approaches and techniques have been included in a wide range of other activities and provision for a more diverse client base.

In an outdoor therapeutic context, mindfulness practices have a key role in establishing interconnectedness with surroundings, people, and nature as well as providing a space for examining thoughts and feelings, for deeper reflection. The conference workshop stressed the importance of personal mindfulness practices and their application in professional and daily life. Through using mindfulness, participants develop their own connection with the natural environment, enhance the experience of their clients and through recognition of interconnectedness develop a more sustainable and environmentally aware approach to the outdoors.

The author has been using these MB approaches with a variety of clients from those with chronic illnesses and pain conditions through to persistent young offenders, incorporating them into activities ranging from rock climbing to the design of spaces for relaxation and contemplation. This paper introduces participants to the broad field of Mindfulness Based Approaches, their source, development and practice, from dealing with behavioural issues to helping people with chronic illness and stress.

Nearly a hundred years ago, Professor J. Arthur Thomson gave the keynote address to the 1914 Annual meeting of the British Medical Association. It was titled "Vis Medicatrix Naturae" or the 'Healing Power of Nature'(Thompson 1914). He opened saying:

> What then do I mean by the healing power of nature? I mean to refer to the way in which Nature ministers to our minds, all more or less diseased by the rush and racket of civilisation, and helps to steady and enrich our lives.

And he went further saying:

> That the healing power of nature is also that associated with *mindful* contact with the animate and inanimate natural portions of the outdoor environment.

It is this 'mindful contact with the outdoor environment' that this paper discusses, including how we can use Mindfulness Based Approaches in Adventure Therapy, to deepen our personal practice and encourage our clients to do the same.

The Negative Impact of Our Disconnection from Nature

Though we know it is important to spend time outdoors, society is more focused on technology, social media and other ways of escaping. Yet how can these technological fixes really compare with the peace of a mountain hike, or the thrill of seeing a kingfisher as you paddle past? Being in nature can contribute to physical, emotional and mental well-being, states, far more than technology, which is essential to the growing epidemics of depression, obesity, diabetes and coronary heart disease.

In fact these NCDs (non-communicable diseases) are the leading cause of death in the world today and are forecasted to have risen by 17% between 2004 and 2015 (WHO 2009). This rise can be seen as demonstrating the mismatch between the way we live and the way our bodies are designed to work, the limits on our capacity to respond and adapt to our modern lifestyles. Yet WHO recommendations on lifestyle changes suggest that 80% of deaths from these causes are preventable, and that lifestyle improvements could have resulted in saving 36M deaths worldwide by 2015. Unfortunately the evidence is that the suggested minimum year on year improvement of just 2% has not happened and the mismatch continues (WHO 2009b).

Some argue that we are trapped in an addictive process where we feel increasingly threatened by nature and more comfortable with our insulated homes and use of technology, with the result that our society is stressed out, overweight, out of shape, depressed, spiritually hungry and suffering from all sorts of disorders (Cohen 2003). That some seek quick fixes in the form of antidepressants, miracle drugs, diet milkshakes, plastic surgery, or temporary relief in the form of smoking, alcohol and / or drugs is undeniable.

While questioning the way we operate from a materialistic, self-centred and disconnected view (MacKinnon 2012) others describe this increased alienation by coining terms such as "nature-deficit disorder." The absence of connectedness and awareness of nature results from fixation on artificial entertainment rather than natural wonders (Louv 2006). Those who are obsessed with computer games or drive by car from activity to activity, miss the restorative effects which come with the nimbler bodies, broader minds and sharper senses that are developed during random running-around in everyday urban existence.

Yet it is also clear that emotional attachment to our natural environment creates more self-awareness, a greater appreciation and valuing of interconnectedness with others, including non-human species and so leads to more sustainable, pro-environmental behaviours (Gosling & Williams 2010). This can be seen in other than western cultures where we can find those that have a greater understanding of nature, a closer relationship to it and through this stronger communities, where the human mind does not exist in separation from the natural world and that our mental well-being essentially depends on our ability to develop a “mature” relationship with our natural surroundings. This relationship is further explained by studies showing that an inspirational place can inspire a person’s life (O’Brien & Kudaibergenova 2012) which can in turn lead to inspiration for a wider community (Urmanbetova & Abdrasulov 2009). This inspiration could also provide a partial answer to crises we face relating to climate and our environment. Lessons learned from indigenous communities are showing us how to deepen the relationship between our environment and physical wellbeing and setting our mental states in an ecological context through the use of ecopsychological approaches (Kampfhammer 2012).

So as outdoor and adventure therapists can we contribute not only to mental health but to a more holistic, whole body approach to health, one that will also encourage a connection between improving personal health and that of communities and our environment? How can we encourage people to look at the spectacular scenery rising above them and see mountains neither daunting nor unfamiliar? How can we encourage them to build their own connections, and how as therapists would we know when they have? It is this building of connections through mindfulness practice that is discussed here.

Mindfulness and Connecting with Nature

First though, what do we mean by mindfulness, how and why incorporate it into our practice? Although emanating from a Buddhist tradition more than 2500 years old, mindfulness has been influenced by other contemplative schools, including Christianity, Islam and Taoism. In the context of outdoor-based practices there is also a strong affinity to aboriginal, and other traditional cultures that cultivate a deep connection with the earth, nature and all aspects of our wider environment. The key is what mindfulness is and how it helps.

Those working in mainstream healthcare settings may recognise that there has been tremendous growth in therapies linking to mindfulness such as Mindfulness Based Cognitive Therapy (MBCT), Mindfulness Based Stress Reduction (MBSR), Mindfulness Based Chronic Pain Management even Mindful Leadership. But for others it may have little meaning, in fact in some cultures there is no word for mind or mindfulness and certainly it is not a word that we may frequently use with our clients.

Working with others, introducing them to mindfulness it can be easier to start with its perceived opposite, 'Mindlessness'. This word which may immediately conjure up images of violence, bad behaviour, unthinking, uncaring and we can see all of these in the outdoors, not necessarily violence, though damage to wilderness is this, but about our failure to protect the environment, to care for our surroundings. Following this as an 'environmental theme of today' how as outdoor and therapy professionals can we teach this care, can and do we exemplify it in our own behaviour?

So whether it is mindfulness as 'moment by moment non-judgemental awareness' (Kabat-Zinn 1990), Goldstein's 'very precise awareness infused with equanimity', or simply a phrase I often use with clients, 'engagement without entanglement', it is here that mindfulness starts this moment by moment awareness, of ourselves, of others, of our environment, our responsibilities, actions and consequences. Not necessarily sitting quietly or being deep in thought though these may obviously be helpful. Importantly it is how we make and how we demonstrate our own connections, our own awareness, including awareness of ourselves and how we enthuse those we work with to do the same.

It may be in the way Goethe taught 200 years ago (Brook 1998), that we, and others, learn to appreciate our landscape by:

- Observing with patience and rigour
- Deepening our sense of wonder of the world
- Using sensual and emotional awareness to experience phenomena as fully as possible
- Attending to connections between phenomena the concept of interconnectedness

We all use activities outdoors to create experiences, give opportunities for activity, thought and reflection but how do we take someone from gaining a skill to developing a connection that will last, one that will influence behaviour, be transformative. When we're leading groups, how often do we give people time to appreciate the view? How often do we stop and stare, especially at scenes that can have an impact? How often are we mindful of our own impact on others, the impression we give when we meet them, how our own feelings and emotions influence our behaviour?

We can look at groups undertaking activities and wonder how we move from the obvious benefits such as skill development, confidence and teamwork to the less obvious but potentially life long connections that will influence their health, their lives and that of the environment we are all part of. What is it that gives the young girl a connection that she takes into adult hood and helps her develop trail running as a means of coping with depressive states rather than excessive diet, drink or drugs?

Or the young man whose connection with the mountains established through a climbing programme leads to coping with anxiety disorder through participating in mountain marathons? What helps turn a troubled teenager with ADHD and consequently few school qualifications into a successful athlete, outdoor instructor and consistently positive adult role model?

The provocative theory "cognitive biophilia" suggested that we use images and symbols of nature to aid communication and this helps us understand thoughts, feelings and emotions, our own and those of others (Lawrence 1993). For children, nature is the richest, most detailed, and most readily available informational context they are ever likely to encounter. Louise Chawla reported that adults almost universally cite the outdoors as one of the most significant settings of their childhood (Chawla 2003). She suggests that adults use these recollections of nature for what the poet Wordsworth called "tranquil restoration,"

Coming back to the 'environmental theme' we have the statement in Roszak's seminal work 'Ecopsychology' that feeling a sense of belonging to the broader natural community may be a prerequisite for increasing environmental protection. He goes on to argue that fostering ecological behaviour through expanding our sense of self is key because 'if the self is expanded to include the natural world, behaviour leading to destruction of this world will be experienced as self-destruction' (Roszak, Gomes, & Kanner 1995).

So we can examine how mindfulness, awareness of self and others, in and of nature will foster individual and community health and well-being and from that how adopting mindfulness practices can enhance the work we're already doing.

METHODS

My work is based on mindfulness teaching and practice with groups, with teachers, therapists and others. Traditionally mindfulness is often taught in 8-week blocks, based in a room full of mats, chairs and cushions. The programmes consist of weekly sessions of 2.5 hours where participants are taught a variety of meditation practices, awareness exercises and techniques such as pacing and mindful movement. A common requirement of those seeking to teach mindfulness is that they do participate in these 8-week programmes.

In taking Mindfulness into an outdoor activity and adventure therapy arena these traditional practices may still be taught, however experience shows that it is necessary to adapt the settings used and the practices themselves to ensure they are relevant to those taking part and to the overall aim of enhancing activities, establishing and deepening connections and contributing to individual wellbeing. This adaptation includes developing new programmes designed to provide shorter or more intensive experiences. Our core programmes therefore consist of a range of activities including:

- Breath awareness
- Mindful Movement including tai chi and chi gung

- Meditation practices including Body Scan, Mindfulness of Breathing, Kindly Awareness
- Mindful Walking
- Sense awareness practices including meditations on individual senses
- Nature awareness
- Body Awareness
- Journeying, especially travelling light
- Solo experiences
- Journaling including use of social media, video, photography, poetry and art
- Bushcraft (for impromptu shelters).

The sessions start with initial meetings, not motivational interviews, but the opportunity to discover more about the individual and perceptions of the programme. These early meetings are followed by experiential sessions as many will never have tried a particular activity. The aim is to identify core activities the participant wants to engage with and a number of supporting ones that can be developed over time. Participants quickly gain responsibility for their own programme, deciding its pace and direction. To date activities have ranged from bird watching in hides through to multi day adventure races, all activities chosen and engaged in by clients.

One element common to all mindfulness programmes is the outdoor instructor or therapist undertakes the same activity. We work together, report in together, share experiences, spend time on solo, discuss shared learning. There is no 'them and us', no white coat / patient, no instructor / student divide, simply all participating with the therapist as guide.

Evaluating the impact of methods including assessing pre and post experience takes places throughout the programmes using well tried and validated tools such as the sensual awareness inventory (slightly adapted), the five facets of mindfulness questionnaire and the connectedness to nature scale.

The sense awareness inventory (Burns 1998) provides a good starting place as it encourages the individual to reflect on their experience. It allows them to highlight aspects of awareness, a particular sense, that could be worked with in more detail and it allows questions such as:

> If these are things that make you feel good how often do you do experience them' and 'what stops you?

These questions are especially relevant when our results show that most are free (hence the slight modification removing the 'activity' column of Burns' original as it was found items in the activity column often involved cost, which may limit the engagement of certain client groups).

Table 1. Mindfulness Inventory

Sight	***Sound***	***Taste***	***Touch***	***Smell***
Sunshine	Waves crashing	Ice cream	Polished wood	Airports
Xmas trees	Laughing	Fruit cake	Pile of leaves	Seaside
waves	Drums	Bacon sandwich	Hugs	Baking
smiles	Rushing river	curry	Rock	Frying
Open fire	seagulls	cheese	Fur	Fresh grass
Falling leaves	Birds singing	dumplings	Icy cold	Salt & vinegar
hawks	Wind	oranges	Wind	Wood burning
Dog wagging tail	Crackling fire	pizza	Warm fleece	
Snowing		coriander	Hot bath	
Breath freezing			Girl friend	

This inventory is used before, during and after a programme and participants are encouraged to use it with family, partners and friends during and after the intervention. Notice that many of the items listed are free.

The 5 facets of mindfulness questionnaire (Baer 2008) was chosen because of its effectiveness across a wider variety of experiences and especially considering pre and post programme issues of apparent mindfulness and what the author refers to as 'experiential mindfulness' i.e. A response once you've got more experience of what mindfulness is and how it manifests itself in your daily life. The questionnaire consists of 39 questions (Likert marked), covering:

- Describing
- Acting with awareness
- Observing
- Non-reactivity to inner experience
- Non-judging of inner experience

Table 2. Pre and Post intervention responses to 5 facet of mindfulness questionnaire

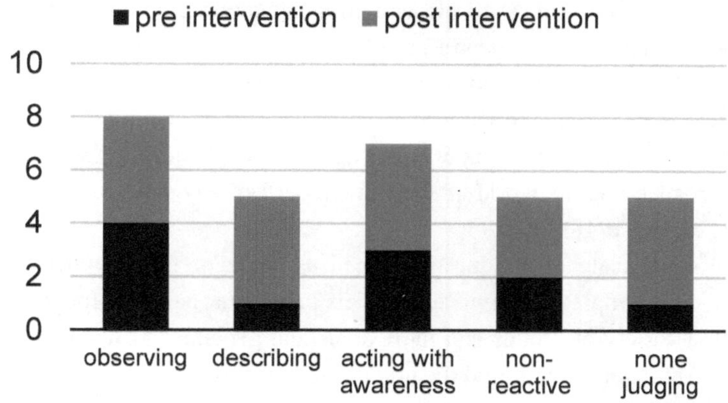

It is ideal for use in nature, the outdoors, as it almost directly follows Goethe's instructions detailed above. It helps people understand, helps emphasise that connections don't need to be about big rugged environments, can simply be noticing bushes and birds in the park.

So far the results of pilot programmes are promising. They show that across a range of activities and programmes we see improvement in all aspects:

- Observing (though here we have the previously mentioned experiential issues of thinking you are mindful or observant because you're not sure what it actually means to be so)
- Describing being able to express thoughts, feelings and emotions more effectively
- Acting with awareness understanding the impact on self, others and the environment of personal actions
- Being able to be less reactive, having the ability to choose how to respond rather than just jumping in
- Being less judgemental, less blaming of themselves and others

As the chart shows, significant improvements are seen in an individual's ability to be observant of life around them, describe their experiences, to act with more awareness of their own impact on self and others and to be less judgemental of themselves. These points can be critical for those with chronic conditions, physical and psychological, helping to remove a 'why me'? or 'it's my fault' reaction. In fact, a key aspect of the whole mindfulness programme is it encourages, allows time for a less reactive, more responsive process. These improvements are the subject of a longitudinal study that will help highlight the statistical significance of the results and influence future programme design.

The connectedness to nature scale (CNS) (Mayer & Frantz 2004) has also been found useful as it is designed to illustrate an individual's experiential connection to nature and how it influences behaviour. Its development follows the sagacious contention more than 60 years ago that people need to feel they are part of the broader natural world if they are to effectively address environmental issues (Leopold 1948).

The CNS scale of 15 questions such as some of those shown here, was chosen as it is simple to administer, predicts behaviour, has been found reliable in use with a variety of groups and individuals and generates provoking discussion relating to thought process, and the mindfulness of actions and consequences.

Sample Questions (again using Likert scale, some are reverse marked):

- I often feel disconnected from nature
- I think of the natural world as a community to which I belong
- I have a deep understanding of how my actions affect the natural world
- My personal welfare is independent of the welfare of the natural world
- When I think of my place on Earth, I consider myself to be a top member of a hierarchy that exists in nature.

The CNS has also shows evidence of value orientation, ecological behaviour, perspective-taking, even identity as an prospective environmentalist and it demonstrates links between personal well-being and feeling connected to nature.

CONCLUSION

In addition to the specific benefits seen with programme participants, a further perspective of this work is that if people feel connected to nature, then they will be more likely to engage with it, to use their connection as part of a 'self-management for health and well-being programme' that doesn't feel as restrictive or controlling as more practitioner led initiatives. In engaging with nature they are less likely to harm it, for harming it would in effect be harming their very self.

However it is worth bearing in mind that many people knowingly engage in self-destructive behaviours e.g. They may believe smoking helps them deal with stress rather than understanding or acknowledging the detrimental and addictive effects of nicotine and smoke. An improved connection to nature may help if it is as readily accessible as a packet of cigarettes, which appreciating a good view maybe, yet if the connection is only through a long solo journey then this will not have an impact on the individual's daily lifestyle.

There is also growing consensus that our modern lifestyles including consumptive behaviours, need to change profoundly to avoid the epidemic of non-communicable diseases mentioned in the introduction. Mindfulness in and of nature, something we are part of rather than separate from, can play a key role in raising the awareness and ability of individuals to create a healthy and an environmentally sustainable society.

For outdoor and adventure therapists practicing mindfulness deepens our own awareness of self and the world around us while enabling us to engage our clients in ways likely to have more prolonged and profound effects. A sustainable solution for them and the environment we are all part of.

REFERENCES

Baer, R.A. et al (2008) *Construct validity of the five facet mindfulness questionnaire in meditating and non-meditating samples.* Assessment 2008; 15; 329 originally published online Feb 29, 2008

Brook, I (1998) Goethean Science as a way to read landscape; *Landscape research,* Vol 23, No. 1

Burns, G.W. (1998) Nature Guided Therapy; Brunner Mazel, Philadelphia

Chawla, L. (2003) Children, Youth and Environments; Vol 13, No.1 (Spring 2003)

Cohen, M. (2003) *The Web of Life Imperative*, Trafford Press, Canada

Gosling, E. & Williams, K.J.H (2010) Connectedness to nature, place attachment and conservation behaviour: Testing connectedness theory among farmers: *Journal of Environmental Psychology*, Vol 30, No. 3, pp 298-304

Kabat-Zinn, J. (1990) *Full Catastrophe Living: Using the Wisdom of your body and mind to face stress pain and illness;* Dell Publishing, New York, USA

Kapfhammer, W. (2012) *Nature, Crisis and Reform among the Sateré-Mawé*; Goethe Institute, Marburg

Lawrence, E.A. (1993) Animal Symbolism as Cognitive Biophilia in Kellert, S.R. & Wilson, E.O. (1993) *The Biophilia Hypothesis*; Island press, Washington D.C.

Leopold, A. (1949). *A Sand County Almanac*: With essays on conservation from Round River. New York: Ballantine Books.

Louv R. (2006) *Last Child in the Woods*, Algonquin Books, Chapel Hill, U.S.A.

MacKinnon, C. (2012) *Shamanism and Spirituality in Therapeutic Practice*, Singing Dragon, London

Mayer, S.F. & Frantz, C.M (2004) The connectedness to nature scale: A measure of individuals' feeling in community with nature. *Journal of Environmental Psychology* 24, 503 515, Elsevier, London

NICE (2007) *Clinical Guideline 23* (amended) Quick reference guide (amended) Depression: management of depression in primary & secondary care. Issued with amendments April 2007; National Institute for Health & Clinical Excellence, London

O'Brien, V & Kudaibergenova, T (2012) *Land, Culture and Everyday Life in Krygyz Villages;* Visible Voice, Manchester

Roszak T., Gomes M.E., Kanner A.D. (1995) *Ecopsychology, Restoring the Earth, Healing the Mind*, Sierra Club Books, San Francisco, U.S.

Segal, Z.V., Williams, J.M.G., Teasdale, J.D. (2002) *Mindfulness Based Cognitive Therapy for Depression*; Guilford Press, New York

Thompson, J.A. (1914) "*Vis Medicatrix Naturae*" Keynote Address at the Annual Meeting of the British Medical Association, 1914.

Urmanbetova, J.K. & Abdrasulov, C.M. (2009) *Sources and tendencies in the development of Kyrgyz Culture*. Ilim, Bishkek

WHO (2009) *Milestones in Health Promotion: statements from global conferences*. World Health Organisation, Geneva, Switzerland

WHO (2009b) *Interventions on diet and physical activity: what works*: summary report World Health Organisation, Geneva, Switzerland

CHAPTER 26

Adventure Therapy through Existentialism

Alexander Rose

INTRODUCTION

Existentialism is a philosophical current born with Søren Kierkegaard (1813-1855) and developed subsequently, among others, by Friedrich Wilhelm Nietzsche (1844-1900), Martin Heidegger (1889-1976), José Ortega y Gasset (1883-1955), Jean-Paul Sartre (1905-1980) or Albert Camus (1913-1960). This paradigm sets out questions about the nature of the human being and the conditions of his existence (Gonzalo Pardo & Pérez Álvarez, 2007).

In our field, only a few articles link existentialism with Adventure therapy (Adams, n.d.; Glass & Jackson, 2009), and only in one of our major guides. Most of them (Davis-Berman & Berman, 2008; Gass, 1993; Gass, Gillis, & Russell, 2012) do not refer to it, in comparison to approaches like Psychoanalysis, Transpersonal theory, Gestalt, Cognitive-behavioural or Systemic.

Thereby, the main objective of the paper is to present Logotherapy and value its paradigm as an alternative-complementary theoretical frame from which to focus Adventure therapy.

HISTORY OF EXISTENTIALISM

Until the apparition of Existentialism, in the 19th Century, one of the mainstreams of philosophy was to question human's "essence" (what is permanent and immutable). Søren Kierkegaard (1813-1855), was the first philosopher who stated that experience (unique and unrepeatable) was more important, and precedes the essence. Kierkegaard, influenced by Georg Hegel, stated that our life is determined by our actions, and previously, by our choices. Therefore, our elections are crucial in our life. We are completely free to choose, we are self-determinant, and therefore, as if we were on the edge of a precipice, we experience *Angst*, anguish or anxiety in our life.

Martin Heidegger (1889-1976), starting from Kierkegaard's postulates, in order to understand our meaning of life, introduced the concepts *"Da-sein"* (to-be-there, in the world) and "*Geworfenheit*" ("throwness", thrown into the world). Emphasizing that one is destined to be (here and now), helpless, with the only certainty of death, both to the life experiences and at the end of our life (Gallego-Pérez, 2012).

> If I take death into my life, acknowledge it, and face it squarely, I will free myself from the anxiety of death and the pettiness of life and only then will I be free to become myself. (Heidegger, 1962)

So, according to Heidegger (1962), there is no more option than to choose in life: to live towards being (the essential way) or towards the things or having (the superficial way).

Other relevant philosophers that belong to this approach and that developed these early theories, divided in pessimists and optimists, are, on one hand Jean-Paul Sartre (1905-1980) or Albert Camus (1913-1960) that had the anguish view of the theory and, on the other, José Ortega y Gasset (1883-1955) and Gabriel Marcel (1889-1973), with their *ratio-vitalism*, had the positive view of self-determination.

Existential Psychotherapy

Existential psychotherapy is a method of therapy that, according to Yalom (1980) operates on the belief that inner conflict within a person is due to the individual's confrontation with the givens of existence. These givens are: the inevitability of death, freedom and its attendant of responsibility, existential isolation and meaninglessness (Yalom, 1980). Apart from the givens, "the principal common point is that all of them stem from a life issues therapy" (Gonzalo Pardo & Pérez Álvarez, 2007).

So, on one hand, Existentialism has originated specific schools like Viktor Frankl's Logotherapy or Irving Yalom's Existential psychotherapy, and on the other, influenced basic psychological and medical paradigms like Karl Jaspers' or other therapies like Gestalt's theory through Gary Yontef's practice and research (Gonzalo Pardo & Pérez Álvarez, 2007).

The different aims and principal procedures and techniques of these above listed Existential schools are summarized below:

Fig. 1. Adapted from Gonzalo Pardo & Pérez Álvarez (2007)

Existential psycho-therapeutic approach	**Main intervention aims**	**Principal procedures and techniques**
Logotherapy (Frankl)	Self-distancing (stop fighting the symptoms and redirect life to other values) and self-transcendence (stop being self-centred) in order to find meaning of life.	Specific therapy for Noogenic neurosis and unspecific therapy for psychogenic neurosis: Paradoxical intention for self-distancing and De-reflection for self-transcendence. Socratic dialogue.
Existential psychotherapy (Yalom)	Acquisition of strength against the anguish of death, taking responsibility facing liberty, learning about solitude and searching for meaning.	Specific techniques like Disidentification or situational restructuring.
Phenomenological-existential therapy (Gestalt) (Yontef)	Expansion of the field of consciousness (uptake from the environment, self-awareness, responsibility for choices, self-acceptance). Integration of all aspects of oneself for the development of their own abilities.	It is characterized by its emphasis on the experiencing of everything that concerns oneself and on the concentration on here and now.

In García-Alandete & Gallego-Pérez´s (2009) the central points of the existential philosophy influencing psychotherapy (Logotherapy) are:

- Human existence consists of being thrown into the world and confronted with the "nothing" (Sartre, 1945), death (Jaspers 1946; Heidegger, 1962), suffering and nonsense, all these "extreme situations" (Jaspers, 1946), which experience the existence from a ground state of fear (Heidegger, 1962).
- This being thrown into the world naked, into existence, implies freedom as the need to choose, as "condemnation" (Sartre, 1945) which can be fatal, because one may fail or succeed in his decisions. Not to choose is impossible; this is already a choice (Sartre, 1945).
- Along with freedom, responsibility, having to answer for one's own decisions in front of others and towards oneself.

- Election either Anguish or Meaning.

LOGOTHERAPY

Viktor Emil Frankl (1905-1997) was an Austrian Jewish neurologist and psychiatrist. He founded the Third Viennese School of Psychotherapy: the Logotherapy. “Logos” is a Greek word that can be translated as “meaning”, “significance” or “purpose”. Logotherapy focuses on significance of human existence, as well as the search of meaning by men. For Logotherapy, the person is considered as a global being, with a biological, psychological, social and spiritual dimension.

Frankl conceived his theory in close contact to Freud’s Psychoanalysis first and Adler’s Individual Psychology, thereafter, collaborating with both successively, but diverging later from their teachings. The reason was, on one hand, the emphasis of Freud and the Psychoanalysis on the fight of oneself to overcome pulsions (impulses) and, on the other, Adler, with its emphasis on solving the inferiority complex, pouring into the social and needing success and power in order to master it, and therefore the lack of space to decide for oneself (García-Alandete & Gallego-Pérez, 2009).

For Freud, motivation appears from the “will to pleasure“, and for Adler from the Nietzschean “will to power“. For Frankl’s Logotherapy, supported on Kierkegaard’s ideas, in contraposition to the prior theories, our first motivation is the fight for finding meaning to our own life. Therefore, noogene neurosis appears when a lack of meaning exists (Frankl, 1979).

> Frankl has devoted his career to a study of an existential approach to therapy, and has apparently concluded that the lack of meaning is the paramount existential stress. To him, existential neurosis is synonymous with a crisis of meaninglessness. (Yalom, 1980)

Frankl was against the psychologism of this period and rejected determinism defending human freedom and its capacity for self-determination (Frankl, 1979; 2000; 2001).The vision of the human being that distinguishes Frankl's Existential Analysis includes phenomenological-anthropological concepts as freedom, responsibility, the ability to self-distancing and self-transcendence, the unique value of being a person, the unconditionality of the meaning of life, the multidimensionality of the being and consciousness as 'body' of meaning. In Frankl´s words (1979), the man is a being, constitutively conscious of itself, free and responsible. Although there are conditioning factors (biological, psychical, social or spiritual), these are not determinant, with oneself always being able to decide. Thus, Logotherapy is not usually concerned with the past, but with the choices to be made in present and towards future (Frankl, 1979; 2000; 2001).

Psychopathology, under Logotherapy, sets psychological diseases in relation to life problems, being meaninglessness the cause and origin for noogene neurosis, and anxiety-depression, for example, only symptoms. It is that the person stays treating anxiety or depression, and not the problem itself (Frankl, 1992). Two basic alterations have been described: augmented self-conscience (hyper-reflexivity) and sense of himself diminished (diminished self-experience) (Gonzalo Pardo & Pérez Álvarez, 2007). The main intervention aims in Logotherapy are self-distancing, accomplished through stopping fighting the symptoms and redirecting life to other values, and self-transcendence, trying to stop being self-centred, in order to find meaning of life (García-Alandete & Gallego-Pérez, 2009).

These objectives are accomplished within specific therapy for Noogenic neurosis and unspecific therapy for psychogenic neurosis. The techniques for working towards resolving psychogenic neurosis are paradoxical intention for self-distancing and de-reflection for self-transcendence. The major tool is, in relation with the patient, Socratic dialogue (García-Alandete & Gallego-Pérez, 2009).

THE USE OF LOGOTHERAPY AS A FRAMEWORK IN ADVENTURE THERAPY WITH ADOLESCENTS

General Considerations

From this paradigm, we deal with patients. This is taken from the Latin present active participle of *patior* ("suffer"): the patient is considered a suffering person. On the other hand, "person" is the product of "what we receive", "what we learn", "what we decide" and "what we project" (Gallego-Pérez, 2012). So, our role as therapists is to try to make aware in our patients that suffering is a partner along our life, and depending how we deal with that we will be complete or not. Therefore, the patient is helped when he manages to be free, and not only when symptoms disappear and he feels good, like in CBT (Gallego-Pérez, 2012).

Adolescence and Logotherapy

Most of the literature of Adventure therapy is related to struggling (and suffering) adolescents (juvenile justice, drug abuse, behavioural problems or others). The period of adolescence can be considered as a vital crisis, occurring changes in their five dimensions: psychobiological, emotional, intellectual, social and transcendental (Papalia, 2005). Logotherapy is a potential frame given that conceives the person as global. Also from the Logotherapeutic paradigm, noogene neurosis appears when meaninglessness occurs. In the existential void proliferate phenomena such as depression, addiction and aggression (Prats Mora, 2001), so common in Adventure therapy clients. This fact and Frankl's assertion that the problem of meaning raised in a radical way can reach subjugate the individual, especially in the period of puberty (Frankl, 1992) make necessary to consider this point of view. In addition, achievement of meaning is a major factor in the construction of identity that corresponds so relevant to adolescence (Gambini & Ronco, 1999).

Adolescence and Choice

Adolescence is the critic period where we settle the learning of the consequences of our elections. From this paradigm, there is always a possibility of choice that is related to freedom and responsibility. Even if there seems to be no freedom, we still can choose our attitude (Frankl, 1979). Using Adam´s words (n.d.), Itin (2005) describes Adventure therapy as one means of confronting clients with their choices. Both paradigms have as an aim to provoke change, but it is Logotherapy that pursues change of attitude. This is one of our major goals: get patients to assume their (free) choices.

Succinctly, Adventure therapy tries to take the client out of his comfort-zone (Gass, 1993) and after a process of debriefing (i.e. using Socratic dialogue), try to enhance personal capabilities in order to create (attitudinal) change. It is our duty as professionals to get our patients reach holistic plenitude, and using as an example a two-axis continuum (fig. 2.) the relationship between challenge and competence needs to be positive. The use of prescript challenge is part of Gass, Gillis, & Russell's (2012) Adventure Therapy definition, but what has to be considered as well is the perception of competence of our patients, closely linked to freedom and responsibility.

Fig. 2. Adapted from Gallego-Pérez (2012).

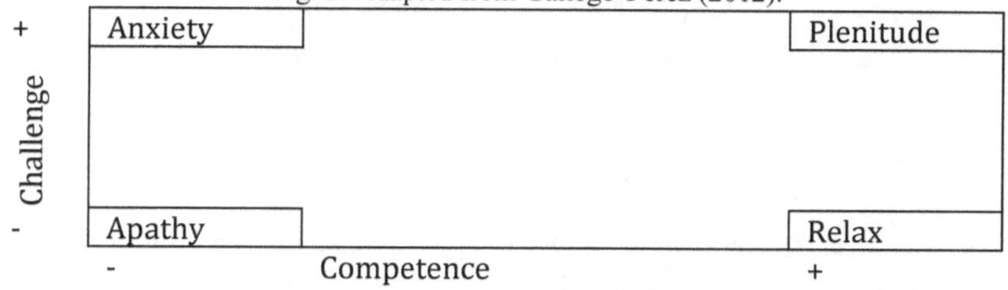

Finiteness of Experience

Helping our patients to understand the finiteness of our provided experiences, will make them focus in "here and now", understanding the responsibility of the election of choices. Many experiences provided from an Adventure or Wilderness Therapy setting can be considered as life changing experiences, and are great opportunities to solve psychic or existential problems, or strengthen prior solutions (Gallego-Pérez, 2012). The concept from physics "Hysteresis", brought to the psychotherapist's argot by Gallego-Pérez (2012) is very helpful to understand this process: a patient changes in an inner level in contact with the experience, similar as ferromagnetic materials do, under influence of an electromagnetic field. There are experiences that change substantially, an irreversible vital learning.

Conclusion

Following Gallego-Pérez (2012) and Gonzalo Pardo & Pérez Álvarez (2007), Logotherapy is said to be propaedeutic both in the fields of research and clinical: the person needs to be considered as a global being, with a biological, psychological, social and spiritual dimension. According also to Glass & Jackson (2009), "using Existentialism as a theoretical basis [...], counsellors emphasize the attainment of a higher self-awareness, authenticity, and the freedom to choose how participants react [...], while encouraging participants to find strength within themselves in order to develop healthy relationships with others. This increased awareness and authenticity is desired so that participants may have a better understanding of purpose or meaning in their lives."

The fundamental aim of this text has been to create, from the beginning, the frame to discuss approaches and paradigms used in our field, in order to value the rich amalgam we develop in therapy and to understand the need to create a "higher" philosophy in which to set our individual interventions.

References

Adams, A. (n.d.). *Existential Psychology How does it Influence Wilderness Therapy*. In http://www.development.tas.gov.au/__data/assets/pdf_fie/0016/4255/00existpsychology.pdf

Davis-Berman, J. & Berman, D. (2008). *The Promise of Wilderness therapy*. Boulder, CO: Association for Experiential Education.

Frankl, V. E. (1979). *El hombre en busca de sentido*. Barcelona: Herder.

Frankl, V. E. (1992). *Psicoanálisis y Existencialismo. De la psicoterapia a la Logoterapia* (5ª reimpresión). México: Fondo de Cultura Económica.

Frankl, V. E. (2000). *En el principio era el sentido. Reflexiones en torno al ser humano*. Barcelona: Paidós.

Frankl, V. E. (2001). *Psicoterapia y existencialismo. Escritos selectos sobre la logoterapia*. Barcelona: Herder.

Gambini, P. & Ronco, A. (1999). *Che senso ha una vita senza amore? Prima applicazione di un test sull'adolescenza*. Attualitá in Logoterapia, 22, 33-44.

García-Alandete, J., Gallego-Pérez, J. F., & Pérez-Delgado, E. (2009). *Sentido de la vida y desesperanza: un estudio empírico*. Univer-sitas Psychologica, 8(2), 447-454.

García-Alandete, J. & Gallego-Pérez, J.F. (2009) (Coord.). *Adversidad, sentido y resiliencia. Logoterapia y afrontamiento en situaciones límite*. Valencia: Edicep.

García-Alandete, J. (2011). *Inteligencia emocional, optimismo y crisis existenciales*. II Congreso de Antropología, psicología y espiritualidad. Ávila: Universidad de la Mística.

Gallego-Pérez, J.F. (2011). *Paradojas existenciales: el vacío fuente de sentido*. II Congreso de Antropología, psicología y espiritualidad. Ávila: Universidad de la Mística.

Gallego-Pérez, J.F. (2012). *Psicopatología Clínica y de la salud en Adultos*. Catholic University of Valencia: Unpublished document.

Gass, M. (1993). *Adventure Therapy: Therapeutic applications of adventure programming*. Dubuque, Iowa: Kend All / Hunt publishing company.

Gass, M. Gillis, H.L. & Russell, K.C. (2012). *Adventure Therapy: Theory, Research, and Practice*. New York: Routledge.

Glass, J. S., & Jackson, J.M. (2009). International Journal for Existential Psychology and Psychotherapy, 2, 1, http://journal.existentialpsychology.org/index.php?journal=ExPsy&page=article&op=view&path%5B%5D=112&path%5B%5D=55

González Pardo, H. & Pérez Álvarez, M. (2007). *La invención de trastornos mentales*. Madrid: Alianza.

Heidegger, M. (1962). *Being and Time*. New York: Harper & Row.

Itin, C. (2005). *Challenge by choice as professional enabling*. Rocky: Newsletter of the Rocky Mountain Region of the Association for Experiential Education, 6(2), 2.

Jaspers, K. (1946). *Psicopatología general*. México DF: Fondo de cultura económica.

Längle, A. (2000). *Viktor Frankl. Una bibliografía*. Barcelona: Herder.

Lukas, E. (2003). *Logoterapia. La búsqueda de sentido*. Barcelona: Paidós.

Papalia, D. (2005). *Psicología del desarrollo*. 9ª edición. Madrid: Ed. Mcgraw-hill.

Pérez Álvarez, M. (2006). *La terapia de conducta de tercera generación*. eduPsykhé, 5, 159-172.

Prats Mora, J.I. (2001). *Logoterapia y adolescencia*. NOUS: Boletín de Logoterapia y Análisis Existencial (5), 35-49.

Sartre, J.P. (1945). *El existencialismo es un humanismo*. Conferencia. http://www.uruguaypiensa.org.uy/imgnoticias/766.pdf

Yalom, I. D. (1980). Existential Psychotherapy. New York: BasicBooks.

Yontef, G. (2002). *The Relational Attitude in Gestalt Therapy Theory and Practice*. International Gestalt Journal 2002, 25/1, 15-34. http://www.igt.psc.br/ojs2/index.php/igtnarede/article/viewFile/1754/2423

EXPLORING

The future is not something we enter. The future is something we create.

-H. Jackson Brown Junior

CHAPTER 27

The Yin Yang of a Wilderness Therapy Experience

Val Nicholls

ABSTRACT

This paper draws on a recent doctoral study that used qualitative methods and a grounded theory research design to explore participants' perspectives of their experience of *Quiet time* within the context of an activity-oriented and challenge-based wilderness therapy program. *Quiet time* is defined as an internal and subjective 'sense' of solitude, independent of a need for physical isolation or communicative separation. The phenomenon of *Quiet time* is described as one way in which participants purposively created opportunity to cope with, savour or process the physical and emotional highs and lows of a wilderness journey.

Participant accounts of some of the short term and longer-term positive impacts of *Quiet time* are identified. The Chinese Tai Chi yin-yang symbol is utilized as a dynamic representation of some of the ways in which the opportunity and experience of *Quiet time* may be appreciated as a natural and significant compliment to the predominately group-focused and activity-orientated approach of a challenge-based wilderness therapy program. The main implication from this research is that the therapeutic potential of challenge-based wilderness therapy programs may be enhanced by promoting opportunities for participant-initiated *Quiet time* through the adoption of an unhurried and process-oriented approach to the wilderness adventure experiences.

INTRODUCTION

Grounded in the philosophy and practices of experiential learning, wilderness therapy programming is increasingly regarded as an effective alternative to more traditional forms of therapy for people identified as 'at risk' or 'vulnerable' (Gass, 1993). Typically, within the context of a small group journeying through remote and natural environments, wilderness therapy utilises adventure activities such as kayaking, caving, abseiling, and bushwalking to promote positive attitudinal and behavioural change. Fundamental to this approach is a philosophy of change grounded in the development of competence and the confronting of internal limits. However, in recent years a number of studies have invited a fresh appraisal of the role of action and challenge in the process of change, and drawn attention to the potential for personal transformation through the experience of relaxation, inactivity and immersion in nature (Leberman & Martin, 2002; Trace, 2004).

This paper reports on findings from a qualitative study that used a grounded theory design that explored concept of *Quiet time* from a participants' perspective. The inspiration for the study derived from the author's personal experience as a facilitator of a challenge-based and activity oriented wilderness therapy programs. Frequent observations of participants indicated that the potential for personal growth and enhanced wellbeing resided not only in the development of competence, the confronting of internal limits and the processing of experience via facilitated group debriefs, but also within experiences of quietude, stillness and silence.

RESEARCH DESIGN

Grounded theory (Strauss & Corbin, 1998) was chosen as an appropriate research design to guide the exploration of participants' experience of relaxed inactivity, stillness and silence. The perceived merit of this decision was based on an understanding that grounded theory is an especially appropriate design in studies in which little previous research has been done (Charmaz, 1995). Its procedures would provide the research with a systematic set of analytic processes to guide the collection, analysis and interpretation of qualitative data in the form of interviews, photographs, journals, field notes and standard program documentation (Creswell, 2005). That grounded theory links well to practice in that it produces theory that is relevant to the context and concerns of practitioners (Locke, 2001).

The Mountain Challenge wilderness therapy program was selected as the site for the study. This program is one of a number of specialist programs offered by

Project Hahn (now known as the Wilderness Program), a Tasmanian-based Government funded provider of wilderness therapy programs. At the time of the study the agency took its name from the founder of the Outward Bound movement, Kurt Hahn, and identified its purpose as promoting personal growth through challenge and adventure.

Sixteen male and two female participants from four Mountain Challenge wilderness therapy programs scheduled between February 2002 and February 2005 participated in the study. All but one of the adult participants came to Mountain Challenge as part of ongoing therapy for drug and/or alcohol addiction. The Mountain Challenge program consisted of a four-day self-sufficient journey that aimed to provide opportunities for participants to experiment with new and positive attitudes and behaviours beyond the support of the rehabilitation centre.

Given that participants' primary focus was the experience of the Mountain Challenge as an adjunct to their ongoing rehabilitation program, it was considered important to minimise the effects of data gathering in the field, and to avoid methods that might engender a sense of surveillance or otherwise interfere with the development of rapport, confidence and trust within the group. Previous experience as a facilitator of the Mountain Challenge showed that as a consequence of illegal behaviour and subsequent interaction with the police force, many participants are familiar with, and distrustful of, methods of observation, interviewing and tape recording. It seemed likely that adopting a participant-observer role could be construed as a form of surveillance or monitoring. With that in mind, a facilitator/researcher role was adopted instead. Guidelines set out by Strauss and Corbin (1990) and Maxwell (1996) to enhance the trustworthiness of the study and to protect from undue bias were adhered to.

Data Collection and Analysis

Semi-structured interviews formed the mainstay of the study, and were scheduled pre and post trip in order to minimise interference with the therapeutic process of the wilderness program. Participants dictated the emotional depth of the interview and were under no obligation to disclose material of a sensitive nature. Interviewees were provided with a transcript of their interview and retained the right to delete any sections they preferred to exclude from the analytic process. Data was also collected in the form of photographs taken by participants, journals, field notes and standard program documentation.

Following the procedures of grounded theory methodology, data collection and analysis occurred in alternating sequences. However, the right to privacy afforded the participants when they left the rehabilitation centre meant that in all but four cases it was not possible to schedule follow up interviews. With this in mind, grounded theory methods were adapted to capitalize on any opportunity to compensate for the unavailability of participants for follow-up interviews. For example, the interview with Charlie (Group 3) was approached with an understanding of emerging categories and concepts, ideas and questions derived from the analysis of interviews with Groups One and Two. Similarly the product of Charlie's interview informed the interview with Mitch (Group 3) and so on. Thus data gathering and analysis occurred in the classic alternating fashion at the micro level within the group and at a macro level between groups. A four phase analytic framework guided the collection and analysis of data. The framework, depicted in Figure 1, derived from a coding paradigm model developed by Strauss and Corbin (1998) and entailed a combination of inductive and deductive categorisation.

Figure 1. The analytic framework for a grounded theory of Quiet time

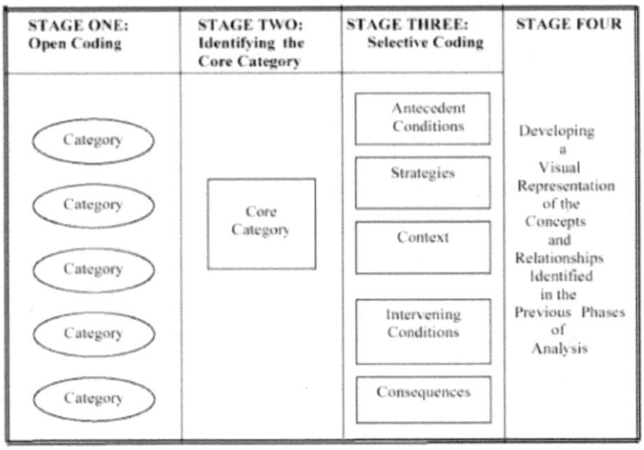

In simple terms, the task at hand during Stage One was to lay the groundwork for subsequent stages of analysis by getting a sense of the data through the process of open coding and initial major category building. The prime intent of data collection at this stage was to scope the concept of stillness as a potential research focus. With these foundations in place, the task at Stage Two was to identify the core category or central phenomenon of the investigation. Stage Three required a return to the database in order to reconsider the core category in terms of its antecedent conditions, the ways in which it is utilised, as well as its context, consequences and some of the intervening conditions that might encourage or restrain its occurrence. The final stage, as detailed above, entailed the development of a visual representation of the concepts and relationships identified in the previous phases of analysis.

RESEARCH FINDINGS

Initial motivation for the study derived from an interest in wilderness therapy participants' experiences of stillness and inactivity, thus at the first stage of the analytic process the concept of *Quiet time* had yet to be identified. However, early in the research process, an interviewee responded to the question 'what was happening for you in those times when nothing particular was going on?' with a detailed description of two instances of what she described as *Quiet time*. It became clear in subsequent interviews that other respondents identified with the use of the phrase. When asked about their experience of *Quiet time*, participants talked spontaneously about incidents of reflection and/or solitude, resting, absorption in nature and gentle conversations around the campfire. From that point, the research inquired about *Quiet time* rather than 'stillness' and welcomed participants' response to, or spontaneous use of, the phrase as marking an event that fell within the parameters of the investigation.

QUIET TIME: A SENSE OF SOLITUDE

Establishing the concept of *Quiet time* as core category or central focus of the study begged the question 'What is at the heart, what is the essence of participants' experience of *Quiet time*?'

The research findings identified *Quiet time* in terms of a sense of solitude; that is a state of being alone but not lonely, a form of privacy rather than isolation. A 'sense' of solitude that, contrary to understandings of solitude as an objective and external condition, was defined by four co-occurring subjective and internal conditions: 1) a sense of being alone, 2) a positive frame of mind, 3) a personal time perspective, and 4) focused attention.

Experiences characterised by three, or less, of the features were not defined by participants as *Quiet time*. For example, within the wilderness therapy program, Mick retreated from the group to distance himself from Sally whom he found irritating. Despite his relative solitude, and focused attention, Mick did not include this experience of sitting alone, immersed in accusatory thinking patterns as an example of *Quiet time*.

Figure 2. Four key elements of Quiet time

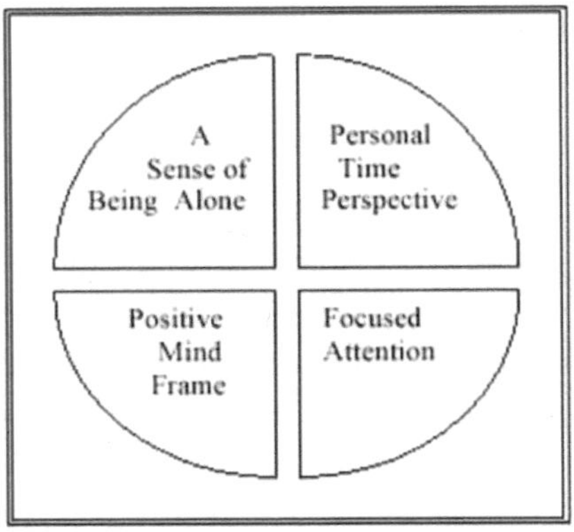

SENSE OF BEING ALONE

The sense of solitude associated with *Quiet time* was expressed in two broad ways. Firstly, all accounts of *Quiet time* were underpinned by a pervasive sense of wilderness solitude. Despite 4WD tracks, mobile phone coverage, the occasional glimpse of townships and an understanding that, at any point, a fit person could access 'civilization' within three hours or so of walking, participants revelled in a sense of physical isolation from the 'shitty life' (Mitch). The relative isolation, seclusion and solitude of the wilderness environment fostered an inner sense of liberation and expansiveness:

> I think, well maybe the isolation we were in would have a lot to do with that because, you haven't got them pressures of what people think of you, all of them were dropped, gone away. (Andy)

Journeying through a natural landscape...

> Sorta, yeah, it took me away from like the shitty life you might as well say, yeah, in such that from where I've just come from, you know what I mean, like yeah it just took all me worries away. (Mitch)

Secondly, most accounts of *Quiet time* were characterized by an additional sense of solitude through the purposeful act of temporarily disengaging from the social context of the group. Contrary to traditional conceptions of solo and solitude, the sense of solitude synonymous with *Quiet time* was experienced, with two exceptions, within two to thirty metres of other participants. Charlie's account of 'my bit of space' is typical, and suggests that solitude of *Quiet time*, is more about social disengagement than physical isolation or communicative separation:

> Yeah, even with a group of five when you're sitting on top of a mountain you only had to move five metres away and you had your own bit of space...you'd think a bit better and not even see the other person...I knew there were people around me, but it was like, it was my bit of space, yeah, equally I thought I could think aloud and it wouldn't have mattered, you know. (Charlie)

The three other defining characteristics of *Quiet time*: a personal time perspective, focused attention and positive mind frame are discussed later in the paper.

Understanding Quiet Time in the Context of a Wilderness Therapy Program

Having developed an appreciation of *Quiet time* as an experience of solitude, stages three and four of the grounded theory procedure involved a reconsideration of *Quiet time* in terms of how, when and why it occurred, the conditions that encouraged or constrained its occurrence, its function and consequences. This process culminated in the development of a visual diagram representing all of these concepts and relationships.

Rather than re-iterate the detail of the visual model provided in Nicholls (2008), this paper invites an alternate and visually simpler model for understanding the phenomenon of *Quiet time* in terms of a relaxed, positive and subjective sense of solitude within the communal context and activity orientation of a wilderness therapy program. This complementary model is based on a framework for understanding solitude proposed by Philip Koch (1994).

Solitude and the Yin Yang Symbol

In his book 'Solitude: A philosophical encounter,' Koch (1994) drew upon the Tai Chi diagram of the yin-yang relationship, to symbolize a conception of solitude that is inextricable from encounter or social engagement. In Chinese philosophy the concept of yin and yang represent complimentary opposites within a greater whole.

From this perspective everything, all aspects of life, have both yin and yang characteristics. Koch (1994) suggested four ways in which the dynamic of the yin yang relationship may be applied to an understanding of the nature of solitude and its place within the whole of a healthy life. From this perspective, Koch interprets the symbol as a visual representation of:

- Solitude and encounter as complementary opposites.
- A timely relationship between the desire for solitude and the desire for social engagement.
- How experiences of solitude and encounter/social engagement impact upon and transform each other.
- The place of solitude in a healthy life.

Figure 3. Yin Yang diagram: Solitude and encounter

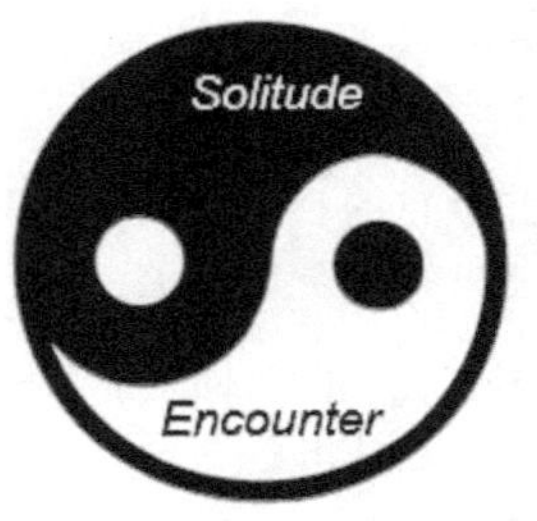

As previously described, participants in the Mountain Challenge equated the concept of *Quiet time* with subjective experiences of a sense of solitude. With this in mind, Koch's interpretation of the yin yang symbol provided an innovative and intriguing framework for exploring some of the findings of this investigation into the phenomenon of *Quiet time*. The symbol also underscores, in a visually simple manner, the advice of Daniel (2005) who, based on his research into the life significance of wilderness solo, cautions that 'Whilst it is tempting to look at (the experience of solitude) in isolation from the rest of the expedition, we may oversimplify our understanding of its significance in doing so (p. 93).

The remainder of the paper is structured by the four interpretations of the yin yang symbol described above and as applied to findings in this study.

Quiet Time and Communal Time as Complimentary Opposites

Participants utilized the relative solitude and cognitive freedom of this personal time in three broad ways: to respond to nature; to reflect; or to relate in an authentic and heartfelt manner.

In contrast to the group context and communal focus of much of the Mountain Challenge program, the solitude of all accounts of *Quiet time* was infused with a personal time perspective described by participants as 'It's time for yourself' (Bec); 'It's My time, MY time' (Pete).

Figure 4. Yin Yang diagram: My time and communal time

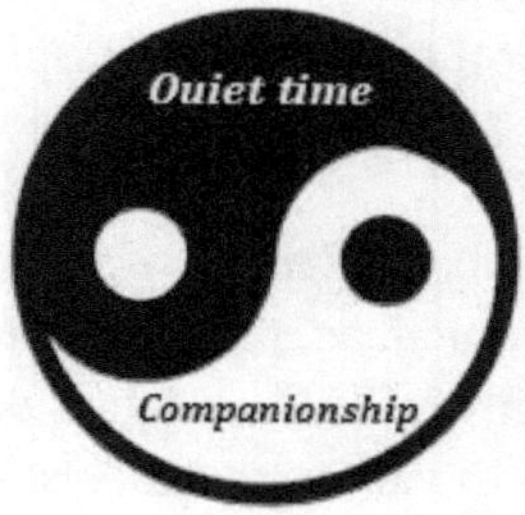

RESPONDING TO NATURE

Although the level of euphoria in the following extract differentiates it from most other *Quiet time* accounts, Dave's experience of relative solitude on top of Mt. Trestle is typical of other *Quiet time*s spent responding to nature. That is, it occurs when Dave is socially disengaged from his companion and is characterised by an intense sense of being alive within the moment. The experience is essentially non-verbal, embodied, sensuous, emotionally charged and difficult to explain:

> The moon was rising, (I was) sitting on top of one of the columns. That was just brilliant. The wind was blowing, damn cold...I definitely felt alive, the tingles, the excitement, the adrenaline, it was fantastic. It's hard to describe really... I've experienced things like that before but they've all been different, this was like 'Wow!'... It had so much more of an edge to it, probably because I was straight, and I had no other thoughts about anything else but what I was doing at that particular moment. That was it, nothing else mattered...There was no concern about anything else apart from what I was doing at the time and getting the most out of it, and, I think I pretty much did that. (I felt) pretty pleased with myself actually, because I was heading towards the end of the program, I felt good about that I'd completed it, and I was nearly there. I was out there enjoying things, with a straight mind, no artificial toxins in me whatsoever, and the feelings that I was getting were great, the jubilation. My chest was pounding. It was great! And I realized 'Hey, wow, you don't need that other crap (laugh) to really enjoy these things. (Dave)

That participants utilise the solitude of *Quiet time* to appreciate nature is also apparent in the way they regard the beauty of their environment as an appropriate reward for physical effort. Gus 'had to have' brief moments of *Quiet time* to savour the view or 'I'd have walked all day and not seen anything'. On attaining a small summit Charlie ripped off his shirt and lay spread-eagled on his back on a large flat rock:

> I just took me shirt off and let the wind blow through... A lot of them Quiet times there was nothing, like I just shut my eyes and I can still see the green glow from the sun, so I just did that so that it was total blackness or pull me cap down, so total blackness. That is just, what, like a total, muscle relaxant or whatever (Charlie leans back in his chair, outstretches his arms his arms and expels the air from his lungs in a manner of total relaxation.) Phew! Letting go. (Charlie)

For someone whose mind is 'always on the go' the relief from physical effort and release or 'letting go 'of tension is difficult to express. Charlie resorts to body language and advises the researcher to 'get a video' as a way of recording his deep sense of relaxation.

Choosing to simply focus on the sights, sounds and feel of the natural world during *Quiet time* gave some participants a chance to stem the tide of novel experience and time to process and adapt to the various physical, emotional and social challenges within the Mountain Challenge. For example, lying by himself under the tarp at night, Col calms his 'racing mind' by focusing on the stars. Joe goes to bed early 'to get that *Quiet time*' by listening to the running water in the creek nearby. In similar vein, staring into the coals of the dying fire provides Gus with an unfamiliar opportunity to still his mind:

> I stayed up on two of the nights, after everyone had gone to bed, with the campfire. I actually went to bed one night then jumped back up, and just sat around the campfire, and I didn't think, I just took some time out and I just stared at the fire, checked out the fire and tried to listen out for some animals around and just took some time out and that was good for me cos' mentally all day I was going, my brain was going, 15 to the dozen... And I haven't done that in so long I probably couldn't even pinpoint the last time I did do that. Just sit, just sit, and stop thinking and relax. (Gus)

Reflecting

In line with conventional expectations some participants used the privacy of *Quiet time* to reflect upon their progress. Charlie explains 'When you get *Quiet time* you can think, I did a good job, like, pulled me own weight and a bit more'.

Participants also used this personal time to ruminate on current concerns outside of the Mountain Challenge and particularly their roles and responsibilities as parents and partners. As a corollary of years of drug and /or alcohol abuse, family life is, for many participants, fraught with significant domestic and custodial issues. The following extract exemplifies the content of participants' reflections and illustrates a ponderous and ruminative style of thinking characteristic of reflective *Quiet time*:

> Yes I went down on the rocks just in front of the hut there and just looked out over Hobart. I tried to put the thoughts of what I'm going through with my kids and their mother out of my head but in fact that's what I ended up basically thinking about. I, and didn't come up with any answers, not any answers at all, but it was clear thinking and after coming away from there I knew inside myself basically where I stood, which is basically the same place that I knew I was but I felt at ease with it, if that makes sense. (Gus)

Participants frequently resorted to metaphor to convey experiences of *Quiet time* that were easier to 'feel' than describe or witness. For example, Col tries to 'suck up the good energy' inside of him, Ben felt someone had 'taken the broom and swept all the shit out of (his) brain', *Quiet time* experiences 'Blew (Gus) away'.

The personal insights and embodied sense of wellbeing frequently accompanying *Quiet time* spent in reflection or responding to nature echo those identified by McKenzie (2003) in a study of the Outward Bound process of change. McKenzie proposes that traditional understandings of reflection as a predominately cognitive and linear process are incomplete and fail to recognize that reflection 'may also be non-cognitive in character and include embodied interactions such as intuitive insights and a sense of 'coming to know' (p. 20). Understanding *Quiet time* as a route to alternate and valid ways of knowing finds support in recent research findings in the cognitive sciences (Claxton, 1997).

RELATING

Andy was the first interviewee to articulate the potential for intimate conversational exchange to be regarded as *Quiet time.* He said:

> The Quiet times are very unique… some of them are with a friend when you're just having a chat and you get onto a certain topic when you can both help each other out and still that is a Quiet time between two people or three people, it doesn't really matter because just by talking to someone they could be saying something you might really struggle with, and, talking about it with someone you get more peace of mind out of it, get more understanding, and it gives you more, you're not just talking about shit, you're talking about things that are heartfelt and things you've done in the past that's not happening now. (Andy)

Quiet time conversations were typically spontaneous, ruminative and characterised by the sparking of ideas thoughts and feelings of one group member to another. That participants' definitions of *Quiet time* might include intimate verbal exchange was an unexpected finding, although Hammit (1982) identified the drive for intimacy and privacy with ones companions as a highly valued dimension of wilderness experience, and Koch (1998) identified the potential for shared intimacy within solitude.

With this in mind, the white spot at the centre of *Quiet time* may be said to symbolize the way in which a sense of intimate community may be part of the experience of *Quiet time.*

Quiet time spent relating in heartfelt conversation was suggestive of the kind of spontaneous and informal peer discussion identified by Burridge (2004) and Russell (2000) as having significant impact on the processing of experience but is, as yet, unaccounted for in the literature.

These findings reinforce the notion that wilderness adventure experiences, including *Quiet time* spent relating in heartfelt and honest conversation yields, amongst other gains, social, emotional and psychological benefits that may extend beyond the life of a program (Ewert, 1989). According to Peck (1987):

> We cannot really be ourselves until we are able to share freely the things we most have in common: our weaknesses, our incompetence, our imperfection, our inadequacy...this is the kind of individualism that makes real community possible. (p. 58)

Figure 5. Yin Yang diagram: Quiet time and companionship

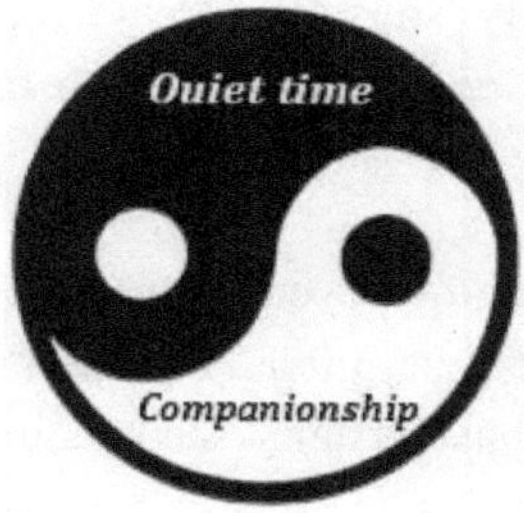

A Timely Relationship between the Desire for Quiet Time and the Desire for Companionship

Wanting Quiet Time

For many of the participants, the communal nature of the wilderness journey generated a number of privacy needs that they met by disengaging from the social context of the group for *Quiet time*. In due course, needs met, they reengaged with the group. In addition to the desire for personal time to focus on nature, reflect or relate, for some, the taking of *Quiet time* was a deliberate self-help or coping strategy. For example, when walking in single file along the track, Mitch periodically allowed himself to fall to the back of the line for some *Quiet time*. In this position of relative solitude he chose to focus on the terrain underfoot in a deliberate attempt for respite from a perceived pressure to make conversation and jokes, or in any other way take up the self-imposed role of congenial group clown. Disengaged from the social context of the group he enjoyed the ease of simply being himself without the need to think about group or the tasks at hand:

> I wasn't thinking about the pain in my legs, going up the hill, I wasn't thinking about who was talking behind me, I was just in some little void that I could get into and there was nothing there and I didn't have to worry about anything...I didn't have to be that sort of funny person to make everyone else laugh, I didn't have to be that clown all the time... I mean it's probably like a rest, a mind rest I guess. (Mitch)

Taking Quiet Time

The yin yang diagram provides a simple reminder, by the way of the black spot of *Quiet time* within in the white of communal / group time, of how, despite the presence of others, participants found ways to respond to their desire for *Quiet time*. For example, Pete simply 'slips off' to his tent; Mick liked to 'just walk off and find (his) own little spot and sit down'. Dean finds opportunity even whilst walking along the track:

> I'd just simply stop and everyone else keeps walking, but they're still all around me and simply be, literally in the middle of everybody and just stop and have, just have a thirty seconds of total alone time right there and then. (Dean)

Although *Quiet time* was predominately a spontaneous, informal and participant-initiated experience, in some instances participants referred to a *Quiet time* that came about in response to a facilitator initiated invitation for a 'Quiet sit'. For some, these opportunities were the only occurrence of *Quiet time* reported. It is interesting to note that the invitation for a 'Quiet sit' was no guarantee of an experience identified by participants as *Quiet time*. Given the imperative for a positive frame of mind and focused attention, opportunity for a sense of solitude initiated and prescribed by a facilitator proved to be highly conditional.

The Duration of Quiet Time

The duration of *Quiet time* ranged from 'just a minute to stop and take it all in' to an hour or so to 'take some time out'. Typically, *Quiet time* lasted between 15 to 20 minutes.

Koch (1994) proposed 'attentive time' rather than chronological time as a measure of the duration of solitude. This concept sits well with the research findings. Focused attention was one of the four key concepts integral to all *Quiet time* accounts. As Koch suggested, when the focus of attention was disrupted or the need for focus fulfilled, awareness of the group recurred and *Quiet time* gave way to social re-engagement.

The concept of 'attentive time' also sheds useful light on why some participants found the 15 minute time frame for a facilitator initiated 'quiet sit', challenging. When Charlie felt the 'sit' was 'getting a bit long' he experienced a mis-match between his capacity to attend and the time frame determined by the facilitator.

Having Time for Time Quiet Time

A temporal and cyclical relationship between *Quiet time* and social engagement was not always at play. Certain intervening variables were found to impede the occurrence of *Quiet time*. Physical, emotional and environmental conditions that challenged participants' basic needs or stirred negative mind frames inhibited the occurrence of *Quiet time*. For example, programs characterized by a focus on physical prowess and individualism, or targets and time frames that precluded, for example, the opportunity to linger on a summit, sit for 'smoko' or take time to examine the depths of a rock pool exacerbated performance anxiety and diminished the sense of 'having time to take time' for *Quiet time*. In contrast, factors such as a stunning vista, overcoming physical challenges, pleasant weather, a campfire and low levels of noise fostered the kind of positive mind frame and focused attention conducive to participants' taking time for *Quiet time*. Most important, according to the study participants, to the occurrence of *Quiet time* was that the wilderness journey be infused by a process oriented and 'no rush' approach.

QUIET TIME AND THE GROUP EXPERIENCE IMPACT UPON AND TRANSFORM EACH OTHER

In commenting on his fatigue and recalling 'that was a buggered stop not a *Quiet time* stop, although everyone did go quiet', Charlie identifies one of a number of intervening conditions at play within the overall context of the Mountain Challenge, that were found to impact upon the incidence of *Quiet time*. They included: 1) individual participant needs, strengths and limitations, 2) environmental factors, 3) facilitator styles, and 4) levels of group development.

For example, Gus frequently took time for reflective *Quiet time*, Mick welcomed *Quiet time* as an opportunity to respond to nature, Pete and Sally enjoyed writing in their journal, and Dave preferred not to. Summits and panoramic views were particularly conducive to *Quiet time* spent attuning to nature and reflecting; campfires and campsites were conducive to *Quiet time* spent relating to others. Facilitator styles that encouraged peer discussion enhanced the potential for *Quiet time* spent 'relating'. No accounts of *Quiet time* were identified within the context of risk, immediate effort, unmet basic needs, or in the early stages of group development when levels of trust and security were low. Concerns, anxieties and social insecurities precluded the kind of positive mind frame integral to *Quiet time*. Once group development evolved towards a sense of security, camaraderie and companionship, incidents of *Quiet time* occurred.

Facilitator styles conducive to an unhurried and process-oriented experience impacted particularly positively on the conditions antecedent to *Quiet time*. *Quiet time* spent relating in heartfelt conversation was dependent on the group having attained high levels of trust and security.

A number of identifiable outcomes arose as a result of *Quiet time*. These outcomes impacted positively on body, mind and spirit in terms of a sense of euphoria or 'natural high', a sense of self-worth, insight, relaxation, peace, 'a mind rest', anxiety reduction, mental clarity and the development of empathy. Whilst it was beyond the scope of the study to ascertain the impact of *Quiet time* on the overall group process, it is conceivable that these kind of outcomes and the sense of reinvigoration of mind, body and/or spirit that participants brought back to the companionship of the group impacted positively at an individual and collective level.

As part of the long-term rehabilitation process participants in the Mountain Challenge attend group and individual therapy aimed at addressing habitual, destructive patterns of thought and behaviour. The findings indicate that participants come to the Mountain Challenge motivated by a desire for personal growth, reinvigoration and refreshment. Against this backdrop it is conceivable that experiences of peace, belonging and other such positive emotions carry especial significance.

The Place of Quiet Time in a Healthy Life

On return to the rehabilitation centre, the participants were unanimous in the sense of wellbeing and accomplishment that they attribute to their Mountain Challenge experience. How much of that positive sense of self can be directly attributable to participants' experience of *Quiet time* is speculative. However, within the data it was possible to identify a number of examples that illustrate clear links between *Quiet time* during the Mountain Challenge and a newly found and sustained appreciation of the place of *Quiet time* in a healthy life.

Prior to entering the rehabilitation centre, at the height of their drug and alcohol abuse, participants typically regarded opportunity 'to be alone' as an experience to be avoided or endured. Lacking the positive mind set characteristic of *Quiet time*, 'being alone' was equated with the kind of confused thinking, negative self-beliefs, anger, shame or feelings of loneliness apparent in the following extracts:

> I didn't like myself that much so I hated being by myself. *(Joe)*
>
> I haven't had any Quiet time I can tell you... it would give me time to think...I deliberately went out of me way not to (be alone). *(Andy)*
>
> I didn't like the person I was changing into… I didn't want to be around anybody 'cos I always felt shameful, like everyone was looking at me and pointing the finger at me. 'Oh she's nothing but an alcoholic' which I was...The shame and the guilt. Even when the children came home from school I still wanted to be on my own, so I wouldn't be very nice to them. Always being a real bad mother because I just wanted to be on my own. Didn't want anyone around me. (Sally)

On return to the rehabilitation centre Dave, Dean, Gus, Col, Charlie and Andy spontaneously commit to the habit of incorporating *Quiet time* into everyday life. They anticipate that *Quiet time* will bring benefits that outweigh any social or personal inconvenience. For example, despite the threat of ridicule by other residents and being labelled 'fucking mad' Gus persists with his regular 'yak' to himself on the balcony as a way of gaining perspective and insight. Despite the effort and challenge of writing, Andy finds that with practice, *Quiet time* spent journaling gets easier and provides him with a new found capacity to acknowledge the positive and take control of destructive thinking patterns.

Dean, a carpenter, draws on his trade to explain the way in which he anticipates his experiences of *Quiet time* during the Mountain Challenge will provide him with 'tools' to deal with 'the dark forces' and support him through the lifelong process of recovery from addiction:

> (Quiet time) is definitely time for me, and I never really knew how to... be able to consciously find my own time. 'Coz I could have gone away for ten minutes every day and I would not have known how, from a bulls roar, how to find my own time and how to do a little bit of soul repairing... So that was excellent, that is a tool that has gone into a tool box that stays with me now. (Dean)

Prior to the Mountain Challenge the same participants regarded solitude as undesirable or unimportant. It is plausible, that for these participants at least, *Quiet time* within the context of the Mountain Challenge provided an experiential opportunity to discover some of the benefits of solitude and, importantly, to develop confidence in their personal capacity to use *Quiet time* constructively.

These participants valued the relaxation and contemplation they associate with *Quiet time* as a self-help and life enhancing strategy and an important part of their path to wellbeing.

Classic and contemporary research affirm that humans have a developmental need to balance the drive for companionship with solitude and that the ability to use and enjoy solitude is a learned skill and correlate of mental health and wellbeing (Buchholz & Catton 1999; Csikzentmihalyi, 1984; Csikszentmihalyi & Larson, 1984; Larson, 1997; Long & Averill, 2003, Maslow, 1971; Winnicott, 1965). Dowrick (1993) wrote extensively on the subject and explained:

> At the heart of many of our difficulties is a lack of conscious understanding that each of us needs closeness with others, and also a knowledgeable, nurturing relationship with our own self. Each of us needs to find a delicate shifting balance between dependence and independence, between being open to others and taking care of ourselves. (p. xxii)

Conclusion

The interrelated, interdependent character of the Chinese symbol yin yang has provided a dynamic representation of some of the ways in which the opportunity and experience of *Quiet time* can be appreciated as a natural and significant compliment to the predominately social focus and active orientation of a challenge based wilderness therapy program.

Understanding *Quiet time* as a participant-initiated response to the need for privacy, and as a self-structured opportunity for reflection, attuning to nature or participating in authentic and heartfelt conversation, provides insight into at least one of the ways in which participants in a challenge-based wilderness therapy program exert agency over their wilderness therapy experience.

In addition to the therapeutic benefits associated with communal living, shared reflective and adventure activities, this study underscores the therapeutic merit of promoting opportunity for the solitude of *Quiet time* through a 'no rush' approach to the wilderness journey.

References

Bobilya, A. J. (2005). Wilderness, solitude, and monastic traditions. In C. E. Knapp & T. E. Smith (Eds.), *Exploring the power of solo, silence, and solitude.* Boulder, CO: Association for Experiential Education.

Buchholz, E. S., & Catton, R. (1999). Adolescents' perceptions of aloneness and loneliness. *Adolescence*, 34 (133), 203 -214.

Burger, J. M. (1995). Individual differences in preference for solitude. *Journal of Research in Personality, 29*, 85-108.

Claxton, G. (1997). *Hare brain tortoise mind.* London: Fourth Estate Ltd.

Csikszentmihalyi, M., & Larson, R. (1984). *Being adolescent*. New York: Basic Books Inc.

Koch, P. (1994). *Solitude: A philosophical encounter*. Chicago: Open Court.

Kimball, R., & Bacon, S. (1993). The wilderness challenge model. In M. Gass (Ed.), *Adventure Therapy: Therapeutic applications of adventure programming* (pp. 11-42). Dubuque, Iowa: Kendall/Hunt

Larson, R. W. (1997). The emergence of solitude as a constructive domain of experience in early adolescence. *Child Development,* 68, 80-93.

Maslow, A. (1971). *The farther reaches of human nature.* New York: Viking.

McKenzie, M. (2003). Beyond the Outward Bound process: Rethinking student learning. *Journal of Experiential Education, 26* (1), 8-24.

Mulvay, E., Arthur, M., & Repucci, N. (1993). The prevention and treatment of juvenile delinquency: A review of the research. *Clinical Psychology Review, 13*, 133 -167.

Nicholls, V. (2008). *Busy doing nothing: researching the phenomenon of Quiet time in a challenge-based wilderness therapy program.* Unpublished thesis. University of Wollongong. NSW. Retrieved on 9/1/09 from: http://ro.uow.edu/thesis/132

Trace, N. (2003). *Complexity, Buddhism and adventure therapy.* Paper presented at the Third International Adventure Therapy Conference, Victoria, B.C. Canada.

Winnicott, D. (1965). *The maturational processes and the facilitating environment: studies in the theory of emotional development.* London: Hogarth Press and the Institute of Psychoanalysts.

CHAPTER 28

Art in the Woodlands: Creating a Holding Environment for Students with Autism

Kevin Burrows

ABSTRACT

My work takes place in a two-acre eco-therapy environment. In this 'Forest School' woodland, students with autism appear to respond positively to being part of creative woodland activities. From experience, I have observed that peoples' perceptions change in natural environments. In such places people appear to learn less by the deconstructive forming of concepts and abstracts, and more from awareness of sensate, experiential and emotional learning. In this paper, I suggest that through contact with the natural world, people within the Autistic Spectrum (AS) can develop their perceptions of self and world view through sensory perception and the senses rather than through the constructed dualistic framework typically perceived by 'neural-typical' people (or people outside of the Autistic Spectrum).

In this work, I seek to explore how creative and natural environments can promote relational experiences to sustain positive behaviour and self-fulfilment. From my view these environments offer more coherent forms of learning that help to inform natural therapy and teaching models, which better meet the needs of people with autism. Observations from my practice indicate that many teaching and therapy methods that rely upon deconstructive analysis and the ability to form abstracts are concepts outside of the cognitive abilities of those with autism. Instead, there is a need to form models, which recognise and reflect on therapy and learning as part of the same relational process.

Ideas about nature-therapy nurture a shift in our contemporary collective unconscious, from controlling to accepting 'wildness'. The potential for 'green' or 'eco-therapy' models of therapy and education that include benefits for people with autistic spectrum perceptions are collectively useful. As practitioners, we have a choice of addressing autistic differences or not. Either we attempt to control the 'wildness' of autistic behaviour (and thus access existing deconstructive models of therapy and education) or we seek new emergent models that are more congruent with the 'wildness' of autistic perception. This paper explores the potential for woodland environments and the creative freedom of art, to nurture positive experiences for those living with autism.

INTRODUCTION

Wilderness and adventure therapy sometimes seeks to take dysfunctional adolescents out of their comfort zone through relational experiences in nature as a kind of 'hero's quest', in order to face and conquer fears, challenge behaviours, and encourage profound experiences in nature. Often, they return to urban environments and are not able to make sense of, accommodate or sustain what has been experienced. Jordan (2009) calls such experiences a psychological 'one night stand with nature'.

Traditionally, the wilderness and the mountain are places of pilgrimage, offering people opportunities for gaining inner strength, knowledge and understanding of self, a place to face demons, to conquer fears, to accommodate life change. At the 'Wilderness and Inner Space Conference' (2009) hosted by the University of Kent, Stanton spoke of wilderness and wildness as 'primal resonance between the raw and wild in nature'. At the same conference Adams spoke about mountains as 'environments of wonder and fear'. I agree that nature offers wild and often dark places of transference, soul searching, awe and wonder, and that it is through this inner-outer perception of self and other that transitional spaces in nature can heal. But I question how this can work for a person who has autism and who therefore has little or no capacity for affective resonance or empathy with place, other than self-formed perceptions through abstracts or metaphors.

Totton (2009) suggested that we have forgone our wildness through our own domestication. For this author, we have come to perceive natural environments through a conceptual framework that separates us from nature, and perhaps includes a necessity for domination over nature. I hypothesis that for people with autism, this relationship with nature becomes anxiety laden. For the person who has autism, I suggest that there already exists a wildness of autistic perception, which is trapped in a civilised, neural-typical world imbibed with domestic rules of separation, judgement, value and isolation.

Jordan (2007) pointed out that when we observe people within the autism spectrum, it is not the autism that we see but a reaction a secondary behavioural manifestation of the condition. Jordan believes people who have autism are under severe stress, severe anxiety, due to their fractured perception of the world. In other words, the person with autism can demonstrate extreme anxiety in environments that are outside their autistic perception of the world. It is not unreasonable to suggest that the world outside of autistic perception that Jordan speaks of, is the same as Totton's civilised, domesticated world. These different perceptions challenge us to critique traditional western concepts of nature and natural environments, and raise questions about our use of adventure therapy when working with clients with autism. [See Appendix 1 for a clinical definition of Autism disorder].

Neurological and Behavioural Theories of Autism

Ozonoff, Dawson, and McPartland (2002) stated that deficits in executive functioning are central to deficits in autism, and are linked to the brain's frontal lobes. Executive functioning deficits affect behaviour through deficits in concepts of inner models of reality. These deficits suggest an inability to empathise or build inner abstracts, or to make conceptual analyses that connect to concepts about outer worlds. 'Theory of Mind' (ToM) is the ability to attribute mental states, beliefs, intents, desires, pretending, and knowledge, to oneself and others, and to understand that others have beliefs, desires and intentions that are different from one's own. Baron-Cohen (cited in Harvey, Fossati & Lepage, 2007) link ToM deficit with damaged prefrontal cortex (part of the brain's frontal lobes). These authors indicate that for the person who has autism, aspects of empathy, transference and projection are flawed.

Frith and Happe (cited in Cumine, Dunlop & Stevenson, 2010) suggested that, unlike neural-typical people, people who have autism might develop a kind of self-consciousness through using intelligence and experiential learning rather than through intuition. Frith and Happe further suggest, that aspects of autistic spectrum (AS) functioning cannot be explained by ToM alone. Frith and Happe propose that people with AS have weak central coherence, and may not contextualise or access the 'whole picture'; yet are very good at defining detail or smaller fragmented parts of the whole. This difference in perception can distort sense of self and inter-relationship in socio-behavioural patterns. Using neurological measured tests against a neural-typical control group, Minshew (1997) found the autism group:

- used more nonverbal visually oriented processing and retained letters as visual-graphical codes;

- relied on lower level visuospatial analysis, had less activation in anterior regions and more in posterior regions associated with visual processing;
- had more activation in right brain hemisphere; and
- had a selective impairment in complex information processing which does not involve visual-spatial processing (Minshew 1997, pp.303-316).

THE TRIAD OF IMPAIRMENT, EXPERIENCE AND SENSATION

In the Diagnostic and Statistical Manual of Mental Disorders IV (American Psychiatric Association, 2000), the impairments of autism have been grouped into three areas of functioning known as the 'triad of impairment':

- Reciprocal social interaction
- Verbal and nonverbal communication
- A restricted repertoire of activities and interests (American Psychiatric Association, 2000).

These differences might also be explained by the concept of the triad of competence (Peter, 2003). The 'triad of competence' offers interest, affect and structure as three pedagogical components that may give rise to AS coherence in learning. Indicators of learning gain might be an emerging triad of competence that facilitates other ways of accessing or substituting an AS deficit in emotional engagement and learning through therapeutic programs.

Another aspect of the AS is sensitive attunement, and its relationship to environment and social functioning. Bogdashina (2003) suggested that environment and sensory perception is basic to many areas of academic, communicative and social functioning or intersubjectivity. Delacato (1974, cited in Bogdashina, 2003) explored concepts of hyper and hyposensitivity in people with AS. The volume of distorted sensitivity and information can affect anxiety and account for all aspects of the AS triad of impairment. Hyper and hypo-sensitivity in people with AS increases sensate overload or shutdown, creates abnormal perceptions, gives rise to anxiety, and sets rigid patterns of behaviour that impair the ability to socialise and communicate (Bogdashina, 2003). All of these can be observed as behaviour (concurring with the triad of impairment), or can be measured neurologically.

I have observed that Forest School environments seem to calm AS students. I hypothesise that this may be explained as reduced hypersensitivity in AS, leading to reducing anxiety, and reducing all aspects of the AS triad of impairment.

During his presentation about 'Hope and therapy' at the seventeenth BACP Research Conference (2011), O'Hara stated 'Frontal lobe capacity shuts down in situations of emotional flooding'. This statement seems to support the view that in both neural-typical and AS mind sets, sensation either influences, or is influenced by, the function of the frontal lobes. In relation to the concept of ToM, damaged or dysfunctional frontal lobes in the person within the AS suggest that sensation and emotion are processed at different rates to those processed by neural-typical people.

Bruner's (1993) findings concerning patterns of narration, scaffolding and story acquisition suggested people with autism have difficulty in seeing the patterning that form archetypes. Furthermore, Morgan (1996) explained that the person who has autism may have difficulty in thinking in anything other than concrete terms, and that the presentation of abstract choices can send them spiralling into anxiety. As individual and worldview is perceived through the senses, people within the AS can develop different (what we might term 'fragmented' or 'distorted') perceptions of self and world, with an inability to construct inner abstracts or perform conceptual analysis. With all this in mind, one can see the confusion the person with autism might experience in trying to exist and perform within educational or therapy models that are based on a reductionist bias that relies on deconstruction to form abstracts, and metaphors to explain our environment and world view.

Animal Sensation in Autism

Drawing on her own autistic experience, Grandin suggested that fear is the main emotion in both animals, and in people with autism. She goes on to suggest that for the person with autism, thinking is based on a non-abstracted world perception of what she terms *seeing in details* (Grandin & Johnson, 2005). In other words, perceptions that are sensory-based, thinking in sounds, thinking in touches, and thinking in pictures. Seeing what is actually there, what is sensed, rather than seeing an abstract projection of inner concepts as the outer world. Similarities between her autistic perception and animal sensate experience have enabled Grandin to create stress-free environments for cattle and other livestock. Grandin has drawn parallels with her own autistic perception of animal sensory-based thinking, environment, and behaviour in her profession as a cattle corral designer (Grandin & Johnson 2005). I suspect there is a commonality of reduced anxiety and stress between a perceived relationship of sensory thinking, sensate experience and environment, in both Grandin's corral designs and the fragmented world perception of those who have autism.

Cozolino (2006) stated that Grandin's AS brain architecture shifts perception from cerebellum-dependant language areas to her visual cortex, enabling her to think in images. There may be neurological compensation between left and right hemispheres of the brain associated with what Grandin refers to as animal sensory based thinking. In their paper 'Are animals autistic savants?' Vallortigara, Snyder, Kaplan, Bateson, Clayton & Rogers (2008) suggested that savant syndrome is often associated with some left brain dysfunction, together with right brain compensation. These notions seem to affirm a shift from language-dependant neural processing to visual image based thinking in AS neural processing. As Grandin points out, not only does AS perception think in pictures, but neural-typical visual processing is selective. For this author, 'inattentional blindness works at a high level of mental processing, meaning that your (neural-typical) brain does a lot of processing before it allows something into the consciousness' (Grandin & Johnson, 2005, p. 66). Perhaps this neural-typical filtering of visual perception can be seen as a reversal of the aforementioned concept of right brain compensation in people with AS (Vallortigara et al., 2008).

A Psychology of Self and Other-than-Self

Object relations theory was pioneered by British psychologists Fairbairn, Klein, Winnicott, Guntrip and Stuart, amongst others (1940 to 1950) and is the process of developing the mind in relation to others in the environment. The 'objects' of the theory are both real others in one's world, and one's internalised image of others.

Winnicott (1971) established the *me and not me* concepts of separation of the self into the inner *me* and the outer *not me.* These concepts can be seen to promote a Cartesian dualism perception of self and other than self. Concepts of the abstracted and separated self are still prevalent in many models of therapy and education. Winnicott's lesser known contemporary Mahler observed the *normal autistic phase*, describing the first period of the infant's life as inward-turned. The infant's next hypothesised developmental stage was *symbiosis*, an experience of self-with-other, a relational rather than dissociative or separating experience (Mahler, Pine & Bergman, 2000).

Mearns and Cooper (2005) cited relationality as the formative natural state of our early development, and expand 'being in relation' to include the human and other than-human (p. 5). This suggests that a holistic and interconnected relationship to the environment is essential to a reciprocal and interdependent behavioural outcome between human and other-than-human. Unlike the Cartesian dualism world model (Totton, 2009), which is anthropocentric, (separating humankind from their connection to nature, with nature considered outside of a person), people with autism have a more connected wild, animal or gestalt perception which can lead them to demonstrate, extremely anxious behaviour (Jordan, 2007).

The Ecological Self

Naess (cited in Sessions, 1985) suggested that we confuse the self with the concept of the ego, and that our *ecological self* transcends the individual ego. The concept of the ecological self-promotes an interrelational, interconnected self, with 'other' as an experience of great breadth and depth. This ecological self is not perceived through the deconstructive separateness of the reductionist objective self as individual ego, but through a reciprocal relationship with the human and other than human environment. For this author, 'there are no boundaries and everything is interrelated. But insofar as we perceive things as individual organisms or entities, the insight draws us to respect all human and non-human individuals in their own right as parts of the whole without feeling the need to set up hierarchies of species with humans at the top' (Sessions, 1985, p.68). The inherent healing capacity of this connection becomes a process of healing our relations to all living beings.

The ecological self's inclusive relationality towards the person with autism invites interconnectedness through many levels of brain function. The question emerges: Do people who have autism function better in a holistic, relational environment of sensate experience and perceived wildness, outside of the neural typical domestic, deconstructed world view?

Autistic perception through the wildness of sensate experience is perhaps relational, from a paradigm outside of language acquisition. In those who have autism, this might be traced to a holistic sense of what is going on, or a heightened holistic awareness. Bogdashina (2003) outlined this concept through what she terms *gestalt perception* an autistic world view where the unprocessed and experiential is simultaneously perceived holistically and in infinite detail. Bogdashina (2003) discussed different perceptual worlds for those who have autism, and how their perceptions (like neural-typical people) are grounded in real experiences.

The Use of Art in Nature

Language is the Cartesian tool of our domestication, deconstructing and separating what is sensed and experienced, and forming the relational into detached cognate abstract and metaphor (Hillman, 1972). The deficiency in the language centres of the brain in those who have autism denies access to this domesticated and projected abstract or a perceived world view of self and other than self. Barrows (cited in Roszak et al., 1995) pointed out 'it is only by constructs of Western mind that we see ourselves as living in an inside, bounded by our own skin, with everything else on the outside' (p.106).

In my work, it is relationality and belongingness in nature that I seek. During a personal experiential 'solo', a short form of vision quest facilitated by Mary Jane Rust and David Key in Knoydart Scotland, I created a drawing entitled 'From the judging stone emerges the green man'. The title reflects the moment of paradigm shift or atunement in my relationship with the Earth. This creative intervention of art in nature formed an interrelated and reciprocal cohesion between wildness, connectivity and sensate experience for me, encouraging a shift that enabled me to sense my ecological wild or feral self, outside of the Cartesian dualism world view of object relation theory, that separates human and other-that-human into self and other.

Perception and language, being tools of connectivity or separation, mean neural pathways offer many routes to how and what is perceived, and through which brain functions. Expressive art therapists Knill, Levine & Levine 2005 offer 'overcoming Cartesian dualism' as a philosophical basis for expressive arts therapy. Husserl saw Cartesian dualism as founded on the method of radical doubt presupposing the existence of the natural world as described in mathematical physics (cited in Knill, Levine & Levine 2005). This suggests that if we suspend notions of the objectivity of the external world, which separates consciousness and nature, we can become free to look at the world and our mental life as they appear in the phenomena of experience. Intimating that Husserl's phenomenological method be seen as 'presuppositionless investigation into the nature of experience as it appears', rather than formulated beforehand, through some theoretical presupposition (Knill, Levine & Levine 2005, pp. 21-26).

Jung's concepts of the *imaginal self* (cited in Hillman, 1972) and *active imagination* (Chodrow 1997; McNiff 2009) are essential components of expressive arts therapy that enable visually oriented processing as a direct experiential process. These concepts may inform inclusive methodologies in AS therapy and learning models.

Hillman (1972) believed that, unlike the Cartesian ego, the imaginal ego forgoes the need to translate or reformulate imaginal speech in a bid to rationalise, interpret, or analyse the imaginal dream or fantasy into abstract or archetype. McNiff (2009) highlighted Hillman's distinction between the symbolic and the imaginal, describing how images as particular phenomena are distinct from symbols, and how the imaginal is central to the expressive arts therapies in that they do not interpret imagery (McNiff, 2009, p.42).

My own reflection of imaginal speech through images is that the drawings made in my Knoydart Solo seemed to fall effortlessly from my pencil without any presupposition. Jung's concept of the imaginal as a primacy of perception (cited in Chodrow, 1997) links to Minshew's aforementioned findings, that people who have autism process better through visuospatial perception. Grandin's comment about 'thinking in pictures', suggests people with autism can form their world view within the primacy of the imaginal. This makes plausible the inclusion of paradigms of therapy and education that recognise imaginal perception as language, through the field of sensate wildness, through the expressive arts.

Chodrow (1997) cited Jung's term *active imagination* as having many overlapping perspectives with the expressive medium of dialectic ritual (of painting, drawing, sculpting, dance and music), with inter-modal relationality between the expressive arts, citing the 'dancing of a mandala' (p.8). Hillman's imaginal self, and the Jungian concept of active imagination have been significantly expanded through therapeutic sand tray methods (Lowenfeld, 2007). McNiff (2004) stated 'play is arts mode of being' (p.153). Creative arts and play therapist List takes sand tray worlds into natural environments and considers *simultaneous perception* (i.e. places of visual, tactile, sensate experience of self and other than-self) as reciprocal relationships 'in the here and now' outdoors of her therapeutic garden (cited in McCarthy, 2008, p.80). These notions help to bring expressive arts therapy dialogue into a relational experience of reciprocity between human and other-than-human, in outdoor natural, holding environments.

WOODLAND AS A NURTURING CONTAINER

In her writings 'Creating restorative ecotherapeutic practices', Watkins stated her therapeutic woodland space is an environment that 'is a holding and sustaining force' (cited in Buzzell & Chalquist, 2009, p.226). Barrows (in Roszak et al., 1995) stated 'nature has always been a holding environment for me' (p.104).

Over time, my work with people who have autism in Forest School woodland environments has come to include an intent of addressing the anxiety and confusion already present in the autistic mind when set in a domestic anthropocentric neural-typical world view. Foregoing the mechanistic deconstructive learning environment of abstract and metaphor, we seek to access the nurturing container of Forest School woodland to hold and reciprocate the wild and sensate perception of an autistic mind-set and the holding capacity of nature.

In regard to natural places as places of learning, Abram (1996) spoke about North American *Vision quest* and the Aboriginal *Walkabout* as ways in which Indigenous oral cultures turn towards the more-than-human earth for teachings to vitalise and sustain the human community. Knight (2009) reflected that there is something magical and enchanting about woodland, 'trees have a magic of their own' (p.94).

In my own European culture, woodland was once the predominant feature of the English landscape. Pockets of which are still in existence today, connect me with the myth and legend of my own Indigenous woodland culture. Stories of *The green man* and *Jack in the green* are thought to date back to wild or feral men of the woodland. Woodland, therefore may be seen as one of my own Indigenous eco schemas. Today these mythical beings or selves may be viewed as metaphor, but it should be recognised there is always a subjective, experiential and sensate origin to all metaphor. Another question emerges: Through sensate phenomenological experience in the woodland, can we sense our former state of wildness?

Being in the traditional and experiential place of the feral self (the traditional proposed setting of The green man, and Jack in the green) and experiencing what presents itself, becomes a phenomenological experience where nature is viewed as experiential and relational rather than a predetermined cognate abstracted from metaphor.

Figure 1. Kevin Burrows: Creative groupwork experience in a natural environment

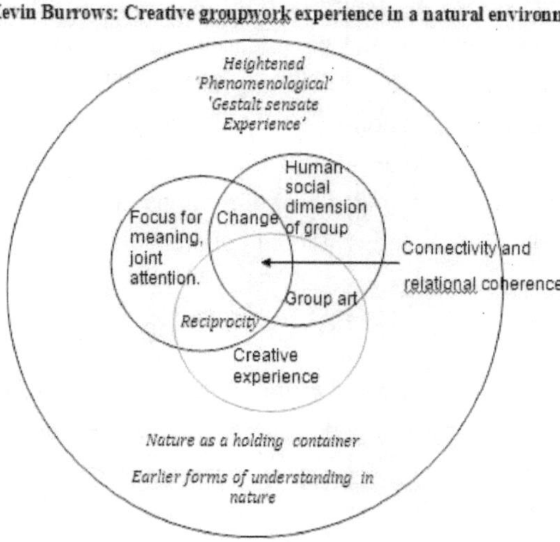

Educationalists Beard and Wilson (2009) discussed the outdoors as places that awaken the senses and increase experiential learning. They suggest that it is the sensate natural rhythmic qualities in nature that meet our experiential learning needs. They describe outdoor spaces of mangrove and forest as places where the senses are more in tune with the natural rhythms of the outdoor environment and a vital part of our ability to create a good experiential learning climate.

Clinical psychologist Burns (1998) commented on the possibility of our psychological and biological hard-wiring being triggered by natural stimuli, and how the environment is much more than a location for experiential learning. Rather, the environment is an integral part of experience. Kaplan and Kaplan (1989) conducted research in nature and conceptualised nature as restorative. They commented that perceptual aesthetic reactions that support effective human functioning indicate the existence of an ancient and far-reaching human behavioural function attuned with unconscious assessment of environments. These authors postulate that humans' reactions to natural environments can be beneficial via restorative qualities. Hartig and Statts (2004) called restorative environments a 'health resource' (p. 273).

Creative Group Work Experience in Natural Environments

From experiences and literature, I developed a model to describe potentials for interaction between human and natural beings in Forest School woodlands (see Figure 1). It is anticipated that working creatively in a natural woodland environment can engage both AS and neural-typical perceptions. In Figure 1, the outer large ring is seen as nature (a holding container), where earlier forms of understanding in nature might be experienced through a heightened sensate, phenomenological or gestalt sensate experience. The three smaller overlapping rings (human social dimension of group, focus for meaning and joint attention, and creative experience) overlap to form three more vectors: change, group art and reciprocity. When blended in the centre of the diagram, these form connectivity, relationality and relational coherence.

To Conclude

Is it the environment that we 'neural typicals' have constructed through our perceived separation from and domination of nature, what people with autism find anxiety laden?

I believe that it is the deconstructed 'self and other' as a concept that has separated much neural-typical world perception into 'me and not me'. This separates many of us from our 'relational selves as beings' in relation to the more-than-human. Combined with the possibility that people who have autism have not lost their ability to engage their gestalt perception of what is going on around them, and are aware of the more than-human world through their relational perception as ecological self, the original hypothesis is supported.

It is this reciprocity between the human and more-than-human world in nature that has the potential for healing actualisation, as relational and connected participants, on many levels of holistic being. This is why I consider that working creatively in woodlands with art is of benefit to people with autism. Based on experience, and backed up by theoretical and empirical literature evidence, it is likely that nature offers a cohesive 'holding environment' and is therefore beneficial for people who have autism. Further, inclusive relational therapy and learning can reciprocate in art and in nature, for both autistic and neural-typical minds sets.

References

Abram, D. (1996). *The spell of the sensuous*. New York: Vintage Books.

Adams, T. (2008). *Wilderness and inner space conference.* Hosted by the University of Kent: Retrieved on 11/5/09 from: http://www.libranches.org/branches/southeast/documents/ConferenceReport_WildernessandInnerSpace.pdf.

American Psychiatric Association. (2000). *Diagnostic and statistical manual of mental disorders. Fourth edition, Text revision.* Washington, DC: American Psychiatric Association.

Beard, C., & Wilson, J. P. (2009). *Experiential learning.* London: Kogan Page.

Bogdanashina, O. (2003). *Sensory perception issues in autism*. London: JKP.

Brunner, J. (1993). *Understanding other minds.* Oxford: Bookcraft.

Burns, G. (1998). *Nature guided therapy: Brief integrative strategies for health and wellbeing.* Philadelphia: Brunner / Mazel.

Buzzell, L., & Chalquist, C. (2009). *Ecotherapy.* San Francisco: Sierra Club Books.

Chodrow, J. (1997). *Jung on active imagination.* New Jersey: Princeton.

Cozolino, L. (2006). *The neuroscience of human relationships: Attachment and the developing social brain.* New York London: W. W. Norton

Cumine, V., Dunlop, J., & Stevenson, G. (2010). *Asperger syndrome: A practical guide for teachers.* Oxon: Routledge.

Delacato, C. (1974). The ultimate stranger. In *The autistic Child.* California: Academic Publications.

Dunn Buron, K., & Wolfberg, P. (Ed.). (2008). *Learners on the autistic spectrum: Preparing highly qualifled educators.* Kansas: Autism Asperger Publishing Co.

Frizell, C. (2008.) *In search of the wider self.* Retrieved on 8/20/09 from http://www.ecotherapy.org.uk/ files/ecotherapy/home/Caroline_Frizell.pdf.

Grandin, T., & Johnson, C. (2005). *Animals in translation: The woman who thinks like a cow.* London: Bloomsbury.

Harting, T., & Statts, H. (2004). Alone or with a friend: A social context for psychological restoration and environmental preferences. *Journal of Environmental Psychology, 24*(2) 199-211, June 2004.

Harvey, P., Fossati P., & Lepage, M. (2007.) Modulation of memory formation by stimulus content:

Specific role of the medial prefrontal cortex in the successful encoding of social pictures. *Journal of Cognitive Neuroscience[online].* Retrieved on 2/28/08 from: http://jocn.mitpress.org/cgi/content/abstract/19/2/351.

Hillman, J. (1972). *The myth of analysis*. New York: Harper Torchbooks.

Husserl, E. (1960). *Cartesian meditations*. The Hague: Martinus Nijhoff.

Jordan, M. (2009.) *Landscapes of the Mind Conference.* Friday 25 – Sunday 27 September 2009. Eden Project. Retrieved on 11/25/09 from: http://www.traydio.com/UserConsole/ViewArticle.aspx?Title=Martin_Jordan_speaking_at_Sept_2009_Confer_conference_on_Landscapes_of_the_Mind&ArticleID=2733.

Jordan, R. (2007). *Rita Jordan on causation.* Retrieved on 1/1/08 from: http://www.education2. bham.ac.uk/webautism/avpreview.html.

Kaplan, R., & Kaplan, S. (1989). *The experience in nature: A psychological perspective.* New York: Press Syndicate of the University of Cambridge.

Knight, S. (2009). *Forest schools and outdoor learning in early years*. London: Sage.

Knill, P., Levine, E., & Levine, S. (2005). *Principles and practice of expressive arts therapy: Towards a therapeutic aesthetic.* Philadelphia: Jessica Kingsley Press.

Lowenfeld, M. (2007). *Understanding children's sandplay: Lowenfleld's world technique.* Eastbourne: Sussex Academic.

Mahler, M.S., Pine, F., & Bergman, A. (2000). *The psychological birth of the human infant symbiosis and individuation*. New York: Basic Books

McCarthy, D. (2008). *Speaking about the unspeakable: Nonverbal methods and experiences in therapy with children*. London: Jessica Kingsley Press.

Mcniff, S. (2004). *Art-based research*. New York: Jessica Kingsley Press.

McNiff, S. (2009). *Integrating the arts in therapy*. Springfield: Thomas.

Mearns, D., & Cooper, M. (2005). *Working at relational depth in counselling and psychotherapy*. London: Sage.

Minshew N. J., Goldstein G., and Siegel D. J, (1997). Neuropsychologic functioning in autism: Profile of a complex information processing disorder. *Journal of the International Neuropsychological Society, 3*, 303-316.

Morgan, H. (1996). *Adults with autism: A guide to theory and practice*. New York: Cambridge University Press.

O'Hara, D. (2010). *Seventeenth Annual BACP Research Conference*. BACP. Retrieved on 5/8/10 from: http://www.bacp.co.uk/admin/structure/files/pdf/6922_saturday%20programme.pdf.

Ozonoff, S., Dawson, G., & McPartland, J. (2002). *A parent's guide to Asperger syndrome and high-functioning autism: How to meet the challenges and help your child thrive*. New York: Guildford Press.

Peter, M., 2003. Drama narrative and early learning. *British Journal of Special Education, 30*(1)22.

Roszak, T., Gomes, M., & Kanner, A. (Eds.). (1995). *Ecopsychology: Restoring the Earth, healing the mind*. San Francisco: Sierra club books.

Sessions, G. (Ed.). (1995). *Deep Ecology for the 21st Century*. Boston: Shambhala Publications.

Stanton M. (2008). *Wilderness and inner space conference*. Hosted by the University of Kent. Retrieved on 11/5/09 from: http://www.libranches.org/branches/southeast/documents/ConferenceReport_WildernessandInnerSpace.pdf.

Totton, N. (2009). *Really wild therapy: Exploring beyond the boundaries of the self*. A keynote address presented at the Fifth International Adventure Therapy Conference. Edinburgh University. Retrieved on 1/2/10 from: http://www.bacp.co.uk/5iatc/Keynotes.php.

Vallortigara, G., Snyder, A., Kaplan, G., Bateson, P., Clayton, N.S. & Rogers L.J. (2008). Are animals autistic savants? *PLoS Biology, 6* (2) 42. Retrieved on 11/1/10 from: www.plosbiology.org.

Winnicot, D.W. (1971). *Playing and reality.* London: Routledge.

Culture 24. (2009). *Woodland mythology: Icons a portrait of England.* Retrieved on 12/20/09 from: www.icons.org.uk

CHAPTER 29

The Interplay between Life and Death: A Narrative from Bushman's Hole

Lourens Human

ABSTRACT

On the 8th of January 2005, Don Shirley and David Shaw, two technical cave divers attempted to retrieve the body of Deon Dreyer from Bushman's Hole, a freshwater cave in the Northern Cape, South Africa (SA). Deon Dreyer had died on a previous caving trip on the 17th of December 1994 during a technical cave dive. During the retrieval cave dive, David Shaw lost his life and Don Shirley survived the cave dive. On the 9th of January 2005, Don Shirley narrated his experience of the fatal cave dive to Gordon Hales, a journalist. This interview is the focus of this paper, which attempts to understand how Don Shirley made sense of the fatal cave dive, through narrative analysis and narrative metaphor. Findings from the narrative analysis found that Don Shirley made sense of the fatal cave dive not according to the stages of normative grieving models, but through his own unique process. In this process he established an interplay between 'life' and 'death' in cave diving, which facilitated his process of making meaning of the fatal cave dive.

The goal of this paper is to portray a research study, and is two-fold in nature: The first goal is to describe how a cave diver made sense of a fatal cave dive in a unique way, and not according to the grieving phases postulated by normative grieving models. The second goal is to transfer what was learned from this process to the context of therapy in general, and to adventure therapy specifically.

INTRODUCTION

The participation of people in adventurous activities like bungee-jumping, paragliding, rock-climbing and sky-diving is increasing (Olivier, 2006; Tomlinson, 2004). Various reasons have been given for the growth of people's participation in adventurous activities in modern times, such as people's desire to seek adventure, the advancement of adventure activity equipment through technology, as well as the portrayal of participation in adventure activities via the media, such as television (Buchan, 2004; Willing, 2008).

Various terminology are used to describe people's participation in adventurous activities, such as: action sports (Bennett, Henson & Zhang, 2002), adventure sports (Buchan, 2004), dangerous sports (Willing, 2008), extreme sports (Brymer, 2005; willing, 2008) and lifestyle sports (Hill, 2002). Although the various terms are often used interchangeably (Buchan, 2004), this study uses the term 'extreme sports', as this research focuses on the narrative of a surviving technical cave diver regarding a fatal technical cave diving operation, in which a fellow technical cave diver lost his life. This is in accordance with the work of Brymer (2005), and Brymer & Odes (2009), who view 'extreme sports' as an activity where the probability of death is high in the context of a poorly managed mistake or accident.

The occurrence of death in sport in general, and adventure sports specifically, is not an uncommon phenomenon (Le Breton, 2000). Examples of studies conducted on death in sport include hockey (Karofsky, 1990), football (Henschen & Heil, 1992) and basketball (Vernacchia, Reardon & Templin, 1997) to name a few. In extreme sports, studies on death have been conducted in race car driving (Wann & Waddill, 2007), scuba diving (Doka, Schwarz & Schwarz, 1990; Smith, 1995; Ozdoba, Weis, Plattner, Dirnhofer & Yen, 2005), as well as cave diving (Byrd & Hamilton, 1997; Petri, Definis-Gojanovic & Andric, 2003).

The reasons for fatalities in diving have also been studied. For example, between 1992- 2005 there were 24 fatalities in recreational scuba diving in Western Australia. It was found that uncertified recreational scuba divers were more prone to fatalities than certified recreational scuba divers. Furthermore, the fatality rate was higher for shore dives than diving from commercial boats amongst recreational scuba divers (Buzzacot, Rosenberg & Pikora, 2009). There were 368 fatalities in cave diving in the United States of America (USA) between 1969-2007, mainly caused by drowning due to cave divers having insufficient air because they got lost or they started diving with insufficient air (Buzzacot, Zeigler, Denoble & Vann, 2009), as well as lack of experience and improper safety procedures (Byrd & Hamilton, 1997).

This paper focuses on a fatality in the extreme sport of cave diving, which has been labelled as one of the most dangerous explorative pursuits of all (Farr, 1991). On the 8th of January 2005 two cave divers, David Shaw and Don Shirley, attempted to retrieve the body of another cave diver, Deon Dreyer. He had died at the age of 20 years during a cave dive on the 17th of December 1994 at Bushman's Hole in the Northern Cape, South Africa (SA). This retrieval operation was undertaken at the request of Deon Dreyer's parents. Bushman's Hole is the third deepest freshwater cave (+/270m) (Zimmerman, 2005). This retrieval operation turned out to be a fatal one. David Shaw died during this retrieval operation, and Don Shirley survived after exiting the cave at Bushman's Hole over 13 hours later (Shirley, 2005). On the 9th of January 2005, Don Shirley narrated his experience of this fatal cave dive to journalist Gordon Hiles. His narrative is the focus point of this paper.

Various normative grieving models have been developed to understand and support people who are going through a grieving process. These models can pertain to people who are confronted by the possibility of their own death, due to for example terminal illnesses (Kübler-Ross, 1969), and/or people who have lost a loved one (e.g. a child, friend, spouse, colleague) through death (Horowitz, 2006). The underlying principle of these models is that people who are grieving go through certain phases in the grieving process. Although these models have value for people who are grieving, as well as for health professionals (e.g. psychiatrists, psychologists, social workers) they can also be limiting. Not all people go through the same grieving phases postulated in these models; instead, they make sense of death in their own unique way. By following the grieving phases outlined within models too strictly, health professionals may fail to 'see' and 'hear' the unique grieving processes people experience. As Bonanno (2009) and Kilcrease (2008) stated, people don't make sense of loss through grieving models, but rather through their own unique grieving process.

There are two goals for this paper: 1) to describe how a cave diver made sense of a fatal cave dive in a unique way, and not according to the grieving phases postulated by normative grieving models; 2) to transfer what was learned from this process to the context of therapy in general, and to adventure therapy specifically.

METHOD

Participants

The surviving cave diver in this research is Don Shirley. He is a European male, who at the time of the fatal cave dive was 48-years old. Don is involved in the South African franchise of the International Association of Nitrox and Technical Divers (IANTD), and was the Director of IANTD in Africa (Zimmerman, 2005). The journalist who interviewed Don Shirley regarding the fatal cave dive on the 9th of January 2005 was Gordon Hiles.

Research Paradigm

In this research, a cave diver narrated his experience to a journalist regarding the fatal cave dive of a fellow cave diver. For this reason, narrative metaphor within the constructivist/interpretive paradigm was adopted as the theoretical position for this research (Terre Blance & Durrheim, 2006; Young & Collin, 2004). Johnson (1993) stated that 'narrative is a fundamental mode of understanding, by means of which we make sense of all forms of human action' (p.11). Broyand (1992) stated 'always in emergencies we invent narratives … we describe what is happening as if to confine the catastrophe' (p.21). Narrative assists people in creating order out of dis-order, and allows bodily beings (*zoe*) to become human beings (*bios*) (Kearney, 2002). Narratives are primarily shaped by history and culture, as narrative is the meeting place of experience, history and culture (Crossley, 2000; Lock, Epston & Maisel, 2004; Sclater, 2003; White & Epston, 1990). This study focuses on the narrative that unfolded between Don Shirley and Gordon Hiles one day after the fatal death of David Shaw.

History implies that when people narrate their experiences they do it by taking pastlived experiences and possible future experiences into account, as past and future fuse into the present narrative (Larner, 1998). 'Since all stories [narratives] have a beginning (or a history), a middle (or a present), and an ending (or a future), the interpretation of current events is as much future-shaped as it is past-determined' (White & Epston, 1990, p.10).

Culture also plays a role in the way people narrate their experiences, as culture is an 'integral part of each individual's psychological flesh and bones … the material objects we create, the ideas we hold and the actions we take are shaped in a fundamental way by the social framework we have been raised in' (Cushman, 1995, p.17-18). 'Culture speaks itself through an individual's story [narrative]' (Riessman, 1993, p. 5). The cultural context of this study was sport in general, and cave diving specifically.

SUBJECT OF NARRATIVE ANALYSIS

The goal of narrative analysis is to understand how people make sense of their experiences through narrative (Langdridge, 2007; Ollerenshaw & Creswell, 2002; Riessman, 1993). The narrative used in this research was generated by means of an interview between Don Shirley and Gordon Hiles. Permission was obtained from both Don Shirley and Gordon Hiles to use the narrative for research purposes.

The narrative can be seen as a form of naturalistic material. The researcher was not present during the narration, which would have taken place irrespective of this research project (Potter, 2004; Potter & Hepburn, 2005). Using naturalistic material has the advantage that the narrative is not biased by predetermined psychological research agendas; that the interactional difficulties between interviewee-researcher relationships (for example rapport building) are avoided; and that the scope of material is not limited to the predisposed context of the research project (Potter & Hepburn, 2005).

Although there are various approaches to narrative analysis (Human, 2008; Ollerenshaw & Creswell, 2002), Riessman's (1993) approach to narrative analysis was employed in this research. This approach to narrative analysis entails the following phases:

- *Attending:* In this study the researcher focused on the lived experience of Don Shirley who survived a fatal cave dive in which David Shaw lost his live on the 8th of January 2005 at Bushman's Hole in the Northern Cape, SA.
- *Narrating:* In this research Don Shirley narrated his experience of the fatal cave dive in which David Shaw lost his life, to Gordon Hiles. As already indicated, this narrative can be seen as naturalistic material.
- *Transcribing:* In this study the researcher transcribed the interview between Don Shirley and Gordon Hiles from a video tape which took place on the 9th of January 2005, a day after the fatal cave dive. Permission was granted by Don Shirley and Gordon Hiles for the material to be used for research.
- *Analysing:* In this research the researcher analysed the narrative through an inductive process (Sparkes, 1999) to understand how Don Shirley made sense of the fatal cave dive on the 8th of January 2005.

FINDINGS

The narrative of Don Shirley leaves the researcher with the impression that it contains two opposing but interwoven secondary narratives, which can be summarized in the words: '*Fighting for life ... in the presence of death*'. In the narrative, Don Shirley creates interplay between 'life' and 'death' in an attempt to make sense of the fatal cave dive in which David Shaw was the victim and he the survivor. The narrative has a beginning '... *in the presence of death*' (Secondary narrative 1), which is followed by a middle '*fighting for life…*' (Secondary narrative 2), and ends by returning to '*...in the presence of death*' (Secondary narrative 1). This relationship is depicted in the Figure 1.

SECONDARY NARRATIVE 1: '… IN THE PRESENCE OF DEATH'

This secondary narrative is characterized by three movements, namely: the presence of death in a conversation between Don Shirley and David Shaw prior to the cave dive; the presence of death in the cave pertaining to the initial part of David Shaw's cave dive; and as the presence of death in the cave due to equipment (computer) failure in the initial moments of Don Shirley's cave dive.

The first movement in the secondary narrative starts with Don Shirley telling Gordon Hiles how he and David Shaw discussed the possibility of them dying during cave diving, before they commenced the retrieval cave dive on the 8th of January 2005. Don Shirley stated:

> Dave and I, discussed it even here, the fact that if something happens we'd [Don Shirley and David Shaw] like to stay wherever [cave] it [body] is … Um, it's like a battle, you know soldiers die in battle, it's a bit of a noble thing, even though a battle is not a nice thing… As far as doing the dive and not coming back, he [David Shaw] would be fine with it, in the same way I [Don Shirley] would be.

Don Shirley emphasizes two things of importance in the above quotation. The first is that both he and David Shaw accept death as an integral part of cave diving and that a cave can be their tomb, as can be seen in the words: '…the fact that if something happens we'd [Don Shirley and David Shaw] like to stay wherever [cave] it [body] is…' Through these words, Don Shirley indicates that he and David Shaw were in accordance that if they died during the cave dive, they would like their bodies to stay in the cave where they had died. The second aspect is depicted by using a military metaphor, in which he states that dying during a cave dive is not a tragedy of life, but something noble. This comment by Don Shirley reflects his and David Shaw's position on death. It is important to note that according to Don Shirley, he and David Shaw saw death as noble and not as a tragedy (which is a common, perhaps dominant viewpoint held in Western society).

The second movement in this secondary narrative depicts Don Shirley telling Gordon Hiles that David Shaw entered the cave first: 'Dave and I were both kitting-up on the surface… and we shook hands and said I'll see you in twenty minutes… and then he went, and then I waited for my count down, and then I went.' During his descent, Don Shirley realized that something was wrong regarding David Shaw: 'I would have expected bubbles by then… Dave would have been on his way up… would have been venting off as he came, and there was nothing… I could see a light in the distance like a lone star, like a real lone star in the dark, in the night'. The term 'venting off' refers to the release of pressure inside the re-breather machine when ascending, which David Shaw should have been doing by that time. The releasing of pressure causes bubbles that move through the water. The absence of these bubbles introduced the possibility of the presence of death during the cave dive. It seemed as if the presence of death did not remain within the boundaries of the conversation between Don Shirley and David Shaw prior to the cave dive, but followed them into the cave.

Figure 1: 'Fighting for Life…in the presence of death'

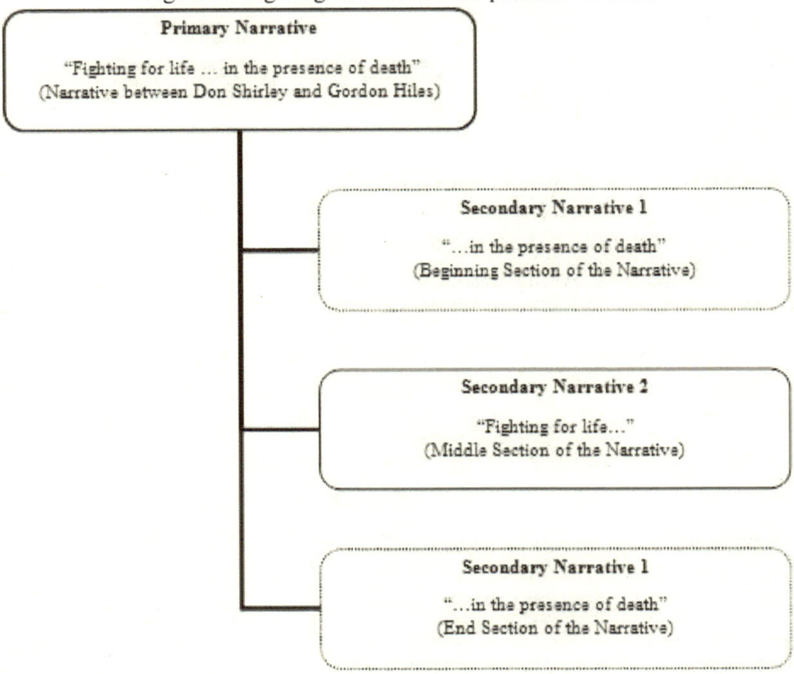

The third movement in the secondary narrative portrays the initial moments of Don Shirley's descent, when he tells Gordon Hiles: 'I passed the 220 line… I heard a 'click' and then a few metres on I heard a 'doef'… my electronics were blown, smashed right across the front of the screen… so I went on to open circuit'. Here, Don Shirley is referring to the equipment (computer) needed for the functioning of his re-breather, which is a complex breathing unit that extracts the Carbon Dioxide that the diver exhales and adds clean Oxygen. The re-breather probably broke due to the high pressure at a depth of 220m in the cave. Once the re-breather's equipment failed, Don Shirley had to go onto 'open circuit', which refers to standard cylinders and regulators that do not re-circulate the breathable air. This shortens the time a cave diver can remain in a cave. Due to the fact that Don Shirley's equipment had failed him, he started moving upwards out of the cave. He stated:

> I started to come up… everything was working fine… the computer was beautiful, I have got a nice new coloured VR 3 that stands out beautifully… I got up to 46m, and then the world started to spin… just like being in a washing machine, I was completely out of it, and I was just running on instinct.

The 'computer' (also called the 'VR 3' that Don Shirley is referring to in this quotation) is necessary for managing a decompression schedule, and is not the same one that caused the malfunctioning of Don's re-breather. The potential presence of death had now left the boundaries of the conversation between Don Shirley and David Shaw prior to the cave dive, and had entered the cave. Don Shirley realized that the potential of death was inherently present in the cave due to the fact that something had gone seriously wrong with the cave dive of David Shaw (as there were no bubbles), while his own equipment that regulated the re-breather had also failed him. He described his ascending as 'going fine' up to 46m in the cave, when he started experiencing vertigo as described through the washing machine metaphor. He started fighting for his life in the potential presence of death, as can be seen in the other secondary narrative.

SECONDARY NARRATIVE 2: 'FIGHTING FOR LIFE…'

In this secondary narrative Don Shirley tells Gordon Hiles of the actions that he took to fight for his life in the presence of death. There were six actions, namely: establishing a compass for himself due to his experience of vertigo; demonstrating a fighting attitude to retain his life; using his cave diving skills in his pursuit for life; doing the things that he needed to do step-by-step; dealing with time 'second-by-second' within the context of 'lumps-of-time'; as well experiencing the support of back-up divers.

The first action was to establish a compass for himself due to the vertigo he was experiencing: 'I was on the roof and um, it's just like being in a washing machine, I could, I knew that something was going wrong, feel it, like you, like you know you gonna faint'. To deal with the vertigo, he established a compass for himself by using the line in the cave. He stated:

> It's like kiddies playing on a washing line, you know they hold the line with their hands like this, and then they twist and hold it forward, and then they twist and hold it backwards. So that's exactly how it felt on this line. All I was concentrating on was grabbing the rope with one hand, and then finding it again with the other. Once I've done that then I move my hand to somewhere else. But I couldn't distinguish direction; I didn't know which was left or right. Um, I wasn't, I didn't even know which was up or down, um, but I knew that the drum was at the one end of the line and the coil was at the other. So I've found myself a compass. So I've found myself a compass, I was back at the drum. And then thought, but I wanted to go the other way, and I went the other way.

It seems that he used the line in the cave as a compass to establish direction for himself in the cave, which he had lost due to vertigo. This also gave him a sense of stability.

The second action pertained to demonstrating a certain attitude, as the presence of death in the cave made him realize that he had to survive this ordeal. He fought for his life through a fighting attitude which can be seen in the following words:

> And it was um, survival thing, you know you're thinking, what do I need to do now, that I need to survive, and it was thoughts just like that, you just saying what do I need to do now to live? There wasn't an option, there was never ever an option in my mind that I wouldn't come out, I did not have that, it wasn't, it wasn't on my option list, it was I will survive I will come out.

Although Don indicated in the opening lines of the narrative that he and David Shaw saw death during cave diving as a noble thing and not as a tragedy, this did not imply that death was accepted passively. Despite the presence of death in the cave and the view that death during cave diving is a noble thing, Don Shirley still decided to fight for his life.

The third action that assisted him to resist the presence of death in the cave was through his cave diving skills. He stated:

> You know, the familiarity with my gear, the fact that I could actually find things by touch, 'cause obviously I was concentrating on the line, I, if I needed a regulator I could find the regulator, I could pull out the appropriate part of the regulator, and breathe it, and, find the pressure gauge so I can actually see what's going on.

It seems that knowing his gear, knowing where the gear exactly was and how to use it effectively assisted him to focus on the compass he had established for himself due to vertigo. Not being familiar with his gear could have had catastrophic consequences by countering his actions to fight for his life and resist death.

The fourth action was to fight for his life in the presence of death by doing things step by-step, as can be seen in the following words:

> It was a case of saying of a, of I now need to breathe, and now I need to exhale, and everything was at that level, it was, there was no, nothing

> automatic about anything… But now, now it was a different story, now I was, surviving, and um, the way I worked it was I just said ok I got um, what's the next thing I must do. You know, breathe in breathe out, check gauge, and um, then I break it down into tasks, I've got to get from here to the *50%'s*.

He was able to fight for his life in the presence of death by focusing on what he needed to do at that moment to survive. Doing things step-by-step kept him from doing more than what was necessary to survive in that moment, which could have distracted his attention from surviving.

The fifth action in fighting for his life in the presence of death pertains to the manner in which he related to time. He stated:

> My time span was just that, that second, and surviving that second, without it being a long, a long drawn out thing. And I knew how long I had to stay, but I'm just thinking lumps of time, it's like I've got to be here, um, for fifty minutes, or I've got to be there for a hundred minutes.

It seems that there are two aspects to his notion of time during the cave dive. On the one hand he was dealing with time in 'lumps of-time', while on the other hand he was surviving 'second-by-second' within those 'lumps-of-time'. This could have assisted in him focusing on the here-and-now, and not on past and/or future events. Focusing on the here-and-now would also have assisted him in doing things step-by-step.

The sixth action that assisted him in fighting for his life in the presence of death was the support of back-up divers and support personnel. For this retrieval cave dive there were back-up divers to support Don Shirley and David Shaw during the cave dive. Once the dive had gone wrong for both Don Shirley and David Shaw, the back-up divers were used to meet with Don Shirley at certain intervals while he was busy decompressing. He stated that a back-up diver came along and 'I wrote the slate, um, basically saying I'm having a bad time and um, have got vertigo, and that I'm vomiting um, and a um, you know, got problems, and he went off with that slate'. He also said:

> The guys [back-up divers] were good, they keep on coming, giving me stuff, moved my hand to places I needed to move it to, and finding things that I needed to find, I'd write them a letter [on a slate], so they'd say, ok, you know they'd go off and get it and come back... doc [medical doctor] was sending down messages saying I should come out and go to

> the chamber, had already sent down some um, some potions and lotions to stop me being sick, but it did not stay down for more than about thirty seconds. So that didn't have much hold, but I wrote back saying I didn't really wanna come out yet, I wanted to get my 6 minute stop out of the way at least.

It seems that the support of back-up divers and support personnel formed an integral part of his endeavour to fight for his life in the presence of death. This most probably created the experience of not being alone in the survival battle and having continuous support from other people. Once Don Shirley had narrated the various actions that he had taken to fight for his life in the presence of death, he returned to the other secondary narrative.

Secondary Narrative 1: '… In the Presence of Death'

In this secondary narrative, Don Shirley once again addressed the phenomenon of dying during a cave dive with Gordon Hiles. He stated:

> What we'll have to debate on that is, Dave, Dave's expressed wish, which he did several times, is to stay where he was, so um, I think that unless his wife countermanded that, um, I would prefer to leave Dave as he is where he is a, end of story. Um, the only thing that would be sad would be future treasure hunters, um, you know Dave sat there in a lot of gear, um, which actually wouldn't deteriorate too much.

From this quotation it seems that three things are of importance. Firstly, he would prefer to leave David Shaw in the cave as his final resting place as this was David Shaw's wish. Secondly, only if David Shaw's wife wanted his body to be retrieved could this wish be overruled. Lastly, he was afraid that in future, 'treasure hunters' would steal David Shaw's gear. Don Shirley concludes the narrative by once again portraying life and death as being integral to cave diving. He said 'I don't see a cave as nasty place… and neither did Dave. A cave is a place where we lived… where life happened, and that would be a fitted end, just like the Egyptian's tomb'.

Discussion

In the introduction to this paper, two goals were stated. The first goal was to describe how a cave diver made sense of a fatal cave dive in a unique way, and not necessarily according to the grieving phases postulated by normative grieving models. But we know more about how he processed the experience of the cave death, and less about how he dealt with his grief. The second goal was to transfer what might be learned from this narrative process to the context of therapy in general, and to adventure therapy specifically.

With reference to the first goal, Don Shirley first made sense of the fatal cave dive by creating an interplay between 'life' and 'death' in cave diving. To him, life and death are equally present in cave diving. Secondly, he saw death as a 'noble thing', and not a tragedy. For many in especially the Western world, a tragedy is something that people try to avoid (due to fear) and therefore keeps them from living adventurous lives; whilst a perspective of 'nobility in death 'allows for exploration and adventure. Thirdly, despite seeing death as a noble thing, he did not accept death passively, but fought actively for his life. This he did through various actions during the cave dive. In this particular narrative, no support was found for a sense-making process through a normative grieving model (Horowitz, 2006; Kübler-Ross, 1969); rather the demonstration of resilience in the presence of death (Bonanno, 2009; Kilcrease, 2008).

With reference to the second goal, this narrative may confront people who are informed by normative grieving models (for example, health care professions such as physicians, psychologists, or social workers). Not only might their normative grieving models be challenged, but they may be invited into an open attitude, and provided with a unique view of life and death, of the relationship between life and death, as well as how they make sense of life and death. Within the field of therapy in general, and adventure therapy specifically, health care professionals must balance an interplay between normative grieving models, while also respecting people's unique way of making sense of death. This principle can also be transferred to other areas in adventure therapy, for example in examining depression and anxiety, and peoples' unique experiences of those phenomena.

This narrative encourages health care professionals to develop their ability to allow people to make sense of their own experiences through narrative, while also being cognisant of normative models of dealing with human behaviour. For therapists, and adventure therapists in particular, the author comments it should be a matter of unique experiences *and* normative models, rather than unique experience *or* normative models.

Conclusion

The narrative of Don Shirley confronts one to examine their own view of life and death. It is possible that seeing death as a 'tragedy' may keep one from living an adventurous life. Perhaps seeing death as something 'noble' does not ask for a passive acceptance of death, but rather an active participation in the journey of life.

Acknowledgement

The author wishes to acknowledge Edrich Smook, a postgraduate counselling psychology student, for his involvement in this research project.

References

Bennett, G., Henson, R., & Zhang, J. (2002). Action sports sponsorship. *Sport Marketing Quarterly, 11*, 174-185.

Bonanno, G. A. (2009). *The other side of sadness. What the new science of bereavement tells us about life after loss.* New York, NY: Basic Books.

Broyard, A. (1992). *Intoxicated by my illness and other writings on life and death.* New York, NY: Clarkson Potter.

Brymer, G. E. (2005). *Extreme dude: A phenomenological perspective on the extreme sport experience.* Unpublished doctoral thesis. University of Wollongong, Australia.

Brymer, E., & Oades, L. G. (2009). Extreme sports: A positive transformation in courage and humility. *Journal of Humanistic Psychology, 49*,114-126.

Buzzacot, P. L., Rosenberg, M., & Pikor, T. (2009). Western Australia recreational scuba diving fatalities, 1992 to 2005. *Australian and New Zealand Journal of Public Health, 33*, 212-214.

Buzzacot, P. L., Zeigler, E., Denoble, P., & Vann, R. (2009). American cave diving fatalities 1969-2007. *International Journal of Aquatic Research and Education, 3*,162-177.

Byrd, J. H., & Hamilton, W. F. (1997). Underwater cave diving fatalities in Florida: A review and analysis. *Journal of Forensic Sciences, 42*, 807-811.

Crossley, M. L. (2000). Narrative psychology, trauma and the study of self/identity. *Theory & Psychology, 10,* 527-546.

Cushman, P. (1995). *Constructing the self, constructing America: A cultural history of psychotherapy.* Reading, MA: Addison-Wesley.

Doka, K. J., Schwarz, E. E., & Schwarz, C. (1990). Risky business: Observations on the nature of death in hazardous sports. *Omega, 21*, 215-223.

Farr, M. (1991). *The darkness beckons: The history and development of cave diving.* St. Louis, MO: Cave Books.

Henschen, K. P., & Heil, J. (1992). A retrospective study of the effect of an athlete's sudden death on teammates. *Omega: Journal of Death and Dying, 25*, 217-223.

Horowitz, M. (2006). Stages of grief models. Retrieved from: http://www.mentalhelp.net.

Hill, L. (2002). *Climbing free.* London, England: Harper Collins.

Human, L. H. (2008). Unique outcomes in professional training in psychology through an adventure experience. *Acta Academia, 40*, 151-174.

Johnson, M. (1993). *Moral imagination: Implications of cognitive science for ethics.* Chicago, IL: University of Chicago Press.

Karofsky, P. S. (1990). Death of a high school hockey player. *The Physician and Sports Medicine, 18*, 99-103.

Kearney, R. (2002). *On stories.* London, England: Routledge.

Kilcrease, W. (2008). Stages of grief: Time for a new model. *Psychology Today.* Retrieved from http:// www.psychologytoday.com.

Kübler-Ross, E. (1969). *On death and dying: What the dying have to teach doctors, nurses, clergy, and their own families.* New York, NY: Touchstone.

Langdridge, D. (2007). *Phenomenological psychology. Theory, research and method.* London, England: Pearson.

Larner, G. (1998). Through a glass darkly. Narrative as destiny. *Theory & Psychology, 8*, 549-572.

Le Breton, D. (2000). Playing symbolically with death in extreme sports. *Body & Society, 6*, 1-11.

Lock A., Epston, D., & Maisel, R. (2004). Countering that which is called anorexia. *Narrative Inquiry, 14*, 275-301.

Olivier, S. (2006). Moral dilemmas of participation in dangerous leisure activities. *Leisure Studies, 25*, 95-109.

Ollerenshaw, J., & Creswell, J. W. (2002). Narrative research: A comparison of two restorying data analysis approaches. *Qualitative Inquiry, 8*, 329-347.

Ozdoba, C., Weis, J., Plattner, T., Dirnhofer, R., & Yen, K. (2005). Fatal scuba diving incident with massive gas embolism in cerebral and spinal arteries. *Neuroradiology, 47*, 411-416.

Petri, N. M., Definis-Gojanovic, M., & Andric, D. (2003). Scuba diver with a knife in his chest: Homicide or suicide? *Croatian Medical Journal, 44*, 355-359.

Potter, J. (2004). Discourse analysis. In M. Hardy & A Bryman (Eds.), *Handbook of data analysis* (pp. 607-624). London, England: Sage.

Potter, J., & Hepburn, A. (2005). Qualitative interviews in psychology: Problems and possibilities. *Qualitative Research in Psychology, 2,* 281-207.

Puchan, H. (2004). Living extreme: Adventure sports, media and commercialisation. *Journal of Communication Management, 9*, 171-178.

Riessman, C. K. (1993). *Narrative analysis*. Newbury Park, CA: Sage.

Sclater, S. D. (2003). What is the subject? *Narrative Inquiry, 13*, 317-330.

Shirley, D. (2005). *Living, dying & diving in South Africa: The David Shaw story*. Retrieved from: http:// www.technicaldivingafrica.com.

Smith, N. (1995). Scuba diving: How high the risk? *Journal of Insurance Medicine, 27*, 15-24.

Sparkes, A. C. (1999). Exploring body narratives. *Sport, Education and Society, 4*, 17-30.

Terre Blanche, M., & Durrheim, K. (2006). Histories of the present: Social science research in context. In M. Terre Blanche, K. Durrheim & D. Painter (Eds.), *Research in Practice: Applied methods for the social sciences* (pp. 1-17). Cape Town, South Africa: University of Cape Town Press.

Tomlinson, J. (2004). *Extreme sports: In search of the ultimate thrill.* Hove, England: Firefly Books Ltd.

Vernacchia, R. A., Reardon, J.P., & Templin, D.P. (1997). Sudden death in sport: Managing the Aftermath. *The Sport Psychologist, 11*, 223-235.

Wann, D. L., & Waddill, P. J. (2007). Examining reactions to the Dale Earnhardt crash: The importance of identification with NASCAR drivers. *Journal of Sport Behaviour, 30*, 94-108.

White, M., & Epston, D. (1990). *Narrative means to therapeutic ends.* New York, NY: Norton.

Willig, C. (2008). A phenomenological investigation of the experience of taking part in extreme sports. *Journal of Health Psychology, 13*, 690-702.

Young, R. A., & Collin, A. (2004). Introduction: constructivism and social constructionism in the career field. *Journal of Vocational Behavior, 64,* 373-388.

Zimmerman, T. (2005). *Raising the dead.* Retrieved from http://www.technicaldiving africa.com.

CHAPTER 30

Creating Reflexive Space: A Utilisation of Art-making in Outdoor Programs

Cathryn Carpenter and Tarquam McKenna

ABSTRACT

The healing capabilities of the arts as a therapeutic tool have long been used to rehabilitate and aid in recovery processes. Most significantly, within the mental health sector, art has been used to help build personal insight, and is central to the work of art therapy. Art-making offers a visual and non-verbal method of communicating peoples' thoughts, ideas and feelings, and also provides an approach that may help reconcile identity conflict. When combined with spending time within a natural environment, art-making can challenge perceptions of an individual's identity, connection to others, as well as sense of place in the world.

This paper discusses ways in which art has been utilised in the outdoors as a process to encourage exploration of a sense of being, becoming and belonging; both internally and externally. The ideas expressed here have evolved through direct practice in the field with both clients and tertiary students, and is reflective of their experiences. This paper documents art-based approaches and processes that enhance the provision of 'reflexive space,' which is central to therapeutic work. The structuring of boundaries, the explicit facilitation of diverse relationships, and the articulation of intention are variables within an outdoor program that if attended to, can strengthen the deepening of one's awareness of self, and create feelings of greater wellbeing.

INTRODUCTION: A MEANINGFUL LIFE

The fundamental premise of our work though perhaps idealistic, is the need to be engaged in a life that has meaning and flow. The intersection of meaning that can occur between experiences in the natural world and the world of art-making can generate outcomes of wellness and wellbeing through processes or encounters that can be transformative, reclaiming and restorative. Reflexivity is our capacity to make sense of our experience, and build on our learning in order to act purposefully into the future. Reflexive space is a space in which people can make positive use of reflection, and develop personal understandings of the environment around them. For any process to be meaningful, each individual needs to invest some time and energy placing their interpretation of new experiences within their own past and future understandings of their world.

In this discussion we aim to share some of the literature and experiences that have influenced and informed the evolution of our approach to utilising art in natural places as a paratherapeutic tool that can deepen and enhance both participants' and practitioners' lives. An individual's sense of wellbeing is a key determinant in improving their health. Furnass (1995) defined wellbeing as:

> Satisfactory human relationships, a meaningful occupation, opportunities for contact with the natural environment, creative expression, and making a positive contribution to human society (p. 6).

This definition clearly indicates that the creative process of making art in the outdoors, especially within a group context, has potential to enhance the health and wellbeing of people participating in the activity. Documenting the personal experience of enhanced wellbeing has been guided by World Health Organization researchers who suggest that:

> In some ways, wellbeing might best be assessed subjectively, as it is strongly associated with notions of happiness and life satisfaction. Thus personal wellbeing might be measured in terms of how happy or satisfied people are with their life or with aspects of their life (their job, health, etc.) (Wilkinson & Marmot, 2003, p.6).

Within this paper we use peoples' art and reflections to enlarge understandings of what is happening in the therapeutic process of making art in nature, and explore how making art in the outdoors can facilitate a reciprocal and cyclic deepening of peoples' connection to place, assist in exploring sensations of belonging, and increase the perceptions of happiness and wellbeing.

The insights provided by the work of Csikszentmihalyi (1975) and Seligman (2011) and others in the development of the Positive Psychology movement maintain that the prevailing model of psychology, with its focus on illness and symptoms, does not reflect an optimal well-adjusted view of human potential. These authors noted that, although the study of mental illness has successfully led to the identification, classification, and treatment of many disorders, it has neglected to account for what has become increasingly evident: that the improvement or absence of psychiatric symptoms does not necessarily increase wellbeing, and that increased happiness is a treatment imperative in and of itself.

According to Duckworth, Seligman and Steen (2005), the relief of suffering does not lead to well-being, it only removes the barriers to well-being. Well-being is a process over and above the absence of depression, anxiety, and anger.

In Csikzentmihalyi' s (1975) seminal work, 'Beyond Boredom and Anxiety' he shared initial findings of his research with diverse populations focusing on what made someone happy and satisfied with life. His subsequent theory of flow has informed and shaped the dynamics of the art-making experiences the authors have provided for participants in outdoor programs. Flow 'provides a key to understanding the strivings of the self and illustrates the human search for an improved quality of wellbeing' (Csikzentmihalyi, 1990, p.153). In many ways the search for an optimal learning environment is a strategy to enhance a participant's ability to access the 'flow' of an optimal human experience. According to Csikzentmihalyi, 'The best moments in our lives…usually occur when a person's body or mind is stretched to its limits in a voluntary effort to accomplish something difficult and worthwhile' (p.3).

Seligman (2002) outlined three domains in which people experience happiness: the pleasant life (pursuit of positive feelings), the engaged life (using your strengths for success), and the meaningful life (using your strengths for purposes beyond yourself) (p. 249). Ryff and Singer (2008) define key aspects of happiness as 'human flourishing' or 'eudemonia' (cited in Seligman, 2011). An approach to health and wellbeing outlining these components is provided in Table 1.

Art making outdoors on an adventure therapy or educational program can be structured to enable participants to have a sense of freedom and self-exploration in pursuit of an alternative understanding of their lives.

OUTDOOR PROGRAMS AND THE UTILISATION OF ART-MAKING TO CREATE REFLEXIVE SPACE

Programs in the outdoors utilise adventures in natural surroundings, within a group context for recreational, educational or therapeutic intent. As the number of these programs has grown, increasing concerns have been raised about the ways in which these programs are implemented. Loynes (2002) along with others, such as Ringer (1999) and Brookes (2003), have questioned the predominance of generic processes and outcomes that take the focus away from the individual capacity to determine what they need or want in a given experience.

Carpenter (2008) articulated a range of approaches available in order to clarify choices facilitators have in the construction of an educational or therapeutic experience. The continuums outlined in Table 2 indicate each paradigm's context and emphasis, building upon the earlier work of Ringer (1999) and Loynes (2002).

This paper discusses outdoor programs that combine a generative approach with the processes of art-making and explicit health and wellbeing objectives. The following sections weave together the knowledge gained from the authors' combined experiences of working with people in outdoor environments, along with various theories that have shaped the processes by which we create reflexive space. These processes include the promotion of permeable boundaries, deep awareness of the physical place, a new interpretation of space and time, and relationships with self, other and the natural world. These sections present artwork created by participants of our outdoor programs to exemplify these concepts.

Table 1: Key aspects of the eudemonic approach to health and wellbeing (Ryff & Singer, 2008)

Self-Acceptance – Long term self-evaluation that demonstrates awareness and acceptance of both personal strengths and weaknesses
Positive Relationships – Ability to love, empathise and are for others
Personal Growth – Realisation of personal potential along with a focus on self-development, growth and becoming
Purpose in Life – Finding meaning and direction in life that can accommodate different stages in life
Environmental Mastery – Capacity to create or control and engage in a surrounding context that suits personal needs
Autonomy – Sense of independence, self-determination and freedom that is not governed by outside influences (Ryff and Singer, 2008)

Table 2: Paradigms of practice (Carpenter, 2008)

Algorithmic – *rational*		**Generative - *intuitive***
Predetermined measurable outcomes	*Outcomes* ⟷	Emergent, creative, based on hope and possibility
Artificially constructed experience that is objectively action and conversation centered. Learning is metaphonic.	*Experience* ⟷	Journeys or reflexive spaces where meaning and value subjectively emerge within the experience. Learning is goal free – a process rather than a solution
Facilitator leads in transactional style with consent and limited choices	*Relationships* ⟷	Facilitator accompanies journey – egalitarian relationships are based on mutuality and trust
Place is the action entre – a resource to be resolved, controlled and co modified.	*Place* ⟷	Place is central critical and ecocentric. A place to be, to relate within community and environment
Progress and Consumption along with leadership and self reliance	*Ethos* ⟷	Politically motivated – social justice, inner congruence and human interdependence

Boundaries

For facilitators aiming to support effective therapeutic learning experiences, understanding the need to provide a physically, emotionally and spiritually safe place from which to expand participants' horizons, is fundamental in the selection of place. When working with marginalised or disadvantaged populations, the provision of this space becomes even more important. As Berman and Davis-Berman (2005) suggest, positive supportive environments are more ethically sound as well as being more conducive to change.

Csikszentmihalyi (1990) emphasised the need for being grounded in a safe and supportive environment to encourage individuals to reach beyond their comfort zones; however this concept remains elusive for many. How does a facilitator structure an experience of a space that will be experienced as being safe and supportive? Attending to the dimensions of space, place and time provides a program with boundaries that can contain and safely shape the learning or therapeutic environment.

Permeability of boundaries has been a characteristic of the work style in groups undertaken in the authors' programs. The external boundaries for containment of the group have malleability: it is the sense of freedom that is one of the core bonds for group members. Whilst we believe it is important to maintain ethical boundaries with participants, we are making a strong call for permeability in these boundaries, and hold to the belief that this is essential for how a group may function, which is key for the development of reflexive space. We have arrived at a place in our work as illustrated below in Image 1, in which there are conscious mechanisms in place to create an open space for knowing. This openness allows for complexity of meaning, and recognises there is qualitatively an invitation to be here as a group member in a space which is safe, open, permeable and not overly regulated.

Image 1. Flow, boundaries and core of self*

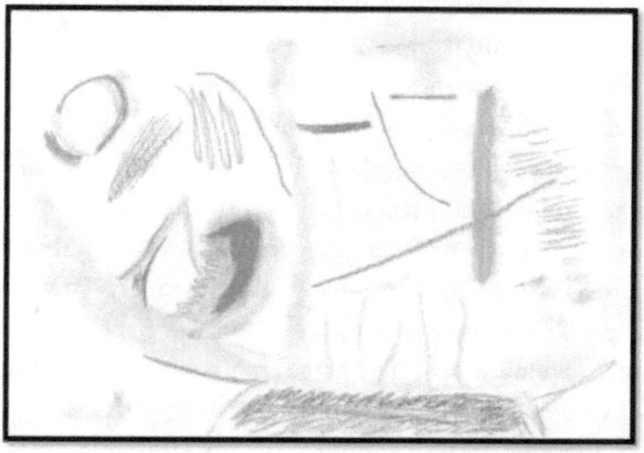

*In this image created by a participant in the outdoors, the artwork becomes a basis for attending to boundaries, interiority and the interior world of patterns, flow and affect. The image assists in locating the psychological as well as phenomenological events across space and time, and is an intimate statement of encounter. The art-making moved the learner across space, place and temporality. The setting of the natural world was an inspiration that enabled a thick, deep and rich contemplation of the environment through the participant's unique personalised art form. There is not the necessity to answer the call for interpretation and analysis. The art has a reflexive capacity drawn from the participant's desire to offer the image to the group. In this immersive, shared space they recognise the lines, shapes and forms they create whilst representations of perception, are realisations of affect.

The Physical Place

The choice to locate our reflexive art processes in the outdoors or natural environments is a deliberate one. Natural environments are usually neutral, without artificial restrictions, and can be selected to support and frame the intentions of the program. Place is traditionally a physical location, as with Tuan's (1977) observation that, 'place achieves concrete reality when our experience of it is total, that is through all senses as well as the active and reflective mind' (p. 56). The place selected for our programs is new to all participants; however, the processes ensure a gradual layering of experiences in the place. As familiarity is increased, so too is an understanding of ways we connect to place.

The physical place is usually an area of visual interest and natural beauty. Natural features can generate a range of emotional responses including awe, curiosity, discomfort and challenge. Kaplan and Kaplan's (1995) research into human relationships with nature, which resulted in the concept of a restorative environment, takes our initial emotional response to 'place' to a deeper level. These authors explained, 'extended time in nature provides a sense of wellbeing, of being renewed, of being restored' (Kaplan & Kaplan, 1995, p.146). The natural environment has health and healing benefits in its own right. A recent review of research literature indicates that contact with nature promotes health and wellbeing in many ways. For example, contact with nature has recuperative qualities and enhances positive outlook on life (Maller, Townsend, St.Ledger, Henderson-Wilson, Pryor, Prosser & Moore, 2008).

Once people develop a sense of place, the subjective experience often also results in the development of a sense of ownership: a territorial sense of safety within that space that may be valuable to maintain. Creswell (2004) indicated that understanding our relationships with place are important, 'Place is not just a thing in the world but a way of understanding the world' (p.11). Getting to know a place, and slowing down and spending time are simple ways that enable our horizons to expand, internally and externally.

Re-experiencing Space and Time

The subjective experience of space determines participants' willingness to explore their perceptions openly with others, and through the process of sharing their artwork, come to a deeper understanding of their internal motivation and thoughts. Creating an open, supportive and non-judgmental space is vital. It must be recognised that the lived experience of the program space changes over time, and that the ideas of 'space' and 'place' require each other for definition. From the security and stability of 'place', we are aware of the openness, freedom and threat of 'space', and vice versa (Tuan, 1977). When trying to convey the importance of the experience of safe space, the Chinese philosopher Lao Tse (traditionally regarded as the founder of Daoism and author of the Dao-te-Ching in the 6th Century) alluded to the significance of the 'essence' within: 'Walls with windows and doors form the house, but it is the empty space within that is the essence of home' (cited in Tuan, 1997, p.6). In this way the virtual structures of the boundaries seem to shape the reflexive space well.

Incorporating what are known as 'kairos' interpretations of time into these types of program is vital. Kairos time involves, moving with the natural rhythms of the day, and allowing an unspecified amount of time to enable activities to draw to a natural conclusion. Knowing the right time to bring the group together, to change focus of an activity or shape a discussion requires the facilitator being attuned to each individual and the group. This approach to the work also requires a period of time for people to slow down and become accustomed to the change in life patterns. In this reflexive space, people are encouraged to take as long as required for the activity rather than be regulated by hours and minutes. The kairos interpretation of time allows participants to better understand the interconnected pathways of nature and their place in the natural world. Image 2, created by a participant, shows how a kairos interpretation of time creates space for playfulness and self-discovery.

Image 2. Pathways: Nature, energy and water*

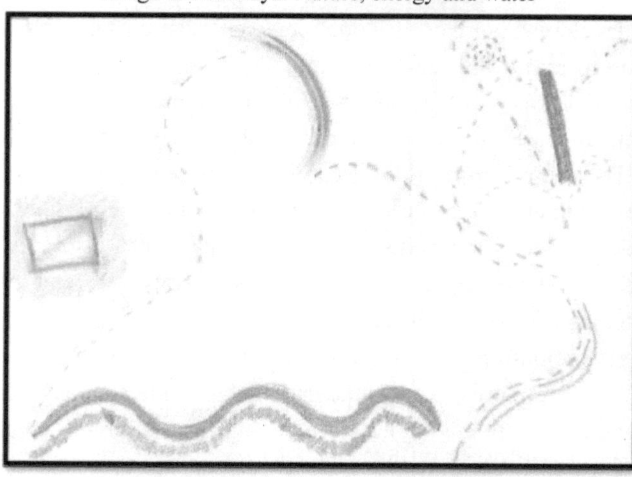

*In this artwork, it is through playfulness and reverie that the learner using art moves to a space of connection with the natural world and her place in it. As Winnicott (1971) wrote, 'It is in playing and only in playing that the individual child or adult is able to be creative and to use the whole personality, and it is only in being creative that the individual discovers the self' (p. 63). Jung (1933) spoke directly to the power of the process of art-making when he said, 'The discipline of drawing endows that fantasy with an element of reality, thus lending it greater weight and greater driving power. And actually these crude pictures do produce effects which, I must admit, are rather difficult to describe... freed from a wretched state of mind by working at a symbolical picture... in this way something invaluable is won, namely a growth of independence, a step towards psychological maturity' (p. 80).

Relationships

Relationships with the environment, with other people and with our past and future selves are further key structures in our development of reflexive space. Seligman's (1996) work explores the human relationship with nature in order to achieve an understanding of perceptions individuals have of the role of the natural environment in their lives. His early work charted the transition of our perceptions of nature from regarding nature as being an external object, through to its being experienced subjectively as part of us. Seligman's (2004) work also explores a more idealised relationship with the natural world by describing the way people feel their interaction with the natural world increases over time. Increased time spent in nature also emphasises the potential for it to become a restorative place, as described by Kaplan and Kaplan (1995).

Beyond their connections with nature, small group sizes in outdoor programs also assist development of critical interpersonal relationships that participants need to come to terms with and negotiate. The social context of the individual within a group is very significant, because the remoteness of the program's location elicits the need for human interaction for the comfort and potentially, the survival of the group. Forsyth (2001) confirms that being part of a group can be 'appropriate treatment for a variety of problems, including addiction, thought disorders, depression, eating disorders and personality disorders' (p. 629). Relationships developed within groups can be therapeutic, and being in the outdoors can magnify both the benefits and the issues.

The final relationship that provides fundamental insight into the construction and experience of reflexive space is the knowledge, understanding and confusion embedded within perceptions of our selves. The construction or exploration of an identity that we are comfortable with is central to the development of a meaningful life. Sociologist Giddens (1991) suggested that self-identity 'has to be routinely created and sustained in the reflexive activities of the individual' (p. 52). This emphasises that it is through interaction with the external world and self-reflection that the individual identity defines itself. Giddens's approach to identity formation credits the individual with the power and ability to shape their future.

The psychological sense of identity that we hold to is characterised and defined by our belief that the deep structure of the self is mediated by and influenced by symbols in society and in ourselves. Thus, the power of the image in the artwork intersects with the symbols, and art-making becomes a means of connecting these internal and external worlds. The artwork is an intermediary to the restructuring of the psychological 'life world' and 'life story'. This form of innovative art-making, during an encounter with the natural world, is an opportunity to articulate experiential knowledge. As the images become imaginative symbols of shifts in insight and shifts in one's sense of the self, the image becomes an intermediate step between the environment and the emergent and ever-changing sense of self-hood for participants (see Figure 3).

Image 3. The centre*

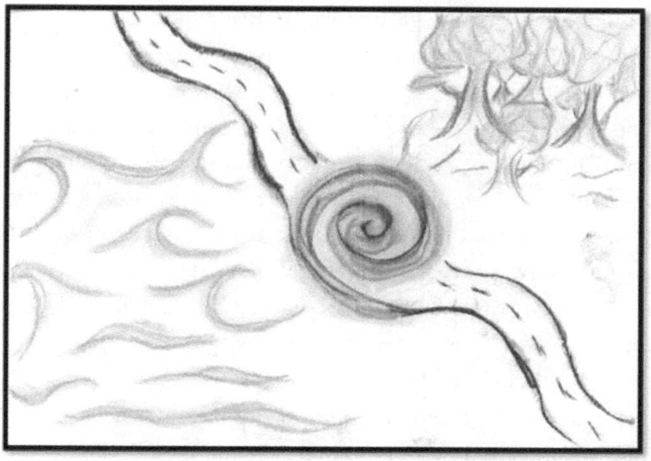

*The students in the bush setting become sensitive to and aware of other ways of knowing. As Case (2007) notes, they can 'recall images, present images, body changes, and feelings [that] are all interconnected in a process of thinking . . . conscious reflection... reverie and play' (p. 113). Case also alludes to the quality of knowing as uncovering their sense of self whilst their 'non-verbal narrative of knowing' sits alongside the verbal and written forms of perception (p.113). The artwork becomes a form of heuristic inquiry. The participant was able to review, re-create and re-invent their sense of self through the encounter with the natural world and the art making process.

There is a permeability and flexibility at the core of this process. The framework of boundaries and relationships within this reflexive space is open and permeable, free and flexible. The collective respectful space enabled the creation of narratively rich art-making experiences.

SELECTING THE ART-MAKING PLACE AND PROCESS

In order to facilitate the art-making process, it is important to be intentional in selecting place and process. Tuning in to common human responses to environments enables us to optimise activities via the selection of location. To enhance an 'inward focus', a natural amphitheatre, or sitting within a treed enclosure or at night around a fire, all seem to assist in channelling of attention inwards. Being on the top of mountains, on cliff faces or beaches tends to broaden the inner horizons and enhance a focus outwards, or on the future. The location also needs to be isolated from other groups or the passing traffic of people in order for the individual and the group focus to be maintained.

Many adventure therapy and education programs are in a state of constant motion within a journey context (for example, bushwalking, paddling, ski touring, etc.) from the beginning to the end, with activity being a dominant spatial factor. Even programs that do not include a longer journey usually entail a short self-contained journey to facilitate the sense of separation from everyday commitments. From the authors' perspective the development of reflexive space is enhanced by stopping for a couple of days in one place. Programming 'stationary space' far enough into the journey for a sense of separation and achievement, but not so close to the end of the program that concerns of returning home dominate the thought patterns is important.

Strategies like having a central point for drinks and snacks where people can attend to their own needs when appropriate enable the facilitator to engage with each person informally, which helps attenuate their sense of the group's needs. Using food breaks as transitions in time are also helpful to encourage people to immerse themselves in the reflexive space being created. All programs are limited by chronological time, however facilitators can reduce the impact of time by creating a space that supports the experience of 'flow' and opportunities to experience and understand the components of a happier and more meaningful life.

When incorporating art-making into the reflexive space, the authors use portable and very practical and pragmatic art materials. The selection of chalks and paper has at the core some principles of simplicity and are manageable for non-artist group members. The spirit of the colours and the emptiness of the large formatted paper on board are noteworthy. These experiences attend to a sense of spirit, as evident in the writing of Farrelly-Hansen (2001). Farrelly-Hansen's 'Contribution to nature: Art therapy in partnership with the Earth' is particularly pertinent to the nature of the work and the sense of group focus we establish using art.

The provision of a range of materials and the invitation to utilise natural materials (within National Park regulations) provide options for creative interpretations and an exploration of textures, colours, and personally-constructed meanings. The inherent characteristics of natural objects like trees, rocks, reeds or root systems to reflect strength, flexibility or alternative paths are incorporated into the process.

The deliberate encouragement to use traditional symbols like circles, arrows, spirals, triangles and squares reduces the expectation that people will attempt to draw or accurately replicate what they can see; the focus can begin to reflect more accurately what they feel.

Intention, Encounter, Engagement

Within the context of this paper any deliberation on intentionality is necessarily limited. That said, we are eager to note several key characteristics that underpin our 'intention' of the art-making process outdoors. The intent is always, in our minds, open and permeable. The reflexive group space is illustrated in Figure 1, where it is noted that there is a permeability of meaning that occurs around boundaries, relationships and the intentions of the work.

The development of a reflexive space utilising the boundaries of space, place, time, the intentions of the program, and the relationship between people and the landscape, are interwoven. The reflexive space for art-making and the capacity to advance a sense of self is discussed later in the paper but the ultimate intention of the work is the move toward 'new ways of knowing' for group members and facilitators. Intention here is ontologically located, and our notion of intentionality is largely predicated on the belief that art making is a symbolic way we can have meaning (Jung, 1933). Intentionality for us is aligned with the belief that all acts of consciousness are physical and mental phenomena. The intent of being with a group in a bush setting and making art is to deepen this sense of self-knowledge in this collection of people or community. The community that is created is unique to this moment of being together, and the quality of *encounter* that the participants have in the *immediacy of the moment* is at the core of the intent of the work together.

Figure 1. Reflexive space within the program space

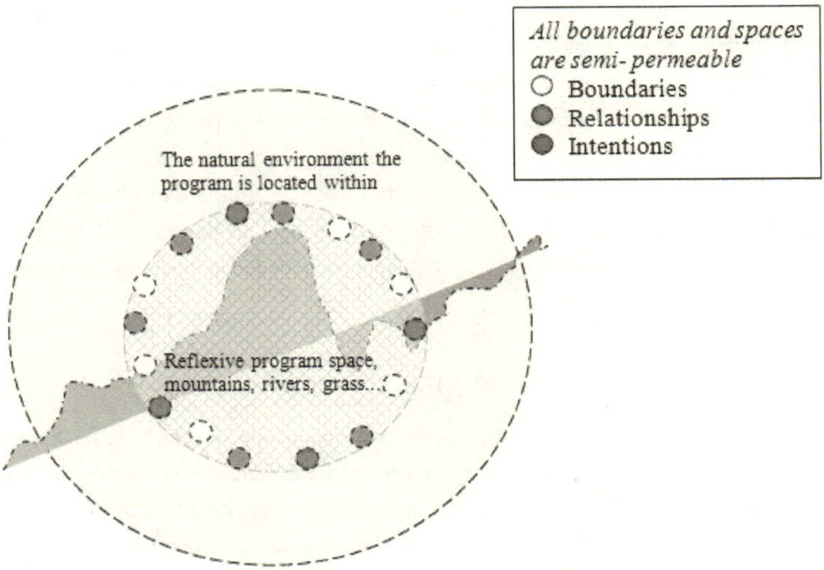

The definition of 'encounter' we hold to is fashioned after Buber (1973), Yalom (1991) and Grotowski (1991) and is a way of being 'alongside' other human beings. This presence is without any qualification or objectification of the other person. Based on this definition, we view encounters for the individual as an act of offering oneself to the landscape. In engagement of the reflexive art-making activity as described here, there is an emergence from oneself that is unique to the open and permeable opportunity of being alongside other group members. Encounter for the group is the quality of relationship that stresses the mutual, holistic existence of our immediacy and self-hood. We hold to the notions that the hermetic space for the encounter is a concrete meeting place with another person. This coming together is as Grotowski (1991) reminds us the 'discarding of masks, the revealing of the real substance, a totality of physical and mental reactions' (p.211).

The quality of engagement we are calling for is modelled after Seligman (2011) which, by his definition, is hopeful, enthusiastic and meaningful. The art-making is significant as it provides a generative and reflexive relationship where the learner is increasingly reflexive and becomes more self-aware as they positively interact with the environment. There is a greater likelihood and capacity that individuals will develop a yearning for meaningful moments in the natural environment using the artful practices described here. In the bush the students and the teacher alike work to re-view, re-create, and re-invent their world sense as the learner, because of the intersection of art in the environment. The artwork becomes a reflexive tool for reflection on both selfhood and the environment. In art-making, which is largely self-directed such as undertaken here, there is a quality of personal empowerment noted, a kind of self-developed sense of self-confidence and self-esteem. The art work sits alongside the environment, and the art is inscribed with the meaning of the learners. The student, the artwork and the environment all intersect as landscapes of possibility, bringing a breadth and depth to the complexity and uncertainty of the learning process.

Being, Becoming, Belonging

The artwork that we make has many ways of being viewed, contested, and critiqued, but in the group making process become a reflexive mode of self-understanding. As part of the group-work these symbols come to represent connectivity between the individual and the group. The earlier comments around the intention and intentionality of this work emphasise the belief that we are all in the space together to experience encounters with one another and the land. These encounters are unique to the specific landscape (in our case the Australian 'bush'). The facilitators of the group aspire to bring a new level of meaningfulness that might not be afforded the group when they are not in 'flow'.

In making the art images in the natural environment, the capacity for self-acceptance, positive relationships, personal growth, purposefulness and autonomy are being moulded and made clearer. Thoughts and feelings generated by contemplating qualities of being, belonging and becoming are explored in detail in the group. Participants are encouraged to explore these ideas in relation to their sense of the immediate or now, by attending to past reflections and future possibilities. We engage deliberately with the meaning of each word, the exploration of a natural sequence of the words that was appropriate for the individual or the group, and the visualisation and creation of a meaningful image.

Within the context of this paper there is limited capacity to reflect fully on the qualities of being, belonging and becoming, but we wish to note that these states of self-hood impact on the sense of self and the wholeness participants experience in the outdoor setting and in their lives. In the encounters and engagements, and through the art-making, the individual and group members develop insight into their existence. Participants consider how nature and the environment as a location impacts on their sense of being. The ensuing artworks are statements of feelings, thoughts, sensations and meanings embedded in the environmental context. The members of the group are called on to draw and symbolically state their experience of the self. They comment on time and space for the self and for others, and report coming to know themselves physically, emotionally, and affectively through the whole experience. This affective knowing is a result of using art as a reflexive tool. The outdoor setting provides the forum to share the characteristics for being and becoming more of their 'authentic self', and is an occasion to discover and to recognise participants' own and others' sense of belonging. Image 4 is both consciously and unconsciously biographical, and moves between these two worlds.

Image 4. Energy, colour and aliveness*

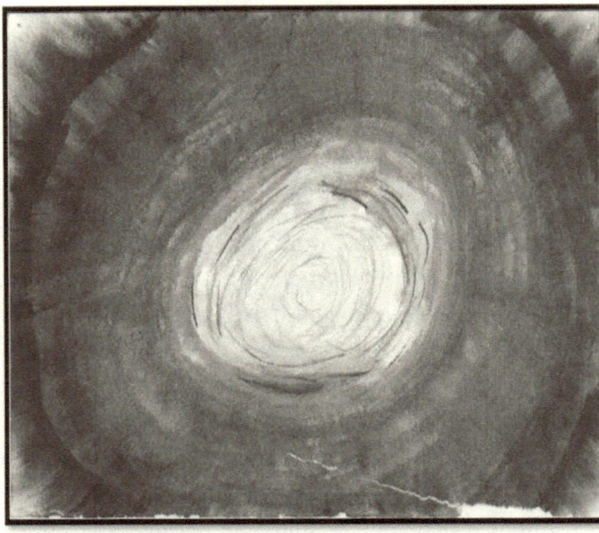

*This piece of artwork created by a participant of an outdoor program demonstrates the ideas of being, belonging and becoming that arise from affective knowing. This affective knowing seems to have produced a piece of art that is full of vitality.

According to Wood (2011), The German word lebendigkeit is normally translated as 'vitality'. Unpacked, lebendigkeit means 'one is in it': in the play (fullness). The term refers to active states of being 'fully alive', incorporating notions of spontaneity vivacity, movement and change. It implies an element of trust in one's own intuition and a full engagement in playfulness, sensual enjoyment, and spontaneity. It can be used to describe the quality of relating to artwork and art-making (p.261).

Conclusion

In essence, the practice of art-making in the outdoors is about the mind, body and soul coming together to achieve a positive sense of self and other. This alone is not so unique, but what is especially relevant, is how the imagining and art-making deepens particular ways of knowing. We can facilitate opportunities to gain a deeper understanding of the self within the world through the creation of a reflexive space in outdoor programs. Clarity around the negotiation of boundaries, relationships, and the intention with each individual within the group enables a learning space to emerge that is challenging, safe, free, and reflective.

Creating awareness through engaging in the art process has been a key feature of the authors' work in outdoor settings. As McNiff (1992) stated, the art-making becomes a 'medicine' for our young people and they take to it openly. Participants symbols, shapes and moments of meaning are deepened by and through the art-making. Their artistic endeavours are framed by their own reflections on what is said through the images about their psychological and physical makeup. The reflexive space allows them to find meaning that is shared by the individual in the group. This intimate dialogue is shared in the group as a spontaneous expression. The authors hold that this expression gives participants the opportunity to affirm the varieties of life. The images lead participants to respond to and be *held by nature*. Using these images as evocative art-making processes, we set out to investigate the social construction of self, by the self, particularly the self of individuals having a multifaceted identity. In the provision of this reflexive space, we are developing a sensitive and gentle approach that makes individuals feel cared for and safe. The resulting growth in knowledge and confidence can empower and motivate participants to seek a more meaningful, happier and healthier approach to life, and a stronger sense of identity.

References

Berman D., & Davis Berman J. (2005). Positive psychology and outdoor education. *Journal of Experiential Education, 8*(1)174.

Brookes, A. (2003). Adventure programming and the fundamental attribution error: A critique of neo-Hahnian outdoor education theory. In B. Humberstone, B. Brown & K. Richards (Eds.), *Whose Journeys? The outdoors and adventure as a social and cultural phenomena: Critical explorations of relations between individuals, 'others' and the environment* (403-422). Cumbria, UK: The Institute for Outdoor Learning.

Buber, M (1973). *Between man and man.* Translated and introduced by Robert Gregory Smith. London: Collins.

Carpenter, C. (2008). *Changing Spaces: Contextualising outdoor experiential programs for health and wellbeing.* Unpublished Doctoral Thesis. Deakin University, Australia.

Case, C. (2007). Imagery in supervision: The non-verbal narrative of knowing. In J. Schavarien and C. Case (Eds.), *Supervision of art psychotherapy: A theoretical and practical handbook* (95-115). London: Routledge.

Duckworth, A., Steen, T., & Seligman M. (2010) *Positive psychology in clinical practice.* Philadelphia, PA: Positive Psychology Center, University of Pennsylvania.

Cresswell, T. (2004). *Place: A short introduction.* UK: Blackwell.

Csikszentmihalyi, M. (1975). *Beyond boredom and anxiety.* San Francisco, USA: Jossey Bass.

Farrelly-Hansen, M., (Ed). (2001). *Spirituality in art therapy: Living the connection.* Philadelphia, PA: Jessica Kingsley.

Forsyth, D. R. (2001). Therapeutic groups. In M. A. Hogg & R. S. Tindale (Eds.). *Blackwell handbook of social psychology: Group process* (628-659). Oxford, UK: Blackwell.

Furnass, B. (1995). *Survival health and wellbeing into the twenty first century.* Proceedings of Nature and Society Forum, Australian National University, Nov. 30-Dec. 1. Canberra Australia: Nature and Society, Inc.

Giddens, A. (1991). *Modernity and self-identity: Self and society in the late modern age.* Cambridge, UK: Polity Press.

Grotowski, J. (1991). *Towards a poor man theatre.* London: Methuen.

Jung, C. G. (1933). *Modern man in search of a soul.* Oxford: Trowbridge & Essher.

Kapln, R., & Kaplan, S. (1995). *The experience of nature: A psychological perspective.* USA: Library of Congress Cataloguing in Publications Data.

Loynes, C. (2002). The generative paradigm. *Journal of Adventure Education and Outdoor Learning,* 2(2)113-205.

McNiff, S. (1992). *Art as medicine.* Boston: Shambhala. Maller, C., Townsend, M., St. Ledger, L., Henderson-Wilson, C., Pryor, A., Prosser, L. & Moore, M. (2008). Healthy parks, healthy people: The health benefits of contact with nature in a park context: A review of current literature (2nd

Ed.). *Social and Mental Health Priority Area, Occasional Paper Series.* Melbourne, Australia: Deakin University Faculty of Health and Behavioural Sciences.

Martin, P. (1996). New perspectives of self, nature and others. *Australian Journal of Outdoor Education,* 1(3) 3-9.

Martin, P. (2004). Outdoor education for human/ nature relationships. *Conference Proceedings International Outdoor Education Research Conference,* July 2004. Bendigo, Victoria, Australia: La Trobe University.

Roman, M., & Euell, J., (1971) Art as a community mental health tool. *Community Mental Health Journal,* 7(2)134-143. Netherlands: Springer.

Ringer, M. (1999). The facilitation of facilitation? Searching for competencies in group work leadership. *Scisco Conscientia, 2*, 1-19.

Ringer, T. M. (2002) *Group action: The dynamics of groups in therapeutic, educational, and corporate settings.* London: Jessica Kingsley.

Ryff, C. D., & Singer, B H. (2008). Know thyself and become what you are: A eudemonic approach to psychological wellbeing. *Journal of Happiness Studies, 9*, 13-39.

Tuan, Y.F. (1977). *Space and place: The perspective of experience.* Minneapolis: University of Minnesota Press.

Seligman, M. (2011). *Flourish: A visionary new understanding of happiness and wellbeing.* London: Free Press.

Wilkinson, R., & Marmot, M. (Eds.). (2003). *Social determinants of health: Solid facts* (2nd Ed.), 1-28. World Health Organization.

Wood, C. (2011). *Navigating art therapy: A therapist's companion.* London: Routledge.

Winnicott, D. W. (1971). *Playing and reality.* London: Tavistock.

Yalom, I. D. (1991). *Love's executioner, and other tales of psychotherapy.* London: Penguin.

CHAPTER 31

Conversing with a Crayfish, Traveling with the Birds: Synchronicity, Immediacy and Reciprocity in Our Relationship with Nature[1]

Nick Hall

ABSTRACT

This is a paper about the nature of our relationship with nature, and the validity of self as a legitimate and accurate measure of what is. As such, some may consider this paper 'art' rather than 'science'. The author invites readers to remain open to wide ways of 'knowing' and 'understanding' as they explore the author's perspective.

INTRODUCTION

In this paper I want to describe some of the observable features of our relationship with parts of our world that are considered to be 'other than human'. I want to put forward the idea that the self, as experiencer of the world, is potentially a fully valid tool for ascertaining and measuring 'what is', as well as for perceiving, observing, and recognising information in the fields of relationship and meaning. We are at present, the only 'tool' we have to experience and validate these realms of science that are as real and concrete as the realms of science for which we have engineered reliable tools and frameworks for measuring and understanding. I want to assert that our relationship with what is considered 'other than human' is as personal and meaningful as our human-to-human relationships, and operates in the same emotional, energetic and practical ways. I have experienced some powerfully helpful and mysterious things when working with nature, particularly in its more undiluted states. To me, these are

[1] This paper is not double-blind peer reviewed.

phenomena that make adventure therapy the useful experience that it is widely recognised to be.

Some Terms

Nature: the parts of the world that are not controlled by humans through use of force.

Meaning: that which creates pleasure, deep unassailable contentment, and clarity of consciousness.

Science: the study and understanding of what is.

Synchronicity: described by Carl Jung as a 'causal connecting principle', this is how I use the word here. With causal meaning being involved in the relationship of cause and effect, causal works differently to this mechanical relationship, and involves a beneficial relationship that operates in a way that is to some extent unknown (and perhaps unknowable); where real interactions and benefits can be observed. The salient feature here is that, whilst there appears to be no explainable functioning of cause and effect, the events are 'synchronised' in a way that is meaningful to the participants.

Immediacy: experiencing and responding to what is happening in the present moment, particularly pertaining to a relationship with the self and that which is perceived and named as being external to the self.

Reciprocity: a balanced relationship of give and take. The balance being provided by the participants' mutual satisfaction with the outcome of an interaction, and/or the outcomes of a continuing series of interactions. This reciprocity is an observable and consistent phenomenon, where balance provides only positive emotional consequences, and imbalance provides negative emotional consequences. Imbalance significantly raises the risk of undesired physical consequences, and balance minimises, but does not eliminate, undesired physical consequences.

How does Nature Communicate with Us?

I believe that nature communicates with us, however not in spoken or written language. My experience is that nature speaks in its own peculiar languages

languages we can recognise, and that potentially have meaning to us. Nature could be said to speak in a range of nuances that ignite sensory recognition and energetic responses in us. We could see nature speaking with things such as temperature, movement, sound and colour. We could see nature speaking with beauty; a fine and emotionally powerful beauty. This is the beauty widely recognised in a colourful sunset, soaring mountains, a long thin waterfall, a wild animal in its home setting, or the fresh and earthy aromas of a rainforest. This beauty is present but less commonly recognised in all experiences of nature. I am not speaking of a subjective beauty that relies on personal taste; I am referring to the beauty that is omnipresent, experienced in all interactions with nature, but not necessarily recognised or acknowledged as such. I am therefore asserting the existence of such a phenomenon.

Nature could also be seen as speaking, curiously enough, in metaphor. Similar to the use of metaphor in literature, natural elements are used to function as metaphors to provide rich connotations of meaning with sensory and literal symbols. To describe how these types of messages can be communicated directly from nature (and perhaps these are the original source of our recognition and use of metaphor), I will provide some first-hand accounts.

They Know Their Truth

The second personal perception/observation I want to share has to do with what I consider to be one of the salient features of truth. One of my roles is as a therapist and counsellor. When I speak with clients that have come to me for support, I speak in English, even when they do not speak English, which is the case with some of my clients who have been refugees from conflicts in Africa and Asia. With these clients I sometimes use an interpreter. This I find to be a complex situation, where accuracy of detail can be difficult to establish. What do I know about the truth of what they are telling me?

African clients come from their different cultures, with different conditions, different agendas, and are non-English speaking. Other clients, particularly those with gang involvements, English speaking, may be telling me wild, exaggerated stories linked in to what and who is important to them.

In both circumstances (to pick two broad examples) it has been my experience that I have no practical or absolutely reliable way of determining the accuracy and honesty of what they are saying to me. What do I know for sure? They know the truth of what they are telling me. They have the capacity to know, cognitively and/or emotionally, the quality of their truth. By quality, I mean what is absolutely clear, what is speculation, what is fantasy, an idea or ideal, what is unknown, and what they are confused about. They are always actively involved in this capacity. They are the one who has the most first-hand information about what they are experiencing and what they have experienced.

If we can agree that this observation is, or even may be, a reliable constant, what happens if we transfer this information to what is happening in our relationship with nature? In much the same way as my human clients, my experience is that the elements of nature are telling me their truth, in their multitudinous and sometimes quite foreign manifestations; and these elements know the truth of what they are telling me.

The Point of No Return

Here I will describe another personal perception/observation. This is a moment that invariably comes up when I am working on an outdoor program, traversing remote places. It's a moment, different for each person, that I call 'the point of no return'. On an individual's journey with the group into the bush, my observation is that they come to a point, simultaneously 'on the track', and inside of themselves, where it is just as big a decision to go forward as it is to turn back. They are aware, in their own way, that they are required to make a decision.

What is happening here? One thing that happens, from my observations and conversations, is that the participant becomes aware of, amongst other things, and to different degrees in different individuals, a set of realisations (personally meaningful observations). These realisations I describe in the following way:

- I have to deal with the wild environment;
- I am changing in the way I relate to nature;
- I am starting to relate to the raw purity of nature;
- I want to change the way I relate to these people I am with; and
- This is different than in the city. Here, I have my simple set of belongings, I am very vulnerable, it is obvious that nature is very powerful and beautiful, and I need to rely on myself and these people I am with.

There is a moment when they may choose to move into the unknown, encouraged by an unusual set of circumstances. I am asserting that one of the active and conscious partners in this relationship is nature.

Some Firsthand Stories of Synchronicity, Immediacy and Reciprocity

The following is an account of synchronicity written by Jung (1952), from his article 'Synchronicity, an acausal connecting principal':

> A young woman I was treating had, at a critical moment, a dream in which she was given a golden scarab. While she was telling this dream, I was sat with my back to the closed window. Suddenly I heard a noise behind me, like a gentle tapping. I turned round and saw a flying insect knocking against the windowpane from the outside. I opened the window and caught the creature in the air as it flew in. It was the nearest analogy to a golden scarab one finds in our latitudes, a common rose-chafer, which, contrary to its usual habits had evidently felt the urge to get into a dark room at this particular moment. (Jung, 1952)

In my work I have had numerous experiences of the same type of phenomenon, both working in the developed landscape and in wild places. Some examples I (and others) experience as subtle and perhaps ambiguous; others, like Carl Jung's example are experienced as clear and emphatic. The following is an account of one of my experiences of synchronicity.

The Crayfish Story

I was co-facilitating an adventure therapy program with a group of young women living with mental illness. On the first day, to help encourage a sense of fun and ease of communication, I introduced a surprise extra member of our group, a realistic looking rubber crayfish that squeaked when you pressed its rubber tummy (stomach). The crayfish wanted to be present at our group discussions, but someone would need to be her voice. The young women understood the crayfish's role and were happy to include her in our group. The toy was adopted as a group mascot and, as I had intended, provided an opportunity for fun and meaningful talk. These were a group of women who struggled with many facets of day to day living, and who experienced, as it would turn out, deep gratitude for the simplest of pleasures.

We walked into the Tasmanian bush with them (not getting very far by normal standards), and camped on a sodden patch of clear ground of their choosing not suitable for camping by many standards but the right distance down the track, and soft to lie on. The next morning after heavy rain the women decided to return the way we had come. As we had almost reached the edge of the clearing (which was everywhere awash with flowing water), I pointed out a small hole in the ground, about ten centimetres across, into which a flow of water was disappearing. I pointed it out because I found it both curious and potentially dangerous if you were to step in it. As we looked into the hole a fresh water crayfish emerged a creature that is most unusual to see, from my knowledge and this one being almost identical in size to our mascot.

Two Birds Story

We were four days into a five-day adventure therapy program. It was the second day of our three-day bushwalk, and we were at a point where we were most remote from the vehicle in which we had travelled to the start point of our walk.

In our group we had a young man who was both Aboriginal, and an inmate of a youth detention centre from which he had made several escapes prior to coming on the program. He had disclosed earlier on in our program that he had decided not to make any more escapes, and to cooperate with his captors for the remaining time of his incarceration.

As the program unfolded, he was showing himself to be the member of our participant group who most often took a leadership role. He was experiencing successes with most of his leadership decisions at times in a way that drew the marked attention and admiration of the rest of our group, including the facilitators.

At a point in the track there was a particularly difficult piece of navigation. It was a feature of our program that our participants were fully responsible (up to the point of serious and immediate danger), for all navigation decisions even if this meant losing the track. Our young Aboriginal man was leading; the rest of the group was letting him lead. After several attempts, he could not find where the track continued, even with the help of some of his fellow participants.

First he became angry and demanded that the facilitators show him which way to go. When this was gently refused, with reminders of our agreement on who was navigating the route, he moved into trying to trick us into revealing which way to go. Over half an hour went by with him persisting with this strategy, and no one else in the group showing that they were attempting to find a solution. He then decided that he would follow me very closely everywhere I went sitting in the grass by the track, going to the nearby stream to fill my water bottle everywhere I went, he was right next to me. In response to this I headed off into the bush, through the scratchiest scrub I could find, in the direction of where we would eventually meet the continuation of the track. As our young man and I made off into the dense vegetation, a forest raven appeared flying slowly above our heads travelling in the same direction. This forest raven was being followed very closely, by a smaller brown coloured bird, chirping and flapping about, side to side behind the raven.

Conclusions

The personal stories I have included in this paper suggest to me that our relationships with non-human beings work in the same way that our human interrelationships work. Nature has the capacity to communicate to us its truth, in direct and meaningful ways. As is the case between humans, there is a possibility of healthy and sustainable relationships with nature. What I mean by 'healthy and sustainable relationship' is as follows: such a relationship is personal and intimate, mutually experiential and meaningful, with a reciprocal level of input and commitment. These features are coupled with an understanding and acceptance that the relationship exists most powerfully in the present moment, and will constantly change.

If this is so, then I suggest that it is reasonable to extrapolate that the same behaviours we find to be wise in our inter-human relationships carry that same wisdom in our relationships with nature. So that what we find to be wise, and what we find to be stupid in our relationships with people also applies with how we behave with nature.

These stories, and the phenomenon of synchronicity, immediacy and reciprocity suggest to me that nature wishes to have a conscious relationship with us.

References

Jung, C.G. (1952). *Synchronicity: An acausal connecting principle.* Bollingen, Switzerland: Bollingen Foundation.

Jung, C.G., Adler, G., and Hull, R.F.C. (1970). *Collected works of C.G. Jung, Volume 8.* Princeton: Princeton University Press.

CHAPTER 32

Should Making a Serious Mistake be a Criminal Act? An Examination of Some Legal Consequences of Gross Negligence in Outdoor Leadership

Peter Kellett

ABSTRACT

Whenever we are operating as professional outdoor leaders, be it in adventure therapy, outdoor education, adventure tourism or recreation, we have a clear duty of care to our clients. In all of these settings, the use of adventure activities implies acceptance of some risk, but duty of care demands that the level of risk is appropriate to the participant and the therapeutic, educational or recreational objectives. Judging that appropriate level of risk is one of the key functions of the outdoor leader. When the level of risk is too high, adventure can quickly turn into mis-adventure and serious injury or death may result.

While the concept of civil liability due to leaders' negligence is well understood by those working in the outdoors, I suggest that few will appreciate that in extreme cases, they may also be charged with criminal negligence and possibly jailed. This paper will explore the appropriateness of judicial punishment in just such situations, where outdoor leaders make significant errors of judgement, resulting in serious harm to those in their care. Using an English case study, the paper will question the various justifications posited for punishment, and for incarceration in particular. The question of wider, systemic culpability will also be examined. Implications have relevance for all outdoor leaders, including adventure therapists.

Introduction

The first case in Britain where a custodial sentence was imposed for 'corporate manslaughter' involved young people on an outdoor activity. This was the well-known Lyme Bay case, which followed the deaths of four students while sea-kayaking near Plymouth in 1993 (Fulbrook, 2005). While the instructors leading the sea kayakers were almost certainly negligent, in this case, it was the company director who was charged, tried and ultimately jailed for three years.

In September 2003, a British school teacher by the name of Paul Ellis was sent to jail for twelve months. He had eventually pleaded guilty to a charge of the manslaughter of Max Palmer, a ten year old boy who died on an outdoor activity that Ellis had organized and led. Ellis was the first teacher to be jailed in Britain for a breach of the Health and Safety Act and regulations (Bennett, 2003; Leckie, 2004).

In sentencing Ellis, the trial judge described Ellis's actions as 'unbelievably foolhardy and negligent' (Wainright, 2003; BBC News, 2003). The judge also commented that he had been considering a sentence of three years, but had reduced this to one year after Ellis changed his plea from not guilty to guilty, was visibly remorseful, had attempted to save the victim at considerable risk to himself, and his career as a teacher was ruined (Bennett, 2003).

At the time of sentencing, Ellis was a 42 year old geography teacher at a secondary school near Blackpool in Lancashire, England. He was married and had three children.

Why was Paul Ellis jailed? Is making a serious mistake as an outdoor leader a criminal act? Should such mistakes be treated similarly to other criminal acts? What might be achieved by imposing this type of penalty? Were there other options? Was there any other culpability? What does this case mean for outdoor adventure activities and for those who work in the field of outdoor leadership, including adventure therapists?

Civil and Criminal Negligence

This paper explores the purposes of punishment in Western society and relates this to the case of Paul Ellis. Some of the unintended consequences of judicial punishment will also be elaborated.

As previously stated, Paul Ellis was charged with negligence manslaughter, the serious criminal offence of causing death due to gross negligence. The law of negligence is more typically applied in civil cases, in those situations where a person (the plaintiff), is seeking some compensation for loss, damage or injury caused by the defendant. To satisfy a finding of negligence there must be a duty of care owed to the plaintiff, and this duty must have been breached in some way by the defendant. Further, the breached duty of care must have caused the loss, injury or damage, and these consequences must have been reasonably foreseeable. In order for there to be a finding of criminal negligence (in this case gross negligence manslaughter), a very high degree of negligence is required.

Bronnit and McSherry (2005) have defined negligence manslaughter as a great falling short of the standard of care that a person should have exercised, involving such a high risk that death or grievous bodily harm would follow that the doing of the act merited criminal punishment. Lord Mackay (in R v Adomoko [1995] 1 AC 187) suggested that:

> The jury must go on to consider whether the breach of duty should be characterised as gross negligence and therefore a crime. This will depend on the seriousness of the breach of duty committed by the defendant...whether having regard to the risk of death involved, the conduct of the defendant was so bad in all the circumstances as to amount in their judgment to a criminal act or omission.

Cases where people are successfully prosecuted for criminal negligence are very rare (Fullbrook, 2005). This paper discusses a British outdoor education case study because to date there have been no such cases (in any form) in Britain or Australia, in the field of adventure therapy. There have been cases of criminal negligence in North America, and perhaps other jurisdictions, but it is beyond the scope of this paper to explore all of these.

While there are differences between British and Australian law, the two systems are more alike than unalike. Both are a combination of statute and case law; the basis of Australia's law was imported with British colonization. While Australian and other Commonwealth courts are no longer bound to follow the precedents set by British courts, British cases may still be cited in their proceedings, and have some influence on the outcomes. In addition, the lessons learnt from a close examination of Ellis's leadership will be relevant wherever there are organised outdoor activities.

The issue of whether Ellis had a duty of care to the victim will be accepted for the purposes of this paper, however, it should be noted that the victim was not one of Ellis's students, did not attend his school, and that the victim's mother was present on the outing and at the scene of the tragedy. In the author's home state of South Australia, the guidelines for conducting camps and excursions produced by the Department of Education and Children's Services expressly state that staff who take their own children on outdoor activities 'take complete responsibility for the care and supervision of their children' (DECS, 2007 p. 40). This situation may vary across the Australian states and internationally.

The Facts in This Case

In May 2002 Paul Ellis, the head geography teacher at Fleetwood High School near Blackpool, England organized and led a weekend trip to Glenridding in the English Lake District. There were twelve year-eight students from the school (aged 12 and 13) under the supervision of three adults: Ellis, another teacher from the school, and Patricia Palmer, a classroom assistant at the school who took along her ten year old son, Max.

Ellis had previously organized a number of similar weekend 'activity trips' to the Glenridding area for Fleetwood students, and the trips were well publicised within the school. The activities included fell (hill) walking, ghyll (stream) scrambling, and on some occasions, rock climbing (if a qualified instructor was available). The centrepiece (highlight) of each trip was 'plunge pooling' into Glenridding Beck (Health and Safety Executive [HSE], 2005). 'Beck' is a local name for a mountain stream. There were photographs of the plunge pool activity on display at the school, so the school's administration was well aware of the typical program and activities. 'Plunge pooling involves jumping from a height into a natural pool, often in a mountain stream' (HSE, 2005, p. 4). In this case, it involved a four metre jump from a rock ledge into Glenridding Beck.

The group stayed overnight at a hostel in Glenridding on the Friday and Saturday nights. It had rained heavily as the group travelled up on the Friday evening, and Saturday was cold, wet and windy. The leader cancelled the outdoor activities he had planned for the Saturday, and instead took the group to the local towns of Ambleside and Keswick. However, the students were still keen to go plunge pooling before returning home the next day.

There was no rain on Sunday morning and Ellis went to look at the beck. He considered that water levels had gone down enough to try the plunge pool, and instructed the group to get ready. The weather forecast for Sunday, apparently not checked by Ellis, indicated rain and a temperature of 5 degrees Celsius at 3000 feet, the approximate summit altitude of Helvellyn, the major hill above Glenridding Beck, and the source of its water. The slopes of Helvellyn are steep and slatey, so water flows into Glenridding Beck are highly responsive to rainy periods.

On route to the pool, the Fleetwood High group met staff and students from another school who were staying nearby. They too had used the plunge pool on previous visits, but decided that on this day, it was too dangerous. This information was shared with Ellis, but, 'he replied that he had a rope and continued towards the pool.' (HSE, 2005, p. 21). The rope was actually in the group's minibus about half a kilometre away.

Ellis jumped in, pronounced it fine to carry on, and the other teacher went down to the exit point to assist students to leave the water. The water temperature was subsequently measured at 8.6 degrees Celsius, 'as cold as the English Channel in February' (HSE, 2005, p. 21).

When ten year old Max Palmer jumped in he panicked and it was immediately obvious that he was in trouble. Ellis jumped in again and tried to save Max, but after a few attempts was so cold that he was unable to do anything other than save himself. He was assisted from the water by the other teacher, and took no further part in rescue attempts. He did not have warm clothing available at the pool.

By now Max's mother had also jumped in, but was unable to help her son and was also overcome by the cold. The second teacher told some of the students to fetch the rope and they ran back to the minibus parked near the hostel. Max and his mother had now been in the water for 20-25 minutes. Fortunately some of the rope fetchers also decided to raise the alarm and three staff from the other school came running with rescue and survival gear.

In the meantime, another of the students jumped in to try to grab the boy, but Max was now washed out of the pool and downstream. The student found Max's mother and was able to save her with the help of the teacher. This student was now very cold and Ms Palmer was semi-conscious. Both were subsequently flown to hospital and treated for hypothermia (HSE, 2005). Some students eventually pulled Max from the water about 150 metres downstream, but he was later pronounced dead at the scene. Throughout the episode the second teacher in the party did his best in the situation, and some of the Fleetwood students acted with great bravery in attempting to rescue Max. They almost certainly saved Patricia Palmer, but were also putting themselves at considerable risk (HSE, 2005).

What are the Justifications for Punishment?

Walker's seminal text on the issue of sentencing in the British legal system, described a range of purposes and justifications for punishing offenders (Walker, 1991). Broadly, these fit into two traditions: the retributive and the utilitarian, the objectives of which will be discussed in turn. Both traditions include one common objective which is quaintly described as 'elimination and incapacitation'.

Since the abolition of capital punishment in England, Australia and most western countries, this typically involves putting serious offenders in prison so that re-offending becomes impossible and the public is protected from them (Walker, 1991).

The retributive tradition is perhaps the more straight-forward. It is based on the belief that punishment for wrong-doing is deserved, and that it incorporates elements of vengeance, penance and atonement. These ideas date back at least to the Greek Classical period, and were later supported by Judaism, Christianity and Islam, all of which encompass some belief that guilt is expiated by suffering (Walker, 1991). The nineteenth century philosophers Kant and Hegel also considered punishment to be an essential part of making good (Walker, 1991). The retributionist knows that 'he is inflicting more or less what the offender deserves' (Walker, 1991 p. 67).

A modern variant of this retributive tradition is known as the 'justice model' of punishment, sometimes also referred to as 'just deserts', which was first clearly articulated by the American criminologist von Hirsch (1976). The justice model has strongly influenced North American, British and Australian legal systems, and has led to more codification of laws and less sentencing discretion for judges. From this perspective, punishment is almost a duty. This belief that wrong-doing should generally be punished in a commensurate manner has also permeated both public and legal opinion in areas where codification has not taken place (Walker, 1991; Tomaino & Kapardis, 2004).

The justice model has attracted strong criticism from supporters of the utilitarian tradition. Duff and Garland (1994) point out that it is backward looking, with the type and degree of punishment being determined by the terms of the past offence. 'From this viewpoint, a form of 'atonement' must occur in the life of the offender regardless of any deterrent effect or rehabilitative counter effect' (Tomaino & Kapardis, 2004, p. 88).

However, the utilitarian tradition of sentencing seeks to achieve much more than mere punishment. It is forward looking, even optimistic, seeking to achieve benefits for both the individual and society, among them being the important one of reducing the likelihood of future offences being committed. In brief, 'It contributes to this by deterring the offender from re-offending, discouraging others from following his example, or putting him [in prison] where he cannot offend any longer' (Walker, 1991, p. 6).

Deterrence can be both specific and general. Specific deterrence discourages the person from re-offending, while general deterrence targets the rest of society by using the offender as an example. 'People are deterred from actions when they refrain from them because they dislike what they believe to be the possible consequences of those actions' (Walker, 1991 p. 13). Walker also suggests that there is an educative function to punishment, extending beyond general deterrence. Under this justification, punishment will have an additional utilitarian purpose, by making it clear to the public that some actions are unacceptable.

However, general deterrence and public education can only be effective if the crime and its punishment are widely known and this relies on the vagaries of the media. Even when cases are widely reported, there is little supporting evidence to show that general deterrence is really achieved (Tomaino & Kapardis, 2004). In addition, the utilitarian tradition is an optimistic one focusing on correction, reform, and rehabilitation. If successful, it brings about changed attitudes and behaviours so that the offender can become part of society once again. It is for this reason that prison systems are frequently called departments of corrections.

Finally, there is the ritual and expressive function of denunciation. This is a formal and official statement of disapprobation aimed at satisfying the victims of the crime and the community as a whole (Walker, 1991). Durkheim (cited in Duff & Garland, 1994) wrote that 'the rituals of punishment serve to reaffirm the core beliefs of the society and reinforce feelings of solidarity amongst the law-abiding' (p. 32). Australian legal commentators agreed:

> A suspended sentence is a good illustration, for an offender may receive a prison term that is not put into operation until there is a breach of a bond's conditions. Therefore, the prison term is a declaratory statement of the inappropriateness of the conduct (Tomaino & Kapardis, 2004, p. 89).

Duff and Garland (1994) asked whether crime must be punished in some material way. 'May censure be enough in self-evident situations, or is greater effect achieved by adding harsh treatment?' (pp. 14-15). The research of Tomaino and Kapardis (2004) suggested that generally it is not.

Walker (1991) suggested that in practice, both the public and sentencers follow both the retributive and the utilitarian sentencing traditions, with their views varying over time. These variations are usually most apparent following political crusades (e.g. getting 'tough on crime' or 'waging war on drugs') in relation to particularly notorious cases which inflame public opinion, or where there has been a series of similar situations and 'crime' seems to be on the increase (Tomaino & Kapardis, 2004).

Walker (1985) suggested that 'sentencers should not strain public tolerance' (pp. 72-73), and noted that, 'in real life most sentencers admit to having some regard to what they believe to be public opinion' (p. 64).

Why was Ellis Jailed?

Did any of these justifications for a custodial sentence apply in Ellis's case? What is achieved by jailing the adventure leader who makes serious errors?

Judges are not always specific about which justification(s) for punishment are influencing their choice of sentence in particular cases. Sometimes it can only be inferred from their summing up or general statements within the judgement. One problem for judges following either or even both sentencing traditions is that they can never know if the punishment in a particular case will have any future benefit, except for temporary elimination and incapacitation where a custodial sentence is imposed.

Ellis was certainly being 'eliminated and incapacitated' for the twelve month period that he spent in prison, but offences such as negligence manslaughter are hardly 'serial'. Ellis was lucky to survive his second time in the plunge pool, and was most unlikely to repeat his errors at Glenridding Beck. He had also lost his job as a teacher, and it was unlikely that that he would ever again be permitted to take a group of young people into the outdoors. In such a case the justification of public safety did not apply.

Did Ellis need to be personally deterred from future foolhardy leadership of young people on outdoor activities? Again, almost certainly not, based on the reasons given above. Had it been shown that Ellis was a person in need of reform, rehabilitation or correction? A teacher for nearly twenty years, a family man, promoted to head of geography, and frequently giving up his weekends to take students on outdoor activities, he was seemingly committed to his profession and his students. In the words of the Cumbria Police, 'We were not dealing with a career criminal here but a teacher who had made a severe error' (Cassidy, 2003).

Was jailing Ellis an attempt to educate the public in general, and outdoor leaders in particular, that risky or dangerous activity with young people was unacceptable, or that poor decision making during these pursuits would not be tolerated?

The decision in Ellis's case, to charge and ultimately to convict and punish, may well have been influenced by context. The death of Max Walker was one of a series of highly publicised cases of young people dying on school outdoor activities in Britain in the preceding decade. In March, 2002, prior to the events being examined here, Phil Revell, an education journalist and ex-teacher wrote a

Guardian article on deaths on school trips, stating that 'a high-profile prosecution would encourage heads and governing bodies to take safety seriously' (Revell, 2002). Just two months later, Max Palmer drowned at Glenridding.

Was Ellis therefore being used as an example for the purpose of warning (deterring) or educating other outdoor leaders? Was there an epidemic of student deaths which needed to be stamped out?

In fact, English outdoor activities as measured by participant student deaths were remarkably safe. There had been 47 deaths over the previous 17 years, an average of less than three per year for an estimated student population of around ten million (Revell, 2002). Moreover, sixteen of these had occurred in a single motorway accident involving a school bus (Fulbrook, 2005), so the average of deaths while students were actually participating in an adventure activity was less than two per annum.

However, there had been six British students killed during outdoor activities in 2001, and another seven in 2002 (Revell, 2002). Nearly all cases had involved drowning, and most of these deaths had also resulted from river activities where teachers and leaders had misjudged water levels and strength (Fulbrook, 2005). Fulbrook also reported that in July 2003, less than two months before Ellis's trial, twelve students and a teacher were fortunate to escape drowning while swimming on the Northumberland coast (Fulbrook, 2005).

Given this series of much-reported incidents preceding the events at Glenridding Beck, and just before Ellis's trial, how much was the trial judge influenced by public opinion or by the desire to 'send a message' to teachers and outdoor leaders?

At the time of Palmer's death in 2002 and Ellis's trial in 2003, there was also considerable discussion among outdoor practitioners in the English Lake District about the increasing number of deaths, injuries and near misses in the British outdoors (C. Batten, personal communication, September 6, 2003). Perhaps the 'time was ripe' for the authorities to make an example of someone like Ellis, to use him as a means of general deterrence and education.

This was not only ethically suspect, but also likely to be ineffective. 'Severe exemplary punishments, where sentencers make an example of a particular offender, do not seem to discourage would-be offenders' (Walker, 1985, pp. 98-99). This view is also supported by Tomaino & Kapardis (2004).The principle of general deterrence raises some important moral issues. Is it right to punish one person in the hope that it may deter someone else from similar behaviour in the future? Should the punishment not relate only to the crime that has been committed, rather than to one or more that may or may not ever be? Some writers have seen general deterrence as treating offenders as a means to educate or deter others, and have cast doubt on its ethical validity. Walker, (1991), Hudson, (1987), and Tomaino & Kapardis, (2004) suggest that under this doctrine in particular, offenders may be more harshly treated than others, and that the degree and type of punishment may exceed what the crime has earned.

In this regard the justice model is less morally ambiguous. It is opposed to:

> the use of draconian penal sanctions for the purposes of general deterrence. Penalties to frighten off would-be-offenders for crimes about which there is heightened concern should never, on the commensurate deserts principle, mean that any one offender receives more severe punishment than the calculus of culpability in the particular instance indicates is warranted' (Hudson, 1994, p. 56). In Kantian terms, the individual has a 'right to be treated as an end and never as a means. (Hudson, 1994 p. 56)

As for the educative function, the death of Max Palmer received wide media attention in Britain, as did the charging and ultimate conviction of Paul Ellis. While media reports condemned Ellis's actions, it was the investigation carried out by the Health and Safety Executive (HSE) and released in 2005 which identified the sequence of errors committed by Ellis and by the education system for which he worked. The HSE report also made a series of recommendations regarding future outdoor excursions, especially for those 'hybrid activities' which involve both water and land activities. The report was widely promoted through HSE press releases (HSE, 2005a; HSE, 2005b) and through the HSE website. In June 2011, the full report was still on the HSE website, available to all who wished to learn from the event.

It is therefore arguable that the function of educating the outdoor leadership community, and those agencies for whom they work, was better achieved by these means than by jailing Ellis. Furthermore, media discussion at the time of his sentencing focused on his jailing rather than on the lessons that could be learned from the tragedy.

Was the trial judge therefore invoking the expressive or ritual function of punishment? Was Ellis convicted and jailed to satisfy the needs of those other victims, Max's parents, especially his mother who was there at the time? Tomaino and Kapardis (2004) suggest that, 'Long sentences can also be justified because they are seen to offer some therapeutic benefit to victims' (p. 94).The statement of Max's father after Ellis was sentenced indicates that he at least may have felt a need for Ellis to be punished. He said it was important that lessons were learned from Max's death so that similar tragedy did not happen again: 'Today, Paul Ellis received 12 months in prison. We have received a life sentence' (Bunyan, 2003).

In sentencing Ellis, Mr Justice Morland said, 'In my judgement the circumstances are so serious that I must pass an immediate prison sentence'. He went on to say that he would be 'failing in his duty' if he gave Ellis a suspended sentence (BBC News, 2003, p. 2). These statements from the trial judge suggest that he was, at least to some extent, following the retributive tradition in sentencing. His use of the word 'duty' even indicates some adherence to the justice model.

The HSE investigation report into Max Palmer's death was published well after Ellis's trial and conviction. In fact, he had already finished his time in prison. It can be argued that the HSE investigation went far more deeply into all the circumstances surrounding the event, in particular the organisational and supervisory procedures of his school and the Local Education Authority (LEA) for which he worked.

The HSE investigation identified two main causes contributing to Max Palmer's death. They were:

- the inappropriate actions of the party leader before and during the event; and
- the weakness of the management systems which allowed an unsuitable leader to be in charge of a party of schoolchildren in a high-hazard environment (HSE, 2005b p. 1).

Legal action against the school and the LEA was considered by the HSE, but did not proceed.

OTHER IMPACTS OF PUNISHMENT

In addition to its effects on the offender, there are some unintended consequences of judicial punishment, some 'collateral damage'. Families are deprived of partners, parents and incomes in the short term, and then have the task of dealing with the stigmatized 'criminal', 'felon' or 'prisoner' upon release (Walker, 1991). In the case under discussion it is not known whether Ellis lost his family, his house or the family car as a result of these events, but pressure on all of them was inevitable.

Paul Ellis also had to twice endure 'trial by media', firstly in May, 2002, when the sad event occurred, and then again in September 2003 when he was convicted. There was even a third, but lesser, episode when the HSE report was released in 2005. Following Ellis's conviction, Britain's second biggest teaching union, the National Association of Schoolmasters Union of Women Teachers (NASUWT) advised its 223,000 members not to take part in school outings (Curtis, 2004). However, the larger National Union of Teachers (NUT) refused to give similar advice (Clare, 2004). The trade magazine 'International Tours and Tourism News' (2003) reported a drop in school outings following the Ellis case.

Conclusions

It seems probable that in sentencing Ellis, Mr Justice Morland was applying a number of the justifications for punishment, drawing from both the utilitarian and the retributive traditions. Almost certainly, Ellis was being used as a means of general deterrence and education for outdoor practitioners, but he was also jailed because the judge thought that his actions deserved severe punishment. Faced with the grieving parents and the high level of media interest, it is probable that he was also applying the ritual of denunciation.

There are serious personal consequences for outdoor leaders, including adventure therapists, who like Ellis, make fatal errors of judgement. These can include deep personal feelings of failure and remorse, wearing the stigma of their own incompetence and negligence, loss of their employment status (especially regarding any career advancement), loss of their job, and even loss of their career.

If greater punishment than this is seen to be warranted, there are a number of non-custodial options open to judges: censure, good behaviour bonds, fines, and community service orders. From the author's perspective, for outdoor leaders, including adventure therapists in outdoor settings, censure, denunciation and the resultant stigma is likely to be punishment enough. If a custodial sentence is indicated due to the severity of the case, then suspending that sentence for people unlikely to re-offend can be an effective option. The ritualistic, educative and deterrent aims are likely to have been achieved. The work of Tomaino and Kapardis (2004) has shown that the severity of punishment has little impact on the frequency of offending.

While the HSE found serious shortcomings in the supervisory and approval systems of the school administration and that of the LEA, it was only the teacher (undeniably incompetent to make a critical safety decision, untrained for the activity, unprepared, but offering an extra-curricular activity in his own time), who was charged, convicted and jailed, who lost his job and career, and whose family also suffered as a result. Had action been taken against the employing bodies, it would have been a civil action for damages or resulted in a fine for breach of safety regulations. The penalties would have been purely financial ones targeting organizations rather than an individual, and paid by those organizations or their insurers.

Deaths during guided adventure activities of any kind are very rare. Outdoor leaders of all kinds, including adventure therapists, will do well to remember that when something goes seriously wrong in the outdoors, it is their leadership decisions and actions which will come under the most intense scrutiny. In cases such as this, where the standard of leadership is found to be exceptionally negligent, they may not only be liable to civil action, but could also face criminal proceedings.

REFERENCES

BBC News. (2003, September 23). *Teacher jailed over drowned boy.* Retrieved on 4/30/08 from: http://news.bbc.co.uk/2/hi/uk_news/england/lancashire/3132102.stm.

Bennett, C. (2003, September 5). Is jail the answer for fatal negligence? *The Guardian*, p. 5.

Bronnit, S. & McSherry, B. (2005). *Principles of criminal law*, 2nd ed. Sydney: Law Book Company.

Bunyan, N. (2003, September 24). *Teacher who let boy jump to death in pool is jailed.* Retrieved on 1/3/04, 2004 from: http://www.telegraph.co.uk/news/main.jhtml?xml=/news/2003/09/24/ nteach24.xml.

Butt, P. (Ed.) (2004). *Butterworth's concise Australian legal dictionary*, 3rd ed. Sydney: Lexis Nevis Butterworths.

Cassidy, S. (2003, September 24). Lakes death teacher is the first to be jailed for manslaughter of pupil. *The Independent.* Retrieved on 2/28/07 from: http://www.independent.co.uk/news/education/education-news/lakes-death-teacheris-the-first-to-be-jailed-for-manslaughter-of-pupil-580985.html.

Clare, J. (2004, February 19). Union tells teachers to end all school trips. *The Telegraph.* Retrieved on 3/1/04 from: http://www.telegraph.co.uk/news/main.jhtml?xml=/news/2004/02/19/nskool19. xml.

Clare, J. (2004, February 16). Don't boycott trips, teachers told. *The Telegraph.* Retrieved 4/24/08 from: http://www.telegraph.co.uk/news/main.jhtml?xml=/news/2005/02/16/ntrip16.xml.

Curtis, P. (2004, February 18). Teacher's union advises against school trips. *Education Guardian*. Retrieved on 3/1/04 from: www.education.guardian. co.uk/schooltrips/story/0,10621,1150846,00.html.

Department of Education and Children's Services. (2007). *Camps and excursions: Guidelines for schools and preschools*. Adelaide: Government of South Australia.

Duff, A. & Garland, D. (1994). *A reader on punishment.* Oxford, England: Oxford University Press.

Fulbrook, J. (2005). *Outdoor activities, negligence and the law.* Aldershot, England: Ashgate.

Health and Safety Executive. (2005a). *Glenridding Beck investigation report.* Retrieved on 5/24/08 from: www.hse.gov.schooltrips/investigation/index.htm

Health and Safety Executive. (2005b). *HSE response to education select committee report into school trips.* Retrieved on 4/23/08 from: www.hse.gov. uk/press/2005/e05019.htm.

Health and Safety Executive. (2005c). *Sharing the lessons learnt-HSE publishes web report on Glenridding school trip tragedy.* Retrieved on 4/23/08 from: www.hse.gov.uk/press/2005/e05034.htm.

Hudson, B. (1987). *Justice through punishment: A critique of the justice model of corrections*. London, England: MacMillan.

Leckie, D. (2004). *Essential legal update: Health and safety.* London, England: Leckie.

Press Association. (2003, September 23). Manslaughter plea could spark end of school trips. *The Guardian*. Retrieved on 1/9/02 from: http://education.guardian.co.uk/schools/story/0,,1048150,00. html.

Revell, P. (2002, March 11). Trips that end in tragedy. *The Guardian*. Retrieved on 11/3/05 from: http://education.guardian.co.uk/schools/story/0,,665392,00.html.

Revell, P. (2005, March 15). Outdoors is great. *The Guardian.* Retrieved on 3/11/05 from: http://education.guardian.co.uk/egweekly/story/0,,1437182,00.html.

Sarre, R. & Tomaino, J. (Eds.) (2004). *Key issues in criminal justice.* Adelaide: Australian Humanities Press.

ITTN. (2003, October). School trips under threat. *International Tours and Tourism News, 2*, p. 4.

Tomaino, J, & Kapardis, A. (2004). Sentencing theory. In R. Sarre & J. Tomaino (Eds.), *Key issues in criminal justice.* Adelaide: Australian Humanities Press.

Von Hirsch, A. (1976). *Doing justice.* New York, USA: Hill and Wang.

Wainwright, M. (2003, September 24). School trips under threat as teacher is jailed for boy's death. *The Guardian.* Retrieved on 1/9/04 from: http://www.guardian.co.uk/uk/2003/sep/24/schooltrips.schools.

Walker, N. (1985). *Sentencing: Theory, law and practice*. London, England: Butterworths.

Walker, N. (1991). *Why punish? Theories of punishment reassessed.* Oxford, England: Oxford University Press.

CHAPTER 33

Contact with Nature as a Research Variable in Wilderness Therapy

Nevin Harper

ABSTRACT

Today's technological and highly urbanized western society has significantly reduced our direct contact with wild nature. This disconnect is suggested to contribute to increasingly compromised human health and wellbeing. If contact with nature a key component of wilderness therapy is an antidote, what theoretical support exists to articulate its use in practice, and how can we empirically demonstrate its effectiveness? This paper encourages a program of research to determine the influences of direct contact with wild nature in wilderness therapy. If found to mediate or contribute to positive psychosocial outcomes, 'contact with nature' could gain acceptance as an evidence-based practice for use across multiple sectors and therapeutic modalities.

INTRODUCTION

The role nature plays in wilderness therapy is poorly understood. Practitioners and academics alike are quick to provide personal expressions, anecdotal evidence and borrowed theories to lay claims to the therapeutic value of nature. Research designed to isolate nature's mediating or confounding impact on therapeutic outcomes will improve the articulation of wilderness therapy's theoretical underpinnings. Considering the link between nature and human development, Kellett (2002) stated:

> The relative absence of published material on this subject may be indicative of a society so estranged from its natural origins it has failed

> to recognize our species' basic dependence on nature as a condition of growth and development. (p. 118)

While wilderness therapy begins to show promise as a treatment option, primarily with adolescent populations, clinical outcomes reported in literature are primarily conceived as the result of clinical interventions that occur outdoors (Clark, Marmol & Cooley, 2004; Bettmann, 2007; Russell, 2003). Nature's inherent healing qualities have been implied in the literature of these and similar studies, but not often described as a directly contributing therapeutic factor (Beringer & Martin, 2003; Taylor, Segal, & Harper, 2010). Norton (2011) highlighted the unique therapeutic environment that the wilderness provides, and her research also describes the positive impact that simply 'being in nature' can provide; however this is relatively unique in wilderness therapy literature.

Beringer and Martin (2003) challenged the dominant adventure therapy theorists as simply using the outdoors and nature 'in principally utilitarian terms' (p. 31), while placing emphasis in defining adventure therapy on the activities and the experience. As an extension of these authors' challenge, it is here argued that supportive research is needed beyond the acceptance and expression of nature's role in adventure and wilderness therapy. This need is not unique to adventure and wilderness therapy. Even eco-psychology as a field of study has asked the question:

> How does ecopsychology hope to persuade others to be interested in its theoretical propositions if it cannot provide data to support its foundations? (Thompson, 2008, p.35). A parallel question is here asked of wilderness therapy.

This paper suggests undertaking research of direct contact with nature in efforts to support outdoor and wilderness-based therapy through the generation of research evidence. A brief exploration of wilderness therapy is provided, followed by musings on cultural history that provide one perspective on what may have brought modern western society to a place where contact with nature is described as 'novel', and implied in the literature to be inherently 'therapeutic'. Theoretical support for these ideas, along with a proposed research approach to test these propositions is offered.

Wilderness as Therapy

Wilderness therapy can be viewed as one approach under the umbrella term of adventure therapy. Adventure therapy theorists have articulated challenge and risk-related activities, experiential learning, and novel settings and experiences as core elements of practice, integrated with conventional therapeutic approaches (Gass, 1993). Further, wilderness therapy is described to include the realities and influences of outdoor living and travel as integral to therapeutic practice (Russell, 2001). Adventure therapy can arguably be practiced in an office setting, while wilderness therapy cannot (unless metaphorically travelling in the 'wilderness' of the mind). As adventure therapy can occur in wild nature, the term wilderness therapy will be treated as inclusive of adventure therapy herein.

The natural environment, in essence, that which separates wilderness therapy from adventure therapy in non-natural settings, may in fact be a therapeutic variable, or at least mediate, yet maybe confound, reported research outcomes (Harper, 2009). If we accept, even just for the sake of argument, that nature itself has an impact on the individual in therapy, we must then look more critically at why, and how, we can then take advantage of these understandings to better serve clients. A critical perspective must first be anchored in historical and practical context. To begin this exploration, I ask, 'how have we come to experience nature as a setting or condition which has an effect on us outside of our daily experience?' That is, how did we come to experience being in contact with nature as novel?

Modern Failure of Human Development

At no time in human history have humans been more physically and psychologically removed from a healthy and intimate relationship with wild nature. Many western nations now report rates of urbanization greater than 80%, and the United Nations stated in 2008 that more than half the world's population is now urbanized. Further, a now-commonly cited study in health research cites that North Americans spend, on average, 90% of their day indoors and an additional 5% in their cars (Klepeis et al., 2001), suggesting western lifestyle patterns of humans primarily living in 'built' versus natural environments.

Urbanization has become more prevalent since the shift toward agricultural societies when the nomadic lifestyle pattern was rapidly replaced by a more static life in ever-expanding settlements. Agriculture has been singled out as one of the most significant acts of our species in altering the relationship between humans and the rest of nature. Offered here is a simplistic explanation lacking depth, and acknowledging that 'any attempt to seize upon a single historical variable to explain the western world's relentless humanizing of the wilderness is intrinsically narrow' and does not account for developing socio-cultural processes (Oelschlaeger, 1992, p. 284). The agricultural argument, covered in depth elsewhere (see Shepard, 1982) does however provide 'legs' for theoretical musings to stand on as to why contact with nature, and surely the wilderness therapy context, may provide a healing or therapeutic experience for the human condition.

With 300,000 years of hunter/gatherer ancestry (those who traveled and modified their lifestyles by the rhythm of migratory paths, climate, geography and tribal and inter-tribal influences) to the planting of crops to sustain permanent settlements only 7,000-8,500 years ago, very little had changed in the human relationship with nature (Davis, 2009). During the acceleration of agricultural practices, and subsequent growth in populations, so the argument goes, a divide was forged between humans and nature (Shepard, 1982). The increasing need to control nature for food production resulted in new constructs such as 'weeds' and 'wild'. This growth in production, the advent of the resource extraction industry, and early signs of large-scale environmental degradation, was well underway as humans entered the Golden and Iron ages. By the time of the Industrial Revolution, wilderness in many parts of the world were exploited and controlled as resources serving human needs. To re-quote Thoreau (1962):

> In wild[er]ness [resources] lies the preservation of the [western] world['s consumptive lifestyle patterns].

Today's technological and highly urbanized western society is severely disconnected from nature. The teaching of basic food production and local knowledge of flora and fauna, let alone excursions into wild nature, are often considered novel and unique experiences. Further, we are also now witnesses to the gravest conditions of global environmental health, from species and cultural extinction to climate change and deteriorating air quality and food security issues. While not hard to rationalize nor demonstrate, ill environmental health has been linked to ill physical health. Harder to legitimize is the relationship between ill environmental health and its negative effect on the human psyche, ill mental health. Eco-psychology theory depicts our psychological health as intricately related to environmental health (Roszak, Gomes, & Kanner, 1995). We may yet come to accept the links between current global environmental problems and increasing rates of mental illness as a society.

Shepard proposed in *Nature and Madness* (1982) that a dualistic relationship between humans and nature is resultant from our failing to become fully mature as a species. This immaturity, he aligns with being stuck in an adolescent stage of development, due in some part to rapid growth in civilization, continued separation from nature as a species and some deeper, illogical, failure of human development, as he suggests – a madness. He points out that the notable social psychologist Fromm (1955) questioned the sanity of society almost 55 years ago, suggesting a significant cataract in the universal vision of our relationship to nature.

With an apparent cultural 'forgetting' of modern western society's earlier relationship with nature, and possible evolutionary preferences being denied, it is easy to conceive that we should be taking action to restore our relationship with wild nature from a psychological and health perspective. If our societal 'madness' has detached us from an equitable and beneficial balance with our environment, what is the antidote, and how does it work? If contact with nature as simply proposed here is the antidote, and a key in the wilderness therapy context, what theoretical support exists to articulate it?

Theoretical Support: Contact with Nature for Therapy

Contact with nature has been demonstrated to contribute positively to human health and well-being (Maller, Townsend, Pryor, Brown, & St. Leger, 2005; Miles, 1987). Studies cited are often backed with conceptual support from attention restoration theory (ART), and contextualised in biological and evolutionary discourse (Gullone, 1997; Kaplan, 1995; Kaplan & Berman, 2010).

ART suggests that contact with nature contributes to restoring our ability to pay attention. The theory has been tested, and has continued to show support in research literature for more than two decades (Berman, Jonides,

& Kaplan, 2008; Hartig, Mang & Evans, 1992; Kaplan, 1995; Kaplan & Berman, 2010; Kaplan & Kaplan, 1989; Laumann, Garling, & Stormark, 2001). Kaplan (1995) described directed attention as that which requires concerted voluntary effort and is 'susceptible to fatigue, controls distraction through the use of inhibition', whereas involuntary attention requires no effort and is therefore presumed to not cause fatigue (p. 170). Involuntary attention occurs when in environments or viewing environments that are unique or fascinating but not requiring direct cognitive effort (think of a calculus lecture versus staring at a campfire), the outcome of increased directed attention is improved cognitive and emotional functioning. Further, the increases in directed attention from time spent in contact with nature have been theoretically linked to increases in executive functioning (decision-making ability) and self-regulation (impulse control and resisting temptations) which are highly valuable resources to the clients and practitioners across education, development or therapeutic settings (Kaplan & Berman, 2010; Kuo & Faber-Taylor, 2004).

Comprising a number of constructs (see Table 1), ART has been explored across varied populations and settings, and has demonstrated improved directed attention along a spectrum from simply viewing nature, to being physically active in nature; important findings for urban planning, health promotion, education and therapeutic sectors alike (see Maller et al., 2002 for an overview of health benefits arising from contact with nature).

'Wild nature' provides a dynamic ever-changing environment in direct contrast to a static indoor 'built' environment. This reality suggests that therapists and clients of wilderness therapy are afforded greater opportunities for heightened sensory, motor and affective responses, thereby offering potentially greater opportunities for the therapeutic process in natural environments. ART provides a readily accessible framework to evaluate the effect of contact with wild nature. From a practice perspective, the constructs of the Perceived Restorativeness Scale (PRS) should inspire critical thinking on how the environmental setting may contribute to their client's outcomes.

Table 1. Constructs of the Perceived Restorativeness Scale (PRS)

Construct	**Description**
Being away	The setting is different or 'novel' relative to your everyday work/life setting; hence, you are 'away' from it
Fascination	Attention is held easily, not requiring concentrated effort, think of staring into a fire or babbling creek
Coherence	The setting 'makes sense' in that things are not confusing or illogical
Scope	The setting provides adequate opportunities for exploration and interpretation
Compatibility	The setting is in alignment with personal (and evolutionary) preferences, skills and knowledge
Familiarity	The setting is 'known' to you, or has traits you are familiar with
Preference	The setting is a 'preferred' place, you would rather be in that setting than others

Notes:

1. Kaplan's original theory had only four constructs: Being away, Fascination, Extent, Compatibility

2. Hartig and others have further developed the theoretical constructs for attention restoration theory, including separating: Coherence and Scope into distinct constructs from Extent, and adding Compatibility and Familiarity (Terry Hartig, personal correspondence, Summer 2009)

Last, evolutionary and biological preferences have been identified and more recently suggested as linked to increased pathology in western society. This provides an interesting perspective on how being in nature may assist or detract from therapy, yet, how our biological realities are tested by rapid technological change and intensive urbanization of lifestyles demands a paper of its own, and cannot be adequately covered here (see Gullone, 2000 for her treatise on the link between reduced contact with nature and increased psychopathology).

Considerations for the wilderness therapy practitioner regarding evolutionary preferences include whether or not specific terrain or weather conditions may be ideal or detrimental to the therapeutic experience of a particular client. Asked here to provoke further research and theoretical explorations, I simply leave the suggestive example that dark caves, mountain ridges, a sunny day at the beach and open prairie wind storms all likely provide unique experiences to those traveling in them, and surely in relation to a combination of lived experiences as well as our collective evolutionary preferences (Verbeek & de Waal, 2002). It is acknowledged that assessing client's compatibility to specific environments may be an idealized level of sophistication for future wilderness therapy research and practice.

Research in the field of wilderness therapy is evolving in the purview of an influential medical model a reliance on outcomes research within the hierarchical evidence-based paradigm (Harper, 2010). Regardless of theoretical orientation and pedagogy of practice, the therapeutic value of contact with nature simply outdoors or in wild nature has been mostly ignored in empirical investigations of this field, leaving outcomes to be interpreted as being reached by clinical intervention alone (i.e. therapeutic approach, activities, group process, etc.). This is not to say that nature has not been expressed as therapeutic in our field, it has (Miles, 1983).

Practitioners and academics generally agree with the premise that nature has inherent therapeutic qualities and likely contributes meaningfully to individual change processes. One scholar-practitioner has more recently been providing a theoretical framework and case study results to support the notion of nature-based therapy (Berger, 2006; 2007; Berger & McLeod, 2006). These efforts are to be applauded, and should be advanced and built upon.

Further, the reality of widespread use of contact with wild nature in wilderness therapy underscores the significant need to provide evidence in support of this approach, especially in times of heightened liability and ethical concerns that often produce barriers to practice, such as 'being outside' for a practitioner in a conventional office setting. The issue lies in the dearth of evidence to support these universal assumptions of the field.

TESTING ART: NATURE AS 'KERNEL' OF EVIDENCE

As adventure therapy and wilderness therapy flirt with the discourse and dominant ideology of evidence-based practice (EBP) in an effort to solidify its standing as a valued therapeutic approach, a number of concerns are present: (1) limitations of the EBP paradigm to capture the ecological contributions of the wilderness therapy process, (2) the lack of theoretical grounding currently articulated in adventure therapy, and (3) the diverse expression of adventure therapy practices (Harper, 2010).

Internationally, the role of EBP in funding of programs and services has become increasingly important, and cause for critical review. Recognizing that numerous political and economic influences drive the EBP paradigm, this paper proposes a judicious methodological approach to EBP research utilizing 'kernels' of evidence in support of one highly significant process variable in wilderness therapy direct contact with wild nature.

Kernels are influence procedures bringing about behavioural change (Embry & Biglan, 2008). One example is the use of peer-mentors in educational settings that has shown to effectively increase desired academic outcomes. Rather than 'proving' effectiveness of a model of practice or therapeutic approach, kernels can be demonstrated by isolating and evaluating effectiveness of a particular variable. In the example given, simply utilizing student peer support as mentors was shown to increase gains in learning. In the case of wilderness therapy, isolating common elements of practice such as contact with wild nature could be utilized in a basic research approach (i.e. random controlled trials across settings). In short, kernels are the behaviorist researcher's new catchy term for 'components', although they specify that a component may be broken down into parts but a kernel needs to be indivisible to qualify. A wilderness therapy 'solo' experience for example, would not be a kernel as it can be divided into smaller units—reflection, alone time, self-care, contact with nature, fasting, journaling etc. It is here cautiously proposed that 'contact with wild nature' may be considered a kernel for outcomes research. That is, a standalone variable to be investigated.

While the reported benefits of contact with nature are broad and supported by a number of theories, research generally supports the premise that it positively influences health and well-being (Kaplan, 1995; Maller et al., 2005). Contact with nature, if demonstrated as an effective kernel, could gain acceptance as an available EBP for use across therapeutic practices and populations. In contrast to research attempting to demonstrate efficacy of therapeutic approaches or program models, kernels of evidence possess higher likelihood of adoption since they can be simple, affordable, and easily delivered across educational, development and treatment settings. This, versus the significant change required to implement an EBP model with its specific training and fidelity issues make kernels attractive to practitioners (Embry & Biglan, 2008). As a developing field of practice, wilderness therapy will be influenced by the EBP paradigm; its researchers and practitioners need to ultimately, determine their participation in it. Contact with wild nature may prove to be a significant variable, clearly setting wilderness therapy apart from residential and institutional treatment settings (Harper & Russell, 2008).

Proposed Research Methodology

A program of research utilizing contact with wild nature as a treatment variable in recognition of ecological influences in wilderness therapy is suggested. Perceptions of potential environmental effect are discussed and suggestions for theoretical development, practice, and future research are offered.

RCT and Contact with Nature

The 'gold standard' approach in EBP research is the double-blind random control trial (RCT), an experimental design in which strong cause-effect inferences are supported (Howell, 2002). The RCT is a key design feature in EBP, demanded by many governmental and fund-granting institutions. Traditional control and treatment group RCT designs have been criticized in human service fields as being unethical (i.e., to delay treatment for control group participants), difficult to maintain fidelity, and impractical due to issues of participant consent, referral support and treatment adherence, among other challenges to internal validity (Victoria, Habicht, & Bryce, 2004). Further, from a practical standpoint, RCT does not tend to provide clinicians with the necessary understanding of how treatment variables effect change or relate to particular client profiles (Davison, 2000). So while published RCTs report outcomes on more or less-effective manualized treatment approaches (Drew et al., 2002; Liddle et al., 2001), they provide limited understanding of more finite treatment variables that may be applied within a treatment approach. Mechanisms of change have seen limited inquiry in the pursuit of 'outcome efficacy' across treatment research, yet they remain the most important understanding needed to improve clinical practice (Kazdin & Nock, 2003).

One evidence-based alternative to conventional RCT experimental design with control (i.e. no treatment) and treatment groups is to maintain the standard treatment approach as the control (i.e. treatment-as-usual, TAU) and alter treatment variables for each treatment group similar to basic experimental research design. TAU in a manualized treatment as a control group allows for research when conventional RCT is deemed unethical or impractical due to acute client needs, costs or logistical issues in participant recruitment. Treatment of high-risk adolescent populations have been successfully studied utilizing TAU in RCT experimental designs (Spirito, Stanton, Donnaldson & Boergers, 2002) and provide a template for research which is ethically defensible and more likely to reduce issues of internal validity while providing increased understanding of treatment variable effects.

Treatment groups in experimental research should be rationalized for comparison, strive to test the theories of specific variables and to clearly express the stage of development that particular field has achieved. It is critical to clearly define the variable 'contact with wild nature' proposed for investigation. Second, it is equally important to articulate its relationship to potential enhancements in the treatment process and improvements in outcome. Current theoretical understandings of nature and wilderness-based treatment is a patchwork of understanding, much borrowed from other social and psychological disciplines. Reference to ART, for example, has been made by authors in adventure and wilderness therapy for decades as an underpinning theory without supportive research from the field (e.g., Davis-Berman & Berman, 1994; Miles, 1987). Further, a theoretical framework on human-nature relationships has been articulated in efforts to encourage use of natural environments for therapeutic ends (Norton, 2009). RCT research directly evaluating 'built' versus natural (direct contact with wild nature) treatment environments will sustain the assertions our field has precariously relied on, increase the strength of inference of field research, and contribute meaningfully to theory development.

METHODOLOGY AND INSTRUMENTATION

The first critical task is to define the settings in which built versus natural treatment environments could be examined. The findings of a study could easily be dismissed without clarity as to how one could replicate the study or implement the kernel in practice. Second, the study would require measures that are designed to reliably capture the data sought; as an example, (a) affective change over time, and (b) whether or not the treatment setting was influential in that change process. The indoor setting would be best identified and described as one that has no influence of wild nature. Obviously, a built environment with large windows overlooking a beautiful park would not do. If the control group experienced treatment in an entirely 'built' environment (imagine an interview room in the interior of a building without windows a human-built space), the outdoor setting would ideally be in wild nature (i.e. with minimal to no influence of human built components). While a park setting may be appropriate, the researcher would want to create a metric for 'greenness' or 'naturalness' that could be easily replicated. For example, if the area were photographed, what percentage of the setting is 'built' versus 'wild nature'? Then of course, people will ask whether a manicured garden is 'natural', relative to wild nature etc. Ideally, do what you can to reduce limitations by increasing rigour in design through clear definitions and research procedures.

To evaluate the effects of setting on treatment, the Perceived Restorativeness Scale (PRS, see constructs above in Table 1), intended to measure ART, could be employed to identify whether participants report on the theorized benefits of the built versus natural setting (Hartig et al., 1991). Obviously there are other instruments available. Alignment between program intent and measures needs to be considered, however, for the sake of this example, the PRS has been chosen for its broad use in ART research.

Treatment outcomes could be measured during the TAU or manualized approach as part of the ongoing assessment and intervention (i.e. measures with clinical treatment goals embedded), preferably instruments with limited intrusiveness yet recognized in treatment realms as valid and reliable. Following treatment, this methodology would leave the researcher with two sets of aggregated data showing (a) treatment outcomes over the chosen study period, and (b) an indication of the impact of the environment in which treatment took place. In effect, an RCT outcome study of built versus wild nature in a manualized treatment could provide insight to the question: 'Does being in nature improve treatment outcomes?' Second, the study will provide a test of ART, in theoretical support for adventure and wilderness therapy. Last, practitioners and researchers could explore the outcomes by construct of the PRS to advance client-specific interventions (For example compatibility will likely vary significantly based on client's previous life experience, suggesting intervention location (topography, weather and other environmental factors) need to be included in treatment planning.

Conclusion

The aim of this paper is to encourage research to address the lack of empirical understanding of the role of contact with nature in mediating or confounding reported therapeutic outcomes within the fields of adventure therapy and wilderness therapy. While contact with nature is common in practice, its growing body of outcomes literature still suffers from the theoretical rationale and supportive research for its use. Questions remain unanswered: Is being in contact with wild nature therapeutic in and of itself? Does the wild nature setting contribute to or confound research outcomes of therapy?

Our relationship with nature has been professed since time immemorial as integral to our health and a sustainable existence on earth. From the philosophies of First peoples worldwide, to nature writers, to ecopsychologists, we are continually reminded of the need to remain in a healthy relationship with the natural world we are simply a part of. It is in this acceptance that humans are nature(al) that society may recognize their innate desire to regain balance. A heightened eco-literacy, and awareness of possible action is needed.

The underlying premise that humans would be healthier if more connected with nature may provide a conceptual frame for adventure and wilderness therapy researchers and practitioners to meaningfully lead broader societal change. This shift can only be realized following a clear and direct articulation of the therapeutic value of being in nature that we currently universally accept with limited empirical support. As argued here, it is critical that one of wilderness therapy's key practices, that is, being in direct contact with nature, is based on sound research, which is replicable and respected in other allied helping and healing fields. In doing so, both adventure therapy and wilderness therapy practice may ultimately gain further acceptance across conventional treatment arenas.

REFERENCES

Berger, R. (2006). Using contact with nature, creativity and rituals as a therapeutic medium with children with learning difficulties: A case study. *Emotional and Behavioural Difficulties, 11*(2)135-146.

Berger, R. (2007). Choosing the right space to work in: Reflections prior to a nature therapy session. *Australian Journal of Outdoor Education, 11*(1)41-45.

Berger, R. & McLeod, J. (2006). Incorporating nature into therapy: A framework for practice. *Journal of Systemic Therapies, 25*(2)80-94.

Beringer, A., & Martin, P. (2003). On adventure therapy and the natural worlds: Respecting nature's healing. *Journal of Adventure Education and Outdoor Learning, 3*(1)29-40.

Berman, M. G., Jonides, J., & Kaplan, S. (2008). The cognitive benefits of nature. *Psychological Science, 19*(12)1207-1212.

Bettmann, J. E. (2007). Changes in adolescent attachment relationships as a response to wilderness treatment. *Journal of the American Psychoanalytic Association, 55*(1)259-265.

Clark, J. P., Marmol, L. M., Cooley, R., & Gathercoal, K. (2004). The effects of wilderness therapy on the clinical concerns (on Axes I, II, and IV) of troubled adolescents. *Journal of Experiential Education, 27*(2)213-232.

Davis, W. (2009). *The Wayfinders: Why ancient wisdom matters in the modern world.* Toronto, ON: Anansi.

Davison, G. C. (2000). Stepped care: Doing more with less. *Journal of Consulting and Clinical Psychology, 68*(4)580-585.

Drew, A., Baird, G., Baron-Cohen, S., Cox, A., Slonims, V., Wheelwright, S., Swettenham, J., Berry, B. & Charman, T. (2002). A pilot randomized control trial of a parent training intervention for pre-school children with autism. *European Journal of Child and Adolescent Psychiatry, 11*, 266-272.

Embry, D. D., & Biglan, A. (2008). Evidence-based kernels: Fundamental units of behavioral influence. *Clinical Child and Family Psychological Review, 11*, 75-113.

Fromm, E. (1955). *The sane society*. New York, NY: Henry Holt.

Gass, M. A. (1993). *Adventure therapy: Therapeutic applications of adventure programming.* Dubuque, IA: Kendall/Hunt.

Gullone, E. (2000). The biophilia hypothesis and life in the 21st century: Increasing mental health or increasing pathology? *Journal of Happiness Studies, 1,* 293-321.

Harper, N. J. (2009). The relationship between therapeutic alliance and outcome in wilderness treatment. *Journal of Adventure Education and Outdoor Learning, 9*(1)45-59.

Harper, N. J. (2010). Future paradigm or false idol: A cautionary tale of evidence-based practice for adventure education and therapy. *Journal of Experiential Education, 33*(1)38-55.

Harper, N. J., & Russell, K. C. (2008). Family involvement and outcome in adolescent wilderness treatment: A mixed-methods evaluation. *International Journal of Child and Family Welfare, 1*, 19-36.

Hartig, T., Mang, M., & Evans, G. W. (1991). Restorative effects of natural-environment experiences. *Environment and Behavior, 23*, 3-26.

Howell, D. C. (2002). *Statistical methods for psychology* (5th Ed.). Pacific Grove, CA: Duxbury.

Kaplan, S. (1989). *The experience of nature: A psychological perspective*. New York: Cambridge University Press.

Kaplan, S. (1995). The restorative benefits of nature: Toward an integrative framework. *Journal of Environmental Psychology, 15*, 169-182.

Kaplan, S. & Berman, M. G. (2010). Directed attention as a common resource for executive functioning and self-regulation. *Perspectives on Psychological Science, 5(*1)43-57.

Kazdin, A. E., & Nock, M. K. (2003). Delineating mechanisms of change in child and adolescent therapy: Methodological issues and research recommendations. *Journal of Child Psychology and Psychiatry, 44(*8)1116-1129.

Kellett, S. R. (2002). Experiencing nature: affective, cognitive, and evaluative development in children. In P. H. Kahn & S. R. Kellert (Eds.), *Children and nature: Psychological, sociocultural, and evolutionary investigations* (pp. 117-152). Cambridge, MA: The MIT Press.

Klepeis, N. E., Nelson, W. C., Ott, W. R., Robinson, J. P., Tsang, A. M., Switzer, P., et al. (2001). The human activity pattern survey (NHAPS): a resource for accessing exposure to environmental pollutants. *Journal of Exposure and Environmental Epidemiology, 11*, 231-252.

Kuo, F. E. & Faber-Taylor, A. (2004). A potential natural treatment for attention deficit/hyperactivity disorder: Evidence from a national study. *American Journal of Public Health, 94*(9)1580-1586.

Liddle, H., Dakof, G. A., Parker, K., Diamond, G. S., Barrett, K., & Tejeda, M. (2001). Multidimensional family therapy for adolescent drug abuse: Results of a randomized clinical trial. *American Journal of Drug & Alcohol Abuse, 27*(4)651-688.

Laumann, K., Garling, T., & Stormark, K. M. (2001). Rating scale measures of restorative components of environments. *Journal of Environmental Psychology, 21*, 31-44.

Maller, C., Townsend, M., Pryor, A., Brown, P., & St. Leger, L. (2005). Healthy nature healthy people: Contact with nature as an upstream health promotion intervention for populations. *Health Promotion International, 21*(1)45-54.

Miles, J. C. (1987). Wilderness as healing place. *Journal of Experiential Eductation, 10*(3)4-10.

Norton, C. L. (2009). Ecopsychology and social work: Creating an interdisciplinary framework for redefining person-in-environment. *Ecopsychology, 1*(3)138-145.

Norton, C.L. (2011). Wilderness therapy: Creating a context of hope. In C. Norton (Ed.), *Innovative interventions in child nd adolescent mental health,* pp. 36-74. New York: Routledge.

Oeslschlaeger, M. (Ed.). (1992). *The Wilderness Condition.* Washington, DC: Island Press.

Roszak, T., Gomes, M. E., & Kanner, A. D. (1995). *Ecopsychology.* San Francisco, CA: Sierra Club Books.

Russell, K. C. (2001). What is wilderness therapy? *Journal of Experiential Education, 24*(2)70-79.

Russell, K. C. (2003). An assessment of outcomes in outdoor behavioral healthcare treatment. *Child and Youth Care Forum, 34*(3)209-239.

Shepard, P. (1982). *Nature and madness.* Athens, GA: University of Georgia Press.

Somerville, M. (2006). *The ethical imagination: Journeys of the human spirit.* Toronto, ON: Anansi.

Spirito, A., Stanton, C., Donaldson, D., & Boergers, J. (2002). Treatment-as-usual for adolescent suicide attempters: Implications for the choice of comparison groups in psychotherapy research. *Journal of Clinical Child and Adolescent Psychology, 31*(1)41-47.

Taylor, D. M., Segal, D., & Harper, N. J. (2010). The ecology of adventure therapy. *Ecopsychology, 2*(2)77-83.

Thompson, M. (2009). Reviewing ecospychology research: Exploring five databases and considering the future. *Ecopsychology, 1*(1)32-37.

Thoreau, H. D. (1962). *Walden.* New York: Time Inc. Verbeek, P. & de Waal, F. B. M. (2002). The primate relationship with nature: Biophilia as a general pattern. In P. H. Kahn Jr. & S. R. Kellert (Eds.), *Children and nature: Psychological, sociocultural, and evolutionary investigations.* Cambridge, MA: MIT Press.

Victoria, C. G., Habicht, J.-P., & Bryce, J. (2004). Evidence-based public health: Moving beyond randomized trials. *American Journal of Public Health, 94*(3)400-405.

CHAPTER 34

Place, Perception and, Placebo: The Healing Power of Nature

Jamie Mcphie

ABSTRACT

As outdoor alternatives to medication and psychotherapy are becoming more common, much of the research on the restorative benefits of nature suggests there is a genetic basis for humans' values of, and positive receptiveness to nature. However, many of these studies do not accurately capture the explanations for the reported effects in settings that most resemble those where the phenomena usually takes place. In my view, these do not acknowledge the full effects of social context or embodied experiences on people's responses, hindering understanding of how perceptions of nature may benefit wellbeing. I suggest that 'expectation', 'association', 'socio-cultural conditioning' and 'embodied placebo effects' demand greater scrutiny than current approaches include. This presentation is based on pilot research undertaken in 2012 as part fulfilment for a PhD. It will attempt to answer how participants experience specific outdoor environments within two outdoor health intervention programmes and what the benefits of nature are within these interventions using interpretive phenomenological methods. A participant observation approach was adopted between the periods of June to July, 2012. My intention is to help inform health professionals on the nature of effective interventions based around natural settings.

INTRODUCTION

The purpose of this pilot study is to explore how participants experience and interpret specific outdoor environments within health interventions and discover if certain perceptions of nature may influence their health and wellbeing. This will inform the main field of work for my PhD as to the most suitable methodological paradigm to use.

A growing body of evidence indicates that anxiety, stress and mental ill-health are becoming more prevalent in modern society (WHO, 2001; Halliwell, 2005; Spedding, 2006; Summerfield and Gill, 2005). The most established treatment for depressive disorders is antidepressant medication although recent research suggests that there is little evidence that they have a specific pharmacological effect relative to pill placebo for patients with less severe depression or in patients with mild or moderate symptoms (Halliwell, 2005; Fournier et al., 2010). Alternatives to medication and psychotherapy, such as exercise and outdoor, 'nature' based therapies are becoming more common, particularly in treating clinical depression (Bandoroff, 2003; Russell and Farnum, 2004; Pryor, Carpenter and Townsend, 2005; Halliwell, 2005), supporting the long-held view in medicine that nature, as well as physical health is essential to mental wellbeing (Ulrich and Parsons, 1992; Warner, 1987; Greenway, 1995). This belief in the healing power of nature is supported by much 'restorative environments' research undertaken since the 1970's. The most prominent theories underpinning this research are: The Biophilia Hypothesis (Wilson, 1984; Kellert and Wilson, 1993); Attention Restoration Theory (Kaplan and Kaplan, 1982; 1989); and the Psycho-Evolutionary Stress Reduction Theory (Ulrich, 1979; 1983; 1991), which all suggest there is a genetic basis for humans' values of, and positive receptiveness to nature, although there is no convincing evidence to support these evolutionary claims.

Furthermore, many of the studies that use such theories as a philosophical foundation rely heavily on assumptions that use positivistic methodologies that do not accurately record and report the reasons for their effects. For example, many studies have attempted to measure the effects of the 'outdoors' on participants' physiological and psychological stress levels by undertaking the analysis 'indoors'. This method of research may present a limited degree of explanation. The data gathered may be affected by the use of a completely different environment and may not mimic accurately the experience of the people within the 'actual' settings. At the very most, this indoor research, much of which uses photographic slides of outdoor environments, may simply suggest that a 'picture' of a person's perception of what they think nature is, may have an influence on their health and wellbeing (suggesting that the perception itself may be enough to trigger a positive response).

Macnaghten and Urry (1998) suggest that there is no singular 'nature', only a diversity of contested natures and each such nature is represented through a variety of socio-cultural processes from which such natures cannot be separated. This constructivist viewpoint emphasises the impact of social context on people's responses and sees landscape as a subjective cultural representation (Cosgrove and Daniels; 1988; Barnes and Duncan, 1992; Macnaghten and Urry, 1998) rather than a singular objective, measurable phenomenon. This representation may influence the ascription of meanings to various environments (Dinsdale and Fenton, 2006). Allying himself to this viewpoint, Tuan (1979, p.89) surmised that landscape is 'a *construct* of the mind and of feeling' (emphasis added).

Conversely, Ingold (2000) argues that by defining landscapes or environments as a set of cultural values, attitudes and meanings, it propagates a series of dualities between culture and nature, similar to that of subject and object or mind and body. In his view, it "is not a picture in the imagination" or "a formless substrate awaiting the imposition of human order" (Ingold, 2000, p.191), but rather it is grounded in embodied perception and is seen as continually developing and elaborating via interactions (Wylie, 2007; Ingold, 2000). For example, there have been a few studies that have discovered significant predictors of positive adult beliefs about the benefits of nature that have developed from childhood (Lester and Maudsley, 2006; Thompson, Aspinall and Montarzino, 2008), suggesting embodied perception to be of crucial importance, yet this concept seems to have largely been left out of current theoretical frameworks. Oelschlaeger (1991) states that the idea and 'thought' of wilderness is not a product of human cognition in social context, but rather this thought has happened 'to us' out of historical and linguistic inevitability.

Supporting these anti-dualistic views, the traditions of phenomenology, process metaphysics, Gibson's ecological psychology and externalism (see Rowlands, 2010 for a detailed description of externalism) all stress that the self is not merely 'within' the world as a separate entity, but it is 'of' the world (Merleau-Ponty, 1964) and corporeal embodiment and extended minds (Clarke and Chalmers, 1998) are the bases of this experience. In other words, the mind (including consciousness) is a process of physical events that bridge the human form and the surrounding environment (process externalism), treating the human as part of the environment rather than separate from it (including human produce). Therefore, the concepts of culture and nature may be seen as elements of the same ecological process and as such, perceptions of nature must surely be embedded within this process.

If certain perceptions of nature really can influence health and wellbeing, it suggests that a sort of placebo effect is in action. If we follow the majority of current thinking about how placebo effects work, they hint at a conscious cognitive (and subjective) construction of nature. However, the placebo effect can be understood in numerous ways depending on the context in which it is used. It is the definition of placebo as a response to a symbolic intervention (Kirmayer, 2011; Price, Finniss & Benedetti, 2008), sometimes called the 'meaning response' (Moerman, 2002), that is relevant to this research. Thompson, Ritenbaugh and Nichter (2009), see an overemphasis on conscious cognitive approaches to understanding placebo and suggest that it is direct embodied experience that takes precedence over meaning-making in the healing encounter. Frenkel (2008) argues that without prior bodily engagement in an activity there is no way of representing it and so a conscious, cognitive representation of an expected outcome should not be necessary for inducing a physiological placebo response (Meissner, 2011).

In a study examining the autonomic effects of placebo, Meissner (2011) found that verbal suggestion may activate association areas that store memories of bodily activities (embodied memories). In other words, placebo effects are dependent on 'lived experience' rather than conscious representations of expected outcomes (Meissner, 2011). The body can directly respond to sensory or affective stimuli and it does not require meaning in any consciously cognitive sense to catalyse a placebo response and as such, responses that enhance healing may be able to be directly (unconsciously) triggered by *places* (Thompson, Ritenbaugh and Nichter, 2009). Frenkel (2008) calls this model, 'implicit affordance' as the practical significance afforded by a placebo can be determined by the degree of the match between the knowledge and the affordance of the situation (Meissner, 2011).

According to Kirmayer (2011), understanding the effectiveness of placebos and other healing interventions requires knowledge of the person's social world, contexts and commitments. Therefore, taking an embodied approach to outdoor health interventions, a person's 'sense of place' may be highly relevant to this research.

To a degree, it is likely that the belief in the healing power of nature is an assumption founded deep within certain Western cultures. Furthermore, these assumptions occasionally lead to the belief that specific kinds of environment are more beneficial than others (Clark et al, 1994), indicating that current prescriptions that many doctors now adhere to, such as exercise or other kinds of outdoor based therapies as a remedy for stress or depression, may be based on beliefs and assumptions that are either grounded in cultural tradition and influenced by social conditioning or based on beliefs that have been embodied and habitualised over time. Therefore, there may be certain constructs embedded within various cultures that either condition people or habitualise people to like certain environments over others and 'believe' that nature has restorative benefits, so much so that this expectation or 'meaning effect' is embodied, reinforcing these beliefs. If this is so, a clearer and more definitive explanation of how they manifest themselves, particularly regarding the relationship to the varying degrees of 'wildness' of nature (McKenzie, 2000; Nichols, 2000), needs to be sought so that we can use this information to further inform medical institutions and professionals.

Critical literature on the experiential nature of outdoor research suggests that most of the research is based on an outcome-orientated, objectivist epistemology that does not complement the subjective nature of experiences and so the experiences of individuals, and the meanings they make of their experiences, are lost when it comes to research, even though they are central to it (Allison and Pomeroy, 2000; Barratt and Greenaway, 1995). Current approaches to the relationship between green space and wellbeing within therapeutic landscapes certainly need a more substantial effort made in research within the areas of landscape phenomenology, socio-cultural conditioning and embodied placebo effects.

The pilot investigation will observe two small, specific restorative outdoor health intervention groups in order to test and develop appropriate methods and develop a more robust paradigm to support the methodological underpinnings. This will add to the current literature base to help inform health professionals on the nature of health interventions based around natural settings.

RESEARCH QUESTIONS

- How do participants experience and interpret specific outdoor environments within health interventions?
- Do perceptions of nature influence health and wellbeing within these interventions?

METHODOLOGY

In order to address the research questions identified above and some of the limitations of previous research on this issue, my methodological approach involved using settings that most resemble where the phenomena usually takes place so that the data will more likely reflect the interpretations intended.

As my ontological approach incorporates a phenomenological perspective, how people make sense of their life experiences, the data collected were collated and scrutinised, loosely informed by interpretive phenomenological analysis (IPA) (Smith, Flowers and Larkin, 2009).

"Employing a phenomenological paradigm of embodiment demands analytical attention toward the ways in which placebo effects are manifestations of somatic nodes of attention," (Thompson, Ritenbaugh and Nichter, 2009, p.129), that is "the culturally elaborated ways of attending to and with one's body" (Csordas 1993, p.138). By undertaking this qualitative research in different environments, using an IPA approach, I hope to better understand the embodied benefits that a perception of nature may provide in order to develop a suitable model to work from for future research.

Methods

The pilot investigation used two small, specific restorative outdoor health intervention groups, practices that use different environmental settings; an urban park within a city (Urban Park) and a community garden within a town on the edge of a rural setting (Rural Garden). These were chosen due to ease of access, timing and the geographical nature of the settings. The names of the groups were kept anonymous for ethical reasons.

I included seven participants in the pilot study, four of whom completed all the methods mentioned below. All seven participants undertook the video interviews. The participants from the Rural Garden named themselves The Green Man, Katherine (the facilitator), Jim and Gideon. The participants from the Urban Park named themselves Bill, Ben and Chris.

Ethical approval was acquired before data collection began between the periods of June to July, 2012 and all participants signed the relevant consent forms.

Although a bricolage of methods were employed in order to capture the emergent constructions (Denzin and Lincoln, 2000), semi-structured individual interviews using a head-mounted video camera and a hand-held video camera was the main method used. Exploring 'place' with walking interviews was informed by Sheller and Urry (2006); Moles (2008); Jones, Bunce, Evans, Gibbs and Ricketts Hein (2008); and Evans and Jones (2011). The use of headcams specifically for research into social experiences was informed by Brown, Dilley and Marshall (2008) and research involving walking with video was informed by Sarah Pink's (2007) work.

I used dual video feedback to record the data, a head-mounted camera for the participant (for ease of use whilst working and to capture the participant's view) and a hand-held camera for myself. The reason I chose to use two cameras was because when spliced together and played back, it showed the reactions from myself and the participant at the same time, enabling us to analyse any physical reactions to each other or the environment as well as to the verbal information.

The video interviews were recorded during two mornings (one morning per group) within the same week and ranged from fifteen minutes to half-an-hour each. I asked the participants to simply carry on with what they would normally be doing whilst I filmed them in order for the data to resemble their usual routine as much as possible. The initial format consisted of open questions such as, '*why do you volunteer here*?' After the opening questions, I invited the participants to take me on a walking tour of their favourite areas within the park/garden whilst I continued to ask more leading questions such as, '*would you say that by coming here it has had a beneficial therapeutic effect on you and if so, how?*' and more free flowing questions that emerged in response to the occasion. However, the volunteers from the Urban Park declined the invitation to walk as they were keen to continue their time constrained schedule that morning so I simply continued to interview them as they carried on working.

One week after the video interviews, during two mornings (one morning per group), participant socio-demographics were recorded to discover if childhood and previous experiences played an important role in their perception as some research suggests (Lester and Maudsley, 2006; Thompson et al., 2008; Swanick, 2009). Mind maps (Tattersall, Watts and Vernon, 2007), mental maps (Lynch, 1960; Orleans, 1994), a comparative sensation chart, photographs taken by the participants and field notes from observations were also recorded on the same morning as part of this bricolage method.

The participant's data were recorded and the information transcribed. Theoretical memos following each interview and throughout the analysis process were recorded and scrutinised for further development. Three weeks after the initial video interviews (to provide the time necessary for editing the video data), participants were asked to interpret the initial data from all the methods with myself in order to reduce errors regarding my subjective interpretations. Throughout the experience, members were asked to verify and clarify verbalizations and actions in order to assure accuracy and authenticity. After initial themes emerged and were coded from this process, I re-read the collaboratively transcribed data, compared it with the existing literature and the finalised themes were developed by myself.

Credibility and confirmability were produced by the participants interpreting the initial data with myself. Dependability was produced through prolonged engagement with the informants and the use of an assortment of various methods to cross check the interpretations.

FINDINGS

The main reason for the pilot study was to inform the choice of methods and methodological paradigm/s for the main study. There were some rich data generated from the feedback, where some general themes emerged from the participant/researcher interpretations which were later coded and finalised (Table 1) in a format that loosely followed IPA. Only the most relevant themes to inform the methodological paradigm will be discussed in this paper.

Table 1. Themes from the Video Interpretation

Finalised Themes
Childhood influences and exposure to rural environments
Sense of altruism, self-esteem and self-efficacy
Sense of time, place and space ecological proprioception
Sense of physical health
Structure
Sense of Community
Perception of wild nature and Landscape

CHILDHOOD INFLUENCES AND EXPOSURE TO RURAL ENVIRONMENTS

The socio-demographics data confirmed much of the research from Swanick (2009), Lester and Maudsley (2006) and Thompson et al. (2008) as childhood influences and exposure to rural environments were stressed as being particularly important for all participants. This suggests that the participants' perceptions of nature are influenced by positive embedded memories that are then recycled and deployed unconsciously as an influential factor, which may act as an embodied placebo.

Every response from each participant is relevant to their personal history and as such should be taken into consideration, as each participant originally came to the initiatives for very different reasons. For example, the Green Man originally volunteered as a "*good way of getting some experience on my CV and possibly getting a job*", and so many of his responses reflected this initial purpose. Gideon was recovering from drug addiction and so 'structure' was particularly important to him with statements such as, "*You need to keep on weeding, it's a never ending journey*" and "*…has kept me focused, gave me some structure to my week*". Jim did not particularly enjoy open rural 'spaces' and some cities due to fear of attack from behind (acquired from previous embodied experience), which emphasises the point that there cannot be a generalizable response to a singular idea of 'nature' (as with the evolutionary claims).

The perception of the colour green seemed an important link to nature and health for two participants but not for Ben. However, Ben was making a point that he volunteered mainly for the physical exercise and for social reasons when he stated, "*Green…not necessarily that important*". Also, Ben's socio-demographics show that he is conservative, church of England ("*both with a small 'c'*") and stated that "*Environmentalists humanise nature far too much*", suggesting that 'identity' may play a role in his perception. As this identity also partly stems from childhood (as Ben suggested it does), it implies that it is embodied and possibly habitualised in the way that he perceives nature. Interestingly, most of the positive comments about green were from Catherine who comes from a left-wing, middle-class, non-religious upbringing where holidays to the countryside (especially involving bodies of water) were usual. She now follows a Buddhist philosophy.

Examples of positive comments about the colour green include; "conscious feeling that green is healthful" *(Catherine)*; "Greenery – Calming" (Bill); "Spent a lot of time cycling in the countryside filling me with the colour green, with no map, no direction, no aims, so very relaxing…literally felt as though green was coming into me as I was cycling along" *(Catherine)*; "Green filling eyes and brain with this colour that is restful" *(Catherine)*; and "Green being minty cool" *(Catherine)*.

Interestingly, these statements relate and blend the concept 'green' with most of the senses, similar to synaesthesia. This is understandable if "perception involves the simultaneous use of the senses" as Tilley (2004, p.14) insists, implying that perception is embodied. This also suggests an 'embodied association' with previous experience rather than any genetic or culturally preconceived cognitive associations.

When asked to take a photograph of a place (or places) where they felt most relaxed and that gave them a positive feeling of health and wellbeing and to mark it on their mental maps, all four participants included a body of water (a lake for both participants in the urban park and a pond for both participants in the rural garden).

There is much research to suggest that viewing water plays an important role in health and wellbeing, especially regarding the biological/genetic theories (for example; Herzog, 1985; Kellert and Wilson, 1993; Rohde and Kendle, 1994; Wilson et al, 1995) but from the evidence gathered in this pilot study, the attraction to the different bodies of water seemed to be embedded and embodied from a young age in each of the participants, especially Catherine as she had most contact with bodies of water which she now associates with holidays and fond family memories. For example, Catherine stated "*Beaches are also restorative*", possibly influenced by her "*memories of childhood, going to beaches for holidays…I value holidays hugely*".

The attraction to bodies of water was linked to social elements, such as family holidays and a sense of community. Gideon stated, "*The pond I like because we all sit there and have coffee*". It does not seem that there are individual parts (or even 'doses') of nature that have special healing properties as 'objects', but it does seem more like the various elements that are perceived to be healing are associated with, and enmeshed in, other, more complex relationships. If, for example, the physical emplacement of the pond 'affords' the opportunity for a sense of community, then the therapeutic benefits would seem as if they came directly from the proximity to, or viewing, the pond. To an extent, this (in my view) supports the theories of implicit affordances and embodied placebo responses.

Sense of Time, Place, and Space Ecological Proprioception

The view from a 'prominent' position came up a few times in both groups, suggesting that rather than perceiving the view aesthetically, it indicated an ecological advantage to being able to see more of the surrounding environment. However, rather than this being thought of as an evolutionary influence, such as prospect-refuge theory (Appleton, 1975), it could also be seen as an unconscious ecological construction, embedded and embodied from previous experience of being high up. Of course this does not mean that only embodied experiences of 'being' in a place affect future perceptions, as experiences of previously viewed pictures that manifest themselves unconsciously may also influence perception. For example, the participants all designed mental maps that viewed the environments as if looking from above even though none of them have actually seen/experienced the Park or Garden from above.

For some participants, their perception was significantly influenced by the pictorial, aerial map. For example, Catherine had seen this aerial map perhaps many times previously but was surprised when I compared the two maps together, side-by-side, showing their likeness. So, it seems that our current perceptions of the environment we are in can be influenced by being both 'in' a place and by experiencing an interpretive picture 'of' a place (that is not at all like the 'actual' place) in order to achieve a 'sense of place'. This suggests an unconscious influence rather than a conscious cognitive one and may indeed support an embodied placebo response to certain environments, especially if the map/picture holds aesthetic appeal.

Casey (1996) infers that ‘place’ is the most fundamental form of embodied experience, a fusion of self, space and time and to be ‘in place’ is to become aware of one’s very consciousness and sensuous presence in the world. On the comparative sensation chart (Table 2), ‘sense of place’ was positive and unstressed for both inside and out but feelings of freedom and ‘space’ were perceived more outdoors compared to a more homely ‘place’ indoors.

When asked to describe their tactile perception indoors, the descriptions were mostly specific to a regionalised points of pressure on their body, as if the sensations were object to object, whereas the description of the outdoor experience seemed to suggest that more general areas of their ‘being’ were affected ‘within’ a sensed environment. Our assumptions about ‘space’ are connected to these perceptions and need further elicitation.

Most of the sensations experienced inside the buildings were generally quite neutral and bland (although not generally negative) in their descriptions compared to a more positive, richer description outside in the park/garden (Table 2). For the main study, I will not use a specific comparative chart like this one as it seems to be very leading, separating the binaries of inside and outside. Instead, I will simply ask the participants to be as descriptive as possible when in all the environments, noting as many sensations as possible.

A sense of time kept reappearing throughout the data as something that seemed important to the participants. “Spending time in nature is less stressful, less competitive, more relaxing in comparison with meeting deadlines, meeting targets…spending time in nature is giving you a break from all of that” *(Catherine)*; “Not clock watching, like at work” *(Ben)* “Time for conversation and ice cream on the beach” *(Catherine). Even comments such as* “sitting and looking at the view” *(Catherine) are perhaps more suggestive of having ‘time’ to do something relaxing rather than simply the aesthetic appeal.*

Senses of time, place, space and freedom, both positive and negative (as themes of vulnerability were attached to open rural spaces and city spaces in Jim’s case), require further scrutiny.

Table 2. Comparative sensation chart.

Sensations	Inside	Outside
Smell (Olfactory Perception)	None, sense too poor, sweat, wooden table	Clean, perfume from plants, cut privet, warm greenery
Taste (Gustatory Perception)	None, tea, heat, coffee, cup of tea	Fresh cool air, aftertaste of biscuits, cool air
Sight (Visual Perception)	Windows, table, view out of window, untidy kitchen	Glare, trees, views, light, pond, distant view, blue sky
Sound (Auditory Perception)	Noise (unobtrusive), Music, kettle boiling, people coming and going	Nature, birds chatter, crows, children playing, pigeons, train, volunteers chattering, rustling leaves
Touch (Tactile Perception)	Too warm, Formica table, perspiration, fly on arm, heat of cup, elbow on table, pencil in hand	Enjoy the elements, cool air on arms and face, wind, chilly, warmth of sun, wind
Sense of Place and Ecological Proprioception	Relaxed, airy and light place (much valued), comfortable, at home, unstressed, contented, relaxed, at ease, unthreatened, familiar	Contentment, sense of freedom, space and no limits, unhurried, undisturbed, happily sat at top of park with views, slightly less at ease (feeling that someone could come up behind), beautiful view

Perception of Wild Nature and Landscape

One reason that the participants from the Rural Garden initiative took me to the 'nature trail' was due to their belief that it was slightly 'more natural' than much of the rest of the place. One such comment came from the Green Man saying that they "*try to keep part of it natural for this nature walk, you know, so it's not too manicured*".

There were some especially interesting comments regarding all the participants' aesthetic perceptions of 'wild' nature, 'managed' nature and the 'right sort' of nature. For example, Ben emphasised the '*tidying up*' of nature to give the park the '*right message*'. Oelschlaeger (1991) reports that the historical humanisation of wild nature that was initiated by the early agriculturists and taken up after the Renaissance by science, economics and a Judeo-Christian perspective as they tried to "transform a base and worthless wilderness into industrialised, democratic civilisation" (p.68). This leads me to believe that the many temporal transformations and transmutations of the idea of wilderness and nature has permeated through society (via a process of an ecological embedding of culture) and has now become a palimpsest of perspectives that influence our perceptions of it. Therefore, this may influence our health and wellbeing through embodied placebo responses (and as Frenkel (2008) posits, 'implicit affordances').

Again, Ben's perception of 'tidy nature' may be due to the influence of his socio-demographics upon his embodied identity (rather than consciously cognitive, self-imposed identity), whereas Jim and Catherine's idea of nature is slightly different, preferring a less tidy, slightly more 'wild', uncultivated look (but not 'too' wild). According to Urry (1990), this slightly romantic idea of wilderness seems to stem from a socialist, white middle class identity that gained momentum during the Romantic period and one that he terms 'the Romantic gaze'.

So, although the relation between identity and the perception of nature may be heavily influenced by embodied childhood experiences, it may, in turn, be influenced by a historical humanisation of wild nature. This process is traditionally thought of as cultural conditioning (or even genetics) and yet seems more likely to be the dual/mixed process of an ecological embedding of culture (that is embodied throughout one's life) and immediate sensual interactions with the surrounding environments (or ecological proprioception).

CONCLUSIONS

The aims of this pilot study are to observe and record how people who enrol (or are enrolled) on two outdoor initiatives experience and interpret 'nature' within specific outdoor environments in order to discover how the effects of being in these particular environments affect the participants. Specifically, I am interested in finding out if the participants' perceptions of nature influence their health and wellbeing within these interventions. The other aims of this pilot study are to inform the choice of methods and methodological paradigm/s for the main study.

All participants perceived the outdoor health initiatives to have beneficial therapeutic effects for them and that 'nature' played a part in their health and well-being during this time. However, each of these therapeutic 'effects' and definitions of 'nature', 'health' and 'well-being' were subjective and had different meanings that seemed dependent on a variety of previously embedded perceptions.

The data generated from the pilot research indicated that senses of place, space and time were mediated through a variety of immediate sensations and embodied memory through both conscious and unconscious associations. Perceptions of the formalisation of nature and the 'wildness' of nature seem very important and may be dependent on the participants' personalities (mostly stemming from previous childhood experiences from direct experience and historically transmitted experience from an ecological embedding of culture) as to how wild nature should be in order for it to have a positive aesthetic and therapeutic appeal.

According to this research, and in agreement with Meissner (2011), it does seem that placebo responses may be dependent on 'lived experience' rather than conscious representations of expected outcomes. Therefore, embodied identity and embodied associations both seem influential to the perception of nature on health and wellbeing. Our perceptions of health and wellbeing may be dependent on the link between embodied memory and our immediate environmental sensations that are mostly unconscious, embodied and extended. The knotted convergences of cognitive, physical and social processes (which, I contend, are the same process) all seem to shape the participants' enactments and behaviours.

This pilot study has found no supporting evidence for biological, evolutionary theories or any sort of cognitive representation that would support a placebo effect based on expectation but does go some way to support some of the theories from embodied placebo responses, implicit affordances and externalist thought.

References

Allison, P. and Pomeroy, E. (2000) How Shall We "Know?" Epistemological Concerns in Research in Experiential Education. *The Journal of Experiential Education,* 23(2), 91-98.

Appleton, J. (1975) *The Experience of Landscape*. London: John Wiley.

Bandoroff, S. (2003) Family Therapy With A Twist…and a Shake and a Shout: Adventure Family Therapy in Practice. In K. Richards (Ed.) *Therapy Within Adventure*. Augsberg, Germany: Ziel.

Barnes, T. and Duncan, J. (eds.) (1992) *Writing Worlds: Discourse, Text and Metaphor in the representation of Landscape.* London: Routledge.

Barrett, J. and Greenaway, R. (1995) *Why Adventure*? Coventry, UK: Foundation for Outdoor Adventure.

Brown, K. M., Dilley, R. and Marshall, K. (2008) Using a Head-Mounted Video Camera to Understand Social Worlds and Experiences. *Sociological Research Online, 13(6)1. doi:10.5153/sro.1818*

Casey, E. (1996) How to Get From Space to Place in a Fairly Short Stretch of Time: Phenomenological Prolegomena. In S. Feld and K. H. Basso (Eds.), *Senses of Place*. Santa Fe: School of American Research Press.

Clarke, A. and Chalmers, D. (1998) The Extended Mind. *Analysis,* 58, 7-19. Reprinted in Menary 2010.

Cresswell, T. (2004) *Place: A short introduction*. Oxford: Blackwell Publishing.

Cosgrove, D. and Daniels, S. (1988) *The Iconography of Landscape*. Cambridge: Cambridge University Press.

Csordas, T. J. (1993) Somatic Modes of Attention. *Cultural Anthropology*, 8, 135-156.

Denzin, N., & Lincoln, Y. (2000). *Handbook of qualitative research* (2nd ed.). Thousand Oaks, CA: Sage.

Dinsdale, E.A. and Fenton, D.M. (2006) Assessing Coral Reef Condition: Eliciting Community Meanings. *Society and Natural Resources*, 19, 239-258.

Evans, J. and Jones, P. (2011) The walking interview: methodology, mobility and place. *Applied Geography,* 31(2), 849-858.

Frenkel, O. (2008) A Phenomenology of the 'Placebo Effect': Taking Meaning from the Mind to the Body. *The Journal of Medicine and Philosophy*, 33(1), 58-79.

Fournier J. C., DeRubeis, R. J., Hollon, S. D., Dimidjian, S., Amsterdam, J. D., Shelton, R. C. and Fawcett, J. (2010) Antidepressant Drug Effects and Depression Severity: A Patient-Level Meta-analysis. *JAMA,* 303(1), 47-53.

Greenway, R. (1995). The wilderness effect and ecopsychology. In T. Roszak, M. Gomes & A. Kanner (Eds.), *Ecopsychology* (pp. 122-135). San Francisco: Sierra Club Books.

Halliwell, E. (2005) Up and Running? Exercise therapy and the treatment of mild or moderate depression in primary care. A report by the Mental Health Foundation. Available from: http://www.mentalhealth.org.uk/publications/?entryid=43026&entryid5=43026&char=U Accessed: 16/02/10.

Herzog, T. (1985) A Cognitive Analysis of Preference for Waterscapes. *Journal of Environmental Psychology*, 5, 225-241.

Ingold, T. (2000) *The Perception of the Environment: Essays on Livelihood, Dwelling and Skill*. London: Routledge.

Ingold, T. (2011) *Being Alive*. London: Routledge.

Jones, P., Bunce, G., Evans, J., Gibbs, H., and Ricketts Hein, J. (2008). Exploring space and place with walking interviews. *Journal of Research Practice, 4*(2), Article D2. Available from: http://jrp.icaap.org/index.php/jrp/article/view/150/161 Accessed:13/05/2012.

Kaplan, S. and Kaplan, R. (1982) *Cognition and Environment*. New York: Praeger.

Kaplan, S. and Kaplan, R. (1989) *The Experience of Nature: A Psychological Perspective*. Cambridge, U.K.: Cambridge University Press.

Kellert, S. R. and Wilson, E. O. (eds) (1993) *The Biophilia Hypothesis*. Washington D.C.: Island Press.

Kirmayer, L. J. (2011) Unpacking the Placebo Response: Insights from Ethnographic Studies of Healing. *The Journal of Mind-Body Regulation*, 1(3), 112-124.

Lester, S. and Maudsley, M. J. (2006). *Play, Naturally: A Review of Children's Natural Play*. London: Children's Play Council.

Lynch, K. (1960) *The Image of the City*. Cambridge MA: MIT Press.

Macnaghten, P. and Urry, J. (1998) *Contested Natures*. London: Sage Publications Limited.

McKenzie, M. D. (2000) How are Adventure Education Programme Outcomes Achieved? A review of the Literature. *Australian Journal of Outdoor Education*, 5(1), 19-25.

Meissner, K. (2011) The placebo effect and the autonomic nervous system: evidence for an intimate relationship. *Philosophical Transactions of the Royal Society,* 366, 1808-1817.

Merleau-Ponty, M. (1964) *The Primacy of Perception: And Other Essays on Phenomenological Psychology, the Philosophy of Art, History, and Politics*, IL: Northwestern University Press.

Moerman, D. E. (2002) *Meaning, Medicine and the "Placebo Effect",* Cambridge: Cambridge University Press.

Moles, K. (2008) A Walk in Thirdspace: Place, Methods and Walking. *Sociological Research Online, 13(4)2,* doi:10.5153/sro.1745.

Nichols, G. (2000) A Research Agenda for Adventure Education. *Australian Journal of Outdoor Education*, 4(2), 22-31.

Oelschlaeger, M. (1991) *The Idea of Wilderness*. New Haven and London: Yale University Press.

Orleans, P. (1994) Mental Maps of LA. In B. Lenon and P. Cleves, *Fieldwork Techniques and Projects in Geography*. London: Collins Educational.

Price, D. D., Finniss, D. G., & Benedetti, F. (2008). A comprehensive review of the placebo effect: Recent advances and current thought. *Annual Review of Psychology*, 59, 565–590.

Pryor, A., Carpenter, C. and Townsend, M. (2005) Outdoor education and bush adventure therapy: A socio-ecological approach to health and wellbeing. *Australian Journal of Outdoor Education*, 9(1), 3-13.

Pink, S. (2007) Walking with video. *Visual Studies*, 22(3).

Rohde, C.L.E., and Kendle, A. D. (1994). *Report to English Nature—Human Well-being, Natural Landscapes and Wildlife in Urban Areas: A Review*. Reading, U.K.: University of Reading, Department of Horticulture and Landscape, and Bath,U.K.: The Research Institute for the Care of the Elderly.

Rowlands, M. (2010) *New Science of the Mind: From Extended Mind to Embodied Phenomenology*. Cambridge, MA: MIT Press.

Russell, K. C. and Farnum, J. (2004) A Concurrent Model of the Wilderness Therapy Process. *Journal of Adventure Education and Outdoor Learning,* 4(1), 39-55.

Sheller M. and Urry J. (2006) The New Mobilities Paradigm. *Environment and Planning A,* 38(2), 207 – 226.

Smith, J. A., Flowers, P. and Larkin, M. (2009) *Interpretive Phenomenological Analysis: Theory, Method and Research.* London: Sage Publications Limited.

Spedding, A. (2006) *Green Exercise*. RuSource: The rural information network.

Summerfield, C. and Gill, B. (Eds.) (2005) *Social Trends No. 35*. London: Office for National Statistics.

Swanick, C. (2009) Society's attitudes to and preferences for land and landscape. *Land Use Policy*, 26, S62-S75.

Tattersall, C., Watts, A, and Vernon, S. (2007). Mind mapping as a tool in qualitative research. *Nursing Times*, *103*(26), 32–33.

Thompson, C. W., Aspinall, P. and Montarzino, A. (2008).The childhood factor: adult visits to green places and the significance of childhood experience. *Environment and Behavior,* 40(1), 111-143.

Thompson, J. J., Ritenbaugh, C. and Nichter, M. (2009) Reconsidering the Placebo Response from a Broad Anthropological Perspective. *Culture, Medicine and Psychiatry*, 33, 112-152

Tilley, C. (2004) *The Materiality of Stone: Explorations in Landscape Phenomenology Volume 1*. CA.: Left Coast Press Inc.

Tuan, Y. (1979) Thought and Landscape: The Eye in the Mind's Eye' in: D. W. Meining (ed.), *The Interpretation of Ordinary Landscapes: Geographical Essays*. Oxford University Press, New York, pp. 89102.

Ulrich, R. S. (1979). Psychophysiological approaches to landscape visibility. In *Visibility Values, Proceedings of the Conference on Visibility Values* (pp. 99-99). USDA General Report W0-18, Fort Collins, CO.

Ulrich, R. S. (1983). Aesthetic and affective response to natural environment. In I. Altman and J. F. Wohlwill (Eds.), *Behavior and the Natural Environment*, New York: Plenum Press.

Ulrich, R. S. (1991). Wellness by design: Psychologically supportive patient surroundings. *Group Practice Journal,* 40(4), 10-19.

Ulrich, R. S. and Parsons, R. (1992) Influences of Passive Experiences with Plants on Individual Well-Being and Health. In D. Relf (ed.), *The Role of Horticulture in Human Well-Being and Social Development*: A National Symposium. Portland, OR: Timber Press.

Urry, J. (1990) *The Tourist Gaze: Leisure and Travel in Contemporary Societies*. London: Sage.

Warner, S. B. (1987) *To dwell is to garden: A history of Boston's community gardens*. Boston: Northeastern University Press.

WHO (2001) *The World Health Report: 2001: Mental Health: New Understanding, New Hope*. Geneva: World Health Organization.

Wilson, E. O. (1984) *Biophilia*. London: Harvard University Press.

Wilson, M., Robertson, L., Davly, M. and Walton, S. (1995) Effects of Visual Cues on Assessment of Water Quality. *Journal of Environmental Psychology*, 15, 53-63.

Wylie, J. (2007) *Landscape*. London: Routledge.

EXPANDING

Your deepest presence is in every small contracting and expanding, the two as beautifully balanced and coordinated as bird wings.

-Rumi

CHAPTER 35

Towards a Profession? A Question of Paradigms

Anita Pryor

INTRODUCTION: WHAT DO YOU SEE?

Since 1997, hundreds of people from many countries have put aside time, found resources, and made efforts to attend five International Adventure Therapy Conferences. Together we've migrated south to Australia, north to Germany, west to Canada, south to New Zealand, back to the northern hemisphere for the fifth conference in Scotland, and over east to the sixth conference in the Czech Republic. A glance at conferences themes demonstrates that as a professional community, we have 'explored the boundaries' (Itin, 1998), 'looked within' (Richards & Smith, 2003), 'continued to evolve' (Bandoroff & Newes, 2004), 'looked at the essence' (Mitten & Itin, 2009) and 'emerged with insights' (Pryor, Carpenter, Norton & Kirchner 2012).

So what are we to make of this series of events, this progression of gatherings, and our evolution as an international community? An intuitive glance at geographical locations and conference themes leads me to suggest our international community has been 'pulsating' - contracting and expanding, geographically and ideologically. Not going around in circles, but moving in a spiral motion, forwards over time. Admittedly, you may need to hold these lists in front of you, semi-close your eyes, nod your head up and down, and form a double-chin to see it my way; but from my perspective, we have been pulsating over time. From a 'pulsation hypothesis', our ideology has expanded outwards in 1997 (we explored the boundaries); turned inwards in 2000 (we examined the therapy within); expanded outwards again in 2003 (we examined our longitudinal evolution); then connected inwards again in 2006 (we reconnected with our essence). In 2009 we again expanded outwards, and considered the merits of becoming a profession.

Confused? That's understandable. You may see things differently. You may wonder what this talk of pulses, circles and spirals has to do with conferences and therapeutic practices. Based on your own observations, you may believe our international community of practitioners has been progressing along a linear pathway towards becoming a profession – you might hold a 'developmental hypothesis' in relation to international adventure therapy. Or believe we have been undergoing a process of refining and defining various sub-clusters within our diverse field of international adventure therapy – perhaps you hold a 'differentiation hypothesis' in relation to our field of endeavour. Alternatively you may have observed that some practitioners are pushing harder for professionalisation than others, and you may be developing a 'validity/credibility hypothesis' to make sense of what you've observed.

But how does this relate to our practice, and do such hypotheses offer us anything of value? How do these questions help with our future aspirations? This chapter attempts to overt a range of linear progressions and spiral pulses occurring within international adventure therapy towards the possibility of a coherent professional community. In an attempt to expand on the breadth of creative, disciplined, artistic, and scientific ideas presented at 5IATC and 6IATC and included within this book, I introduce some ways to identify our place, and consider our shared path ahead. This chapter addresses the diverse community of practitioners and practices that collectively, internationally, orbit around the terms adventure and therapy.

A History of Continuums

Back in 1993, Gass provided a framework for examining adventure therapy practice called the 'Depth of intervention' continuum (an expansion of the work of Gillis et al. 1991). For Gass, the factors that influence the depth of therapeutic adventure experiences include: the specific needs of the client; the complexity of the client's therapeutic issue(s); the background training and therapeutic expertise of the adventure therapist; the length of time the adventure therapist has to work with the client; the context the client came from and will return to after the adventure experience; the presence of after-care or follow-up treatment following the adventure experience; the availability of adventure experiences; and the therapist/s' limitations in using adventure experiences in his/her treatment approaches (Gass, 1993, p.74).

As is well documented, along this continuum, recreation experiences offer an engaging 'one-shot' adventure experience in a single time-frame to accomplish an objective; enrichment adventure programs purposefully address common issues/problems related to a client's treatment; adjunctive therapy focuses on the therapeutic issues of a client, but this is done alongside or in addition to (rather than in place of) other treatment interventions; and primary therapy replaces more traditional methods as a means of reaching treatment objectives.

In 1994, family therapists Curtis & Sibberas listed variables they believe influence the adventure experience, including: 1) purpose of the adventure (recreation-enrichment-therapy); 2) level of actual risk (low-high); 3) level of perceived risk (low-high); 4) venue for the adventure (indoors-outdoors-wilderness); and 5) participant groupings (individual-couple-family-group) (Curtis and Sibberas, 1994). This list provided yet another means of organising adventure therapy services.

Figure 1. Gass: Depth of intervention continuum (1993)

Recreation	**Enrichment**	**Adjunctive therapy**	**Primary therapy**
Lesser depth of intervention←======→Greater depth of intervention			

In 1995 Abbott stated: 'As in many aspects of human awareness, it is easy to view the options as black and white, that people are either mentally ill or they are not, and that we are doing therapy or we are not' (1995, p.29). Abbott proposed three continua to help explain the differences and similarities between adventure education and adventure therapy.

Figure 2. Abbott: Adventure therapy versus adventure education (1995)

a) The continuum of the problem/need:

- Psychosis
- Neurosis
- Specific issues such as drug and alcohol issues
- At risk of having problems (e.g. youth at risk)
- Need for specific life skills (such as assertiveness)
- High functioning but seeking enrichment

b) The continuum of the process: (adapted from the work of Gass, 1993, p.74)

- Highly focused therapy (primary)
- Adjunctive therapy
- Corrections
- At risk (youth)
- Life skills
- Enriching broad-based personal growth

c) The continuum of outcomes:

- Reduced maladaptive symptoms
- Clarification of personal issues
- Life skills development
- Self-esteem enhancement
- Self-actualization (Abbott, 1995, pp. 29-30)

Rather than a 'graduated continuum' of practice, Crisp (1997) stated it was more useful to highlight distinctions based on the presence or absence of therapeutic procedures, such as assessment and diagnostic formulation, specificity of treatment objectives that relate to causative processes, and the use of an individual treatment plan (p.58): 'By my definition, either something is therapy or it is not. What should differentiate the two is whether therapeutic procedures are instituted (therapy) or not (enrichment)' (p.62). Crisp preferred to use the terms uni-modal therapy and multi-modal therapy rather than adjunct therapy and primary therapy. Uni-modal therapy was where only adventure or wilderness therapy were used to treat a problem, whereas multi-modal therapy used a combination of adventure or wilderness therapy along with other therapeutic modalities, either concurrently or in series (for example combining individual therapy or group therapy within the program, or individual or family therapy prior to or following a wilderness intervention) (p.62).

In 2004, Williams recommended delineation between programs which provide therapy and those that are 'merely therapeutic' (Williams, 2004, p.195). For Williams, a therapist is trained to treat an identified dysfunction.

Before and since these examples, adventure therapy practitioners, researchers and academics have offered a range of perspectives for ways in which we might map, organise or differentiate international adventure therapy practices. Examples drawn from previous International Adventure Therapy Conference Proceedings include: Itin, Ringer, Gillis, Handley, Bunce, Pickard, Richards, Priest, Gilsdorf, Ewert, Carpenter, Bandoroff, Russell, Mitten, Adams, Berman and Davis-Berman, to name a few.

In 2005-2009 the author undertook a PhD study to examine adventure therapy in Australia with a view to building an evidence base for these forms of practice in the Australian context. In an exploration of historic and contemporary practices in Australia, the following continua were found to be useful:

1) Wellbeing target
2) Depth of intervention

3) Intensity of experience

Wellbeing Target

Adapted from Mrazek and Haggerty's (1994) 'Mental health intervention spectrum', the *Wellbeing target continuum* highlights the importance of having a full range of wellbeing interventions for a given society, including *preventive* strategies for whole populations; *early interventions* for at risk communities, families and individuals; and *treatment* and *continuing care* strategies for individuals identified as experiencing a health and/or wellbeing disorder. This continuum has relevance for adventure therapy services operating in a range of settings, including those operating in mental health settings but not exclusively. According to the study, adventure therapy services already have a role across this spectrum of interventions in the Australian context towards a range of wellbeing aims (including mental, physical, social, and cultural wellbeing aims for examples) (Pryor, 2009). A noteworthy extension to Mrazek and Haggerty's spectrum is the addition of *palliative care*, utilised with individuals and groups who are nearing death, and/or grieving the imminent loss of a friend or family member. This adapted continuum offers a population-wide approach to define discrete adventure therapy practices. The range of adventure therapy services are categorised within this continuum according to: a) the rationale for the intervention; b) the nature of the intervention; c) the aims and approach used by the practitioner; d) the needs and vulnerabilities of participants; and e) the point at which an individual chooses to address the need for change in his or her life.

Figure 3. Wellbeing target continuum for adventure therapy

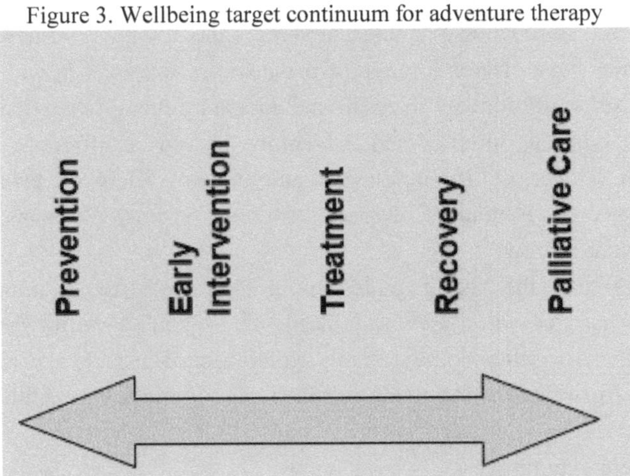

Depth of Intervention

The *Depth of intervention continuum* is an extension of the work of Gillis, Gass and others who have attempted to describe the level of personal 'work' occurring within a given adventure therapy experience. A key difference between the work of Gass and this adapted continuum is that this continuum allows all 'depths' to include therapy –either tacitly or overtly. In the adapted continuum, Gass' *primary therapy* is replaced with the term *treatment*. Treatment has an overt aim of therapy, which may include clinical components such as assessment, problem identification, personal goal-setting, counselling, therapeutic group work, and proactive referral pathways. In the new continuum, all adventure therapy 'depths' may be delivered in collaboration with other services, meaning that any or all may be also be called *adjunct therapy* (Gass, 1993). From this perspective, all depths of intervention involve skilled facilitation to ensure personal safety of staff and participants (across physical, psychological, social and cultural domains) to maximise opportunities for personal meaning-making (including attitudinal or behaviour change if desirable). Within the adapted continuum, definitions of *recreation, enrichment* and *treatment* generally match Gass' definitions (with 'treatment' translating to Gass' 'primary therapy'). An examination of twenty Australian programs in the aforementioned PhD study demonstrated that several additional levels of 'work' occur in the Australian context, including*: respite, training, education,* and *palliative care*. Definitions of these additional 'depths' are provided:

Respite adventure therapy services support people by taking them out of their normal environments to provide 'time out' for a friend, family member or service provider (carer). As such, respite experiences are of mutual benefit to both the adventure therapy participant and their carer. In addition to recreation, respite adventure therapy services tend to include independence-building activities tailored to the needs of each individual. *Training* refers to an intentional program of skill-building, tailored to the specific training needs of individuals in a group context. In the Australian context, adventure therapy training experiences tend to include sequential programs linked with specific vocational aims and outcomes (for example, horticulture) and focus on training relating to social, cultural and economic domains of wellbeing, based on participants' needs. *Education* refers to a deeper level of intentional learning, and includes education 'for life' (in addition to vocation). Adventure therapy education experiences may incorporate pedagogical, philosophical, and epistemological content, and provide opportunities for participants to explore their own perceptions in relation to a range of curricula, towards personal learning. *Palliative care* refers to adventure therapy services that aim to maximise quality of life for people experiencing severe, chronic, ongoing and/ or deteriorating symptoms (such as psychological, physical, spiritual, and/or cultural symptoms) that place participants in the position of needing to contemplate life and death, with the likelihood of imminent death. Palliative adventure therapy programs focus on end-of-life matters, including a focus on family, spirituality and existential domains of wellbeing. These experiences may be considered the deepest of all.

This adaption of Gass' adventure therapy continuum means that in the Australian context, those interested in experiencing 'clinical adventure therapy' (for example, those who wish to engage in primary therapy or have a personal dysfunction 'treated') can choose to participate in *treatment.* Those services, programs, practitioners and participants who may be reluctant to focus on pathology, deficit, or dysfunction (and on the remediation, or rehabilitation of any of these problems) may choose instead to deliver or receive adventure therapy in other more strength-focused ways. With a desire to experience therapy, yet a resistance to engage in 'treatment', people can choose to engage in personal work focusing on mental health and wellbeing, wholeness, wellness, and quality of life via a range of other means, which may also lead to intentional clinical outcomes in psychological, physical, behavioural and social domains. To reiterate, for services, programs, practitioners and participants who wish to focus on remediating a specific personal issue (including a pathology or set of dysfunctions), *treatment* tends to be the adventure therapy experience of choice.

Figure 4. Depth of intervention continuum for adventure therapy

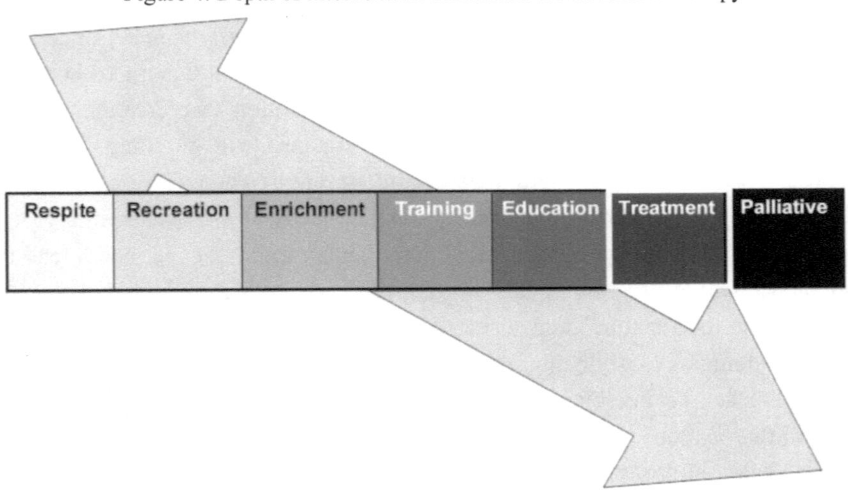

Intensity of Experience

The *Intensity of experience continuum* recognises that each adventure therapy experience supports an individual at a specific point in their wellness trajectory (wellbeing target); may support an individual in a specific area of personal work (depth of intervention); and may also require a specific level of commitment (intensity of experience) from participants. 'Intensity of experience' relates to the frequency, duration and level of commitment required of adventure therapy participants within a specific adventure therapy experience.

In this continuum, commitment levels span from *tasters* through to *ongoing and integrated experiences. Tasters* ready participants for greater involvement, such as longer or more difficult one-off experiences, or even overnight experiences. Of course each of these levels of intensity may have a central focus on respite, enrichment, therapy or palliative care (or other 'depths') – the difference lies in the intensity of the experience for participants. Another style of programming recognises that *day activities* may be placed in an order of increasing intensity (and challenge), in sequential order, to ready participants for the intensity of an extended, remote and highly committing *expedition*. Again, expeditions may be tailored to a range of aims (such as enrichment, therapy, palliative care, etc.). *Ongoing/integrated* experiences offer an ultimate level of intensity and commitment. Either in the form of *residential* ('live-in') environments, or seamlessly integrated with a participant's *community* (again, a live-in environment), these adventure therapy experiences are more intense and committing 'parts of life'. An example of this in the Australian context is an adventure therapy service that operates as part of the daily life of a remote Indigenous community – it is 'part of things'.

Figure 5. Intensity of experience continuum for adventure therapy

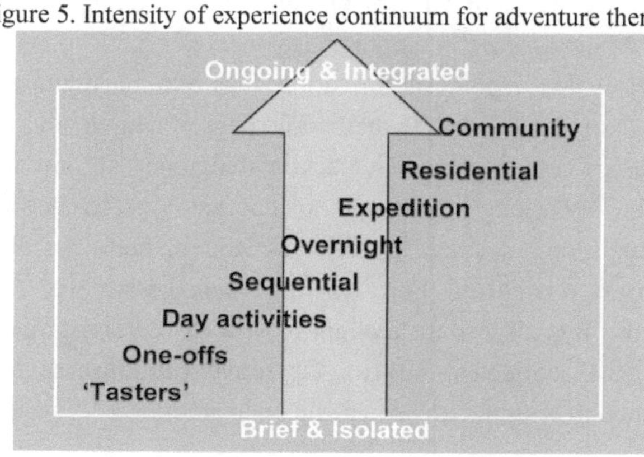

It is acknowledged that these three continua arise within socio-cultural contexts found in Australia and may not have relevance in other settings.

Perhaps as many adventure therapy continua exist as adventure therapy contexts exist. An example of the limitless of this possibility became apparent at the 5IATC. Within an experiential keynote address, facilitators Christian Itin and Cathryn Carpenter asked delegates to 'place' their work along a continuum according to a range of questions. Delegates took a personal position in relation to the strength of their agreement or disagreement with each given question. For each question, the subsequent delegate line repeatedly spanned over 20 metres of floor space – all delegates had a distinct reason for choosing where they were on a given continuum!

My aim in presenting these continua is not to provide a definitive set of frameworks; rather, I hope to convey how our continua change over time and across contexts. No doubt additional sets of continuums, matrices, frameworks, maps and spectrums have been discussed and are yet to be discussed, documented, published or imagined in the minds of practitioners across diverse cultures within the international adventure therapy community.

Art and Science

> If you want security, look towards science; if you want to be confronted, seek art. (Source unknown).

> And if you want to be even more freaked out look even deeper into science. (Source not provided).

True science is a process of curious exploration, a seeking of knowledge and understanding. Mainstream contemporary science as practiced within modernist cultures, tends to value hypothesis formation, bias minimisation, development of transparent and replicable trial methodologies, documentation of research outcomes (findings/ conclusions) and acknowledgment of limitations, towards greater collective knowledge. Although science has a preference for objectivity and clinical conditions, science is also practiced in non-clinical settings, and inherent biases are recognised. For Abbe, true science is never speculative and never adopts the hypotheses as though they were demonstrated propositions (c1900, cited in Goodquotes, 2011a). Objective cautiousness and scepticism appear to be inherent within many scientific endeavours.

True art, it could be argued, is never conventional. Much art pushes boundaries, stretches conventions, evokes personal responses, and necessitates subjective interpretation. For Einstein, true art was characterised by an irresistible urge in the creative artist (c1920, cited in Goodquotes, 2011b). Passions, motivations and subjectivities appear to be inherent within many artistic endeavours. Yet in its multitude of forms, art is also sometimes aesthetic (therefore highly acceptable), and may be used to perpetuate traditions, therefore can be strikingly conventional.

In his 5IATC keynote address, Keith Russell spoke of an emerging dualism within adventure therapy – represented by what he called the *body* and *soul* (see chapter Provoking). Russell observed that contemporary adventure therapy may be divided between these two competing paradigms. In his hypothesis, the body includes theory, research and practice which appears to be seeking validation and acceptance by mainstream behavioural and mental health service systems. In North America, this includes movement towards research outcomes, best practice, licensure, and accreditation. Russell suggests that this process of emphasising and strengthening the body means that adventure therapy in North America may be at risk of losing its soul. Of course these shifts are occurring in many arenas surrounding adventure therapy, such as in healthcare and education. (From a philosophical perspective, body can be considered an expression of residual modernist choices being made within industrialised cultures – cultures that in many other ways are post-modernising in favour of subjective truth and 'soul').

Naturally, most practitioners in the adventure therapy arena include elements of both body and soul within their work. Because we operate within broader political contexts we are often required to utilise body; yet in work that involves relationships with people, it is difficult to contribute anything of worth without some degree of soul. Indeed, both paradigms are reflected in the work of authors included in this book. At a glance, more body-focused papers are included in Chapter 5 (Adapting), and more soul-focused papers are included in Chapter 6 (Exploring). Here, I will list the kinds of content that I consider connects more strongly with either body or soul, or both. The lists are based on my understanding of Russell's dualism, and my interpretation of the content of papers included in this book.

Authors connecting more strongly with the 'body' of adventure therapy include contributions relating to a need for: recognition, validation and effectiveness; articulation of mental health outcomes; establishment of best practices; development of research-based evidence; delivery of evidence-based tertiary courses; and identification of discrete research variables.

Authors connecting more strongly with the 'soul' of adventure therapy include contributions relating to: the importance of country, culture, family and community; cultural roots; respect for individual experiences and emerging realities; uses of storytelling; uses of art; and mysterious lessons in nature.

While most adventure therapy authors and practitioners incorporate elements from both paradigms, some authors appear to more clearly work towards the 'whole'. Contributions that appear to bring together both body and soul include: explorations of theoretical roots; reflections of adventure therapy in light of practices, theories and broader systems; and the need to balance activity and quiet within adventure therapy experiences. Of course these interpretations are wide open to scrutiny.

Related to this discussion of dualism, is an experience that occurred in the process of undertaking the aforementioned PhD study (Pryor, 2009). The aim of the study was to focus on the history, practices, and outcomes of adventure therapy practices in Australia. Early on in the study I came across a significant dilemma - some services were reluctant to call their work 'therapy'. Even services that delivered therapy by any comprehensive or clinical measure refused to use that term. Because of this, I decided to use the term *outdoor adventure interventions* (OAI) (instead of adventure therapy) for the remainder of the study. OAI became a useful way of opening up dialogue about Australian adventure therapy practices without alienating services.

Being new, OAI offered a paradigm-friendly term that encompassed both those adventure services comfortable with use of the term 'therapy', and those services that did not wish to be aligned with therapy. In order to explain this terminology dilemma it should be noted that in Australia, in some settings, therapy implies 'treatment', synonymous with the act of a therapist 'expert' fixing an unwell or dysfunctional individual. As a result, many people have experienced disempowerment in 'therapy'. A number of adventure therapy practitioners applying a wide variety of therapeutic modalities prefer terminology that reflects the practice of encouraging individuals to be their own 'expert', whereby a practitioner's job is to support participants towards their own self-directed healthy change aims. A tension in the Australian context is that both of these groups undertake similar (and different) work, with similar (and different) target groups, towards similar (and different) aims. To only include those programs and practitioners that identify their work as 'therapy' is to miss a number of programs and practices that in essence, by any other measure, deliver adventure therapy.

Due to stigma and perceptions of powerlessness experienced by participants within medicalised systems in Australia, particularly within mental health and behaviour change settings such as juvenile justice centres and drug treatment settings, some participants intentionally avoid 'therapy' services. Therefore, although a service may deliver therapy by trained therapists and meet clinical measures of safety, intent, and outcomes, it may not necessarily be in the interests of the service to use that term. As a result, OAI was found to be very useful for services operating in educational, rehabilitative and community settings in the Australian context.

People may justifiably ask 'If the participant is not asking for therapy, and the service is not stating they provide therapy, then how can another person call the experience therapy?' The answer has to do with cultural context, meaning, and perception. Just as in some contexts, 'adventure' is synonymous with bungee jumping, adrenalin and expensive holidays; in some contexts, the term 'therapy' is synonymous with disrespect, powerlessness and stigma.

To provide further explanation, a similar dilemma occurred in Australia in the broad arena of therapeutic arts practices in the 1990's. As the collective community of Australian arts practitioners began to move towards common practices, training, research, and increased credibility within mainstream services, a tension began to mount between body and soul. The 'professionalisation' process underway (body) led some arts practitioners to voice loyalty to the creative and relational essence of their work (soul) leading to a split in their field of practice. Along the way, some art practitioners began to call their work 'art therapy'; whilst others chose to align with what became known as 'community cultural development' (CCD) arts practice.

Arts practitioners who sought to establish a set of validated, standardised art therapy methods, with an identified accredited professional pathway appeared to choose 'art therapy'; whereas those who recognised a personal preference for using a wide range of creative mediums, having participants 'at the centre' of the therapeutic process, and contextualising art practices within a given place and time, moved towards CCD practice (Marsden & Thiele, 2003). In this case, progression towards professionalisation brought about a split in the professional community that had previously orbited around the terms art and therapy.

Adventure therapy practitioners and authors in other settings have presented further dualisms. For example, Loynes (2002) presented an overview of algorithmic (rational) versus generative (intuitive) paradigms. Carpenter (2008) expanded on this dualism, and discussed philosophical differences in relation to outcomes, experiences, relationships, place and ethos. Gilsdorf (2003) offered a dualism of 'experiential adventure therapy' versus 'controlled adventure therapy', and wrote about a focus on 'effectiveness' versus a focus on 'process and theoretical developments' (p.12). Handley (2003) wrote about the dualism of 'mechanistic learning' in adventure therapy versus 'learning perception' (natural education based on tension and intuition) (p.14).

At risk of presenting one too many dualisms, I share one more example of contrasting paradigms: Positivistic and Naturalistic paradigms. From my interpretation, positivist practices reflect Russell's body and Loyne's algorithmic paradigm; and naturalistic practices more closely reflect Russell's soul and Loyne's generative paradigm.

Positivistic (body) practices follow a scientific, structural, reductionist approach, where the adventure therapy experience can be broken down into segments, parts, components and processes. Within this paradigm, the complexities occurring within an intervention experience can be explained and studied as a cause-effect or linear process. Positivistic (body) practices are well-suited to being described in the language of a structural framework and examined through a behaviourist lens. In line with conventional methods of scientific enquiry, staff and programs utilising positivist practices tend to identify a dysfunction, prescribe a treatment regime or strategy, facilitate an intervention or series of interventions, and expect a predicted outcome based on the original hypothesis. Participants of positivist experiences have a greater chance of knowing what they can expect within their experience prior to participation; intended outcomes tend to be predetermined by staff and program aims as much as by participants themselves. From the author's observations, adventure therapy practitioners working in positivist contexts (for example in mental health treatment and detention settings) tend to push more strongly for 'body' approaches – perhaps out of necessity.

Naturalistic (soul) practices follow more of a traditional (pre-scientific), post-modern (social constructivist), intuitive, place-based, relationship-focused, community-based approach, where the complexities of the intervention experience refuse to be broken down or spread along a linear cause-effect pathway. Rather, the experience clusters and merges, flows and happens according to the rhythms of the group, the setting, the activity, and the adventure that is unfolding. A relational or 'spiral' approach is a better way to describe, investigate and articulate practices operating within a naturalistic (soul) paradigm. Naturalistic approaches sit more comfortably in a postmodern context, where subjective interpretation and personal meaning-making are recognised to be at work in the perceptions of both practitioners and participants. Within naturalistic practices, although the experience may involve a set of intentional processes with an embedded comprehensive psycho-social safety net, participants can expect high levels of choice and decision-making, and a co-participatory experience. From the author's observations, adventure therapy practitioners working in naturalistic contexts (for example in community settings and alternative education settings) tend to push more strongly for 'soul' approaches – perhaps out of necessity.

Which paradigm are you the reader more attracted to, which do you tend to align with, which do you wish to move towards? And how do these dualisms come together within a whole? Or do you have little interest in paradigms and dualisms?

Einstein believed the most beautiful thing we can experience is the 'mysterious' and that mystery is the source of all true art and science (c1920, cited in Albert Einstein Site, 2011b).

So where do science (body) and art (soul) meet, and what role do they play in the international adventure therapy arena? What is the common ground between these two areas of emphasis?

A Landscape of Services

Based on the aforementioned study on Australian adventure therapy practices (Pryor, 2009), it appears that at least three distinct types of adventure therapy experiences exist in the Australian context. They are presented here, in order to both provoke and nurture further discussion about similarities and differences in international adventure therapy. Do they have relevance for international adventure therapy? The reader is invited to judge.

Brief adventure therapy experiences have a start and an end, they are more easily identified as having cause and effect pathways, and are more suited to positivistic (body) frameworks. Brief adventure therapy experiences take people out of 'normal life' for a brief intervention experience. Because these experiences are easier to set aside, break down into their constituent parts, and be replicated, brief adventure therapy experiences more easily invite a 'clinical' or 'structural' approach to programming, language, research and evaluation. (Another way of describing brief adventure therapy services is 'boxed').

Integrative adventure therapy experiences ebb and flow with peaks and troughs of intensity but are on-going – they happen 'along the way'. Like brief experiences, integrative adventure therapy may have a start and an end, but are clearly part of a larger purpose - they are one option, one event within a broader process that may have its own start and end. Integrative adventure therapy may be reduced into constituent parts, but must be viewed within a larger whole. Integrative adventure therapy more easily invites an emphasis on relationships, which are more complex to examine, and require more flexible programming. (These adventure therapy services may be described as 'out of the box').

Socio-ecological adventure therapy experiences have no start or end, and are almost seamless or unnoticed within the life of a given community; they are 'part of things'. Like the 'whole-of-community' approach used in one remote Indigenous community (Pryor, 2009), socio-ecological adventure therapy practices occur as part of daily life; they are part of the health maintenance of a given community and assist to sustain the whole community. Of value within socio-ecological adventure therapy practices are the acknowledgement of culture and context, the story, the subjective, the verbal, the experienced and the shared. (These adventure therapy services may be described as 'life').

Figure 6. Paradigms of practice in adventure therapy

Positivistic (BODY) paradigm	**Naturalistic (SOUL) paradigm**
Problem identification and Solutions identification	
• Practitioners attempt to be objective unbiased and value free	• Practitioners acknowledge subjective biases and values
• Diagnostic/ Prescriptive predetermined hypothesis verification	• Emerging / Evolving creation of a working hypothesis
• Rationalist practice	• Interpretive practice
• Reductionistic/ linear structure	• Holistic / circular structure
• More likely a brief intervention	• More likely an integrative intervention
• Practitioner as expert	• Participant as expert
• Nature as clinic	• Nature as co-therapist
• Adventure outcomes are predicted	• Adventure outcomes are unknown
• Outcome oriented	• Process oriented
• Emphasis on the measurable (verbal, physical, cognitive and behavioural)	• Emphasis on the subjective (relational, emotional, social and cultural)
• A clinical approach	• A relational approach

-- Holistic wellbeing positively impacted --

Figure 7 provides a pictorial demonstration of these differences and relationships as they exist in the Australian context. The typology of practice for adventure therapy invites the reader to consider how you see things, where you belong, and where do you wish to belong.

From the author's observations, adventure therapy practitioners working in positivist settings are more attracted to body (perhaps out of necessity) and tend to prefer clinical approaches (i.e. the top left quadrant). On the other hand, practitioners working in naturalistic settings appear most attracted to soul approaches (perhaps out of necessity) and tend to emphasise the importance of relationships, including whole-of-community approaches (i.e. the lower right quadrant).

Figure 7. Typology of practice for adventure therapy

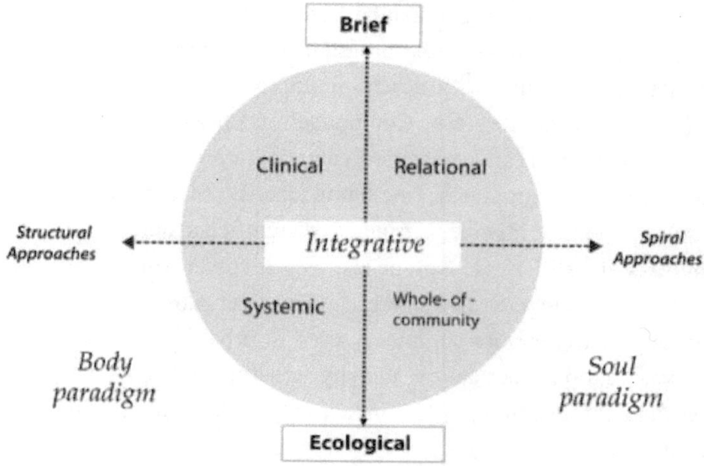

Spiral approach – Within this typology, spiral refers to a circular motion over time. A spiral (whether 2 or 3 dimensional) passes the same way again and again but never in exactly the same place, enabling a fluid and flexible process that enables an adventure therapy experience to become part of things. Spiral approaches naturally match the ebb and flow of kairos time ('appropriate' time) for participants and staff, and tend to be more relevant to *relational* and *whole-of-community* approaches. Relational adventure therapy services tend to focus on the development of relationships between the service, staff and participants; the adventure therapy experience emerges out of conversations and common experiences - based on the needs of individuals and the group, and a given place and time. From the author's observations, these services are often reluctant to be called a 'program'. Whole-of-community adventure therapy occurs naturally within the life of a given community. If the adventure therapy experience was removed, a part of the community life would be missing. In the Australian context these approaches are more commonly used in rural or remote settings. I suggest that adventure therapy practitioners who value spiral approaches (and kairos time) may be more interested in the 'soul' of international adventure therapy.

Structural approach – Within this typology, structural refers to the relatively planned, framed and linear forms of adventure therapy including services that value chronological timelines and distinct (compartmentalised) program components. Program components are usually included based on a research evidence-base in relation to that component, and are included for a specific prescribed intent using a manualised approach (for example, uses a one-hour assessment interview following a standardised format, to be undertaken with all participants at a specific time in the program, in a specific setting, based on an identified theoretical framework). Structural approaches tend to be most relevant to *clinical* and *systemic* services. Components such as assessment, diagnosis, treatment plan, treatment, and outcome evaluation are common within structural approaches. Systemic structures (including family therapy approaches) may embed a role for family members, friends or significant others in the adventure therapy process. In structural approaches, this involvement is undertaken in a planned way rather than naturally emerging. From the author's observations these approaches appear to be more commonly used in urban or metropolitan settings. From my observations, adventure therapy practitioners who value structural approaches (and chronos time) will more actively seek to strengthen the 'body' of international adventure therapy.

Conclusion: Emerging Insights

Are we pulsating in circles, arcs, pendulums or spirals, or are we moving on a linear pathway towards becoming a recognised profession?

Since 1997, we have expanded and connected, migrated north, south, east and west. We have gained a momentum, we're on our way. We are getting to know each other. Within and beyond our international community, insights have been emerging about the nature, characteristics and efficacy of international adventure therapy - but much remains unknown. We are clearer about certain things, but we are clearly not yet a homogenous field of endeavour. We may be a coherent whole, but we are different within.

It is possible that like the strength of surface tension on a pond of water, our ideological tensions hold us together. Differences in perspectives – equally subjective, equally valid – may be helping to maintain our interest in each other. Or we may be about to explode.

Attempts to identify differences and commonalities help to make more explicit the fluctuations and tensions within our shared evolution – but are we moving towards becoming a profession? And should we be moving towards becoming a profession?

To speak of becoming a recognised profession is to raise questions about motivation, belonging, and a role for adventure therapy within local, regional, and global political processes. Each of our personal responses to this possibility will illuminate the crux of our personal, professional, cultural and philosophical differences. Why? Because questions of profession provoke further questions: If we are to become a profession, who is to be included, and who is to be excluded? And what are we to profess? The conversation is different for each of us. Being social in nature, the possibility of social inclusion and social exclusion poke at sensitivities in all of us, perhaps even raise existential anxieties in some ('Am I in, or am I out? Do I want to be in or out?'). Whether in the context of family of origin, school, neighbourhood, community, society, or professional field of endeavour, the risks and opportunities associated with social inclusion and social exclusion are highly personal. Given our differences, is there anything that we wish to collectively profess?

At the very least, the international adventure therapy community can agree that adventure and therapy are essential elements in our shared field of endeavour. Ironically, this statement may also be the *most* we can collectively profess about our work. Conversations that begin to add depth and detail to our 'commonness' (for example, about what forms of adventure therapy exist, what styles are practiced, with whom, towards what aims, and with what outcomes) – leads our collective 'nod' to become a collective 'flutter' of explanations, clauses, definitions, criterion, models, credentials, contexts, client groups and training pathways. We are left conversing rather than professing.

So, can we collectively profess anything? I suggest 'yes' – but not much. Across cultures, we can profess that an intentional use of adventure and therapy in the service of human wellbeing is a worthy endeavour. But if a 'profession' implies narrow training pathways, agreed best practice principles, shared standards, an understood evidence-base, mainstream credibility, and the formation of institutions, I respond 'no'. I suggest we are an international community of professionals, but we are a long way from being a profession. Our only common profession at this stage is very basic: We see merit in a use of adventure and therapy in our work with people.

Should we, an international community of practitioners, researchers, trainers, academics, students, and interested onlookers consider moving towards becoming a profession? Perhaps yes, but in doing so, we may have more to lose than to gain.

To seek professionalisation without the wisdom of 'readiness' is to make decisions about inclusion and exclusion prematurely. I suggest that when we reach a point in time when we are collectively professing that we are a profession we will be one. Until then, smaller factions, quadrants, sub-cultures, and sub-clusters will continue to profess a range of things. And these discrete 'professions' will remain dependent on a range of paradigms, philosophies, values, cultural contexts, ideologies, preferences, and pragmatic decisions.

From my observations, adventure therapy practitioners who work in positivist-clinical settings (the upper left quadrant in the typology) appear most keen for progress towards professionalisation. Yet if just one quadrant of international adventure therapy practitioners pushes ahead towards professionalisation (without other quadrants), we risk losing either body or soul, or both.

Until we are each able to express the views of our most 'different' adventure therapy colleagues with mutual satisfaction, I feel we must be content to call ourselves an international community. Progress towards professionalisation is no doubt useful in some nations, contexts, settings or with some client groups (particularly, those working in medicalised mental health treatment settings towards mental health aims). Yet in other settings, the outward appearance of a 'profession' may undermine efforts to engage specific client groups in a therapeutic change process (for example those working with youth at risk or in cultural settings). I suggest that at the current developmental stage of our international community's evolution each quadrant still has much to learn from the others; to split without understanding what holds body and soul together may be to spilt before maturity. I suggest that on an international level, a premature move towards professionalisation may undermine the strength and momentum of our shared progress to date (see Figure 8).

Figure 8. Risks of premature 'professionalisation'

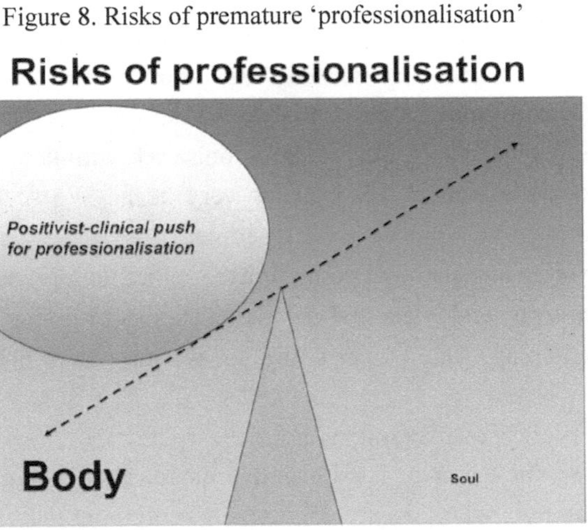

Emerging insights suggest that no one group, quadrant, type, model, program, service, approach, methodology, gender, culture or language can adequately delineate the outer boundaries of international adventure therapy. And I suggest that is a good thing.

International adventure therapy provides a cross-cultural methodology and medium through which a range of service types may contribute to healthy change. Based on anecdotal, theoretical and empirical evidence, adventure therapy offers both a stand-alone or complimentary effective therapeutic endeavour, with potential benefits across the range of physical, mental, emotional, social, cultural, economic, spiritual and environmental wellbeing domains (see Pryor, 2009). Our diverse range of adventure therapy methodologies adds value to service aims in diverse settings, and borrowed methodologies from other practices add value to our own work.

Perhaps our shared strength and sustainability depends upon a deepening knowledge of ourselves, each other, those we are working with, and a use of both body and soul to ensure our practices are effective. If we believe adventure therapy is a useful methodology – an innovative therapeutic medium – our primary task is to focus on doing that well. In cyclical fashion, I take us back to a statement Martin Ringer made back in 2003:

> We need to build collaborative tribal collectives, where many different tribes can co-exist in creative tension and where change and continuity are both present… In short, we need to develop a pan-tribal culture of critically-aware and self-reflective practitioners in the service of our work, and our ability to work together. (Ringer, 2003, p.295)

Adventure therapy collaborates with a range of professional services striving for and delivering intentional wellbeing aims in diverse communities. Whilst the scientist asks adventure therapy practitioners to attend to theory, logic and outcomes of adventure therapy experiences, the artist invites practitioners into healthy relationship with self-awareness and creative expression.

Figure 9. demonstrates the role international adventure therapy may have in assisting individuals, families and communities towards wellbeing via a common use of adventure and therapy.

Connecting across paradigms requires us to nurture respect for divergent perspectives. In order to consolidate a coherent field of practice, a growing appreciation of divergent philosophies, theories, strategies, relationships and program models is required. As international adventure therapy moves towards the outward appearance of a profession, a key challenge will be the development of frameworks, typologies and languages that nurture respect for cross-cultural practices. Attempts to honour differences within the growing profession will require a respectful collaboration of the artist, the scientist and perhaps the listener in each of us.

ACKNOWLEDGEMENTS

The author acknowledges the cultural custodians of Edinburgh lands (Edinburgers) and Czech paradise, 5IATC and 6IATC Conference organisers and hosts, ATIC, twenty Australian outdoor adventure intervention programs upon which some findings of this paper are based, and participants who keep telling us that adventure therapy is a useful methodology.

Figure 8. An international adventure therapy profession

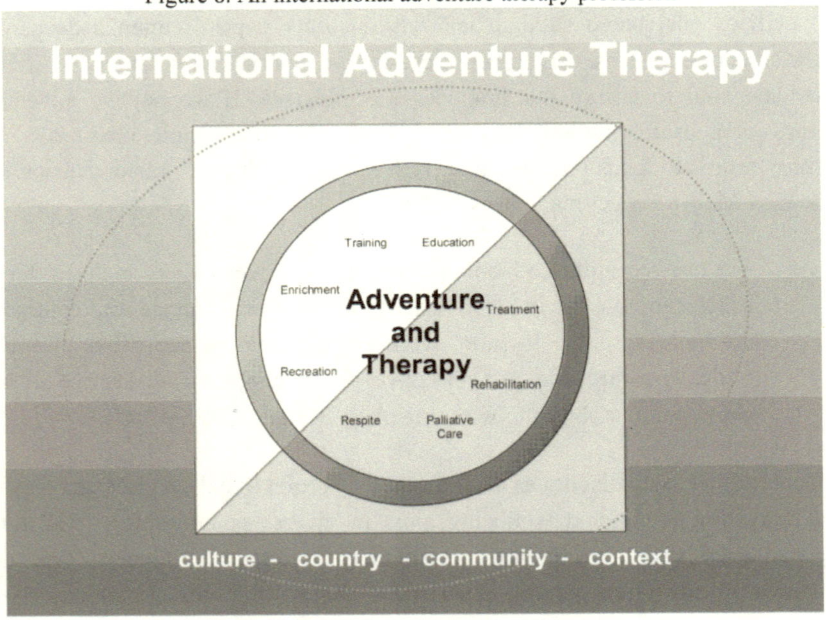

REFERENCES

Abbott, C. (1995). You don't have to be sick to get better: Adventure education, adventure therapy and personal growth. In C. Abbott, & M. Ringer, (Eds.). *Adventure therapy: Proceedings of the 1995 pre-conference workshop.* Ninth National Outdoor Education Conference: Pushing back the frontiers of outdoor education. Southport, Australia: Victorian Outdoor Education Association.

Albert Einstein Site. (2011). *Albert Einstein: Biography.* Retrieved on 9/1/11 from: www.alberteinsteinsite.com/quotes/einsteinquotes.html.

Bandoroff, S. & Newes, S. (Eds.) (2004). *Coming of Age: The evolving fleld of adventure therapy.* Third International Adventure Therapy Conference. Boulder, CO, USA: Association for Experiential Education.

Carpenter, C. (2008). *Changing Spaces: Contextualising outdoor experiential programs for health and wellbeing.* Unpublished Doctoral Thesis. Australia: Deakin University.

Crisp, S. (1997). International models of best practice in wilderness and adventure therapy. In C. Itin (Ed.). *Exploring the boundaries of adventure therapy.* First International Adventure Therapy Conference. Perth, WA Australia: Camping and Outdoor Education Association of Western Australia.

Curtis, R. & Sibberas, J. (1994). *Adventure: A catalyst for enhancing family life.* Unpublished Thesis. Victoria Australia: La Trobe University, Lincoln School of Health Sciences and Bouverie Family Therapy Centre.

Gass, M. A. (1993). *Adventure therapy: Therapeutic applications of adventure programming.* Dubuque, Iowa, USA: Association for Experiential Education, Kendall/Hunt Publishing Co.

Gillis, H.L., Gass, M.A., Bandoroff, S., Rudolph, S., Clapp, C. & Nadler, R. (1991). Family adventure survey: Results and discussion. In C., Birmingham (Ed.), *Proceedings Journal of the Nineteenth Annual AEE Conference.* Boulder, CO, USA: Association for Experiential Education.

Gilsdorf, R. (2003). Experience-Adventure-Therapy: An inquiry into professional identity. In K. Richards & B. Smith (Eds.) *Therapy within adventure.* Second International Adventure Therapy Conference. Germany: Ziel.

Goodquotes.(2011a). *Cleveland Abbe quotes.* Retrieved on 9/1/11 from: www.goodquotes.com/ quote/cleveland-abbe/true-science-is-never.

Goodquotes.(2011b). *Albert Einstein quotes.* Retreived on 9/1/11 from: www.goodquotes.com/ quote/albert-einstein/true-art-is-characterized.

Handley, R. (2003). Matching process with practice: Stage based change as a framework for adventure therapy. In K. Richards & B. Smith (Eds.) *Therapy within adventure.* Second International Adventure Therapy Conference. Germany: Ziel.

Itin, C. (Ed.) (1998). *Exploring the boundaries of adventure therapy.* First International Adventure Therapy Conference. Perth, WA, Australia: Camping and Outdoor Education Association of Western Australia.

Loynes, C. (2002). The generative paradigm. *Journal of Adventure Education and Outdoor Learning, 2*(2)113-205.

Marsden, S. & Thiele, M. (2003). *Engaging art: The Artful Dodgers studio.* Melbourne Australia: Jesuit Social Services.

Mitten, D. & Itin, C. M. (Eds.). (2009). *Connecting with the essence of adventure therapy.* Boulder, CO: Association for Experiential Education.

Mrazek P.J. & Haggerty R.J. (1994). *Reducing risks for mental disorders: Frontiers for preventive intervention research.* Washington, USA: Institute of Medicine, National Academy Press.

Pryor, A. (2009). *Wild adventures in wellbeing: Foundations, features and wellbeing impacts of Australian outdoor adventure interventions (OAI).* Unpublished doctoral thesis. Burwood, Australia: School of Health and Social Development, Deakin University.

Richards, K. & Smith, B. (Eds.) (2003). *Therapy within adventure.* Second International Adventure Therapy Conference. Germany: Ziel.

Williams, I. (2004). Adventure therapy or therapeutic adventure? In S. Bandoroff & S. Newes (Eds.), *Coming of Age: The evolving fleld of adventure therapy.* Third International Adventure Therapy Conference. Boulder, CO, USA: Association for Experiential Education.

CHAPTER 36

The Hidden Adventure: Group Projective Identification in the Practice of Adventure Therapy

Luk Peeters and Martin Ringer

INTRODUCTION

Adventure Therapy programs are most often being organized within a group context. This might be in the form of an existing group (from the same institute or treatment facility) or from an open enrolment program being organized by the therapy provider.

The group is often used as a supportive environment for personal growth and change. As a result of their participation in such groups, participants are able to experience that it is not only them suffering from life, they find fellow companions and supporters. On a group level the identification with an Adventure Therapy group can, as part of a social construction of self, add to one's identity (Stapley, 2006).

At the same time the group could also be considered as a micro reproduction of daily life where participants enact their typical patterns of relating to their world. The essential difference is that in this group therapeutic context the participants will receive feedback and insight from peers about the effect of their habitual coping styles and as such create plenty of opportunities for growth and change.

Some theorists even argue that the group is the major therapeutic agent (Ettin, 2002; Neri, 1998; Foulkes and Anthony, 1965; Bion, 1961; Whitaker and Lieberman, 1964) and that the primary function of the therapist is to take care that the group can fully achieve this task. That is because the group as a whole not only plays an important role in influencing the behavior of its different members but at the same time group behavior will reflect shared individual concerns and issues of its participants. In that same sense an individual's behavior might also provide a way for a group to deal with certain issues it is not otherwise capable of working through on a group level. In that case, the individual behavior provides us with information about group themes and concerns and might not be reduced just to issues affecting the individual. Furthermore, that participant might be seen as the messenger of the group (Whitaker, 2001).

Classical Group therapy theory has paid a lot of attention to some of these group mechanisms; mainly those from a Psycho-analytic and Psychodynamic background (Agazarian, 1997; Boyd, 1991; Brown, 2000; Ettin, 1999; Gillette & McCollom, 1995; Whitaker, 2001) but these insights have not often been translated into Adventure Therapy practices or in guidelines to help to facilitate the individuals' therapeutic process (Ringer, 2002).

In an attempt to bridge this gap we take some anecdotes from episodes in Adventure Therapy practice to link different group phenomena with some theoretical principles and possible approaches. Note that details of the stories were changed in order to protect privacy of the concerned.

Two Stories

The first story is about an adolescent who improves in a significant way during a long term Adventure Therapy program for adjudicated youngsters but then 'regresses' on the last day into a very recalcitrant behavior that is extremely vexing and distressing for the facilitators and the special teachers present on the program.

The situation is even worsened by the fact that supporting technical staff members report that on checking the program equipment, some items are missing. They suspect theft but since what is missing does not have a lot of direct or 'market' value for those youngsters but a lot of attractive expensive material that was readily accessible, has not been stolen. This seems rather strange; more like a kind of attack or act of defiance. But relations with the kids were very good until then so the whole situation has a mysterious air about it.

The program ends in a very unpleasant way, with a lot of disappointment, disbelief and frustration on the part of the facilitators and a fair amount of frustration and anger from the part of the participants towards the 'offender'.

The second anecdote is drawn from a therapeutic program for adults where the group engages in a six-day backpacking trip. During the fourth day of the hike one of the therapists (let's call him Jack) becomes aware of a growing urge to act in a rebellious way and to intrude into the groups 'decision-making process. He notices a tendency within himself to disobey the decisions taken by the leader-of-the-day[1], to start questioning the group's decisions and to defy the existing group norms. As he pays attention to those signals and explores their possible meaning in relation to the group, he shares this with his colleague during the next stretch of the hike. Both try to connect this urge with the dynamics in the group but without success and the colleague does not recognize the same tendency within himself. So they decide to keep alert for how this might develop.

Half a day later the colleague shares his observations and interpretations with Jack. He noticed how Jack was approached by the group in a way, as to provoke deviant behavior. He was (playfully) called out when risking to step out of the single file line they agreed to form while walking along a roadside verge, while the same behavior by other members was left unchallenged. When going over some safety issues the leader-of-the-day especially mentioned that those regulations also applied to Jack and later during the hike when Jack was picking some blueberries along the track another participant questioned if he was crossing a line by doing this.

The Common Underlying Theme

What the previous stories have in common is the underlying unconscious psychological mechanism that influences an individual to behave in a certain way fulfilling a group need. At the same time, the 'chosen' individual acts out an issue that remains unresolved in his or her psyche. This is referred to as group-level projective identification. In summary, if a group is not yet able to deal with a theme that is important to them, they will unconsciously try to play it out by focusing that issue on an individual group member. For example, the aggressive tendencies of group members can be unconsciously directed so that only one member ends up acting excessively aggressively.

Using this lens to focus on our two stories we suggest that the individual behavior of the adolescent from the first story could tell us something about what is happening in, and needed by, the group as-a-whole. Furthermore, that the visible behavior is only a symptom of a perhaps more important and widespread common issue on a group level.

---

[1] The 'leader of the day' is a different participant each day who carries the responsibility for route-finding and most elements of leadership. The program staff maintain power of veto in the case of issues where emotional or physical safety might be compromised. This system minimizes the level of rebellion that participants direct onto staff and maximizes the real-life responsibility of participants.

Projective identification functions not only on group members themselves, but also with outsiders or leaders. These people may even be a more attractive or satisfying target externalizing the 'badness' threatens the group's identity much less.

This links to the second vignette where one of the two therapists (Jack) could perhaps sense and recognize the pressure that the group unconsciously tried to lay upon him in order to produce a behavior that is needed in the group itself, but cannot be dealt with (yet).

Let us look at the described mechanisms more closely and in-depth before we analyze the two vignettes from this perspective.

An Exploration of the Mechanisms Involved

Group Projective Identification is the combined appearance of the mechanisms of projection and that of identification in a way that involves the group-as-a-whole.

Firstly, projection:

> Projection ... occurs when we unconsciously *cannot tolerate aspects of ourselves.* In this case we disown what we do not like by failing to see those aspects in ourselves but projecting the disowned part of ourselves onto others and therefore seeing these characteristics in others. The shorthand for this is 'splitting and projection. (Ringer, 2002).

And furthermore:

> Projection is a process by which an individual reduces his or her anxiety by unconsciously disowning a part of him or herself and imagining that the unwanted feeling or characteristic belongs to someone else. As for most concepts that have been derived from psychoanalytic fields, the word 'projection' is used by different authors to mean different things. Tyson captures the basic elements of projection in the following passage: Projection is an intra-psychic [intrapersonal] event whereby a person unconsciously splits off and gets rid of a bad feeling or an unacceptable aspect of their personality by attributing it to another person or, in some cases, an object. Projection can also involve the splitting off and projecting of positive feelings. In either case, the other is said to be the 'container' for the split-off and projected material. As this process occurs at the unconscious level of fantasy [phantasy], with both projector and container unaware of the process, it is difficult to

detect, yet it may have a profound influence on interpersonal behavior. (Tyson, 1998, cited in Ringer, 2002)

In its simplest form projection involves three conditions all being met:

1) The person projecting believes that another person is experiencing some kind of emotion or has some kind of characteristic or behavior.
2) The other person is not actually experiencing that emotion or does not have that characteristic.
3) The person doing the projecting does have that same emotion present or does have that characteristic but it is pushed out of their awareness.

The term 'projection' implies that the person doing the projecting has disowned and projected (as in throwing a projectile) the unwanted emotion 'onto' the other. It is still a projective process when the other is not aware that the person doing the projection has this inaccurate expectation of them" (Ringer, 2002, pp.134-135).

An adventure therapy group provides a wonderful rich environment for projection to occur, firstly because of the level of anxiety caused simply by being in a group and secondly because of the level of anxiety created by taking part in 'challenge' activities. For every group member, other group members as well as the leaders are potential 'screens' upon which the participant can project disowned elements of him/herself. Each group member with their great variety of valences provides a constant source of stimuli for other group members projections. Great learning can occur for participants when they start to notice repetitive patterns in their projections. For instance, one participant may regularly make remarks to a number of different group members that he/she finds their sense of humor to be cruel. If this is examined in the group, it enables the person who regularly perceives cruelty or persecution to reflect on why he or she experiences this when others in the group do so to a much lesser extent. And it provides an opportunity for those upon whom the group member projects his/her feelings of persecution to reflect on to what extent they are actually cruel or persecutory. Nonetheless, facilitating such reflective conversations calls for quite high levels of skill on the part of the group leaders.

And conversely, when one group member experiences him/herself as regularly being named as having a certain characteristic – such as withdrawal – then that participant may reflect on to what extent that feels true. And each group member who says that they experience that group member as withdrawing can reflect on to what extent they are avoiding to face up to their own tendency to withdraw. Exploring the patterns in one's own projection onto others as well as exploring one's own tendency to be recipient of particular kinds or projections helps all parties to re-integrate their projections and can provide powerful growth opportunities. This tendency to attract projections of a certain type is known as valence, and it can also lead to the participant strongly identifying with certain particular other participants when they display the characteristics with which the first participant most strongly identifies.

Projection is one element of projective identification and identification is the other.

In its simplest form, identification is the unconscious process whereby we lose the distinction between self and other. When we cry at the movies or when reading a sad story it is because we identify with the protagonist who is suffering. At an unconscious level we 'are' the protagonist of the story. We feel 'as if' we were that person. Identification is also a key element of empathy. If we cannot identify with the other, we cannot be empathic with him or her. However in groups, identification combined with projection can form destructive patterns. Another manifestation of identification supports learning vicariously through role modelling:

> The function of a role model is to provide a sustained opportunity for us to identify with another so that we can gradually become what we perceive them to be. We identify with this talented person and so gradually imitate their talents until finally we have introjected the talents and possibly no longer need the role model. Jacques Lacan believed that the first development of a baby's sense of self occurs through identification with others (Leader and Groves 1995). Yet another form of identification occurs when the television news shows a person who has been persecuted or treated unjustly. We may feel the outrage for the other person though a[n unconscious] phantasy that we are that person. At a conscious level it is possible to rationalize the strong feelings by saying things like, 'We can't let that sort of thing happen. What if it happened to us?' However, seeing the television report creates the phantasy that this terrible event has already happened to us – through the unconscious process of identification. (Ringer, 2002, p.136)

The simultaneous functioning of projection and identification at the level of the group-as-a-whole is referred to as projective identification. Bullying and scapegoating in groups are extreme forms of group-level projective identification. They occur when a participant is continually the recipient of projections of weakness, usually because of a valence or predisposition to believe themselves to be weak. The power and repetition of these projections means that they are internalized by the protagonist (hence the word 'identification') so they reinforce that person's original feelings of weakness. Other group members then 'see' weakness in this person and because of their fear of weakness, attack the weakness in the other through directly attacking the person – verbally or physically. So the two self-reinforcing patterns in this process are firstly group participants disowning and projecting their own weakness onto a(n unconsciously) chosen victim and then group level collusion to attack this person – whereby these group members unconsciously attack the weakness in themselves. This pattern reinforces destructive projections rather than helping people to deal with their issues with weakness. The power of this dynamic can be so great that even if a victim of bullying is effectively driven out of a group, very quickly the group finds another victim and starts to repeat the pattern.

Marrone Views Projective Identification as Occurring in Four Steps:

> Step 1 is the subject's projection of a part of himself on to another person. Step 2 is an interpersonal interaction whereby the projector actively pressures the recipient to think, feel and act in accordance with the projection. In Step 3 the recipient complies with the pressure exerted on him to fulfil the projector's expectations and behaves accordingly. A further step, often described, is that the subject reinternalizes the projection, after it has been processed by the recipient. These processes can also be observed in small groups, between the subject and part of the group or the whole group. (Marrone 1998, p.132)

Some authors view the projection/identification dynamic as the most significant influence on the development of all groups (Wells 1995, Bolten 1998). This is perhaps because the group setting creates the perfect conditions for the kind of regression that leads to projection and identification. Also, because of the inevitable diversity of make-ups and valences amongst group members there is a great potential in any group for multiple 'projectors' and multiple 'identifiers' for each 'projector'(see further in this article as well).

However, bullying and victimization and other forms of projective identification, when discussed openly in the group in their early stages provide a wonderfully rich source of potential growth for all concerned. And on the other hand if patterns of projection, identification and projective identification in groups are not explored, they can undermine the therapeutic intent of the adventure therapy group. Even worse, they can result in psychological and emotional damage that goes along with reinforcing unhelpful behaviors and patterns of attribution. A tragic extreme of this is when cyber-bullying drives the victim of bullying to suicide. The collective unconscious aggression is introjected so strongly that he or she enacts the ultimate aggression against a person – murdering him/herself.

Agazarian (1989) refers to the appearance of the abovementioned mechanisms by stating that the maturity of a group can be measured by its ability to deal with deviant behavior on a group level. If the group is not (yet) able to, that behavior will then be projected elsewhere; that might be on an external figure (e.g. director, external therapist), a leader (therapist) or another group member. Although many 'containers' can be suitable the so-called projection screen is not chosen randomly.

The potential for an individual to be 'used' as a recipient for group projective identification depends on his or her 'valence'. A person can have different, even opposing valences. In one group a person may enact one valence whilst in another group that same person may display a completely other valence. Even in the same group a single participant might have the potential to fill in different unconscious roles and likewise more than one group member can have the same valence. It is important to notice that it is not the person who has the most of the characteristics for taking this role or living-up those projections, but the person who is most capable to do so for the 'benefit' of the entire group, that will most likely take the needed position or acting out of the behavior. It often suits a therapy group to have an 'identified patient', so that all the worries and concerns and work can go towards that person but at the same time that person must show that he or she can carry that load and not collapse and really starts needing special care.

Not only certain themes or behaviors can be projected, but also internal conflicts that exist within most of the clients can be projected within a 'preferred' individual, who then takes one side of that conflict and as such allowing the rest of the group to fix themselves in the opposite pole. Or the group can even project the conflict onto a 'selected pair' and then witness how they bring the conflicting poles to the open, making it visible and tangible.

A classic example is the internal tension often present within an individual between structure and creativity. In some groups, this gets highlighted by the ever-recurring conflict between two participants, who describe each other as boring and rigid versus chaotic and impulsive. Like on stage in a theatre play, they perform their role, at the same time supported and disapproved by the other group members who report that they like both persons but are fed up with their everlasting conflict. A further exploration often brings clarity and ownership in the form that most of the participants then recognize within themselves this conflicting polar tendency.

Considered in a process of group development and maturation the mechanism of projecting thoughts, behavior, needs and feelings that are not yet in the capacity of the group could be considered as a healthy one as long as the split is temporary and that there is a sort of re-integration in a next phase of the groups' growth. But it is important to note that the group leaders and facilitators must recognize and deal effectively with such dynamics if they are to be harnessed in the service of healing and growth.

Some authors even argue that the real formation/creation of a group is only possible through the consequences of the construction of a web of projections and identifications (Bolten, 1998). This is very visible in the exaggerated and sometimes even confabulated search for similarities in order to belong that is so typical in the first phase of the development of a group. But also in later phases the splitting and projecting can provide a group some provisional relief. Then, when a participant successfully contains projections for a while, this decreases the anxiety in the group and provides a role model to others on how to integrate projections in themselves and on a group level.

A New Understanding of the Two Stories

With the abovementioned theoretical background in mind, the two described situations present themselves with a novel meaning and new challenges and opportunities to facilitate.

The adolescent might voice and act out the pain that comes along with 'ending'. The end of a successful and heart-touching program is likely to be affecting every group member. Perhaps the facilitators/therapists have not donated enough attention, time and energy to this crucial phase of the group development and the adolescent is signalling this – albeit unconsciously. That is, in the absence of a structured way or meaningful ritual to deal with the loss and grief, the participants themselves sought for a way to deal with this theme.

> At one level the theft may have been an action to secretly look for an object to symbolically help carry the program experience with them (hence the 'stolen' or disappeared technical materials). This was done secretly, because due to the characteristics of the group, combined with the vulnerability and sensibility of dealing with grief and sadness, this could not be voiced directly by the participants. (Eisold, 2009)

On the other hand this triggers a group projective identification mechanism, where the participant with the highest valence for this behavior, was supported to act-out the needs of the rest of the group whilst at the same time being discounted for doing so.

In the other vignette Jack had already shown that he could deal with some conflict and withstand aggression from one of the key-participants of the group, in the beginning of the program.

So he was chosen in favor of the other therapist, who perhaps could have taken this role as well, but had not shown this potential until then.

The urge that Jack felt to start acting in a rebellious and confronting way reflected – in the projective identification perspective the need of the group for differentiation and conflicting viewpoints in order to mature and grow.

One participant had earlier left the program after a rather unclear and confusing conflict between therapist and that specific participant. This incident could have created the phantasy that conflict is dangerous and leads to emotional outbursts and hence should be avoided in order to survive as group.

However, conflict and differentiation *are* necessary in order to promote group development and the group may have been seeking a way to get out of this dilemma by trying to 'use' one of the therapists for that purpose. It should be repeated though, that this is an unconscious tendency on a group-level and out of awareness of the individual participants.

The challenge for the therapist is that, as we saw in this example, he or she is also a part of the group and so is as susceptible as other group members both to project onto others and to be the container for projections from the group members. All of this occurs unconsciously so it is only by paying attention to the 'evidence' that therapists can work against colluding with projections and projective identification. Working in pairs and comparing notes with another therapist is a particularly powerful way of doing this. One therapist might find André to be aggressive, but another not. This difference provides excellent information for both therapists to explore what it is about their own functioning that has one of them possibly not noticing aggression when it exists, or on the other hand, the other one perceiving aggression when it is not there.

In the example above of the leader who stepped out of line while walking along the road, there was clearly a difference between the two therapists experience which was clearly evidence that they needed to look for projective processes in the group.

AND NOW? SOME POSSIBLE ALTERNATIVE INTERVENTIONS

So what could the therapists have done differently or how could they use this information in their following interventions?

In the first story a possible alternative intervention could have been that the therapists started to acknowledge that the ending of a program is often a difficult phase to deal with, hereby sharing their own experiences in this group as a role model, and a way of decreasing the fear of being vulnerable by showing these emotions. At the same time they could honor the participant with 'deviant' behavior for bringing that theme in the groups' awareness and as such reducing the possible scapegoating towards that person. Inviting the other participants to share how they feel and what they normally do in order to deal with loss and grief might reconnect that specific boy with the group again and bind everyone around a common theme. An appropriate ritual and a souvenir with symbolic value to the lived experience could add to the transition to daily life and reduce the chances of more 'losses' of material.

In the case of the six-day hike there are several possible directions to move into, depending on the readiness of the group to tackle this theme.

As therapists, Jack and his colleague could have tried to share their observations and interpretation in a non-threatening way and explore with the participants how they as well might recognize their attraction towards rebellious and conflicting behavior and in a next step look at what is withholding them and how they could overcome this in a constructive way, taking into account the value of the opposing force, that of harmony.

If this was too much of a step another set of interventions could have been that Jack, now with full awareness and supervised by his colleague, would temporary take the assigned position and role but without getting immersed in it. At the same time and in doing so the therapists could ease and clear the way so the participants could gradually get a feel and a taste for that position and the advantages it might have for them to take it as well. In that perspective it is of major important that the role-taking has a temporary character and that role fixation is avoided by slowly removing it from the therapist toward the different group members and in this way becoming a non-threatening part of their behavioral repertoire.

Given that there are no recipes for dealing effectively with every individual situation occurring in a group that involves projection, identification and projective identification, we might ask "How can we learn how do this?" There is overwhelming evidence that the practitioners who are best able to 'harness' these unconscious dynamics are those with a highly developed capacity for self-awareness, attunement to their own emotional worlds, and who have highly developed capacity to deal with the emotional ups and downs that they experience in the process of leading and facilitating.

Conclusions

The behavior of an individual in a group is not completely his or her own responsibility and contains a lot of fascinating information about other participants' wellbeing and about important issues within the group-as-a-whole as well. Using this knowledge in a skilful way can on the one hand defuse the tendency towards blame of the individual and on the other hand provide a gateway to heighten the responsibility of the other group members and direct the whole system towards increased learning and healing opportunities.

Projection, identification and projective identification are ubiquitous unconscious phenomena that potentially provide rich source of material to supplement the already powerful healing in growth that occurs in adventure therapy programs. Hence it behooves us as practitioners to develop our attunement, self-awareness and emotional maturity to levels where we can harness these phenomena to enrich the work we do.

References

Agazarian, Y.M. (1989). The invisible group: and integrational theory of group-as-a-whole; the 12th annual Foulkes Memorial Lecture. *Group Analysis*, 22(4), 74-96.

Agazarian, Y. M. (1997). *Systems-centered therapy for groups*. New York: Guilford Press.

Ashbach, C. and V. L. Schermer (1987). *Object relations, the self, and the group*. London: Routledge.

Bolten, M. (1998). *De groep en projectieve identificatie*. In: Handboek Groepspsychotherapie. Houten, Bohn Stafleu van Loghum.

Bion, W.R. (1961). *Experiences in groups*. London: Tavistock.

Boyd, R. D., Ed. (1991). Personal transformation in small groups: A Jungian perspective. *International library of group psychotherapy and group process*. London: Routledge.

Brown, R. (2000). *Group processes*. Malden, MA: Blackwell Publishers.

Eisold, K. (2009). *What you don't know you know: Our hidden motives in life, business, and everything else.* New York: Other Press.

Ettin, M. F. (1999). *Foundations and applications of group psychotherapy.* London: Jessica Kingsley Publishers.

Foulkes, S.H. and Anthony, E.J. (1965) *Group Psychotherapy: the psychoanalytic approach.* 2nd Ed. Baltimore: Penguin Books.

Gillette, J. and M. McCollom, Eds. (1995). *Groups in context: A new perspective on group dynamics*. Lanham, Maryland: University Press of America.

Marrone, M. (1998). *Attachment and interaction.* London: Jessica Kingsley Publishers.

Neri, C. (1998). *Group.* London: Jessica Kingsley Publishers.

Ringer, T. M. (2002). *Group action: The dynamics of groups in therapeutic, educational and corporate settings*. London: Jessica Kingsley Publishers.

Stapley, L. (2006). *Individuals, groups, and organizations beneath the surface.* London: Karnac Books Ltd.

Whitaker, D.S. and Lieberman M.A. *Psychotherapeutic Change through the Group Process.* Transaction Publishers: New Brunswick.

Whitaker, D. S. (2001). *Using groups to help people.* London: Brunner-Routledge.

CHAPTER 37

Supervision and Adventure Therapy: Fighting Burnout and Providing Emotional First Aid for Practitioners

Elspeth Schwenk and Stephan Natynczuk

ABSTRACT

The work of the outdoor and adventure therapy practitioner is both rewarding and challenging. Outdoor practitioners are generally not therapists yet frequently work therapeutically, but without the support therapists receive through regular supervision. This paper combines theory with practice and will present and explore how some of the constructs of supervision can be adapted from the field of counselling and psychotherapy, and can contribute toward best practice within outdoor and adventure therapy, delivering a duty of care and wellbeing for both client and practitioner. Taking account of several models, but drawing upon a solution focused model of supervision, we will provide a combination of both casework and experiential opportunities to enable participants to work with this model and recycle their learning through a contribution of feedback, discussion and participation. Drawing upon the British Association for Counselling and Psychotherapy's Ethical Framework for Good Practice, we will consider issues of best practice alongside examining how supervision can be adapted to deliver emotional first-aid and the prevention of practitioner burn-out.

INTRODUCTION

According to 2012 United Kingdom Government statistics, one in five people suffers from workplace stress in the UK, with some half a million people reporting they have become ill as a result of this stress. Despite the healing properties of nature and the ambience of the wilderness, outdoor and adventure practitioners are not exempt from stress in their workplace, and have few mechanisms in place to support them, or respond to their state of wellbeing. In this article, based on our presentation at the Sixth IATC in Prague, 2012, we will examine the issue of stress within the professional world of Outdoor and Adventure Therapy, and introduce the concept of supervision and how it can potentially prevent emotional burn out and enhance practitioner wellbeing and best practice.

Background—Where Be Began

At the Fifth International Adventure Therapy Conference in Edinburgh, Scotland, 2009, the focus of the conference centered on: 'Adventure therapy as an emerging approach: Towards a profession', encouraging practitioners to critically evaluate their industry and its approach to, and place within psychological therapy. The IATC committed itself to "ensuring that the appropriate knowledge and practice infrastructures are robustly developed and put into place in order to achieve that recognition" (Richards, 2009, p.8). This particular conference was co-hosted by the British Association for Counselling and Psychotherapy (BACP) – the leading professional body for counselling and psychotherapy in the UK, providing a strong platform of support and recognition of adventure therapy as a "legitimate therapeutic approach" (ibid p.8). At that time, the BACP's mission was to enable access to ethical and effective psychological therapy by setting and monitoring professional standards in its efforts toward the vision of an "emotionally healthy society.

Within counseling and psychotherapy, one of the key aspects of securing and maintaining ethical and effective psychological therapy, and monitoring professional standards is undertaken through the medium of regular supervision. However, very little, if anything, is mentioned about this valuable resource and its potential contribution to adventure therapy and the wellbeing of its practitioners.

In her overview of the 5IATC proceedings, Richards (2012) asks some fundamental questions regarding "the psychological process of change and the benefits of adventure therapy approaches" (ibid p.9). She asks: "How do we know what kind of adventure therapy intervention works best for what client and when? How can we ensure ethical practice and maintain professional standards? How can we understand the change process in action and develop theoretical models? How do we build the knowledge and practitioner base of adventure therapy that ensures it is an effective approach? How do we engage policy makers, clients, professionals, and the public in this emerging knowledge-base?" (ibid p.9). In establishing adventure therapy's value and contribution toward an emotionally healthy society, we would do well to keep these questions at the forefront of our minds.

In this article we consider the process and potential of supervision within adventure therapy as one tool that can assist not only with practitioner wellbeing but also contribute in the endeavour to answer these challenging questions. Set alongside the exciting developments in the field, supervision has much to offer in establishing and demonstrating ethical practice, practitioner wellbeing, and the professional stance of the work being undertaken in all its various forms. Briefly establishing the background of supervision within the UK, we examine its role, purpose and contribution within counselling and psychotherapy today, several models of supervision and what supervision can offer both practitioners and adventure therapy as an emerging industry today.

We will also engage in the debate around resistance to supervision, the tension the concept of supervision can create, and some of the suspicion and challenges to introducing supervision to adventure therapy.

Supervision: What Is It and Where Did it Come From?

Within the UK, supervision has become an integral part of any therapeutic undertaking. The British Association for Counselling and Psychotherapy (BACP) regards the on-going provision of supervision as an essential aspect of good ethical practice, and requires supervisors to enable and facilitate a regular routine of critical reflection with practitioners. At the outset, the BACP's Ethical Framework for Good Practice (2010) establishes the difference between supervising and managing: "There is a general obligation for all counsellors, psychotherapists, supervisors and trainers to receive supervision/consultative support independently of any managerial relationships" (BACP, date, p.7) in order to: "enhance good practice... and protect clients from poor practice" (BACP, date, p.8).

In considering the continuing development of outdoor and adventure therapy, it is expedient to examine the value and role of supervision and its potential contribution toward good practice and ethical mindfulness. There has, however, long been confusion and hesitancy regarding terminology where supervision is concerned. In many parallel fields, supervision is more closely aligned with management and this has created an unfortunate association, and has no doubt contributed to the hesitancy and resistance toward this concept in some quarters within Outdoor and Adventure Therapy. However, despite the confusion, no real effective replacement terminology has been found. This said, the concept has advanced and now not only underpins all psychological therapeutic work within the UK, but is a requirement for practice.

According to Corey et al. (2010) "Supervision has been part of the helping professions from the beginning, but it is only in recent years that supervision has come to be seen as a separate and distinct field with its own set of skills and tools" Since the early days of psychoanalysis, supervision has been an integral part of therapy, and Freud himself provided supervision to fellow analysts through both conversation and letters according to Wheeler and Richards (2007). It is generally agreed that practitioners in training should receive supervision but, beyond that, it varies across nations as to how long it is considered essential to ensure best practice. Within the UK, it is understood that ongoing supervision is a key element of practice and some professional memberships such as the BACP, and now also, the UK Register of Counsellors and Psychotherapists require it, providing a guide that confirms: "Supervision is a value of the Ethical Framework, and the Register requires that all registrants agree to engage in supervision appropriate to their practice. Supervision offers the practitioner a reflective space in which to develop practice and as such benefits client safety" (BACP, 2012).

There is a growing body of literature regarding supervision that examines the topic from a number of perspectives. Carroll and Holloway (1999) take a broad sweeping contextual view that takes a tour of supervision through consideration of racial and gender issues, to working with disabilities or sexual orientation. They also examine supervision and organisation issues--including medical and educational settings, school and workplace, religious and uniformed settings. Other authors have taken a closer look at some of the ethical practice and legal issues that are part of any therapeutic undertaking that they consider should be included within a supervision session (e.g. Falvey, 2002; Mitchels & Bond, 2011). There are a range of supervision models that authors such as Hawkins and Shohet (2006), Carroll (2012), Page and Wosket (2001), Inskipp and Proctor (2001) to list but a few, have developed over the years. None to date have been specifically been designed for Outdoor and Adventure Therapy, but each has much to offer. Feltham and Dryden (1994) take a closer look at the supervision relationship itself and explore the supervisory alliance and relationship, its foci and methods along with some of the potential developmental opportunities supervision has to offer. They note its strengths and weaknesses and also the protective value it offers both the profession as a whole, and the client and practitioner in particular. In 2007, Wheeler and Richards undertook a systematic review of the literature regarding the impact of clinical supervision on all stakeholders in the therapeutic relationship. The findings of this review indicate that supervision has positive impacts on the supervisee, whereby supervisees grow and develop through supervision (Wheeler & Richards, 2007).

Within supervision rests a unique triadic relationship between a supervisor, a supervisee (the practitioner) and his or her clients. While the supervisor and supervisee meet on a regular basis, the client never attends but is always 'in the room', and this activity is in place to ensure his wellbeing as well as the supervisee's. But what happens in supervision and how does it work? There are many definitions, to correspond with the varying contexts and countries where it is undertaken. What can be said is that it is a formal relationship in which there is a contractual agreement that the therapist will present their work with clients in an open and honest way that enables the supervisor to have insight into the way in which the work is being conducted (Wheeler & Richards, 2007), and both parties being held accountable to a formal professional body. A couple of generally accepted definitions are as follows:

> A working alliance between the supervisor and counsellor (practitioner) in which the counsellor (practitioner) can offer an account or recording of her (his) work; reflect on it; receive feedback and, where appropriate, guidance. The object of this alliance is to enable the counsellor to gain in ethical competence, confidence, compassion and creativity in order to give her best possible service to the client. (Inskipp & Proctor, 2001)

In contrast is a definition given by Bernard and Goodyear (1992, p. 2004) reflects more of the US approach: "Supervision is an intervention provided by a more senior member of a profession to a more junior member of that same profession. This relationship is evaluated, extends over time and has the simultaneous purposes of enhancing the professional functioning of the more junior person, monitoring the quality of professional services offered to the clients seen and serving as a gatekeeper for those who are to ender the particular profession" (2004, p. 8).

Moving beyond definitions, perhaps it is easier to think about the function of supervision. In her introduction, Henderson (2009) offers four main functions which are most commonly identified: educative, supportive and creative and lastly, managerial. By educative, Henderson is referring to: "encouraging the development of supervisee's skills, abilities, understanding, personal awareness, and academic knowledge." (ibid, p.xix). This is self-explanatory and can readily be adapted to parallel therapeutic fields. The second function is perhaps a little more obscure in that it encourages the practitioner to look within, and explore their own personal issues and life events and, most importantly, to consider how this might impact upon the relationship and therapeutic work with their client. In the world of adventure, it is acknowledged and generally understood that both the therapist and the client take something away from the experience, and it is very important that the practitioner is given time and space for personal reflection. This enables the practitioner to differentiate his/her material from the client's, to consider the impact of the event or activity, the client, and their work together upon his or her own life. Henderson (2009) also highlights the necessity for the practitioner to be able to identify what is happening within her own life--to be self-aware and thus, better placed to bracket off personal material from her therapeutic work. Understanding the nature and remit of roles and duties can also be addressed within this function. Henderson also discusses the managerial function, whereby practitioners or supervisees have the opportunity to safely explore their work within the expectations of their profession, the ethical codes of conduct they subscribe to, the agency and context within which they work, the collegial relationships, organisational or legal requirements. It is important to clarify here, that this last function should not be interpreted as line management, but management with a small 'm', that addresses the areas mentioned above.

Corey et al. (2010), discuss the goals of supervision, and identifies four goals of promoting supervisee growth and development; protecting the welfare of the client; monitoring supervisee performance and act as gatekeeper for the profession and lastly, empowering the supervisee to self-supervise and carry out these goals as an independent professional. The promotion of internal or self-supervision enables a practitioner to be in the moment and to be self-aware but does not preclude the need for an external supervisor for later reflection. Within the United States, ongoing supervision is not widely practiced, and practitioner independence is more the norm for licensed practitioners. Supervision is often seen as the domain of junior or trainee practitioners, which is in contrast to the UK in particular, where it is recognised as a highly beneficial ongoing activity for experienced and senior practitioners throughout their career.

MODELS OF SUPERVISION

Over the years, supervision has developed and become a specialty field with its own set of unique competencies (knowledge and skills), theories, methods, evaluations, and legal and ethical duties and obligations (Corey et al, 2010). There are now a range of supervision models, some related to a particular theoretical model e.g., person centered or cognitive behavioural approaches to supervision, and others taking a more generic approach.

What they all endeavour to do is provide a structure that identifies the roles, tasks and responsibilities of supervision alongside some of the dynamics related to process, development and context. Stoltenberg and Delworth's (1987) development model, for example, sets out the concept and framework that suggests practitioners have different needs depending upon their particular stage of development. This can also have a parallel within the supervisor's own professional development journey. Using the analogy of an apprentice, the practitioner moves through four stages; from being a novice (trainee), through to Master Practitioner--where the relationship may have a more collegial tone to it. According to Ronnestad and Skovholt (2013, p.60) "Supervisors have a major impact in the Beginning Student Phase. The dependence and vulnerability of the beginning student, in combination with the intense need for confirmation and guidance, combine to make supervision an important learning arena." There is much to learn at this early stage, and a clear argument can be made for a high level of support, as therapists, and this includes Outdoor and Adventure Practitioners, engage with the complexity of human nature and their role in the change process. In contrast to this, Roonestad and Skovholt (2013 p.71) identify five developmental tasks of the Advanced Student or Intern, the first three being closely akin to those identified for the Student Practitioner:

1) To learn more complex conceptual knowledge that meets the criteria set by the training institution
2) To demonstrate procedural competence; that is, sufficient mastery of assessment and therapeutic skills as assessed by supervisors in particular
3) To maintain an openness to information and theory at a meta-level, while also engaging in the "closing off" process of selecting therapy/counselling theories and techniques to use
4) To modify unrealistic and 'perfectionistic' images of psychotherapy and counselling and of the role of the practitioner
5) To manage the bewilderment that comes from seeing psychotherapy/counselling as increasingly complex.

While this is directed toward counselling and psychotherapy practitioners, parallels can easily be drawn with Outdoor and Adventure Practitioners, and again, it is clearly evident that supervision forms a highly influential element of the practitioner's development. From this level of competence onwards, there is "more at stake" as Ronnestad and Skovholt point out, and certainly for experienced and senior Outdoor and Adventure Practitioners, this becomes the case as they take on both clients and activities of an increasingly complex nature. For more experienced practitioners, one of the key elements that supervision has to offer is not only around career development and support, but also practitioner wellbeing and resilience against stagnation and burnout.

Alongside these developmental aspects of supervision, are models such as Hawkins and Shohet's (1989; 2006): Supervision in the helping professions, and age and Wosket (2001) cyclical model. Both models focus on the process of supervision, while Carroll (1996) explores the tasks associated with supervision and also brings into sharp focus the element of context. Together, Holloway and Carroll (1995) examine the systemic (organisational & context) issues that can arise. Proctor and Inskipp (2001) focus on the relationship process that underpins supervision, and Clarkson (2003) also picks up on this crucial element in her relationship model.

Beyond these models are those related to a particular theoretical stance such as Tudor & Worrall (2007) who discuss a Person-centered approach to supervision. Waskett (2009) also reflects upon a solution-focused approach to supervision, which we will discuss in greater length. Taking that perspective a step further, Briggs & Miller (2008) discuss Success Enhancing Supervision, exploring "strategies and practices that enhance clinicians' sense of themselves as competent and successful professionals." Their goal in supervision is to: "facilitate the development of a competent therapist, which ultimately affect his/her efficacy with clients" (Briggs & Miller, 2008, p.200).

How Can We Adapt Supervision and Make It Our Own?

To date, there is little written and identified as a supervision model that is tailor-made to suit Outdoor and Adventure Therapy, and it is timely to consider what the profession needs to ensure both practitioner and client wellbeing. There are many elements that are directly transferrable. While there is certainly room for more than one model to emerge, according to the needs of the practitioner, the context and/or agency of their work, and nature of the therapeutic work they undertake.

Given that supervision is there to promote the development and wellbeing of both practitioner and client, it is important to consider the needs of both parties and begin to explore a more bespoke model that accommodates the particular needs of this developing profession. Natynczuk & Schwenk (in process) began this work by presenting some of the following key ingredients directly transferrable to Outdoor and Adventure Therapy.

KEY INGREDIENTS

As previously stated, supervision provides a point of regular reflection and an opportunity for professional development and support. It ensures a duty of care is extended to both participant (client) and the professional. In order to deliver these ingredients, it is important that supervision has some form of structure and format and is undertaken on a regular and mandatory basis. It should be both personal and professional in offering a safe, reflective space while preferably not being seen as line management, and ideally, should offer a critical appreciation of the factors associated with 'adventure' and 'therapy'.

According to Scaife (2012) supervision is an "instance of thoughtful practice" (p. 2). She continues: "reflective practice involves thinking from a bird's eye view about an event and/or aspects of my practice. The perspective includes myself, encompassing my behaviour, thoughts and/or feelings in relation to my practice, with the implication that the reflection will impact on, although not necessarily alter, my practice" (p. 3). We can begin to assemble some components of supervision: it provides an opportunity for a more 'distanced' perspective (a stepping back or helicopter viewpoint), there is a purpose towards analysis and challenge, and a focus on social, ethical and process--all of which may incorporate aspects of personal assumption, belief, judgment and cultural orientation.

Supervision is an on-going journey of professional exploration and development. It is not a random occurrence – indeed, its very regularity forges a relationship bond between practitioner and supervisor that brings trust and collaborative development to the endeavour. While not undertaken in a vacuum – it does offer a more 'removed' perspective in which reflection, expression and processing can occur and this, in turn, is re-cycled back into the practitioner's therapeutic world Scaife (2010).

Scaife (2010) draws our attention to the multi-dimensional aspect of reflection:

- the process of active awareness about what we are thinking, feeling and doing in the here and now;
- the process of review, taking an observer's perspective of that occurrence; and lastly,
- the concept of 'anticipatory reflection' – put forward by Conway (2001) and Van Manen (1990) and, as Scaife writes, "highlighting the circularity of the reflective process when it informs subsequent practice" (2010, p.5).

For most Outdoor practitioners, the work of Schon (1983) will be very familiar and can be argued as espousing a similar perspective on the reflective process to that outlined by Scaife (2010). Schon (1983) writes about the reflective practitioner and coins the terms: 'reflection-in-action' and 'reflection-on-action. Reflection in Action is something that is in the moment, in the here and now. It is about what else is going on for you. While Reflection on Action is a process carried out *after* the session, possibly in writing up notes, de-brief with a colleague, in supervision, or through the use of Interpersonal Process Recall. The purpose of reflection after the event, is to explore why you did what you did, the process between you and your client (interpersonal) and within you (intrapersonal). The third element is Anticipatory Reflection, which provides a forward-looking perspective and the opportunity to pause and examine hopes and intentions, requirements and potentially unforeseen areas for oneself, one's colleagues and especially for the client(s), set against the context of the anticipated activity.

Considering all three dimensions, this provides with a useful cycle of reflection or reflective continuum for supervision:

See Diagram 1 below.

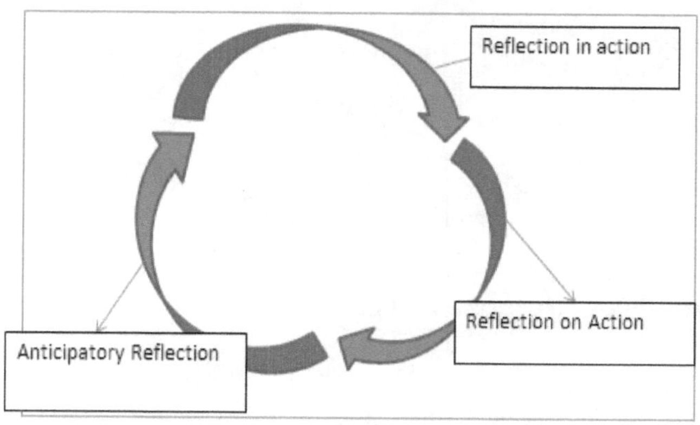

In addition to this reflective continuum, are the following key ingredients presented at the 6IATC (2012). These ingredients form the concentric rings of our model of supervision for Outdoor and Adventure Therapy (Natynczuk and Schwenk, 2012, In process Diagram 2) that continues to be researched and refined. Taking each of the rings, and working from the outside toward the centre, we will briefly expand upon their relevance and contribution to supervision.

There are other models of reflective practice in the outdoors (e.g. Hickman 2011; 2012) that say similar things and, because directly related to outdoor work, may be useful to consider. In addition to this reflective continuum, are the following key ingredients presented at the 6IATC (2012). These ingredients form the concentric rings of our model of supervision for Outdoor and Adventure Therapy (Natynczuk and Schwenk, 2012, unpublished Diagram 2) that continues to be researched and refined. Taking each of the rings, and working from the outside toward the centre, we will briefly expand upon their relevance and contribution to supervision.

See Diagram 2 below:

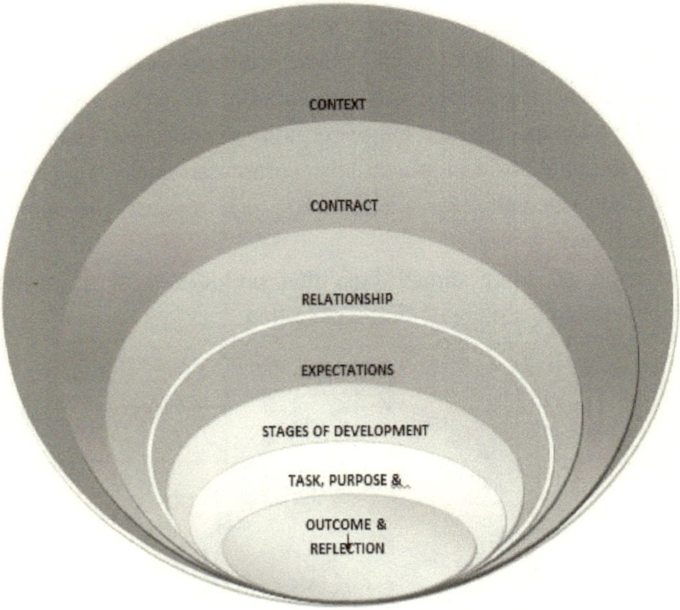

1. Context: Vision, Purpose and Setting

Context is everything: it is essential for the supervisor to be clear regarding the context within which the adventure therapy is to occur. Context refers to the agency and its personnel, the vision of the 'agency' and their particular ethos in delivering adventure therapy. Context also refers to the setting and purpose of the adventure therapy i.e., how it intends to draw upon and utilise adventure, what is meant by the terms 'adventure' and 'therapy', and to what extent adventure is used e.g., climbing, caving, canoeing etc. for therapeutic purposes.

Other key elements of Context are the issues of: Ethics, Responsibility & Boundaries. Working within an organisational context, that draws upon multi-disciplinary teams involves working with difference and respecting issues of equality and diversity, and managing organisational dynamics. Any supervisory work undertaken on behalf of the Agency needs to be cognizant of Agency's Mission and Vision. Ethics refers to the Ethical Framework for Good practice (2010) or Codes of Practice of the associated professional bodies linked to Adventure Therapy e.g. BACP (British Association for Counselling and Psychotherapy), and other professional bodies associated with the various adventure activities undertaken, thereby providing an over-arching framework of ethical practice and standards. Associated with this set of guidelines for good practice are the organisation's own policies and procedures, and principles of legal Responsibility and Boundaries – that relate in particular to the role of adventure therapy practitioners in relation to their clients, and referring agencies, and in working practice within the team itself.

Given the above, it is essential for all supervision participants (supervisee/adventure therapist/practitioner), supervisor and organisation, to determine the role and scope of both Adventure Therapy and supervision. These ingredients are all part of the Contract Agreement.

2. Contract: Expectations and a Duty of Care

Taking a closer look at this contract, it is essential to be transparent regarding the contractual arrangements between the Agency and Adventure therapist/practitioner, the client, referring agencies and the supervisor. All parties need to be clear about what has been agreed, what is to be delivered and the associated methods of delivery i.e., walking, climbing, caving, canoeing, high ropes, bush craft etc. and the embedded purpose or intention for the activity. Written consent needs to be in place to ensure all parties fully understand the risks associated with adventure therapy both from an adventure and therapeutic perspective. Supervision and the agency contractual arrangements enable the adventure therapy practitioner to be clear about these core ingredients.

Carroll (1996) established five roles the supervisor undertakes when working within an organisational context or setting: Firstly, to help supervisees work within and satisfy the contractual demands of the organisation. This may include consideration of values and practice, ethical dilemmas, and areas of responsibility. The second role is to enable supervisees to control and be mindful of the flow of information within the organisation. The third task centres more on the healthcare of the practitioner within the organisation while the fourth task supports the supervisee in their working interface with the organisation and finally the fifth task is to ensure the supervisee looks after themselves while delivering a service to the client on behalf of the organisation.

3. Relationship: Ethics and Responsibilities, Power and Autonomy

In any therapeutic undertaking the relationship rests at the heart of its success. Both the practitioner and client bring the present and also the impact of past relationships into the here and now of their therapeutic relationship, and this is replicated in supervision. In addition, the interplay of peripheral relationship dynamics e.g., client's family (past & present), practitioner's own family (past & present) together with their experience of the organisation or agency with whom they work, and the supervisor's relationship experiences, all interact to form the current context of the relationships. It is particularly helpful therefore, to draw upon systems theory when examining the relationships within adventure therapy.

See Diagram 3 below:

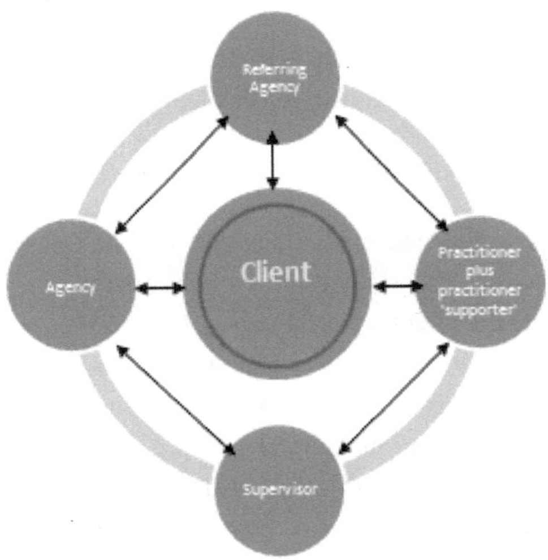

The supervisory process enables practitioners to consider the inter-relatedness of their work, the opportunity and necessity of co-dependence between practitioner and client, the implicit and explicit contract between agency and agency. The potential for parallel process and transference, counter-transference is more than likely as client material (and occasionally practitioner material) becomes less inhibited and the practitioner-client relationship becomes more intense.

Disequilibrium is a key component of adventure therapy and is dependent upon the levels of trust within the therapeutic alliance. To promote safe practice, the adventure therapist often works with another therapist or field staff, who becomes an adjunct to the therapeutic process. Their role in relation to the Adventure Therapist and client needs to be fully explored. The question regarding supervision of this individual would also need to be explored – especially if either the therapeutic process or the adventure aspect became traumatic or personally disturbing.

Once again, Ethics and Boundaries play a key part in ensuring not only 'adventure' safe practice but also therapeutic good practice. This necessitates ongoing professional development for the practitioner and the ability to make key decisions on behalf of the client when the situation dictates. This calls into play the issues of Power and Autonomy and the ethical principles of beneficence and non-maleficence (wellbeing – least harm) set against encouraging and facilitating the client's sense of self and right to be self-governing. In some situations, often quite isolated and intense, the inter-relationship among participants may become easily blurred. Supervision offers an opportunity for reflection (before and after) whereby a practitioner can review and prepare for what happened or should happen, and make sense of the situation, gain some learning and insight into themselves and adventure therapy and better understand and work with the client. Some of these paras are useful, and well-written but I still think writing a 'why do we need it' article maybe more appropriate at this point.

4. Expectations and Duty of Care

According to Gabriel and Casemore (2009, p.112) "The therapist has a responsibility to act on the basis of the principle of beneficence or welfare, in order that the therapy is of benefit to the client. In legal terms, this would translate as the therapist owing a duty of care to the client." Clearly this is an area that needs to be fully explored and agreed upon. The organisation and its Adventure Therapy Practitioners need to be clear and concrete regarding relevant aspects of the law and any child and Vulnerable People Protection issues. Supervision and the Agency can work together to ensure these areas are constantly revisited and woven into the fabric of any contract and delivery of adventure therapy. These safeguarding issues reflect best practice for all parties concerned.

Everyone needs to know who will do what and when and how, and who has professional responsibility and the extent of that responsibility. Creating an atmosphere where expectations can be voiced and explored simply models good practice when working with clients in any setting. This also applies to establishing awareness around the practitioner's stage of development and recognising their particular on-going professional development needs and aspirations, set alongside the agency's expectations of the practitioner.

5. Stage of Development: Training and Development Needs of Both Practitioner and Client

This is an area frequently overlooked and yet brings a valuable dimension of understanding both from an adventure therapy practitioner's perspective and also from the client's perspective. Supervision offers a safe space within which to explore the practitioner's own sense of competence (capability vs limitations) to both develop as a practitioner and deliver the contractual agreement. Because supervision is not line management, there is sufficient safety in exploring what went well and what did not, what skills were required and how competent the practitioner felt in deploying them, and what has surfaced as a potential area for future training and development.

This focus can also be directed toward the client's level of personal, physical, emotional and cognitive development, enabling the practitioner and supervisor to form a starting point and to review the outcome of any interventions. Understanding the client's stage of development enables the practitioner to be realistic, yet appropriately challenging, in his/her work with the client. It informs the practitioner about what life issues/stages the client may be experiencing, for example, and provides a backdrop of developmental context in which to establish and mutually agree some of the tasks, purpose and limitations of the work with the client.

6. Outcome: Task, Purpose and Limitations

Raising this aspect of the work in supervision enables the practitioner to become much clearer both with the client and agency about the why and how they are going to work together and to engage in a discussion regarding the Task, Purpose & Limitations as key aspects of the contract. This generates greater clarity about who the contract is for, any hidden agenda (e.g. desired outcome of the referring agency, or any other third party), potential areas of client concern and/or resistance, client preference and viewpoint, creating a shared realistic expectations and issues regarding power and autonomy within the adventure therapy relationship.

A key element of supervision within adventure therapy is the necessity to review practice and issues related to the activity itself e.g. health and safety, preparation, procedures, and the skills and qualifications or fitness to practice (although it is the Agency who is the employer) necessary to do the job. It is important that practitioners remain competent, insured, with ongoing professional development in appropriate fields to expand their development both in terms of their own personal adventure experiences and developments in best practice. Accompanying in the role of the 'third person' can enable practitioners to refresh their skills and gain additional training. Doing risk assessments is an ongoing process in adventure therapy as the variables can change from moment to moment, taking into account not only the client's willingness and ability to engage and continue with the tasks, but the conditions associated with the activity itself e.g., geographic location, weather conditions, physical and mental wellbeing of all participants, standard of kit etc. Whilst probably discussed frequently in supervision, this also remains Agency responsibility.

7. Outcome and Reflection: Solution-Focused, Generative Support

In adventure therapy something happens for everyone! Supervision enables the practitioner to reflect upon the contract, the client, the relationship, the activity, what went well, what was unexpected, how things could be done differently etc. It offers a 360 review and de-brief and a way to capture and consider the event and process.

Supervision, while upholding an ethical stance, is a form of generative support. It encourages the practitioner to look inwards (a process encouraged for the client) and to think about what is going on for them – how they feel about themselves, in relation to the client, the 'third person', the contract, the outcome and so forth. Adventure Therapy is shrouded in challenge and new experience and for the practitioner, it is important to give sufficient time to reflect on what has happened – to pause and catch up with the experience and discuss the journey. This brings new insight and learning and personal development for the practitioner which can only serve to enhance their work and ensure Best Practice.

Taking a closer look at a solution focused model of supervision adapted to work within Outdoor and Adventure therapy (Natynczuk, this volume) we are especially concerned with identifying what the supervisee does well, where their strongest competencies are, how they cope when things do not go well, and what they, their colleagues and clients notice when they are at their best. It must be remembered that the solution-focused model is a model for change and not for risk assessments. In areas of high risk any muddling of change and risk assessment may be dangerous to the client and supervisee. As with using solution focused techniques for therapy, the supervisor and supervisee co-construct a future where the problem(s) being discussed in supervision are no longer present or are being coped with (solutions are good enough). A solution focused conversation done well is particularly good at exploring the fine details of practice and identifying small changes, easily enacted, that will make a difference. It also helps staff become more aware of their own significance in influencing situations; more aware of their own skills, strengths and resources and more aware of how to avoid getting stuck with a piece of work. In this model the supervisor avoids giving advice and takes care to work with the supervisee's own situation avoiding solutions that involve other people.

Typical questions are:

- How will you know that supervision is helpful to you?
- What situations are hardest for you and how will you know you are moving forward?
- What will tell you that you are working with this client's agenda and keeping the client's safety in mind?
- What will you be pleased to notice about how you address the company's concerns in a way that informs the client and encourages their co-operation?
- How will you know that your work is becoming more productive?
- Imagine that you do become more hopeful about this piece of work. What will you be noticing that will be helping you to feel different about it?

These questions form part of a constructive supervision session that invites and enables the supervisee to explore issues of concern and celebration. It provides a backdrop of generative support, and building upon an effective working alliance that is open rather than collusive, facilitates the practitioner's wellbeing and development.

Stress in the Workplace

Despite working in often enviable, outdoor environments, and doing work that yields both personal and professional gratification, this work is not without its own set of stressors. The hours are often unsociable, including long trips away from home and the family potentially spending more time with clients than with loved ones. Weekends can easily get consumed, and for some, the work commitments mean being away from home from a few nights to even a few weeks. Research undertaken by Marchand, Russell and Cross (2009) "confirmed a high turnover rate of instructors and high challenges experienced with non-work related issues, particularly in sustaining romantic personal relationships." They also identified three constructs related to difficulty levels experienced on the job: a) time and schedule constraint; b) emotional anxiety and stress-related issues;

and c) physical and mental challenges. The authors of this paper discuss some interesting factors, related to instructor age, and the impact of having a spouse or partner also in the profession or related activity. Tenure in a position was another factor the authors highlighted would benefit from additional research, looking at career progression and opportunities for development within the field. Gass (1993) also believed additional research regarding personal relationships for outdoor and adventure instructors would be beneficial. Certainly, maintaining significant relationships, in addition to managing general obligations and attending to personal matters, while away for long or frequent stays in backcountry environments is a challenge. Marchand, Russell and Cross (2009) believe these ingredients may have a significant impact upon job retention in this industry.

Unlike counseling, psychotherapy, social work or many parallel fields, outdoor and adventure therapy work can mean living at quite close personal quarters with clients, where the boundaries become blurred and relationships more intense. Since something is happening for everyone, practitioners are as much part of the process as clients and not exempt from their own material being drawn out into the open once more. The sense of being 'on duty' can feel stressful when it extends into 24-7.

Often the nature of the activity can draw upon and utilise a co-dependency, not only amongst the professionals within the group but, on occasion, toward the clients also. Indeed, this may even be a strategy to enable the client(s) to develop and gain a stronger sense of self through achievement and identity. Or it could occur during an emergency when additional help is required. This can be a stressful occurrence, and requires practitioners maintain a clear sense of their role, responsibilities and boundaries. Keeping in mind the numerous responsibilities can also become overwhelming when other things are on our mind. Maintaining a high level of focus during any extreme sport activity requires considerable mental stamina.

Another stressor is concerning the provenance of the work. In examining the rich diversity of outdoor and adventure therapy, there is an underlying hint of uncertainty about where and how the work comes. Contracts are often variable and/or seasonal and it is not unusual for practitioners to need a backup stream of income. The high level of unpredictability in work can have a serious impact upon practitioner wellbeing. A line manager may well have tremendous empathy for the practitioner, but may also have to choose who to give work to if there is limited work available, or assign practitioners to work with one another when there is unvoiced discomfort within the team. While these issues should be explored within management, practitioners might need to carefully tease out the issues and use supervision as a safe place in which clarify the situation in their minds first.

Outdoor and adventure practitioners are frequently passionate about the environments within which they work, and enthusiastic about the activities they undertake. However, combining work with pleasure can easily lead to burnout and practitioners can experience the inspiration of their work, as well as the desperation. Practitioners can also feel personally responsible for the outcome of the client's experience and again, it is essential that the practitioner draws upon supervision to gain insight into their work.

How Can Supervision Provide Emotional Support and Help Prevent Burnout?

Protecting employee's health and safety in a physical sense with appropriate and good use of ropes, buoyancy aids, harnesses and helmets etc. goes without argument in the UK. Protecting employees' mental health is not as widely accepted and often the provision for supervision falls at the first hurdle for funding. Burnout is a chronic problem in the outdoor industry especially within the sector working with challenging youth. Contributing factors include when organisational expectations are far greater than a worker's ability to satisfy them, when working relationships with colleagues and clients become stressful, or when roles are under resourced. Some organisations provide supervision through their line management. It is unlikely that such a hierarchical arrangement will provide a forum based on mutual respect, openness and honesty which allows one to talk free from fear of an unfavourable job appraisal, or fear of not being re-employed when freelance contracts come around again. Good supervision gives an opportunity to unburden oneself of emotional baggage collected during expeditions, to guard against transference and counter transference issues whereby emotions are transferred or projected between client and therapist.

Good supervision should leave the worker feeling competent, valued, capable, supported, enabled, and confident in their abilities with a sense of moving forward in their work. All of which is more helpful than being left to fend for oneself with the risk of taking unresolved and unexamined problems and difficulties home where partners, family and friends might understand and might be able to help.

Beyond the benefits to client work; where having a regular space within which to unpack the outcomes and process of our work, and where the emotional and psychological aspects of health and safety and client wellbeing can be fully explored, supervision has much to offer the Adventure Practitioner In Summary, supervision helps the practitioner by:

- Providing a safe place in which to debrief
- Establishing clear contracts and boundaries
- Creating opportunities to discuss one's practice with another professional outside of line management
- Exploring what works well
- Exploring the supervisee's strengths, abilities and resources to move forward in their work and/or cope with difficulties
- Discuss any need for further support and to help staff become more aware of their own significance in influencing situations

In offering a reflective space, supervision encourages us to stand back from the work, to separate ourselves from the entanglement of intense engagement with our clients, and look to our own needs as well as those of the client. This has a tremendous bearing on preventing burnout, or identifying practitioner needs and addressing them in good time.

Resistance to Supervision within Outdoor and Adventure Therapy

Outdoor adventure instructors tend to be self-reliant and used to working and playing in difficult conditions where events have to be endured. Some undergraduate students of adventure leadership even expect to have periods of burnout. When burnout does come, instructors will find employment outside the industry or take extended leave, perhaps never to return to working with challenging youth. There is undoubtedly a culture of accepting things as they are and being tough enough to see it through. Organisations that invest in their employees and provide supervision see a very high retention rate for staff (source) and it follows that adventure organisations would expect less disaffected behaviour from staff, less absenteeism and increased presenteeism, with a concomitant improvement in quality of adventure provision from cared for, and motivated, staff.

Suspicion and resistance to supervision is not restricted to adventure instructors (Cottrell 2002). Instructors who are clear that they are involved in facilitating therapeutic adventures might be receptive to supervision when it is part of being a professional in a better defined aspect of working outdoors (Adventure Therapy) whereby instructors are working within parameters of a therapeutic model which they understand rather that making it up as they go along because of some vague notion that doing adventures is good for personal development. Given that supervision is a requirement for working as a counsellor within the UK, the authors hope that when practitioners of therapeutic adventures are eventually recognised as professionals, supervision will be just as much of a requirement to practise as a current first aid certificate is needed to validate National Governing Body Awards for adventure sports leadership and coaching.

WHERE DO WE GO FROM HERE?

As the field of Outdoor and Adventure and Therapy expands in all directions it is timely for supervision to become a natural and fully integrated component of this activity. The challenge that lies before us is twofold: to develop new models of supervision that best fit the needs and requirements of Outdoor and Adventure Therapy and secondly, to overcome the resistance that prevents practitioners from embracing this tool. These two aspects go hand in hand: Supervision is a concept and activity that can easily be adapted to suit practitioner needs as its flexible nature lends itself to a multimodal approach. Perhaps one of the pathways to overcoming resistance is to take supervision out into the field and 'give it a go'. By recycling the knowledge that comes from this experience, adaptions may occur that develop into more appropriate bespoke formats or models. There are endless possibilities with supervision and its potential is only hampered by our reticence and resistance, lack of courage and vision.

REFERENCES

Bernard, J. M. & Goodyear, R. K. (1992). *Fundamentals of clinical supervision.* London: Pearson.

Bernard, J. M. & Goodyear, R. K. (2004). *Fundamentals of clinical supervision.* London: Pearson.

Bond, T. (2010). *Standards and ethics for counselling in action.* London: Sage.

Briggs, J. R. & Miller, G. (2008) Success Enhancing Supervision, *Journal of Family Psychotherapy*, 16:102, 199-222.

Carroll, M. (1996). *Counselling supervision: Theory, skills and practice.* London: Cassells.

Carroll, M. (1999). Training in the tasks of supervision. In E. Holloway & M. Carroll (Eds.), *Training, Counselling, Supervision* (pp. 44-66). London: Sage.

Carroll, M. & Holloway, E. (1999) *Counselling supervision in context*. London: Sage.

Carroll, M. & Tholstrup, M. (2001). *Integrative approaches to supervision*. London: Jessica Kinglsey.

Carroll, M. & Walton, M. (Eds.). (1997). *Handbook of counselling in organisations.* London: Sage.

Clarkson, P. & Wilson, S. (2003) *The therapeutic relationship*. London: Whurr Publishers.

Conway, P. F. (2001). Anticipator reflection while learning to teach. From a temporarily truncated to a temporally distributed model of reflection in teacher education. *Teaching and Teacher Education*, 19(1), 89-106.

Cottrell, S (2002). Suspicion, resistance, tokenism and mutiny: Problematic dynamics relevant to the implementation of clinical supervision in nursing. *Journal of Psychiatric and Mental Health Nursing*. (9), 667-671.

Dempsey, R. (2012). Supervising in organisations. *Healthcare Counselling and Psychotherapy Journal, 12*(1), 4-10.

Falvley, J. E. (2002) *Managing clinical supervision: Ethical practice and legal risk management*. Pacific Grove, CA: Brooks/Cole.

Feltham, C. & Dryden, W. (1994) *Developing counsellor supervision.* London: Sage.

Gabriel, L. & Casemore, R. Ed. (2009). *Relational ethics in practice: Narratives from counselling and psychotherapy*. London: Routledge.

Gass, M. A. (1993). *Adventure therapy: Therapeutic applications of adventure programming.* Dubuque, IA: Kendall/Hunt.

Inskipp, F. & Proctor, B. (1994). *Making the most of supervision*. London: Cascade.

Inskipp, F., & Proctor, B. (2001). *The art, craft and tasks of counselling supervision, Part 1: Making the most of supervision* (2nd ed.). Twickenham: Cascade.

Hawkins, P., & Shohet, R. (2006). *Supervision in the helping professions.* Maidenhead: McGraw-Hill.

Henderson, P. (2009). *Supervisor training: Issues and approaches.* London. Karnac.

Marchand, G., Russell, K. C. & Cross, R. (2009). An Empirical Examination of outdoor Behavioural \healthcare field Instructor Job-Related Stress and Retention. *Journal of Experiential Education,* **31** (3): 359-375.

Masten, A. S. (2009). Ordinary Magic: Lessons from research on resilience in human development (PDF). *Education Canada, 49* (3): 28–32.

Mitchels, B. & Bond, T. (2011). *Legal issues across counselling & psychotherapy settings.* A Guide for Practice. BACP in association with London: Sage.

Natynczuk, S. & Schwenk, E. (In process). *Adventure therapy and supervision.* Manuscript in preparation for submission.

Page, S. & Woskett, V. (1994). *Supervising the counsellor.* London: Routledge.

Page, S. & Wosket, V. (2001). *Supervising the counsellor: A cyclical model.* Hove: Routledge.

Richards, K. (2009).In A. Pryor, C. Carpenter, C.L. Norton (Eds)., *Emerging insights: Proceedings of the Fifth International Adventure Therapy Conference 2009.* Prague: European Science and Art Publishing.

Ronnestad, M. H. & Skovholt, T.M. (2013). *The developing practitioner: Growth and stagnation of therapists and counsellors.* New York:Routledge.

Scaife, J. (2010). *Supervising the reflective practitioner: An essential guide to theory and practice.* London: Routledge.

Schon, D. A. (1983). *The reflective practitioner.* Jossey-Bass: San Francisco, CA.

Stoltenberg, C. D. & Delworth, U. (1987). Supervising counsellors & therapists: A developmental approach. San Francisco: Jossey Bass.

Van Manen, M. (1990). *Researching lived experience: Human science for an action sensitive pedagogy.* Albany, NY: State University of New York Press.

Wheeler, S. & King, D. (Eds.) (2001). *Supervising counsellors – Issues of responsibility.* London: SAGE Publications.

Wheeler, S., & Richards, K. (2007). The impact of clinical supervision on counselors and therapists, their practice and their clients. A systematic review of the literature, *Counselling and Psychotherapy Research, 7*(1), 54-65.

CHAPTER 38

Adventure Therapy and Natural Environments

Alan Ewert

ABSTRACT

This paper discusses the influence that natural environments can play in the field of Adventure Therapy. Various theories and concepts are discussed that highlight the potential ways that natural environments can be effective in both therapy and overall human health. More specifically, is there a connection between adventure-based therapeutic programs that occur in natural environments and human health? This presentation argues that the answer to this question is unequivocally "yes." The extant literature and personal experience suggests that adventure therapeutic programming is positively associated with issues related to human health, and this connection is greatly strengthened when these programs occur in natural and outdoor environments. Moreover, there are three reasons why adventure therapeutic programming can be effective in promoting health and wellness: (1) the environment in which most adventure activities take place, (2) the activities themselves that typically require physical activity and movement, and (3) participation in adventure activities often help develop social networks and support, that is conducive to personal health.

INTRODUCTION

Is there a connection between adventure therapy (AT) programs that occur in natural environments and human health? This paper suggests that based on the extant literature, a substantial number of empirically-derived studies, and personal experience, the answer to this question is unequivocally "yes." Moreover, the extant literature, past research efforts, and personal experience consistently suggest that AT can be positively related to human health, and this relationship can be greatly enhanced when these programs occur in natural and outdoor environments. There are three reasons why AT in natural environments can be effective in promoting health and wellness: (1) the natural environment serves as a setting where most AT take place, (2) natural environments often necessitate activities that typically require physical activity and movement, and (3) participation in natural environment-based AT often facilitate the development of social networks, reflection, and a personal connection that are conducive to personal health.

To further the argument that natural environments can augment the effectiveness of AT, this paper involves the following parts. First, we start with a brief description of the terms natural environment and health. This is followed by a synopsis of natural environments and the values that society places on them. We expand on this thinking by moving to a summary of some of the major theories underlying the belief that nature can be a particularly important variable in various aspects of human health. These theories include the biophilia hypothesis, psychoevolutionary theory, and attention restoration theory. Following this, the specific benefits of adventure programming as related to health and wellness are discussed. Finally, we explore the concept of Intentionally Designed Experiences (IDEs). It is through these IDEs that adventure programming can serve as a particularly effective catalyst in promoting behaviors that lead to positive human health.

HEALTH, NATURAL ENVIRONMENTS AND SOCIETAL VALUES

Definitions

Health is now thought of as more than simply an absence of disease. Rather it takes on a much more comprehensive perspective that includes the psychological, sociological, spiritual, and cognitive, as well as the physical. Accordingly, health is defined using the statement made by the World Health Organization,

> Health is the state of complete physical, mental, and social well-being and not merely the absence of disease or infirmity.

In a similar fashion, natural environments can also be defined using a variety of terms and concepts. For the sake of this paper, natural environments are thought of as natural surroundings, all living and non-living things that take place in a natural manner on earth or on a particular part of it.

Obviously, the value society places on health is self-evident but not always behaviorally regulated. That is, most of us would place a high value on being in good health; many individuals, however, do not follow a set of behaviors that are always beneficial to our personal health.

Societal Values

While the value placed on good health is self-evident, what about the value society places on natural environments (NE). Natural environments (NE) have long been considered special areas for a variety of important reasons, including providing ecological baseline data for the establishment of protected zones, understanding impact analyses, and other tangible and intangible values (Hendee & Dawson, 2008). Some would argue, however, that a more important value offered from natural landscapes is the potential for human growth and transformation. That is, these areas provide avenues, either through the landscape itself or the types of activities typically engaged in these settings, to change human attitudes, belief systems, and behaviors. Consider the following quote from the perspective of a wilderness user:

> I'm a city person, born and raised in New York City. My interest in outdoor environments and wilderness seems to stem from a primordial hunger to get back to roots, to nature, to peace and quiet . . . I have a deep conviction that the source and strength of our lives is in the wilderness, that it is a place of renewal physically and psychically . . . The wilderness, like music, touches something universally felt and experienced by people and perhaps has the power to heal them and bring them together. (Sydney Fine, Wilderness Psychology Newsletter)

There can be little argument that society places value on different components associated with nature and natural environments. While historically this worth was measured in the form of "goods" such as board feet of timber, cubic feet of free flowing water, or tons of a particular mineral, this worth has now extended to other, less tangible, benefits. In addition, natural settings provide a substantial number of functions related to ecosystem processes such as the absorption of pollutants and nutrient recycling. However, beyond the obvious material outputs provided by natural environments, there also exists a number of values that are often linked to natural environments that are either ethereal or difficult to measure (Harmon & Putney, 2003).

For example, individuals often place a high value on many of the functions that are inherently performed by naturally functioning ecosystems, such as the fresh air or fresh water that all of us, both need and enjoy. There are some values, however, that present a more complicated picture in that they represent both intrinsic and extrinsic worth. For example, natural environments are "valued" by some individuals because of the therapeutic impacts they may have on individuals (Bandoroff & Newes, 2004). For example, many report that a walk in the local park or visit to a natural area experienced a sense of restoration and revitalization (Johansson, Hartig, & Staats, 2011). And herein rests the two assumptions underlying the argument that natural environments are connected to human health, and ultimately to adventure therapy. First, it is posited and supported by a substantial amount of past and on-going research that natural environments have the capacity to promote health and wellness in societies across the globe (Frumkin, 2003). Second, while nature by itself can be good for you, structured programs such as those offered through adventure therapy can make it even more effective. Following these assumptions, what then are health-related benefits associated with natural environments and the corresponding theoretical constructs explaining the accrual of these benefits?

Benefits Associated with Nature

> The enjoyment of scenery employs the mind without fatigue and yet exercises it; tranquilizes it and yet enlivens it; and thus, though the influence of the mind over the body, gives the effect of refreshing rest and reinvigoration to the whole system. (Frederick Law Olmstead)

In the above quote, Frederick Law Olmstead (1822-1903) alluded to the fact that viewing scenes depicting nature was extremely beneficial to individuals, and more collectively, to communities and groups (aesthetic value). Yet, beyond the aesthetical quality and tranquillity associated with a beautiful natural scene, do natural environments have any redeeming qualities and contributions relative to adventure therapy and human health and wellness? Thus, three questions provide the logic train for understanding the influence of natural environments on human health:

1. Is nature beneficial?
2. How is it beneficial?
3. Why is nature beneficial?

The literature follows what most of us have already suspected, namely, that nature provides individuals with positive and beneficial experiences (Hartig et al., 2011). Moreover, natural environments mediate these experiences in essentially five ways:

1. Recovery from stress and attention fatigue
2. Encouragement of physical activity
3. Facilitating social contact
4. Encouraging optimal development
5. Providing opportunities for personal development and sense of purpose

Of the five mediating factors listed above, recovery from stress and attention fatigue has received the most research attention (Bowler, Buyung-Ali, Knight, & Pullin, 2010) followed by increased physical activity (Kaczyski & Henderson, 2007). Within the contexts of stress and attention fatigue, three theories serve to provide the explanatory foundation, and include the Biophilia Hypothesis, Psychoevoluntionary Theory, and Attention Restoration Theory.

Biophilia Hypothesis

The Biophilia Hypothesis, first described by E. O. Wilson (1984, 1993), states that there is innate tendency to affiliate with natural things and that this mind-body connection reacts fully to nature. Thus, when humans are exposed to natural objects or views, a response is elicited within the physiological, psychological, and emotional domains. There is a wide range of emotions experienced when individuals are placed in natural environments including, attraction, aversion, peacefulness, and fear-driven anxiety. Kellert (1993) elaborated on this thinking by suggesting that people have a biological need to feel connected to the natural world. As a result of this linkage, the response to a nonthreatening natural environment stimulus has a positive effect on an individual's emotional state, which, in turn, affects their physiological activity levels and autonomic responses (Berto, 2007).

Psychoevoluntionary Theory

The psychoevoluntionary theory emphasizes the connection between natural environments and their effect on issues such as stress (Ulrich, 1983). The underlying premise of the theory is that because of our ancestral direct connection to natural landscapes, humans can experience immediate reactions to natural environments well before they have had a chance to analyze these environments through cognitive processes. For example, stress connotes a physiological response to situations that threaten well-being and is often manifested in physiological indictors such as increased autonomic arousal (e.g., increased heart rate or elevated blood pressure). A generalized model of stress is illustrated in the following:

Task Demand → Abilities/Resources Unable to Meet Demand →
Stress Reaction → Impaired Performance

Conversely, stress recovery occurs in settings that evoke interest, pleasantness, and calm. And this is where biophilia and psychoevoluntionary theory tend to come together. That is, humans are attracted to natural environments and this attraction helps reduce negative factors such as stress. Indeed, natural landscapes can contain a number of dimensions that are associated with restoring scenes, including:

1. Moderate complexity
2. A focal point
3. Natural contents, most notably, vegetation and water

Thus, natural environments serve as stress recovery settings and involve a number of important outcomes for humans under stress. These dimensions involve replacing negative affect with positive feelings, inhibiting negative thoughts, and decreases in autonomic and cortical responses such as fight, flight, or freeze. Psychoevolutionary theory can be conceptualized in the following way:

Stressor
↓
Exposure to Nature
↓
Shift Toward a Positive Emotional State
↓
Positive Changes in Physiological Systems
↓
Moderately High Levels of Sustained Attention
↓
Restoration

One of the most salient studies supporting the concept of the pychoevolutionary theory, investigated the impacts of viewing nature on recovery rates of surgery patients. After randomly assigning surgery patients to either a room with a view of nature or a hospital room without such a room, Ulrich (1984) found evidence that the patients with the view of nature had shorter recovery times, required less pain medication, and had lower incidents of medical issues associated with their surgery, when compared to the patients without the view of nature. Ulrich (1981) suggests the results from this study point to a proposition that people benefit most from visual contact with nature, as opposed to urban environments lacking nature. Thus, for individuals experiencing stress or excessive arousal, nature views appear to reduce arousal more effectively than urban scenes, and hence are more beneficial in a psychophysiological sense.

When considering the AT situation, it becomes clear that natural environments can serve as not just a "personal testing ground" but also can exert a calming and centering impact from which the individual student, patient, or client emerges better able to deal with the negative input from life such as time pressure, work/school-related stress, or social disconformities (e.g., not adjusting to the social group).

Attention Restoration Theory

Attention Restoration Theory (ART) posits that individual attention is either voluntary or directed (involuntary). Directed attention requires effort, plays a central role in achieving and maintaining focus, is usually under a cognitive-control process, controls distraction through the use of inhibition, plays a central role in problem-solving, and is susceptible to fatigue. It is this susceptibility to fatigue that forms the underlying role of natural environments in ART. Essentially, the ART theoretical model assumes these components:

Directed Attention Requires Effort to
Maintain Focus and Avoid Distractions

↓

Directed Attention Fatigues and Results in Difficulty
in Focusing, Irritability, and Distraction

↓

Involuntary Attention Results in a Replenishment
of Directed Attention Mechanisms

According to Kaplan and Kaplan (1989), restorative settings, as provided through natural environments, can be effective in aiding in the recovery of directed attention fatigue through the following properties:

1. *Fascination* - engages attention effortlessly thus allowing directed attention to rest
2. *Being away* - physically or conceptually different from one's usual environment
3. *Extent* - setting is rich and coherent enough to engage the mind and promote exploration
4. *Compatibility* - implies a good fit between one's inclinations/purposes and the activities supported by the setting

Moreover, fascination can take two forms: hard fascination and soft fascination. Hard fascination refers to experiences or activities that are intense, riveting, and limited space or time for reflection or cognitive activity. Soft fascination involves activities or experiences that are moderate in intensity and can focus an individual's attention while allowing for reflection and cognition. Peaceful, natural settings are often thought to be good locations for experiencing soft fascination.

A substantial amount of research has demonstrated the efficacy of the attention restoration construct. For example, people exposed to natural settings generally report better performance on attention demanding tasks (Taylor, Kuo, & Sullivan, 2001; 2002). Natural views from home are positively related to effective functioning and feeling at peace and negatively related to distraction (Kaplan, 2001). People living near nature report improved interpersonal relations and effectiveness at handling major life issues (Kuo, 2001). Exposure to natural environments may be related to improved self-control, reduced ADD symptoms, and improved care in treating dementia (Bossen, 2010). Thus, natural environments can elicit an attention refocusing and sense of restoration through the mechanism described by Attention Restoration Theory. Having explored how natural environments can influence human health, what then are some of the processes through which adventure therapy can interact with the natural setting to produce a more therapeutic venue?

The Health Benefits of Adventure Therapy

The literature and my own personal experiences generally point to a connection between human health and natural environments. Does the same connection carry over to experiences and activities associated with adventure therapy (AT)? For example, aspects of quality of life (QoL) that are often influenced by natural environments include: perceived safety, physical health and exercise, emotional well-being, a sense of community, social interaction, enjoyment, appropriate levels of stimulation, and a sense of autonomy and control. Beyond the obvious fact that most adventure activities occur in natural or outdoor environments are there some underlying commonalities that link AT, natural landscapes, and human health?

In this paper adventure therapy (AT) is defined as "a variety of therapeutic activities and experiences utilizing a close interaction with the natural environment, that contain elements of real or apparent risk, in which the outcome is uncertain, but can be influenced by the participant and/or circumstance" (Ewert & Voight, 2012). Several terms have emerged that seek to better describe the type of therapeutic venue being utilized and include: wilderness therapy, adventure based-counseling, or adventure therapy (Gass, Gillis & Russell, 2012). Often inherent in these programs is to use an underlying clinical approach, couched within an "APIE" (Assessment, Planning, Implementation, and Evaluation) process or structure (Bullock & Mahon, 2001). Usually each client or participant is assessed on an individual basis for purposes of goal setting. The *assessment* of a client then becomes the foundation for treatment and in the *planning* of an appropriate therapeutic experience, often in the form of an "individual treatment plan." The treatment plan directs the interventions or activities which are then *implemented* and the client is observed and assessed for improvement or, in some cases, re-assessment. The outcomes of the treatment plans, or therapeutic interventions, are measured through *evaluation* at the end of participation in the adventure activity or program (Groff & Datillo, 2000). Despite the plethora of AT programs, Baldwin, Pershing, and Magnuson (2004) posit that there are some commonalities across many of these experiences, including the following items:

1. Planned and purposive use of adventure-based activities with specific goals
2. Real-life learning contexts
3. Participant becomes agent of change
4. Goal-directed challenges necessitating the use of individual or group generated solutions.
5. Outdoor or natural environment setting
6. Small group (usually ten or less) context
7. Structured facilitation

In addition, McKenzie (2000) attributes these outcomes to four characteristics common to many adventure education experiences: (a) the unfamiliar nature of the physical environment, (b) the incremental and progressive sequencing of the challenges presented through the adventure education experience, (c) the "processing" of the experience in order to identify and organize meaning for the participant, and (d) the use of small groups to facilitate issues such as reciprocity, group cohesiveness, interpersonal relationships, and the balance between group belongingness and individual autonomy. In addition to the four components described by McKenzie, the adventure education experience also provides opportunities for outdoor physical activity, facing concrete challenges while being part of a small team, and being part of a shared experience that can facilitate future dialogue and discourse. Thus, many of the attributes associated with adventure program activities and experiences are similar to those attributed to healthy lifestyles or behaviors.

Research has demonstrated a strong link between physical exercise and human health (Pretty, et al., 2007). In addition, there are a number of physiological health-related benefits linked to participation in adventure programming. For example, Russell and Phillips-Miller (2002) found that hiking and physical exercise were critical components in a wilderness therapy program. Jelalian, et al., (2006) found that an adventure therapy program patterned after Outward Bound served as an effective adjunct therapy for reducing weight in adolescents. In a similar fashion, Caulkins, White, and Russell (2006) report that physical exercise plays an important role in wilderness therapy for adolescent women.

It seems clear that a number of variables consistent with most AT programs, such as fitness, aerobic training, and balance, are also linked to contributing to human health. However, the often short term and episodic nature of these activities suggests that the true power of AT in natural environments lies, not just in the physicality of the activities, but also in the promotion of health-enhancing behaviors. For example, Bowler, Buyung-Ali, Knight, and Pullin (2010) found less consistency in the evidence supporting the idea of natural environments impacting variables such as blood pressure, hormone levels, or immune functioning, and much more consistency in positive changes in self-reported variables such as revitalization, reductions in anger and anxiety, levels of attention, and lower depression. Marcus and Forsyth (2009) suggest that the most important variables related to health behaviors such as physical activity include self-efficacy, a sense of achievement, and social support systems. Thus, the true value of AT may lie in the affective outcomes it often produces in addition to the movement and activity inherent in the experiences.

INTENTIONALLY-DESIGNED EXPERIENCES (IDEs)

How can these AT experiences and programs be enhanced beyond simply doing them in natural settings? Another way of enhancing the relationship between humans and natural environments and creating subsequent health benefits, however, is through the active use of Intentionally Designed Experiences (IDEs) (Sheard & Golby, 2006). Similar to Mitten's (2009) idea that wilderness programs may serve to focus the benefits of nature, the idea of IDEs is that programming in the natural environment can, and should be, purposeful in its planning and implementation in order to achieve specific benefits. In this way, natural environment-based programs become a type of vector to achieve the psychological and physical benefits of nature offered through theoretical constructs such as ART and PET (See Figure 1).

Figure 1. Intentionally designed experiences and human health outcome model.

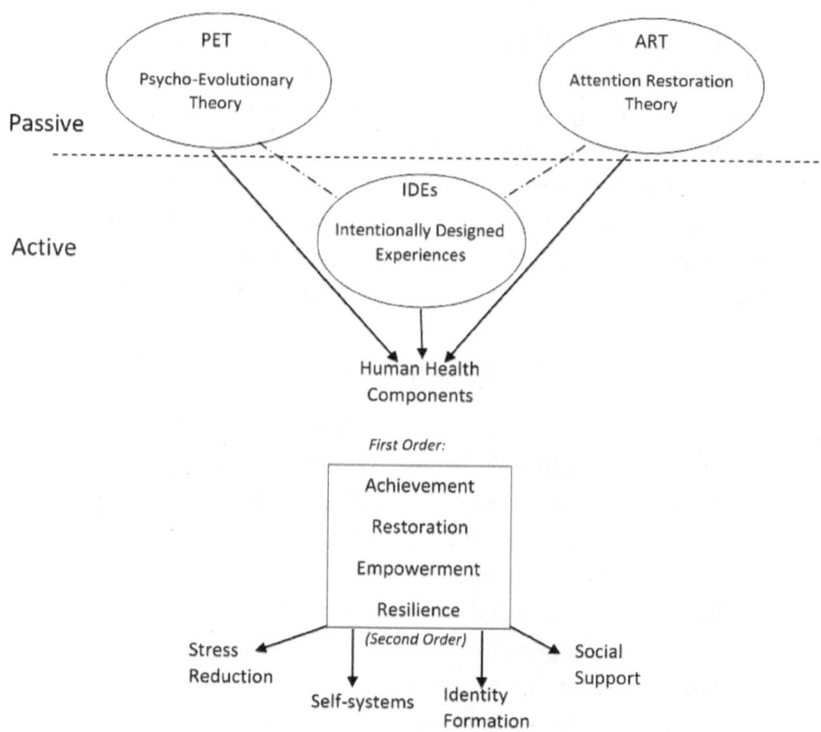

Moreover, Intentionally-Designed Experiences can be separated into two orders or levels. First order benefits can be considered major outcome variables (often health-related) that occur from participation in an IDE and include achievement, restoration, empowerment and resilience. Second order benefits emerge from the occurrence of these first order outcome variables and include benefits related to self-systems (e.g., esteem, concept, awareness, efficacy), stress reduction, identity formation and social support.

The idea of the IDE posits that the purpose, type, and specifics of the program, as well as the type of clients all impact the outcome. The IDE is an active mechanism that, depending on its design, incorporates many of the theoretical underpinnings of the human-nature benefit interaction involving constructs such as ART and PET into a program or experience that ultimately contributes to health and/or quality of life.

Thus, it is very possible that many of the benefits that result from adventure therapeutic IDEs are due, in part, to the natural environments in which they take place. Knowing this, allow us to more fully harness or focus the power of nature through intentional design. For example, Stringer and McAvoy (1992) suggest that programs might set aside more structured reflection time, allow for group discussion on the spiritual nature of the experience, provide for emotional challenge and the testing of personal limits, teach more about the natural history of an area in which a group is travelling, and facilitate personal connections among group members. A greater understanding of how AT can promote the acquisition of specific types of benefits, such as the transcendent experience, stress-reduction, or sense of well-being coupled with a greater understanding of the ways in which IDEs can help to facilitate those benefits may ultimately result in enhanced adventure experiences for those who participate.

CONCLUSION

Adventure therapy offers a powerful avenue for enhancing components for both the intervention based on specific issues and an individual's general health. The popularity of these types of activities and experiences, with many of the subsequent benefits being linked to personal growth and development, strengthening family and social relationships, and increased physical activity. In addition, when formally facilitated and structured, AT can play a vital role in the health of the individual, particularly through its therapeutic and rehabilitative properties. Therapeutic uses of adventure have led to the establishment of myriad adventure therapy programs to bring about personal change within an individual. Inherent in this process are the unique components of a natural setting, risk and challenge, and uncertain outcomes that can be influenced by the individual.

The reason AT can be effective in promoting positive health-related attitudes and subsequent behaviors lies in the ability of these types of experiences to strengthen and build principally on first order outcomes such as empowerment, resilience, sense of achievement, and restoration. As a result of these initial outcomes, second order outcomes, or benefits, often occur which include self-system variables such as self-esteem, stress-reduction, increased physical activity and social support. Organizations such as Outward Bound have long espoused adventure activities and programs as a conduit for enhancing self-systems, creating personal change and greater resilience through the purposive use of challenge and risk. Far from being simply activities and experiences sought out by the dare-devil or individual seeking an adrenalin-rush, adventure therapy, through its use of intentionally designed experiences, restorative qualities, and structured activities in natural environments can enhance the wellness, health, and quality of life for many of our students and clients.

REFERENCES

Baldwin, C. Persing, J., & Magnuson, D. (2004). The role of theory, research, and evaluation in adventure education. *Journal of Experiential Education, 26*(3), 167-183.

Bandoroff, S., & Newes, S. (2004). *Coming of age: The evolving field of adventure therapy.* Boulder, CO: Association for Experiential Education.

Berto, R. (2007). Assessing the restorative value of the environment: A study on the elderly in comparison with young adults and adolescents. *International Journal of Psychology, 42*, 331-341.

Bossen, A. (2010). The importance of getting back to nature for people with dementia. *Journal of Gerontological Nursing, 36*(2), 17-22.

Bowler, D. E., Buyung-Ali, L. M., Knight, T. M., & Pullin, A. S. (2010). A systematic review of evidence for the added benefits to health of exposure to natural environments. *BMC Public Health, 10*, 456.

Bullock, C., & Mahon, M. (2001). *Introduction to recreation services for persons with disabilities: A person-centered approach* (2nd ed.). Champaign, IL: Sagamore.

Caulkins, M. C., White, D. D., & Russell, K., C. (2006). The role of physical exercise in wilderness therapy for troubled adolescent women. *Journal of Experiential Education, 29*(1), 18-37.

Ewert, A., & Voight, A. (2012). The role of adventure in enhancing health-related variables. *International Journal of Health, Wellness, and Society.* (in press).

Gass, M., Gillis, H.L., & Russell, K. (2012). *Adventure therapy: Theory, research, and practice*. New York: Routledge.

Groff, D. & Dattilo, J. (2000). Adventure Therapy. In J. Dattilo (Ed.), *Facilitation techniques in therapeutic recreation*, (pp. 13-37). State College, PA: Venture.

Harmon, D., & Putney, A. D. (Eds.). (2003). *The Full Value of Parks: From Economics to the Intangible*. Boulder, CO: Rowman & Littlefield Publishers, Inc.

Hartig, T., et al., (2011). Health benefits of nature experience: Psychological, social and cultural processes. In K. Nilsson et al., (Eds.). *Forests, Trees and Human Health* (pp. 127-168). New York: Springer.

Frumkin, H. (2003). Healthy places: exploring the evidence. *American Journal of Public Health, 93*(9), 1451

Hendee, J. C., & Dawson, C. P. (2008). Wilderness management: Stewardship and protection of resources and values (4th Ed). Golden, CO: Fulcrum Publishing.

Jelalian, E., Mehlenbeck, R., Lloyd-Richardson, E. E., Birmaher, V., & Wing, R. R. (2006). 'Adventure therapy' combined with cognitive-behavioral treatment for overweight adolescents. *International Journal of Obesity, 30*, 31-39.

Johansson, M., Hartig, T., & Staats, H. (2011). Psychological benefits of walking: Moderation by company and outdoor environment. *Applied Psychology: Health and Well-Being, 3,* 261-280.

Kaczynski, A. T., & Henderson, K. A. (2007). Environmental correlates of physical activity: A review of evidence about parks and recreation. *Leisure Sciences, 29*, 315-354.

Kaplan, R., & Kaplan, S. (1989). *The experience of nature: A psychological perspective.* Cambridge, UK: Cambridge University Press.

Kellert, S. (1993). The biological basis forhuman values of nature. *The biophilia hypothesis*, 42-69.

Marcus, B. H., & Forsyth, L. H. (2009). *Motivating people to be physically active.* Champaign, IL: Human Kinetics.

McKenzie, M.. (2003). Beyond the 'Outward Bound Process': Rethinking student learning. *Journal of Experiential Education, 26*(1), 8-23.

Mitten, D. (2009). Under our Noses: The Healing power of nature. *Taproot Journal 19*(1), 20-26.

Pretty, J., Peacock, J., Hine, R. Sellens, M, South, N., & Griffin, M. (2007). Green exercise in the UK countryside: Effects on health and psychological well-being, and implications for policy and planning. *Journal of Environmental Planning and Management, 50*, 211-231.

Russell, K. C., & Phillips-Miller, D. (2002). Perspectives on the wilderness therapy process and its relation to outcome. *Child and Youth Care Forum, 31*(6), 415-437.

Sheard, M., & Golby, J. (2006). The efficacy of an outdoor adventure education curriculum on selected aspects of positive psychological development. *Journal of Experiential Education, 29*(2), 23.

Stringer, L., & McAvoy, L. (1992). The need for something different: Spirituality and wilderness adventure. *Journal of Experiential Education, 15*(1), 13-20.

Taylor, A., Kuo, F., & Sullivan, W. (2001). Coping with ADD: The surprising connection to green play settings. *Environment and Behavior, 33*(1), 54.

Taylor, A., Kuo, F., & Sullivan, W. (2002). Views of nature and self-discipline: evidence from inner city children. *Journal of Environmental Psychology, 22*(1-2), 49-63.

Ulrich, R. (1981). Natural versus urban scenes: Some psychophysiological effects. *Environment and Behavior, 13*(5), 523 – 556.

Ulrich, R. S. (1983). Aesthetic and affective response to natural environments. In: I. Altman & Wohlwill, J. F. (Eds.). *Behavior and the Natural Environment* (pp. 85-125). New York: Plenum Press.

Ulrich, R. S. (1984). View through a window may influence recovery from surgery. *Science*, 224, 420-421.

Wilson, E. O. (1984). *Biophilia:[the human bond with other species]*: Harvard University Press Cambridge.

Wilson, E. O. (1993). Biophilia and the conservation ethic. In S. Kellert & E. O. Wilson (Eds.), *The Biophilia Hypothesis*. Washington D.C.: Island Press.

CHAPTER 39

Community-based Participatory Research and Realist Evaluation: Complimentary Approaches for Aboriginal Health and Adventure Therapy

Stephen D. Ritchie, Mary Jo Wabano, Jackson Beardy, Jeffrey Curran, Aaron Orkin, Dave Vanderburgh, Karen Born and Nancy L. Young

ABSTRACT

Community-based participatory research (CBPR) and realist evaluation (RE) seem to be complimentary frameworks for Aboriginal health, and they appear to be useful approaches for adventure therapy. CBPR is a collaborative approach to program development and research that is gaining currency as an effective way to meet the needs of individual Aboriginal communities. Often specific community needs are unique and localized, and they may not be addressed by generalized approaches, government programs, and large-scale initiatives. RE is a theory drive approach to evaluation that is particularly effective for understanding the multiplicity and interconnectivity of factors that may influence the outcomes in a particular program. RE allows evaluators to work collaboratively and explore causality, since there are numerous factors that could interact and influence a particular program or project. This paper outlines two Aboriginal health research projects that utilized CBPR and RE as complimentary methodological approaches. The Wikwemikong Outdoor Adventure Leadership Experience (OALE) is a therapeutic adventure program designed for Aboriginal youth ages 12-18 years from one community. The Sachigo Lake Wilderness Emergency Response Education Initiative (SLWEREI) is an emergency response training program designed for lay members from one community. CBPR and RE seem to be complimentary methodological approaches well suited for collaborative projects with specific populations such as Aboriginal communities; and they appear to be robust frameworks that may have broader applicability for program development, research and evaluation in adventure therapy contexts.

INTRODUCTION

Principles and practices of adventure therapy (AT) appear to fit well within the worldview of many Aboriginal communities across Canada. Many of these communities have a holistic view of health and life that includes the individual, their community, and nature. Aboriginal views of health often reflect a balance of mental, physical, emotional, and spiritual health (Hill, 2006; Isaak & Marchessault, 2008). This view also reflects a communal context with other people, and inclusive of the entire created world (Hart, 2000; Hunter, Logan, Goulet, & Barton, 2006; Parkes, 2011). This view aligns with the core elements of many AT approaches: (1) the well-being of the individual; (2) the social milieu; (3) interaction in nature (Gass, Gillis, & Russell, 2012). Interestingly, the Aboriginal perspective of health, and the key elements of AT are also not that much different from the longstanding World Health Organization definition of health: "a state of complete physical, mental and social well-being and not merely the absence of disease or infirmity" (Word Health Organization, 1948).

There are major disparities in health status between Aboriginal and non-Aboriginal Canadians, and Aboriginal populations and communities throughout Canada have challenging and unique health needs (Canadian UNICEF Committee, 2009; Health Canada, 2005; National Collaborating Centre for Aboriginal Health, 2012; The First Nations Information Governance Centre, 2012). The Aboriginal population in Canada is also growing six times faster than the non-Aboriginal population (Statistics Canada, 2008). Despite the growing numbers of children and youth, there is still a significant disparity in health status: "Aboriginal peoples generally have poorer health than the non-Aboriginal population, particularly in terms of maternal, fetal and infant health; child health; certain communicable and non-communicable diseases; mental health and wellness; violence, abuse and injury; and environmental health." (National Collaborating Centre for Aboriginal Health, 2012, p. 4). Many of these disparities can be linked to a long history of colonial policies (Loppie-Reading & Wien, 2009; National Collaborating Centre for Aboriginal Health, 2009b), sub-standard socio-economic conditions (National Collaborating Centre for Aboriginal Health, 2012; The First Nations Information Governance Centre, 2012), and issues related to the provision of and access to services for rural and remote communities (Minore et al., 2005; National Collaborating Centre for Aboriginal Health, 2012).

Most of the health data related to the Aboriginal population in Canada is aggregated on a national level (National Collaborating Centre for Aboriginal Health, 2012), as such there is a dearth of health data at the community level (National Collaborating Centre for Aboriginal Health, 2009a). The Aboriginal population in Canada includes First Nations, Inuit and Métis people. There are 615 First Nations communities in Canada, representing over 50 distinct cultural groups and languages (Aboriginal Affairs and Northern Development Canada, 2013). A large number of these communities are in rural and remote locations. Hence, many First Nations communities have limited access to health related services and programs (Minore, Boone, Katt, Kinch, & Birch, 2004; National Collaborating Centre for Aboriginal Health, 2012), coupled with urgent health related needs and priorities (National Collaborating Centre for Aboriginal Health, 2012). Given both the context of major health disparities and needs, as well as remote locations, there are numerous opportunities to address specific health needs with relevant programs and services developed within each community. However, many health care providers, health promoters, social workers, and health scientists lack an understanding of the cultural nuances necessary to conduct successful research in collaboration with Aboriginal communities.

There are two related purposes of this paper. The first purpose is to present two complimentary approaches to health related research with Aboriginal communities: (1) Community-based Participatory Research (CBPR); and (2) Realist Evaluation (RE). The second is to share how these approaches could be applicable for adventure therapy (AT) program development, evaluation, and research. CBPR is a broad approach to health research that focuses on creating a collaborative partnership between researchers and community members. RE is a comprehensive approach to program evaluation reflecting a particular sensitivity to context and culture. These two approaches are appropriate for program development and evaluation within Aboriginal communities, and they may be relevant for AT. This paper will describe these two approaches, and then highlight two recent projects that were informed by these frameworks: (1) the Wikwemikong Outdoor Adventure Leadership Experience, a therapeutic adventure program; and (2) the Sachigo Lake Wilderness Emergency Response Education Initiative, a first aid training program.

Community-based Participatory Research (CBPR)

CBPR is a collaborative approach that is gaining currency as an effective way to meet the needs of individual communities that may not be addressed by generalized approaches, government programs, and large-scale initiatives. CBPR has been described as a "partnership approach to research that equitably involves, for example, community members, organizational representatives, and researchers in all aspects of the research process" (Israel et al., 2008, p. 48) CBPR positions all stakeholders, including participants, as program designers, implementers, and evaluators. CBPR usually reflects a long-term commitment and a substantive investment of time and resources for all parties involved. It is built on a reciprocal trusting relationship across the research team (Maiter, Simich, Jacobson, & Wise, 2008). Advocates of CBPR often use the abbreviation "co" before the various aspects of a health related research project to emphasize the cooperative nature of the alliance: co-design, co-develop, co-facilitate, co-analyze, co-present, and co-author.

There are many recommendations and principles in the literature for practicing effective CBPR (Community-Campus Partnerships for Health, 2013; Israel et al., 2008; Israel, Schulz, Parker, & Becker, 2001; Tandon et al., 2007). Israel, Schulz, Parker, and Becker (1998) originally identified nine principles or characteristics that capture the key elements of a CBPR approach (Israel, Eng, Schulz, & Parker, 2005; Israel et al., 2008). CBPR has also become increasingly popular for conducting health research with Aboriginal communities. This has resulted in a growing literature base describing challenges, lessons learned, and recommendations (Caldwell et al., 2005; Lardon, Drew, Kernak, Lupie, & Soule, 2007; Maar et al., 2011; Minore, et al., 2004; Mohammed, Walters, Lamarr, Evans-Campbell, & Fryberg, 2012). LaVeaux and Christopher (2009) synthesized the literature on CBPR with Aboriginal communities, and then critiqued the nine principles originally identified by Israel and colleagues since they did not reflect important elements of the Aboriginal cultural context. From this work, nine additional principles were identified for conducting CBPR with Aboriginal communities (Christopher et al., 2011; LaVeaux & Christopher, 2009). Box 1 outlines the nine principles identified by Israel et al. (2005; 1998), and Box 2 outlines the nine principles adapted from Christopher et al. (2011). These principles of CBPR seem to also reflect the tenets of RE.

Box 1
General Principles of CBPR[a]

1. Recognize community as a unit of identity
2. Build on strengths and resources within the community
3. Facilitate collaborative, equitable partnerships in all research phases and involve an empowering and power-sharing process that attends to social inequalities
4. Promote co-learning and capacity building among all partners
5. Integrate and achieve a balance between research and action for the mutual benefit of all partners
6. Emphasize public health problems of local relevance and also ecological perspectives that recognize and attend to the multiple determinants of health and disease
7. Involve systems development through a cyclical and iterative process
8. Disseminate findings and knowledge gained to all partners and involve all partners in the dissemination process
9. Focus on a long-term process and commitment to sustainability

[a]Adapted from Israel et al. (2005; 1998; 2008).

Box2
Principles of CBPR With Aboriginal Communities[a]

1. Acknowledge historical experience with research and health issues and work to overcome the negative image of research
2. Recognize traditional sovereignty
3. Differentiate between band and community leadership
4. Understand community diversity and its implications
5. Plan for extended timelines
6. Recognize key gatekeepers
7. Prepare for leadership turnover
8. Interpret data within the cultural context
9. Utilize indigenous ways of knowing

[a]Adapted from LaVeaux and Christopher (2009) and Christopher et al. (2011)

Realist Evaluation (RE)

Realist Evaluation is an approach to evaluation that was first introduced by Pawson and Tilley in 1997. Since that time, there have been numerous applications and an evolution of this approach within the social sciences and health research literature (Astbury & Leeuw, 2010; Greenhalgh et al., 2009; Jackson & Kolla, 2012; Ogrinc & Batalden, 2009; Taylor, Jones, O'Reilly, Oldfield, & Blackburn, 2010; Wong, Greenhalgh, Westhorp, & Pawson, 2012). RE is rooted in scientific realism: a philosophy of science that embraces the complexity of the social world, suggesting that scientific truths are always embedded in a structure or context (Dunn, 2012; Pawson, Ray & Tilley, 1997; Sayer, 2000). Realism is positioned in contrast to the positivist notion that particular variables can be isolated in order to establish truths about an outcome. From a realist perspective, variables and programs don't cause outcomes in isolation (Wong, et al., 2012), and in fact "one of the most distinctive features of realism is its analysis of causation" (Sayer, 2000, p. 13). When one considers causality through a realist lens, one views a multiplicity and interconnectivity of causes for a particular effect or outcome. This is the *realism* of a complex *real* world.

Realist Evaluation has been described as a theory driven evaluation (Astbury & Leeuw, 2010; Coryn, Noakes, Westine, & Schröter, 2011). There are three essential elements that form the conceptual backbone for realist evaluation: *contexts, mechanisms, and outcomes* (Astbury & Leeuw, 2010; Pawson, Ray & Tilley, 1997) (Jackson & Kolla, 2012). Outcomes are either the intentional or unintentional effects of a program; hence there are multiple outcomes resulting from any program. Mechanisms are the factors related to specific elements of a program that bring about the effects or outcomes. Astbury and Leeuw (2010) summarized a typology of mechanisms in RE and cautioned against confusing mechanisms with program activities or variables. A particular factor may act in multiple ways; hence one mechanism may function differently with different people resulting in multiple outcomes. Contexts describe the features of the social conditions within which the mechanism of a program operates. Contexts aid in addressing and understanding for whom, and in what circumstances, a program may be effective. According to Pawson and Tilley (1997), these three elements combine in a "context-mechanism-outcome-configuration". In other words, a specific outcome is achieved when there is a particular alignment (configuration) of context, mechanism, and outcome (CMO). Specific examples of the CMO interactions of the RE process are provided in the following sections for the OALE and SLWEREI projects.

The Realist Evaluation (RE) framework is comprehensive and holistic, and is a fitting companion for CBPR. It allows community-based evaluators to work collaboratively and explore causality, since there are numerous factors that could interact and influence the particular program or project being evaluated. CBPR is a broad approach used to develop many Aboriginal health related projects and programs, and RE appears to be a useful approach for evaluating those same initiatives.

The Wikwemikong Outdoor Adventure Leadership Experience (OALE)

The Wikwemikong Outdoor Adventure Leadership Experience (OALE) is a 10-day program designed to promote resilience and well-being for youth ages 12-18 from Wikwemikong Unceded Indian Reserve in northern Ontario Canada (Ritchie et al., 2010; Ritchie et al., 2012). The OALE was developed using a CBPR approach over several years (2008-2011). The collaboration involved community leaders from Wikwemikong, and researchers from Laurentian University in Sudbury, Ontario Canada. Promoting resilience and well-being were community identified needs. The program development process involved focus groups, community meetings, interviews with Elders and community leaders, working sessions, and training exercises in Wikwemikong and at Laurentian University. Early in the relationship, a signed formal research agreement outlined expectations and deliverables, and a community research steering committee provided ongoing support and guidance to the CBPR process.

The OALE involves a wilderness canoe expedition that follows a historical travel route through the traditional territory of the community. The route includes many natural challenges (such as rapids, waves, portages, and route finding), and also passes through many areas of cultural significance such as harvesting areas (hunting, fishing, and berry picking), old battle sites commemorated by pictographs, sacred burial grounds, and abandoned village sites. Program designers utilized the Outward Bound Process Model (Walsh & Golins, 1976) and the Medicine Wheel as developmental frameworks. The Medicine Wheel reflects an Aboriginal helping or social work perspective (Hart, 2000), and it is also one of the most common frameworks of Aboriginal health in Canada (Waldram, Herring, & Young, 2006). The OALE includes many program elements such as day leadership responsibilities, daily themes reinforced by experiential activities, evening talking circles (debriefs), and a half day solo experience. There are also culturally relevant elements included such as ceremonies at departure and homecoming, Elder teachings, offering tobacco, smudging, and prayers to the Creator.

Since 2009, approximately 25% of the Wikwemikong population ages 12-18 years have completed the OALE. The program is well established in the community and it appears to be successful and effective (Ritchie & Marrone, 2013; Ritchie, et al., 2012). In the spirit of CBPR, the collaborative team recently completed a 5 year program review (2008-2012) using principles of RE (Ritchie & Marrone, 2013). RE was selected as an appropriate framework since it was comprehensive and particularly sensitive to context and culture. The review process involved the collection of data from numerous sources: field observations in 2012; key informant interviews (with Elders, community leaders, and OALE staff and participants); minutes of meetings; program manuals and research reports; and findings from earlier research in 2009 and 2010. The evaluation process also involved two participatory review meetings to discuss preliminary findings with community leaders. The final report included numerous findings and 70 recommendations.

Two examples of how the RE complimented the CBPR approach to help reflect the realities of culture and context with respect to the OALE were: (1) understanding syncretic spirituality, (2) recognizing the significance of water. Understanding syncretic spirituality was important because the OALE program reflected and embraced multiple perspectives of spirituality and spiritual health. Duggan (2002) described many Anishinaabe people from the area as demonstrating a spiritual *sense of universality*, sustaining a dualism and dialogue between their Anishinaabe spirituality and their commitment to Catholicism. Most of the Wikwemikong community self-identify as Anishinaabe, and their heritage is linked to the Three Fires Confederacy which is a historical alliance between the Ojibway, Odawa and Pottawatami nations. Beyond Catholicism, there is also a strong Evangelical Christian presence in the community. This means that different families and individuals in Wikwemikong are raised in a wide variety of spiritual belief systems. Given that spiritual health is a targeted outcome of the OALE, the spiritual and religious beliefs and affiliations of the community are important to the program. This example reflects a critical understanding of the context (C) within a RE framework. It also has implications for the mechanisms (M) of change within the OALE since a particular program element, such as prayer to the Creator, may have had a different meaning for each youth, leading to different outcomes (O) related to spiritual health. Thus, findings and recommendations from the RE process in this area were carefully worded to be inclusive and syncretic so as not to imply that a singular spiritual belief was more important than another.

The significance of water was less obvious initially. It required the passage of several years, and the insight of Elders in the community, to fully realize the relevant CMOs. Since the OALE involved daily travel on water, there are numerous references in the research data related to water (canoeing on it, playing in it, swimming through it, jumping into it, drinking it, traveling over it, etc.). Through field observations, as part of the RE process, there were also several water-related safety and risk management issues noted with respect to swimming, cliff jumping, wearing Personal Flotation Devices, and crossing long sections of open water in a canoe. In the early stages of the RE process, the targeted outcomes (O) of the OALE (resilience and well-being) were over-shadowed by a pre-occupation with outcomes (O) related to water-related safety. For instance, restrictive protocols for swimming and prohibiting cliff jumping were considered as recommendations. However, based primarily on Elder insights and guidance, the research team realized that the significance of water was related to the targeted outcomes with important considerations related to context (C) and mechanisms (M) for change. Within the community, water symbolizes the beginning of a new life, since the youth began life in water in their mothers' wombs. During the OALE, water was a key element operating in an important introductory context (C) to the experience since it was a soothing presence that helped each youth connect nature experiences and activities together. Essentially, water helped the youth begin their new *program life* together. The water context (C) was also related to important mechanisms (M) such as interacting with others and having fun through activities such as swimming and cliff jumping. Through the RE process, this realization led to recommendations that were structured to be more tolerant and supportive, rather than restrictive and prohibitive, of water related activities such as swimming and cliff jumping.

The Sachigo Lake Wilderness Emergency Response Education Initiative (SLWEREI)

The Sachigo Lake Wilderness Emergency Response Education Initiative (SLWEREI) is a health systems training program targeting community level capacity-building in the area of emergency medical response (Born, Orkin, Vanderburgh, & Beardy, 2012; Orkin et al., 2012). The SLWEREI was developed over several years (2009-2012) using CBPR as a framework informing the research design and methods. The collaboration involved community leaders from Sachigo Lake, and an interdisciplinary team from outside the community. The SLWEREI involves the delivery of a 5-day emergency response training program to community members in Sachigo Lake. The program was developed specifically for the realities of living in a remote fly-in community over 400 km (250 miles) from the nearest urban centre. Principles of wilderness emergency management influenced the curriculum development, however many modifications addressed the realities and relevance of living in Sachigo Lake. Program development and delivery was primarily coordinated in the community by the Health Director, a key research partner. The program was delivered initially in the community in the fall of 2010 and then again in the spring of 2012.

During the program revision and delivery of the SLWEREI in 2012, principles of RE were used as a complimentary framework to accompany CBPR. Recruitment of course participants was led by community leaders. Participants included members of the First Response Team and the Canadian Rangers, as well as health staff, school staff, and community members. The interdisciplinary team from outside the community included two physicians, medical trainees, university researchers and graduate students, and curriculum developers with extensive experience in paramedicine and teaching wilderness first aid.

The interaction of CBPR and RE as frameworks provided for a comprehensive and inclusive environment for the program and research processes. Participants were encouraged to share stories of their personal experiences with emergency response in the community so that the curriculum and program could be modified in *real-time* to respond to actual events that had occurred. Research data collection was also conducted *real-time* so participants were able to reflect on their experience through interviews and focus groups that were built into the course agenda during each day. The training delivery process included relevant practical scenarios such as a plane crash and snowmobile accident. At the request of the community, an entirely new module was developed and implemented on mental health first aid. CPR protocols were revised to reflect the unique pre-hospital situation in Sachigo Lake. At appropriate times, the training program expanded to include dialogue related to emergency response systems in the community. Since Sachigo Lake is a remote community without a permanent physician living in the community, the access to physicians for such an extended period of time was novel; this resulted in a rich learning environment where specific medical questions could be addressed. The hallmarks of the second course were flexibility, adaptability, inclusivity, and relevance, which are also important characteristics of both CBPR and RE.

The interaction of CBPR and RE in the SLWEREI project were different than in the OALE project, since the RE framework was embedded in the CBPR process. Two specific examples of how CBPR complimented the RE approach in the SLWEREI were: (1) understanding the definition of team and community, and (2) implementing daily program response reviews. Throughout an ongoing dialogue, the interdisciplinary team grappled with the context of the research setting, team, and community. Since the program was primarily developed and delivered by a team that was from outside the community, it seemed that there was a development and research team separate from the community. However, defining the research team separately from members of the Sachigo Lake community as research participants was a direct challenge to CBPR and the realist paradigm. Principles of CBPR and RE helped the team resolve and embrace the complexities involved in a collaboration involving geographical, contextual, and cultural challenges.

The development and delivery of the SLWEREI was in a context (C) that included a complex combination of cultures and perspectives since it involved leaders and course participants from a distinct cultural community interacting with a diverse inter-disciplinary team from outside the community. This meant that there were a multitude of complex mechanisms (M) and outcomes (O) that would result. Since the primary intended course outcome (O) was to build capacity, it was implied that this may refer to an outcome defined something like: "community members from SL with the knowledge and skills to respond to health related emergencies". However, this singular perspective ignored many other important mechanisms (M) and outcomes (O). For instance, the highly interdisciplinary research and delivery team included the involvement of medical and graduate learners. This meant that the integrated education of professionals was embedded within a project that was about community education. This brought the realist and CBPR perspective to the fore, with the recognition that all participants learn and develop together, even if they are learning and developing in different ways. The RE paradigm in particular, helped provide insight and understanding to a definition of team and community that was broad and inclusive.

During the delivery of the 5-day SLWEREI, the interdisciplinary team implemented daily program response reviews. These reviews occurred each evening after curriculum delivery and data collection were complete. This format recognized and embraced the complex context (C) surrounding the SLWEREI. In other words, the reviews provided voice to each member of the team who would offer personal reflexive comments (about their own learning), and also unique perspectives and observations about the course delivery and research data that was collected. This resulted in a flexible and responsive program and research agenda that was hyper-sensitive to context (C) and mechanism (M). Since the desired outcome of the program was to deliver relevant training each day, the review process allowed the team to discuss mechanisms such as learning formats, content delivery format (i.e. lecture or demonstration) and order, and relevant scenarios, that would be most likely to work within the context. Since the desired outcome of the research was to understand the mechanisms through which the course may develop capacity and resilience in the community, the review process allowed for the team to share observations and reflect on comments from interviews and focus groups. Not only did this provide a rich format for ongoing data analysis in the field, it also functioned in a synergetic way to influence course content and delivery plans for the following day. In other words, the realist lens allowed the team to review and dissect the program and research together (rather than separately) each day, since the process was recognized as a complex inter-connected network of contexts, mechanisms, and outcomes. Implementing daily program response reviews was a conscious decision that reflected the realist sensitivity to understanding CMO's, and it helped operationalize the collaborative principles of CBPR.

Discussion and Implications for Adventure Therapy

The OALE is a therapeutic adventure program designed for First Nations youth ages 12-18 from Wikwemikong. It involves intentional programming targeting specific health related outcomes (resilience and well-being), and it utilizes wilderness expedition travel in a small group context. The SLWEREI is a health services training program designed for lay members from Sachigo Lake. It is not an AT program or intervention, however some aspects of the program do reflect AT approaches in a few ways. For instance, it involves a philosophy of experiential education that embraces learning through practice, scenarios and simulations; and it uses outdoor settings to guide curriculum development. The OALE and SLWEREI are short-term health-related training programs collaboratively designed and delivered to meet targeted needs identified by specific Aboriginal communities. They are both relevant examples that utilized these methods effectively, but in different ways. In the OALE, the RE framework was used in an evaluation process that was distinct and followed from the CBPR process used through the initial development of the program. In the SLWEREI, the RE was embedded within the CBPR approach during the planning and delivery of the second course.

CBPR and RE: Complimentary Approaches

The primary purpose of this paper is to present CBPR and RE as complimentary approaches to health research, particularly with Aboriginal communities. There has been a trend in the literature towards an increased discussion around evidence-based practice and evaluation with respect to community health promotion (Springett & Wallerstein, 2008). This has led to various approaches to the evaluation of CBPR. One of the main approaches refers to evaluating the effectiveness of a particular program through the use of *participatory evaluation* tools and techniques (Scarinci, Johnson, Hardy, Marron, & Partridge, 2009;

Springett & Wallerstein, 2008). Eng et. al. (2005) described the origin and characteristics of action-oriented community diagnosis (AOCD), which is an approach to evaluation that incorporates community within a broader understanding of the social determinants of health. There is also a tendency towards evaluating the effectiveness of the CBPR process and partnership (Israel, Lantz, McGranaghan, Kerr, & Guzman, 2005) separately from the evaluation of the program or intervention. Nevertheless, one of the central questions in the evaluation of CBPR is the definition of community (Eng et al., 2005), leading to a question about who should be included as part of the evaluation process.

The SLWEREI project was an example where community was defined broadly, and the process included the partnership, process and program; all were evaluated concurrently in a complex contextual environment with numerous inter-connected mechanisms producing myriad outcomes. For instance, there were relevant mechanisms and outcomes related to the effectiveness of the SLWEREI in terms of building community capacity to handle medical emergencies. However, there were also important mechanisms and outcomes related to the collaboration (partnership), such as the participation of medical learners and a graduate student. During the OALE evaluation process, the focus was primarily on evaluating the effectiveness of the program, rather than the effectiveness of the team, since the RE was implemented as a summative process reviewing a five year history of development and implementation. This implied a somewhat narrower definition of community (although broader contextual factors could not be ignored). Thus, principles of RE appear to provide a flexible framework that can be used to evaluate a CBPR program, process, or partnership either separately or together.

Beyond RE, a realist review (RR) expands the realist paradigm to include a systematic method for research synthesis (Pawson, Ray, Greenhalgh, Harvey, & Walshe, 2005; Wong, Greenhalgh, & Pawson, 2010). RR can be defined as "an interpretive theory-driven narrative summary which applies realist philosophy to the synthesis of findings from primary studies that have a bearing on a single research question." (Wong, et al., 2012, p. 93) Pawson et al. (2005) suggested that RR "is well suited to the study of complex social interventions" (p. 32). The sensitivity and flexibility of the realist paradigm with respect to various contexts and applications (i.e. RE and RR) is perhaps its greatest strength. However RE and RR do have limitations (Wong, et al., 2012), and they are not without criticism. RE has an intuitive appeal that often overshadows a complexity that is difficult to operationalize as clear steps in an evaluation process (Rycroft-Malone, Fontenla, Bick, & Seers, 2010; Tolson, McIntosh, Loftus, & Cormie, 2007).

Tolson and colleagues (2007) described RE as an emerging methodology and noted "that the development of meaningful CMO requires skill and processes of deduction to tease out what may be very complex psychosocial interactions…" (p. 194) Rycroft-Malone, Fontenla, Bick, and Seers (2010) were critical of RE, despite claiming that in their study it was an "extremely useful framework for helping us develop explanations and present them in a meaningful way" (p. 12). Their critique highlighted several issues. The main issue related to the challenge of being able to complete a full realist synthesis given funding constraints. Instead, they described their process as using principles of RE, and their conclusions as more general propositions rather than specific findings. A second issue related to defining and differentiating between contexts and mechanisms so that they could classify and analyze factors consistently. These methodological issues seemed to be linked to their description of the iterative nature of the analysis which required abundant time for discussion and debate. In conclusion, they confirmed that RE is best situated as an interpretive rather than deductive evaluation process.

The use of RE as a framework in the OALE and SLWEREI projects resulted in similar key learnings to that of Rycroft-Malone and colleagues (2010). RE was very helpful as an explanatory framework, but challenging in many ways such as: identifying and differentiating between specific contexts and mechanisms; and completing a full comprehensive analysis given budget, time, and resource constraints. Instead, principles of RE were followed rather than a comprehensive realist synthesis identifying all of the CMO's in each project. In both projects (OALE and SLWEREI), the collective description of a CMO was easier to identify than the differentiated description of isolated contexts (C), mechanisms (M), and outcomes (O) that interacted in a multiplicity of CMO's. RE functioned as an approach that helped paint a picture of what was happening at a given point in time.

CBPR and RE seem to be compatible and complimentary approaches that are well-suited for health research with Aboriginal communities. However, they are not inherently designed for replication. In both the OALE and SLWEREI, they were used as principles or frameworks rather than prescriptive methods. RE is a comprehensive exploratory and interpretive approach that is not only useful for the comprehensive evaluation of a program, but it can also be helpful to evaluate the impact and interaction of multiple processes and factors (variables), and to understand the complex nature and influence of partnerships and research team (community) environment. Funded programs in health must often justify their ongoing existence in order to receive funding. Aboriginal health and AT are no exceptions.

CBPR AND RE: IMPLICATIONS FOR AT

The secondary purpose of this paper was to explore the relevance of CBPR and RE as methods to consider for AT research. In 1985, Outward Bound Canada founded the Giwaykiwin Program to address a recognized need for culturally appropriate programming for Aboriginal students from different communities across the country (Lowan, 2008). Lowan, a former Métis instructor who taught in the Giwaykiwin program, completed a thesis exploring how the program impacted the participants, and how the findings could help improve the program. He concluded that the "overarching theme that seems to run through all the findings of this study is the importance of grounding Indigenous education programs as much as possible in the culture and traditions of specific communities" (Lowan, 2008, p. 134). Perhaps not surprisingly, the original Giwaykwin program no longer exists. Yet, the need for culturally appropriate mental health promotion programming for Aboriginal youth continues to increase in Canada (First Nations Inuit & Aboriginal Health, 2003; Government of Canada, 2006; Kirmayer, Simpson, & Cargo, 2003; Mental Health Commission of Canada, 2012; National Collaborating Centre for Aboriginal Health, 2012). It is also a compelling need in other countries (Durie, Milroy, & Hunter, 2009; Hunter, E. & Harvey, 2002; Purdie, Dudgeon, & Walker, 2010). Principles and practices of AT seem to be relevant approaches to address this need, and CBPR and RE are relevant methods that could be used to collaboratively engage, develop, and implement local mental health promotion programs for specific Aboriginal communities.

Gass and colleagues described the black box effect in research and evaluation of AT as a tendency towards not reporting what actually occurred in the intervention to achieve the outcome. They recommended: "it is important for researchers, evaluators, and consumers of research to do the best they can to report, describe, and ascertain the key aspects of the intervention being reported or discussed" (Gass, et al., 2012, p. 288) AT interventions are incredibly complex phenomena that may involve a plethora of factors such as prior participant knowledge, skills and attitudes; various adventure activities selected; numerous unique challenges and problems experienced and resolved; continuous and evolving small group interaction; ongoing relationship development (participant to participant and participant to therapist); and contact with nature including both positive and possibly negative aspects (e.g. inclement weather). Clearly this list is only a fraction of the factors or variables involved. It is very difficult to conceive of a research design that is able to isolate and control or isolate these variables or factors in order to better understand the interactions related to the outcomes of interest. Rather than attempting to isolate particular factors, RE helps researchers focus on how various factors interact to produce an outcome. Perhaps more than coincidentally, Astbury and Leeuw (2010) described the mechanisms of RE as a process of *unpacking black boxes* in programs. The RE approach seems to not only recognize the complexities inside the black box (mechanisms), it acknowledges and even tries to understand variables and influences (contexts) outside the black box. The focus of RE on the interaction of factors (contexts, mechanisms and outcomes) seems to be particularly well suited to address the black box effect in AT research.

Gass, Gillis, and Russell (2012) listed 15 meta-analyses and reviews of literature in AT completed since 1979. They also used the Outward Bound Process Model (Walsh & Golins, 1976) as a framework to outline seven process factors containing 30 ingredients that helped them describe and explain some of the mechanisms for change in AT research (Gass, et al., 2012). However, they also acknowledged that there were key questions for future research such as whether all elements of the AT process were necessary, which factors or ingredients were more likely to lead to change, and how the program elements may work together (Gass, et al., 2012). The realist researcher asks the foundational question: "What works, for whom, in what circumstances, in what respects, and why?" (Wong, et al., 2012, p. 93) AT researchers are asking the same question. RE provides a useful framework for answering this question. RR may also be a useful tool that could be used to further analyze a singular research question about a particular process factor or ingredient.

Conclusion

There are several learnings that emerged through the planning, preparation and writing of this paper. These learnings arose from the execution and evaluation of analogous programs from inside (OALE) and outside (SLWEREI) the AT field. For instance, CBPR may provide a useful framework for planning and developing new AT programs for homogenous populations, such as specific Aboriginal communities. However, the reality for many existing AT programs is that they include broad heterogeneous populations from a wide variety of communities. Given the complex interactive factors in these programs, RE and RR may be useful approaches to consider for research and evaluation. CBPR and RE may not be a perfect match, but they do appear to be complimentary approaches well suited to health related programs and research in Aboriginal communities. CBPR and RE are not the solution for research and evaluation with all AT programs, but they may also be useful for particular AT programs within clearly defined communities.

References

Aboriginal Affairs and Northern Development Canada. (2013, 2010-09-15). Author. *First Nations*. Retrieved January 16, 2013, from http://www.aadnc-aandc.gc.ca/eng/1100100013791/1100100013795

Astbury, B., & Leeuw, F. L. (2010). Unpacking black boxes: Mechanisms and theory building in evaluation. *American Journal of Evaluation, 31*(3), 363-381. doi:10.1177/1098214010371972

Born, K., Orkin, A., Vanderburgh, D., & Beardy, J. (2012). Teaching wilderness first aid in a remote First Nations community: The story of the Sachigo Lake Wilderness Emergency Response Education Initiative. *International Journal of Circumpolar Health, 71*, 1-7. doi: 10.3402/ijch.v71i0.19002

Caldwell, J. Y., Davis, J. D., Du Bois, B., Echo Hawk, H., Erickson, J. S., Goins, T., . . . Stone, J. B. (2005). Culturally competent research with American Indians and Alaskan natives: Findings and recommendations of the First Symposium of the Work Group on American Indian Research and Program Evaluation Methodology. *American Indian & Alaska Native Mental Health Research: The Journal of the National Center, 12*(1), 1-21.

Canadian UNICEF Committee. (2009). *Canadian supplement to the state of the world's children. Aboriginal children's health: Leaving no child behind.* (0-921564038-4). Toronto, ON: UNICEF Canada. Retrieved from http://www.nccah-ccnsa.ca/myfiles/SOWC Canada 2009 Post release Summary June 2009 _4_.pdf.

Christopher, S., Saha, R., Lachapelle, P., Jennings, D., Colclough, Y., Cooper, C., . . . Webster, L. (2011). Applying indigenous community-based participatory research principles to partnership development in health disparities research. [Research Support, N.I.H., Extramural]. *Family & Community Health, 34*(3), 246-255.

Community-Campus Partnerships for Health. (2013). Author. *Principles of good community-campus partnerships*. Retrieved January 16, 2013, from http://depts.washington.edu/ccph/principles.html principles

Coryn, C. L. S., Noakes, L. A., Westine, C. D., & Schröter, D. C. (2011). A systematic review of theory-driven evaluation practice from 1990 to 2009. *American Journal of Evaluation, 32*(2), 199-226. doi: 10.1177/1098214010389321

Duggan, J. F. (2002). Aspects of Anishnabe Catholic spirituality. In M. Mbonimpa, G. Bonneau & K.-R. Bonin (Eds.), *Mysticism: Select essays: Essays in honour of John Sahadat*. Sudbury, ON: Éditions Glopro.

Dunn, J. R. (2012). "Explanation," philosophy and theory in health inequalities research: Towards a critical realist approach. In P. O' Campo & J. R. Dunn (Eds.), *Rethinking social epidemiology: Towards a science of change* (pp. 23-42). New York, NY: Springer Netherlands.

Durie, M., Milroy, H., & Hunter, E. (2009). Mental health and the indigenous people of Australia and New Zealand. In L. J. Kirmayer & G. G. Valaskakis (Eds.), *Healing traditions: The mental health of Aboriginal people in Canada* (pp. 36-55). Vancouver, BC: UBC Press.

Eng, E., Strazza Moore, K., Rhodes, S. D., Griffith, D. M., Allison, L. L., Shirah, K., & Mebane, E. M. (2005). Insiders and outsiders assess who is "the community": Participant observation, key informant interview, focus group interview, and community forum. In B. A. Israel, E. Eng, A. J. Schulz & E. Parker (Eds.), *Methods in community-based participatory research for health* (pp. 77-100). San Francisco, CA: Jossey-Bass.

First Nations Inuit & Aboriginal Health. (2003). *Acting on what we know: Preventing youth suicide in First Nations (the report of the Suicide Prevention Advisory Group)*. Ottawa, ON: Health Canada. Retrieved from http://www.hc-sc.gc.ca/fniah-spnia/pubs/promotion/_suicide/ prev_youth-jeunes/index-eng.php.

Gass, M. A., Gillis, H. L., & Russell, K. C. (2012). *Adventure therapy: Theory, research, and practice*. New York: Routledge.

Government of Canada. (2006). *The human face of mental health and mental illness in Canada*. (Cat. No. HP5-19/2006E). Ottawa, ON: Public Health Agency of Canada.

Greenhalgh, T., Humphrey, C., Hughes, J., Macfarlane, F., Butler, C., & Pawson, R. (2009). How do you modernize a health service? A realist evaluation of whole-scale transformation in London. *Milbank Quarterly, 87*(2), 391-416.

Hart, M. A. (2000). Seeking mino-pimatasiwin (the good life): An Aboriginal approach to social work practice. *Native Social Work Journal, 2*(1), 91-112.

Health Canada. (2005). *A statistical profile on the health of First Nations in Canada for the year 2000*. (Cat. H35-4/30-2000). Ottawa, ON: Her Majesty the Queen in Right of Canada.

Hill, D. L. (2006). Sense of belonging as connectedness, American Indian worldview, and mental health. *Psychiatric Nursing, 20*(5), 210-216.

Hunter, E., & Harvey, D. (2002). Indigenous suicide in Australia, New Zealand, Canada and the United States. *Emergency Medicine, 14*(1), 14-23. doi: 10.1046/j.1442-2026.2002.00281.x

Hunter, L. M., Logan, J., Goulet, J.-G., & Barton, S. (2006). Aboriginal healing: Regaining balance and culture. *Journal of Transcultural Nursing, 17*(1), 13-22.

Isaak, C. A., & Marchessault, G. (2008). Meaning of health: The perspectives of Aboriginal adults and youth in a northern Manitoba First Nations community. *Canadian Journal of Diabetes, 32*(2), 114-122.

Israel, B. A., Eng, E., Schulz, A. J., & Parker, E. (2005). Introduction to methods in community-based participatory research for health. In B. A. Israel, E. Eng, A. J. Schulz & E. Parker (Eds.), *Methods in community-based participatory research for health* (pp. 3-26). San Fransisco, CA: Jossey-Bass.

Israel, B. A., Lantz, P. M., McGranaghan, R. J., Kerr, D. L., & Guzman, R. (2005). Documentation and evaluation of CBPR partnerships. In B. A. Israel, E. Eng, A. J. Schulz & E. Parker (Eds.), *Methods in community-based participatory research for health* (pp. 255-277). San Fransisco, CA: Jossey-Bass.

Israel, B. A., Parker, E. A., Rowe, Z., Salvatore, A., Minkler, M., Löpez, J., . . . Halstead, S. (2005). Community-based participatory research: Lessons learned from the Centers for Children's Environmental Health and Disease Prevention Research. *Environmental Health Perspectives, 113*(10), 1463-1471.

Israel, B. A., Schulz, A. J., Parker, E. A., & Becker, A. B. (1998). Review of community-based research: Assessing partnership approaches to improve public health. *Annual Review of Public Health, 19*, 173-202.

Israel, B. A., Schulz, A. J., Parker, E. A., Becker, A. B., Allen, A. J., & Guzman, R. (2008). Critical issues in developing and following CBPR principles. In M. Minkler & N. Wallerstein (Eds.), *Community-based participatory research for health: From process to outcomes* (2nd ed., pp. 47-66). San Francisco, CA: Jossey-Bass.

Israel, B. A., Schulz, A. J., Parker, E. P., & Becker, A. B. (2001). Community-based participatory research: Policy recommendations for promoting a partnership approach in health research. *Education for Health: Change in Learning & Practice, 14*(2), 182-197.

Jackson, S. F., & Kolla, G. (2012). A new realistic evaluation analysis method: Linked coding of context, mechanism, and outcome relationships. *American Journal of Evaluation, 33*(3), 339-3349. doi: 10.1177/1098214012440030

Kirmayer, L. J., Simpson, C., & Cargo, M. (2003). Healing traditions: Culture, community and mental health promotion with Canadian Aboriginal peoples. *Australasian Psychiatry, 11*(Supplement), S15-S23.

Lardon, C., Drew, E., Kernak, D., Lupie, H., & Soule, S. (2007). Health promotion in rural Alaska: Building partnerships across distance and cultures. *Partnership Perspectives, 4*(1), 125-132.

LaVeaux, D., & Christopher, S. (2009). Contextualizing CBPR: Key principles of CBPR meet the indigenous research context. *Pimatisiwin: A Journal of Aboriginal and Indigenous Community Health, 7*(1), 1-26.

Loppie-Reading, C., & Wien, F. (2009). Health inequalities and social determinants of Aboriginal peoples' health. Prince George, BC: National Collaborating Centre for Aboriginal Health.

Lowan, G. E. (2008). *Outward Bound Giwaykiwin: Wilderness-based indigenous education.* (Master's thesis). Available from Proquest Dissertations and Theses database.

Maar, M. A., Lightfoot, N. E., Sutherland, M. E., Strasser, R. P., Wilson, K. J., Lidstone-Jones, C. M., . . . Williamson, P. (2011). Thinking outside the box: Aboriginal people's suggestions for conducting health studies with Aboriginal communities. [Research Support, Non-U.S. Gov't]. *Public Health, 125*(11), 747-753.

Maiter, S., Simich, L., Jacobson, N., & Wise, J. (2008). Reciprocity: An ethic for community-based participatory action research. *Action Research, 6*(3), 305-325. doi: 10.1177/1476750307083720

Mental Health Commission of Canada. (2012). Changing directions, changing lives: The mental health strategy for Canada. Calgary, AB: Author.

Minore, B., Boone, M., Katt, M., Kinch, P., & Birch, S. (2004). Addressing the realties of health care in northern Aboriginal communities through participatory action research. *Journal of Interprofessional Care, 18*(4), 360-368.

Minore, B., Boone, M., Katt, M., Kinch, P., Birch, S., & Mushquash, C. (2005). The effects of nursing turnover on continuity of care in isolated First Nation communities. *Canadian Journal of Nursing Research, 37*(1), 87-100.

Mohammed, S. A., Walters, K. L., Lamarr, J., Evans-Campbell, T., & Fryberg, S. (2012). Finding middle ground: Negotiating university and tribal community interests in community-based participatory research. [Research Support, N.I.H., Extramural]. *Nursing Inquiry, 19*(2), 116-127. doi: http://dx.doi.org/10.1111/j.1440-1800.2011.00557.x

National Collaborating Centre for Aboriginal Health. (2009a). Child and youth health: The importance of disaggregated data (fact sheet). Prince George, BC: Author. Retrieved from http://www.nccah-ccnsa.ca.

National Collaborating Centre for Aboriginal Health. (2009b). Culture and language as social determinants of First Nations, Inuit, and Métis health. Prince George, BC: Author. Retrieved from http://www.nccah-ccnsa.ca.

National Collaborating Centre for Aboriginal Health. (2012). State of knowledge of Aboriginal health: A review of Aboriginal public health in Canada. Prince George, BC: Author. Retrieved from http://www.nccah-ccnsa.ca.

Ogrinc, G., & Batalden, P. (2009). Realist evaluation as a framework for the assessment of teaching about the improvement of care. *Journal of Nursing Education, 48*(12), 661-667. doi: http://dx.doi.org/10.3928/01484834-20091113-08

Orkin, A., Vanderburgh, D., Born, K., Webster, M., Strickland, S., & Beardy, J. (2012). Where there is no paramedic: The Sachigo Lake Wilderness Emergency Response Education Initiative. *PLOS Medicine, 9*(10), 1-5 e1001322. doi: 10.1371/journal.pmed.1001322

Parkes, M. W. (2011). Ecohealth and Aboriginal health: A review of common ground. Prince George, BC: National Collaborating Centre for Aboriginal Health. Retrieved from http://www.nccah-ccnsa.ca.

Pawson, R., Greenhalgh, T., Harvey, G., & Walshe, K. (2005). Realist review--a new method of systematic review designed for complex policy interventions. *Journal of Health Services Research & Policy, 10 Suppl 1*, 21-34.

Pawson, R., & Tilley, N. (1997). *Realistic evaluation.* Thousand Oaks, CA: Sage.

Purdie, N., Dudgeon, P., & Walker, R. (Eds.). (2010). *Working together: Aboriginal and Torres Strait Islander mental health and wellbeing principles and practice.* Barton, ACT: Australian Government Department of Health and Ageing (Common Wealth of Australia).

Ritchie, S. D., Wabano, M. J., Young, N., Schinke, R., Peltier, D., Battochio, R., & Russell, K. (2010). Developing a culturally relevant outdoor leadership training program for Aboriginal youth. *Journal of Experiential Education, 32*(3), 300-304.

Ritchie, S. D., & Marrone, D. (2013). *Five year evaluation and review report (2008-2012): The Wikwemikong Outdoor Adventure Leadership Experience (OALE).* Internal confidential report. Wikwemikong, ON: Tchigehgamig Wikwemikong Health Centre.

Ritchie, S. D., Wabano, M. J., Schinke, R., Peltier, D., Restoule, B., Russell, K., . . . Young, N. (2012). The Aboriginal youth resilience study: A look at promoting resilience and well-being through outdoor adventure leadership experience. In A. Prior, C. Carpenter, C. L. Norton & J. Kirchner (Eds.), *Emerging insights: Proceedings of the 5th International Adventure Therapy Conference 2009* (pp. 145-161). Prague: European Science and Art Publishing.

Rycroft-Malone, J., Fontenla, M., Bick, D., & Seers, K. (2010). A realistic evaluation: The case of protocol-based care. *Implementation Science, 5*(1), 38.

Sayer, A. (2000). *Realism and social science.* Los Angeles, CA: Sage Publications.

Scarinci, I. C., Johnson, R. E., Hardy, C., Marron, J., & Partridge, E. E. (2009). Planning and implementation of a participatory evaluation strategy: A viable approach in the evaluation of community-based participatory programs addressing cancer disparities. [Research Support, N.I.H., Extramural]. *Evaluation & Program Planning, 32*(3), 221-228.

Springett, J., & Wallerstein, N. (2008). Issues in participatory evaluation. In M. Minkler & N. Wallerstein (Eds.), *Community-based participatory research for health: From process to outcomes* (2nd ed., pp. 199-220). San Francisco, CA: Jossey-Bass.

Statistics Canada. (2008). *Aboriginal peoples in Canada in 2006: Inuit, Métis and First Nations, 2006 Census*. (Catalogue no. 97-558-XIE). Ottawa, ON: Minister of Industry. Retrieved from http://www12.statcan.ca/english/census06/analysis/aboriginal/index.cfm.

Tandon, S. D., Phillips, K., Bordeaux, B. C., Bone, L., Brown, P. B., Cagney, K. A., . . . Bass, E. B. (2007). A vision for progress in community health partnerships. *Progress In Community Health Partnerships: Research, Education, And Action, 1*(1), 11-30.

Taylor, J., Jones, R. M., O'Reilly, P., Oldfield, W., & Blackburn, A. (2010). The Station Community Mental Health Centre Inc: Nurturing and empowering. [Research Support, Non-U.S. Gov't]. *Rural & Remote Health, 10*(3), 1411.

The First Nations Information Governance Centre. (2012). First Nations regional health survey (RHS). Phase 2 (2008/10) National report on adults, youth and children living in First Nations communities. Ottawa, ON: Author.

Tolson, D., McIntosh, J., Loftus, L., & Cormie, P. (2007). Developing a managed clinical network in palliative care: A realistic evaluation. *International Journal of Nursing Studies, 44*(2), 183-195.

Waldram, J. B., Herring, D. A., & Young, T. K. (2006). *Aboriginal health in Canada: Historical, cultural, and epidemiological perspectives* (2nd ed.). Toronto, ON: University of Toronto Press.

Walsh, V., & Golins, G. (1976). *The exploration of the Outward Bound process*. Unpublished Manuscript. Denver, CO: Colorado Outward Bound. Retrieved from http://www.wilderdom.com/theory/OutwardBoundProcessModel.html

Wong, G., Greenhalgh, T., & Pawson, R. (2010). Internet-based medical education: A realist review of what works, for whom and in what circumstances. *BMC Medical Education, 10*, 12-12. doi: 10.1186/1472-6920-10-12

Wong, G., Greenhalgh, T., Westhorp, G., & Pawson, R. (2012). Realist methods in medical education research: What are they and what can they contribute? *Medical Education, 46*(1), 89-96. doi: http://dx.doi.org/10.1111/j.1365-2923.2011.04045.x

Word Health Organization. (1948). Preamble to the Constitution of the World Health Organization as adopted by the International Health Conference, New York, 19-22 June, 1946; signed on 22 July 1946 by the representatives of 61 states (Official Records of the World Health Organization, no. 2, p. 100) and entered into force on 7 April 1948. Retrieved January 8, 2013, from http://www.who.int/about/definition/en/print.html

This book was developed with contributions from:

- Adventure Therapy International Committee (ATIC)
- Association for Experiential Education (AEE)
- AEE Therapeutic Adventure Professional Group (TAPG)
- European Science and Art Publishing (EUSAPUB)

Reviewers:

Sandy Allen-Craig, MEd; Katie Asmus, MA; Judy Atkins; Almut Beringer, Ph.D.; Eric Brymer, Ph.D.; Fiona Cameron, MEd.; Simon Crisp, DipEdPsych, MPsych, DPsych, MAPS; Michael Gass, Ph.D.; Lee Gillis, Ph.D.; Tonia Gray, Ph.D.; Nevin Harper, Ph.D.; Helen Hooper, PhD, Sean Hoyer, M.A., LCSW; Christian Itin, Ph.D.; Chris Jansen, MEd.; Andrea Knepper, LCSW; Chris Loynes, Ph.D.; Denise Mitten, Ph.D.; Sandy Newes, Ph.D.; Val Nicholls, Ph.D.; Barbara Parker-Bell, Ph.D.; Luk Peeters, Ph.D.; Kaye Richards, Ph.D.; Martin Ringer, Ph.D.; Stephen Ritchie, BPE, MBA; Paul Stolz, BTh, MTh, Dip Ed.; Anita Tucker, Ph.D.; Andy Umbers, BA, BSW; Ian Williams, Ph.D.; Allette Willis, Ph.D.

Special thanks to Catherine Hardin in the College of Applied Arts at Texas State University for her editing and formatting assistance.

www.ingramcontent.com/pod-product-compliance
Lightning Source LLC
LaVergne TN
LVHW100245210926
848480LV00003B/829
9781612297736